Farm Animal Metabolism and Nutrition

_____

Farm Animal Metabolism and Nutrition

Edited by

J.P.F. D'Mello

Biotechnology Department
The Scottish Agricultural College
Edinburgh
UK

CABI *Publishing*

CABI *Publishing* **is a division of CAB** *International*

CABI Publishing	CABI Publishing
CAB International	10 E 40th Street
Wallingford	Suite 3203
Oxon OX10 8DE	New York, NY 10016
UK	USA
Tel: +44 (0)1491 832111	Tel: +1 212 481 7018
Fax: +44 (0)1491 833508	Fax: +1 212 686 7993
Email: cabi@cabi.org	Email: cabi-nao@cabi.org
Web site: http://www.cabi.org	

A catalogue record for this book is available from the British Library, London, UK.

Library of Congress Cataloging-in-Publication Data
Farm animal metabolism and nutrition : critical reviews / edited by J.P.F. D'Mello.
    p. cm.
  Includes bibliographical references.
  ISBN 0-85199-378-8 (alk. paper)
    1. Animal nutrition.   2. Livestock--Metabolism.   I. D'Mello, J. P. Felix.

SF95 .F32 2000
636.08′5--dc21
                                             99-048241

ISBN 0 85199 378 8

Typeset by Columns Design Ltd, Reading.
Printed and bound in the UK by Biddles Ltd, Guildford and King's Lynn.

Contents

Contributors

Albright, J.L.   *Department of Animal Sciences, Purdue University, West Lafayette, IN 47907, USA*

Anderson, D.B.   *Research and Development, Elanco Animal Health, PO Box 708, Greenfield, IN 46140, USA*

Buckley, W.T.   *Agriculture and Agri-Food Canada, Brandon Research Centre, Brandon, Canada R7A 5Y3*

D'Mello, J.P.F.   *Biotechnology Department, The Scottish Agricultural College, West Mains Road, Edinburgh EH9 3JG, UK*

Drackley, J.K.   *Department of Animal Sciences, University of Illinois, Urbana, IL 61801, USA*

Drochner, W.   *Institute of Animal Nutrition, Hohenheim University, D-70573 Stuttgart, Germany*

Ellis, W.C.   *Department of Animal Sciences, Texas A&M University, College Station, TX 77843–2471, USA*

Fan, M.Z.   *Department of Animal and Poultry Science, University of Guelph, Guelph, Ontario, Canada N1G 2W1*

Forbes, J.M.   *Centre for Animal Sciences, School of Biology, University of Leeds, Leeds LS2 9JT, UK*

Gahr, S.A.   *Division of Animal and Veterinary Sciences, West Virginia University, PO Box 6108, Morgantown, WV 26506–6108, USA*

Grant, R.J.   *Department of Animal Science, University of Nebraska, Lincoln, NE 68583–0908, USA*

Hancock, D.L.   *Research and Development, Elanco Animal Health, PO Box 708, Greenfield, IN 46140, USA*

Jessop, N.S.   *Institute of Ecology and Resource Management, The University of Edinburgh, West Mains Road, Edinburgh EH9 3JG, UK*

Marais, J.P.   *Biochemistry Section, KwaZulu-Natal Department of Agriculture, Private Bag X9059, Pietermaritzburg, Republic of South Africa, 3200*

Matis, J.H.   *Department of Statistics, Texas A&M University, College Station, TX 77843–2471, USA*

Matthews, J.C.   *Department of Animal Sciences, University of Kentucky, Lexington, KY 40546–0215, USA*

McNab, J.M. *Roslin Institute (Edinburgh), Roslin, Midlothian EH25 9PS, UK*

Michalet-Doreau, B. *Département Elevage et Nutrition des Animaux, Unité de Recherches sur les Herbivores, INRA Theix, 63122 Saint-Genès-Champanelle, France*

Moody, D.E. *Research and Development, Elanco Animal Health, PO Box 708, Greenfield, IN 46140, USA*

Mosenthin, R. *Institute of Animal Nutrition, Hohenheim University, D-70573 Stuttgart, Germany*

Nozière, P. *Département Elevage et Nutrition des Animaux, Unité de Recherches sur les Herbivores, INRA Theix, 63122 Saint-Genès-Champanelle, France*

Officer, D.I. *NSW Agriculture, Agricultural Research and Advisory Station, Grafton, NSW, Australia*

Parker, D.S. *Department of Biological and Nutritional Sciences, Faculty of Agriculture and Biological Sciences, University of Newcastle, Newcastle upon Tyne NE1 7RU, UK; Present address: Novus Europe s.a./n.v., Rue Gulledellestraat 94, B-1200 Brussels, Belgium*

Poppi, D. *Department of Agriculture, The University of Queensland, Brisbane, Queensland 4072, Australia*

Rathmacher, J.A. *Metabolic Technologies Inc., Ames, IA 50010, USA*

Reeves, J.B., III *Nutrient Conservation and Metabolism Laboratory, Livestock and Poultry Sciences Institute, Agricultural Research Service, USDA, Beltsville, MD 20705, USA*

Russell, R.W. *Division of Animal and Veterinary Sciences, West Virginia University, PO Box 6108, Morgantown, WV 26506–6108, USA*

Sauer, W.C. *Department of Agricultural, Food and Nutritional Science, University of Alberta, Edmonton, Alberta, Canada T6G 2P5*

Schofield, P. *Department of Animal Science, Cornell University, Ithaca, NY 14853, USA*

Seal, C.J. *Department of Biological and Nutritional Sciences, Faculty of Agriculture and Biological Sciences, University of Newcastle, Newcastle upon Tyne NE1 7RU, UK*

Preface

There is, once more, a need for an advanced textbook in animal biochemistry and nutrition that covers the specialist requirements of final year undergraduates and new postgraduate students. The existing books have long become out of date, and currently my students are directed to reviews published within the proceedings of various symposia and workshops. However, this approach is less than satisfactory as the reviews are distributed in diverse books and journals that are both physically and financially out of reach of these students. Increasingly these days, libraries resort to restricted lending of journals containing up-to-date reviews and, furthermore, the common practice of holding single copies of conference proceedings is of limited value to the large groups of students we have to teach. Moreover, students still have the problem of consulting different issues of journals and conference proceedings to acquire a comprehensive picture.

In *Farm Animal Metabolism and Nutrition*, I have attempted to overcome most if not all of these limitations by providing a graduated and structured series of critical reviews by international experts, at an affordable price. Current programmes for final year undergraduate and MSc courses at Edinburgh form the basis of the topics selected for this book. In addition, my choice of subjects has been based on experience in teaching final year students at Edinburgh who have at times expressed difficulty with or particular interest in specialist topics. The needs of our commercial clients have not been ignored either, as will be seen from my choice of authors and review topics. In the rapidly changing and expansive fields of farm animal metabolism and nutrition, the limitations of existing general texts are all too evident. No single author can be expected to keep abreast of innovation in all aspects of these fields. I have attempted to overcome these problems by selecting authors who are actively publishing refereed papers and who have an enviable track record in their respective specialisms. Furthermore, my collaborating authors have been selected from major teaching and research establishments around the world.

Farm Animal Metabolism and Nutrition is divided into three sections to reflect major developments. The first section comprises eight chapters within the theme of 'Absorption and Metabolism of Nutrients'. The second section on 'Feed Evaluation Methodologies' contains six chapters, while the third section on 'Intake and Utilization' is based on five chapters. Every book attracts both favourable comments and criticism. Fortunately for me, most reviews of my previous titles have been positive, and these have been much appreciated. While I accept the occasional negative review as an occupational hazard, I am keen to learn from past failings. As regards *Farm Animal Metabolism and Nutrition*, I accept that important areas have not been reviewed. Clearly, for example, the whole issue of quantitative nutrition comprising analytical and predictive models also needs attention, but this may well form the basis of a further volume. In the meantime, current books in the CAB *International* stable should serve to bridge this gap. Selected titles will be found on the rear cover of this book.

As always, I am indebted to my team of authors who have made this book possible and who have invested so much of their valuable time in writing, proofreading and preparing the index, sometimes under difficult conditions. Their enthusiasm for the entire project has been salutary and I hope that the book will provide inspiration to students the world over.

Finally, this book contains references to various commercial products including computer software, which are given in good faith. No endorsement of these products is implied or should be attributed to the editor or CAB *International*, and we cannot assume responsibility for the consequences of their use.

J.P.F. D'Mello

Part I

Absorption and Metabolism of Nutrients

Chapter 1

Amino Acid and Peptide Transport Systems

J.C. Matthews

Department of Animal Sciences, University of Kentucky,
Lexington, Kentucky, USA

Introduction

All cells require a continuous supply of amino acids to meet their metabolic demands. A primary concern of animal nutritionists is the need to understand what the capacity for α-amino acid absorption is, in order that diets can be formulated to provide adequate, but not excessive, amino acids for a given production state. The literature is replete with the characterization of free and peptide-bound amino acid transport systems that are expressed by laboratory animals and humans. By comparison, little research has been conducted to identify the presumably analogous transport systems in farm animal species. Given the economic importance of these species, and the high rates of growth and protein production currently demanded by producers, the lack of knowledge regarding specific farm animal transporter physiology may be limiting our ability to formulate the diets and to design feeding strategies that optimize protein synthesis and retention. Due to the wealth of information regarding amino acid and peptide transport systems and proteins being generated by biomedical research, and the similarities that appear to exist among

animals species, a unique opportunity exists to identify and characterize the function of livestock species-specific free and peptide-bound amino acid absorption mechanisms.

This chapter begins with a general discussion of transport protein (transporter) absorption theory that is germane to amino acid and peptide absorption, proceeds by describing the biochemical and molecular mechanisms that have been characterized for the transport of free and peptide-bound amino acids, and concludes with a description of what is known about these processes in chickens, pigs, sheep and cattle. Unless noted otherwise, the standard three-letter abbreviations for amino acids are used for peptides, and the L isomer is implied for both free and peptide-bound amino acids. Due to the limited number of references allowed for this chapter, the author apologizes in advance for his inability to credit the many researchers who have contributed to the information presented.

Transporter Theory

Mammals have >100 different types of cells. Therefore, as might be expected, considerable variation exists in the amino acid requirements of these cells and in the complement of 'transport systems' that are expressed to meet these requirements. Transport systems (or activities) generally are defined as that protein which recognizes and transfers a selective group of substrates across cellular membranes, whether acting singly or in combination with other proteins. Although best characterized in the plasma membranes of non-polarized cells (e.g. muscle and endothelial), and the apical and basolateral membranes of polarized epithelial cells (e.g. enterocytes and hepatocytes), free (amino acid) and peptide-bound (peptide) amino acid transport systems also mediate the passage of substrates across the membranes of cell organelles (lysosomes, mitochondria, nucleus, etc.).

Transport proteins allow the cell (or organelle) selectively to bind and acquire compounds from a milieu of other substrates. The physiological importance of transporters is usually discussed in terms of their relative ability to recognize and bind a substrate molecule (affinity), and the amount and rate of substrate translocation through the membranes (capacity/velocity). Typically, transport systems that demonstrate relatively low affinities for substrates have large capacities for transport, whereas those that display high affinities have low capacities. The general process of transporter-mediated passage through membranes, however, is the same for all transporters: (i) the substrate(s) binds to the recognition domain of the transporter; (ii) the substrate(s) is translocated through the membrane interior into the cell interior (cytoplasm); (iii) the substrate(s) dissociates into the cytosol; and (iv) the substrate-binding and translocation domain(s) of the transporter is reoriented for future substrate binding.

Eventually, the process of transport requires the expenditure of respiration energy. The coupling of energy to drive transporter function typically is described as direct (primary) or indirect (secondary and tertiary) processes. Primary transporters are energized by the direct transfer of chemical energy stored in high-energy phosphate bonds of ATP (adenosine 5'-triphosphate), as ATP is hydrolysed to ADP and inorganic phosphorus. In contrast, secondary transporter function is not coupled directly to ATP hydrolysis. Instead, secondary transport systems derive the energy to translocate substrates across membranes by harnessing the differences in the transmembrane electrical and chemical gradients of substrates and (sometimes) co-transported ions (Na^+, K^+, Cl^- and H^+). In mammals, amino acid and peptide transport occurs by indirect processes. For example, Na^+-dependent amino acid transport systems are secondary transporters that energize substrate translocation by coupling the transfer of amino acids to the large extracellular-to-intracellular Na^+ (e.g. systems A, ASC and B) and Cl^- (systems IMINO and GLY) gradients (Table 1.1). The cell then pays for the 'free' ride of the solutes down their electrochemical gradients by expending ATP to fuel the function of primary transporters (Na^+/K^+ ATPase and H^+ ATPase), which re-establish the extracellular-to-intracellular concentrations of the co-transported driving ions. One amino acid transport system, system X^-_{AG}, uses both the extracellular-to-intracellular Na^+ gradient and the intracellular-to-extracellular K^+ gradients to energize the transport of anionic amino acids.

Tertiary systems also utilize the energy derived from the electrochemical gradient of a co-transported ion(s), but, in essence, exchange the driving ion for another ion that is a substrate for a primary transporter. For example, H^+ ions are co-transported with small peptides across the apical membranes of enterocytes and released into the cytoplasm by the H^+/peptide co-transporter (Table 1.2). The H^+ then is pumped out of the cell by the apical membrane-bound Na^+/H^+ exchanger (driven by the extracellular-to-intracellular Na^+ gradient), thereby re-establishing the extracellular-to-intracellular H^+ gradient. The extracellular-to-intracellular Na^+ gradient is then re-established by the basolateral membrane-bound Na^+/K^+ ATPase. Hence, the H^+/peptide co-transporter is a

Table 1.1. α-Amino acid transport systems that have been identified in selected tissues, cells, and apical (Ap) and basolateral (Bs) membranes.

Transport system	Coupled ions	Substrates	Fibroblast[a]	Skeletal muscle[b]	Hepatocytes[c]		Enterocytes[d]		Placental scyncytia[e]		Pancreatic acinar[f]	
			Plasma	Plasma	Bs	Canalicular	Ap	Bs	Ap	Bs	Ap	Bs
A	Na$^+$	All neutrals, Pro	X	X	X	X		X	X	X	X	X
ASC	Na$^+$	Neutral (pH 7.5), Anionic (pH 5.5)	X	X	X	X		X	X	X		
asc		Neutrals			X			X			X	X
B (NBB, B^o)	Na$^+$	Most neutrals					X					
B$^{o,+}$	Na^{+g}	Neutrals and cationics			X			X	X^h	X^h		
b$^{o,+}$		Same as B$^{o,+}$			X			X				
y$^+$L	Na^{+i}	Neutrals, cationics, but not cystine							X	X		
y$^+$		Cationics	X	X	X			X	X	X		X
L		Large branched neutrals	X	X	X^j	X^j		X	X	X	X	X
N	Na$^+$	Asn, Gln, His		X^k	X	X			X			
X$^-_{AG}$	Na$^+$, K$^+$	D-,L-Asp, L-Glu	X	X	X^l	X	X		X	X		
x^-_c		Anionics, cystine	X		X^m						X	X
GLY	Na$^+$, Cl$^-$	Gly			X							
IMINO	Na$^+$, Cl$^-$	Pro, hydroxy-Pro		X	X			X				
T		Tyr, aromatics			X							

[a]Kilberg and Haussinger, 1992; [b]Mackenzie *et al.*, 1992; [c]Mailliard *et al.*, 1995; [d]Ganapathy *et al.*, 1994; Mailliard *et al.*, 1995; [e]Matthews *et al.*, 1998b; [f]Mailliard *et al.*, 1995.
[g]May also be Cl$^-$ dependent (Munck, 1997).
[h]Present in rat but not human placentas.
[i]Neutral amino acids only.
[j]In rat hepatocytes, system L has both high-affinity (L1) and low-affinity (L2) components. Adult rats demonstrate primarily L2 activity in canalicular and basal membranes whereas L1 activity predominates in both membranes in suckling pups.
[k]Muscle variation of liver system N.
[l]Primarily pericentral hepatocytes.
[m]Primarily periportal hepatocytes.

tertiary transporter in terms of energy expenditure (Ganapathy *et al.*, 1994).

Most primary, secondary and/or tertiary transporters can accumulate substrates against substrate concentration gradients. In contrast, 'facilitative' transporters (transporter-mediated absorption that is driven by the osmotic gradient and/or electrical charge of the substrate) usually are not capable of concentrating substrates. Instead, facilitative transporters mediate the 'downhill' passage of substrates across membranes. For example, amino acid transport systems asc, L and x^-_c do not couple the transport of substrates with ions, and therefore are not considered to require the expenditure of respiration energy in order to function. Although not usually discussed in these terms, facilitative transport also depends on the generation of membrane potential energy for transporter movement within the membrane. This is because the amount of electrochemical energy required to reactivate the transporter is thought to be derived from the membrane potential, which is a function of the steady-state non-equilibrium ion gradients that are generated by primary transporters (Na$^+$/K$^+$ ATPase, H$^+$ ATPase and Ca^{2+} ATPase) and the antagonistic functioning of transmembrane leak channels (Na$^+$, K$^+$, H$^+$, Ca^{2+},

Table 1.2. Affinity constants for mediated peptide transport in animal cells and tissues.

Animal	Tissue	Experimental model	Co-transport substrate	Substrate	K_t (mM)
Hamster	Jejunum	Everted rings	H+	Val–Val	9.6
				Gly–Sar	6.1
				Leu–Leu	5.6
				Gly–Gly	5.2
				Ala–Ala	3.2
Rabbit	Small intestine	BBMV[a]	None	Gly–Sar	17.3 ± 1.4
			H+	Gly–Sar	19.5 ± 2.0
Rabbit	Jejunum	BLMV[b]	H+	Gly–Pro	2.0 ± 0.20
Tilapia (fish)	Intestine	BBMV	None	Gly–Phe	9.8 ± 3.5
	Intestine	BBMV	H+	Gly–Sar	0.56 ± 0.08
		BLMV	H+	Gly–Sar	13.3 ± 3.8
Rat	Kidney: outer medulla and cortical	BBMV	H+	Gly–Leu	0.101 ± 0.0209
			H+	Gly–Gln	0.003 ± 0.0001
Human	Colon: Caco-2 cells	Apical	H+	Bestatin	0.34
		Basolateral	H+	Bestatin	0.71
Human	Colon: Caco-2 cells	Apical	H+	Gly–Sar	1.1 ± 0.17
Rat	Lung: type II pneumocytes	BBMV	H+	D-Phe–L-Ala	2.0
Rat	Liver pneumocytes	Lysosome MV	H+	Gly–Gln	4.67 ± 0.8
Human	Fibrosarcoma	HT1080 cells	H+	Gly–Sar	11.4 ± 3.3
Rabbit	Small intestine	PepT1 expressed in Xenopus laevis oocytes	H+	Cephalexin	4.20
				Cyclocillin	0.137
Rabbit	Small intestine	PepT1 expressed in oocytes	H+	Gly–Sar	1.90
			H+	Gly–Leu	0.08
			H+	Gly–Glu	0.22
			H+	Gly–Lys	2.40
			2 H+	D-Phe–L-Glu	0.94
			H+	Gly–Gly	2.51
			H+	Gly–Gly–Gly	5.10
			H+	Gly–Gly–Gly–Gly	24.0
Human	Small intestine	PepT1 expressed in HeLa cells	H+	Gly–Sar	0.29
Human	Kidney	PepT2 expressed in HeLa cells	H+	Gly–Sar	0.074
Sheep	Omasum	poly(A)+ mRNA expressed in oocytes	H+	Gly–Sar	0.40
Sheep	Duodenum	BBMV	H+	Gly–Pro	0.005 ± 0.001

[a]Brush border membrane vesicles; [b]basolateral membrane vesicles.

HCO_3^- and Cl^-). Therefore, the energy for all facilitated transport ultimately depends on cellular respiration. How energy is coupled from the transmembrane potential to drive reactivation of the transporter is not understood.

Amino acids and peptides can be absorbed without the aid of transport proteins. However, because cell membranes are relatively impermeable to these charged hydrophilic molecules, the non-mediated absorption of amino acids and small peptides occurs by diffusion through membrane-spanning channels and paracellular pathways, and/or by endocytosis (membrane envelopment). Diffusion is a substrate concentration-dependent event, whereas endocytosis may additionally involve substrate recognition. Typically, the rate of non-mediated amino acid and peptide absorption is much lower than that by transporter-mediated processes. However, at any given time, the relative contribution that transporter-independent absorption makes to the total absorption of amino acids and peptides by a cell depends on extra- and intracellular substrate concentrations, the magnitude of signals affecting membrane endocytosis and structural protein function, substrate size and charge (relative to protein channel charge and size) and intracellular energy levels. A thorough discussion of cellular mechanisms by which transporter-independent substrate absorption can occur is available (Gardner, 1994).

Biochemically Characterized Amino Acid and Peptide Transport Systems

Amino acid transporters

The study of how cells absorb α-amino acid nitrogen historically has followed the study of free or peptide-bound amino acids. The work of Halvor Christensen and colleagues (Kilberg and Haussinger, 1992) has resulted in the characterization of a number of separate amino acid transport systems in epithelial and non-epithelial cells (Table 1.1). These transport activities typically are categorized according to their required energy sources, substrate specificities and kinetics of absorption. The characterization of amino acid transport processes has resulted in the paradigm that translocation of free α-amino acids across cellular membranes occurs by multiple transport activities, often with overlapping substrate specificities for amino acids of the same and/or different class (cationic, anionic or zwitterionic). For example, lysine and leucine are each recognized by at least four biochemically distinct α-amino acid transport systems, with three of these transport systems ($B^{o,+}$, $b^{o,+}$ and y^+L) recognizing both substrates. α-Amino acid transport systems display varying degrees of substrate specificities, ranging from

system IMINO, which is specific for proline, to system $B^{o,+}$, which accepts most dipolar and cationic amino acids. Free α-amino acid transporters, however, do not recognize β-amino acids (e.g. taurine). Recognition of amino acids by transport proteins is thought to be dependent on the α-amino or α-imino group (for proline) and a carboxyl group, with the size, charge and/or configuration of the side chains acting as important determinants for substrate transport (Christensen, 1984).

It is clear from reported free amino acid transport activities of mammalian fibroblasts, skeletal muscle, hepatocytes, enterocytes, placental trophoblasts and pancreatic acinar cells (Table 1.1) that the expression of transporter activities differs among types of cells (e.g. B, $B^{o,+}$, N and y^+L) and between the membranes of cells (e.g. asc, B and $B^{o,+}$). It is also apparent that several transport activities are expressed in most types of cells (A, ASC, y^+, L and X^-_{AG}). Part of this heterogeneity in amino acid absorption capacity appears to be associated with substrate supply. For example, only the intestinal lumen-facing brush border membranes of enterocytes and the bile-facing canalicular membranes of hepatocytes do not express systems A and ASC and, instead, rely on systems B and $B^{o,+}$ to absorb dipolar amino acids. Additionally, the expression of system $B^{o,+}$ confers an added capacity for cationic amino acid transport, as compared with other cells and membranes which only express system y^+. Interestingly, enterocytes also express system IMINO for the absorption of proline in the apical membrane, which is readily transported by system A in the basolateral membrane and in cells other than enterocytes. System L, a predominant Na^+-independent transporter of large hydrophobic dipolar amino acids, also is not expressed in the apical membrane of enterocytes, but is in the basolateral membranes.

Peptide transporters

As with free amino acids, the absorption of peptide-bound amino acids is a universal phenomenon in single-cell and complex organisms. The study of peptide-bound amino acid absorption was initiated with the proposal by Fisher in 1954 that 'peptides, rather than amino acids, may be the protein currency of the body' (as reviewed by Matthews, 1991). Thanks in large part to the pioneering work of David Matthews (Matthews, 1991) and Siamak Adibi (Adibi, 1997), it is now understood that dietary and plasma proteins do not need to be completely hydrolysed to their constituent amino acids for absorption to occur across the apical membranes of intestinal and kidney tubule epithelia. Data collected from many studies designed to understand the quantitative importance of free versus peptide-bound amino acids indicate that peptide-bound amino acids can account for the majority of amino acids absorbed by enterocytes from the intestinal lumen (Matthews, 1991; Seal and Parker, 1991; Webb and Matthews, 1998). A representative list of peptide transport substrates and affinity constants as measured in the tissues, cells and membranes of various species is presented in Table 1.2. The use of hydrolysis-resistant peptides (β-alanylhistidine; carnosine; and glycylsarcosine, Gly-Sar) in whole tissue and brush border membrane (BBM) vesicle experiments has shown that the transport of intact peptides is independent of peptidase or amino acid transport activities and that concentrative peptide uptake is coupled to co-transport of a proton(s) (Ganapathy et al., 1994; Adibi, 1997). In apical (brush border) membrane transport systems, such as enterocytes and kidney tubule epithelia, an extracellular-to-intracellular H^+ gradient energizes the transport of di-, tri and/or tetra-peptide substrates. In isolated intestinal loops, the pH of the transport environment additionally is reported to affect the affinity of the low-affinity, high capacity transport system (Lister et al., 1997).

Three generalized peptide transport systems have been characterized biochemically in mammals: (i) a low-affinity transport system highly expressed in the apical membranes of differentiated enterocytes, which also is weakly expressed in the microvillus membrane of kidney tubule epithelia; (ii) a high-affinity transport capacity expressed primarily in the apical membranes of kidney proximal tubules epithelia; and (iii) a low-affinity system on the basolateral membranes of polarized cell types that displays a more limited range of binding capacity than the low-affinity apical transporters. Consequently, the generalized model that has resulted for the transport of small peptides across mammalian polarized epithelia involves: (i) the recognition and absorption of peptides by the low-affinity, high-capacity transporter; (ii) transport across the apical membrane into the cell cytosol, and hydrolysis to free amino acids; and/or (iii) the passage of intact peptides into the blood by a high-affinity, low-capacity basolateral membrane transporter (Ganapathy et al., 1994; Adibi, 1997; Steel et al., 1997). In fish, a similar model has been proposed, except for the presence of both high- and low-affinity transport systems in the apical membranes and the presence of a low-affinity, high-capacity basolateral transport system that displays a broader range of substrate recognition than that of the apical transporters (Thamotharan et al., 1998).

Consistent with the relatively few transport systems that have been identified for peptide transport, recognition by these 'promiscuous' transporters has been proposed to be achieved with an oligopeptide of four or less amino acids that contains at least one peptide bond, a C-terminal L conformer amino acid, and an overall net positive charge of <2 (Boyd, 1995). Accordingly, β-lactam and cephalosporin antibiotics are substrates for peptide transport systems. A recent report suggests that the peptide bond may not be required for substrate binding by either the low- or high-affinity peptide transport systems (Ganapathy et al., 1998). Although any of the three characterized peptide transport systems recognize many more substrates than does any given amino acid transporter, not all small peptides are recognized, substantial differences do exist in the relative affinities for substrates among peptide transport systems, and at least one peptide transport system (PepT1, see below) is capable of distinguishing between *cis* and *trans* conformers (Table 1.2; Brandsch *et al.*, 1997, 1998). The similarities and differences in the affinities of peptide transport systems have been of practical importance to the pharmacological industry in the development of peptidomimetic drugs. Whether these differences can be exploited to enhance the absorption of specific amino acids as peptides, in nutritionally significant quantities, remains to be determined.

Molecular Characterization of Transport Proteins

The interpretation of biochemical studies designed to characterize transporter activity is complicated by the recognition of multiple amino acids by transporter systems. The recent generation of a number of complementary DNA (cDNA) clones that encode proteins with specific transport activities, and the functional expression of their corresponding mRNAs in various expression models (Malandro and Kilberg, 1996), has clarified a number of questions regarding the specificity, function and expression of transporter activities. A list of the cloned α-amino acid and peptide transport proteins is presented in Table 1.3, except for the family of brain-specific neurotransmitter transporters. Knowledge of the molecular structure of proteins capable of α-amino acid transport has allowed evolutionary and taxonomic relationships to be established based on primary amino acid sequence homologies and predicted membrane topologies (see below). In addition, the gene structure of several of the amino acid transporters has been determined. An important understanding gained from knowing the gene structure is that different mRNAs can be transcribed from a single gene. The transcription of mRNAs that encode different proteins from a single gene occurs by alternative gene promoters or alternative splicing of transcripts and results in a

greater diversity of transporter isoforms and functional characteristics. A good example is the production of CAT2 (high-affinity system y^+ activity) and CAT2a (low-affinity system y^+ activity) proteins from the *CAT2* gene (MacLeod *et al.*, 1994).

The identification of cDNAs has also allowed the amount of mRNA expressed to be quantified (Northern analysis) and the site of mRNA expression to be determined (*in situ* hybridization analysis). Based on the sequence of the cDNA, the amino acid sequence of the protein can be predicted, thus facilitating the generation of antibodies to transport proteins. With antibodies, the amount (immunoblot/Western blot) and site-specific expression (immunohistochemistry) of proteins can be determined. Based on the known cDNA sequence of one species, the cDNA isoform from another species can be identified by hybridizing oligonucleotides that are predicted to bind to regions of shared homology. If oligonucleotides are designed that encompass the whole protein-coding sequence of the cDNA, then the region can be amplified by polymerase chain reaction (PCR), resulting in the cloning of species-specific 'full-length' cDNA. These techniques also can be combined to identify the mRNA of transporters that share homologous regions.

CAT family of cationic amino acid transporters

The Na^+-independent transport of the cationic amino acids arginine, lysine, ornithine and that portion of histidine molecules that is positively charged is known as system y^+ activity. Even though system y^+ transport is not coupled directly to transmembrane-driving ion gradients, system y^+-mediated substrates can be accumulated against their concentration gradients because of the difference between their positive charge and the relatively negative charge on the cytosolic side of the membrane. Currently, four cDNAs have been identified that encode system y^+ activity (*cationic amino acid transport*;

Table 1.3. Free and peptide-bound α-amino acid transport proteins for which there are cDNA clones[a].

Clone	Alternate names	Deduced length[b]	Transport system	Substrate specificity	Substrate affinity	Ions coupled
CAT1	—	622–629	y^{+c}	Cationic	μM	—
CAT2	CAT2a	657–658	y^+	Cationic	μM	—
CAT2a	CAT2b	657–659	y^+	Cationic	mM	—
CAT3	—	619	y^+	Cationic	μM	—
EAAT1	GluT, GLAST	543	X^-_{AG}	D,L-aspartate L-glutamate	μM	Na^+_{in}, K^+_{out}, $OH^-/HCO_3^-_{out}$
EAAT2	GLT, GLAST2, GLTR	573	X^-_{AG}	D,L-aspartate L-glutamate	μM	Na^+_{in}, K^+_{out}, $OH^-/HCO_3^-_{out}$
EAAT3	EAAC1	523–525	X^-_{AG}	D,L-aspartate L-glutamate	μM	Na^+_{in}, K^+_{out}, $OH^-/HCO_3^-_{out}$
EAAT4	—	564	X^-_{AG}	D,L-aspartate L-glutamate	μM	Na^+_{in}, K^+_{out}, $OH^-/HCO_3^-_{out}$
EAAT5	—	561	X^-_{AG}	D,L-aspartate L-glutamate	μM	Na^+_{in}, K^+_{out}, $OH^-/HCO_3^-_{out}$
ASCT1	SATT	532	ASC	Neutral (pH 7.5) Anionic (pH 5.5)	μM	Na^+_{in}
ASCT2	ATB[o]	553	ASC	Neutral	μM	Na^+_{in}
NBAT	Naa-Tr, D2	683	$b^{o,+}$	Neutral cationic and cystine	μM	—
4F2hc	—	529	y^+L	Neutral and cationic	μM	Na^+_{in} (for neutral)
PepT1	—	707–708	H^+/peptide	Di-, tri-, tetra-peptides and Ab[d]	mM	H^+_{in}
PepT2	—	729	H^+/peptide	Di-, tri-, tetra-peptides and Ab[d]	μM	H^+_{in}

[a]Does not include members of the family of brain-specific neurotransmitter transporters (PROT, GLYT1a, GLYT1b, GLYT1c, GLYT2; Malandro and Kilberg, 1996).
[b]Predicted number of amino acids.
[c]In mice, also acts as the recognition site for murine ecotropic leukaemia virus.
[d]β-Lactam and cephalosporin antibiotics.

CAT1, CAT2, CAT2a and CAT3). Of these, CAT1, CAT2 and CAT3 cDNAs encode high-affinity cationic amino acid transport (micromolar K_m values). Based on hydrophobicity profiles, all three transporters are predicted to possess 12–14 membrane-spanning domains. CAT1 mRNA is ubiquitously expressed, being present in all tissues tested except for the liver (Deves and Boyd, 1998). In mice, CAT1 protein is the recognition receptor for infection by the murine ecotropic leukaemia virus (MacLeod et al., 1994). That mice have not evolved to eliminate this source of viral recognition suggests that CAT1 is indispensable in its role of supplying cells with the essential amino acids arginine, lysine and histidine. In humans, CAT2 mRNA is expressed less widely than CAT1, with the highest levels of mRNA expressed in skeletal muscle, placenta and ovaries, followed by lower expression in liver, pancreas, heart and kidney. CAT3, however, is only expressed in significant amounts in the brain.

The liver is the only tissue not known to express significant amounts of high-affinity cationic amino acid transport activity. Instead, the liver demonstrates low-affinity cationic amino acid transport, which is encoded by CAT2a, an alternatively spliced variant arising from the *CAT2* gene. Generally, CAT2a displays an apparent affinity for arginine uptake that is nearly tenfold lower (millimolar K_m values) than that of the other CAT family members. The low-affinity, but high-capacity transport of CAT2a well matches its physiological role of absorbing the relatively large amounts of cationic amino acids from dietary and endogenous sources that enter the liver through portal vein drainage of the intestinal tract.

EAAT family of anionic amino acid transporters

System X^-_{AG} activity is defined as the high-affinity, Na$^+$-dependent, K$^+$-coupled, D-aspartate-inhibitable transport of L-glutamate or L-aspartate. Currently, five glutamate/aspartate family members have been cloned from mammals that are capable of system X^-_{AG} activity. In humans, the proteins are referred to as EAAT1–5 (*e*xcitatory *a*mino *a*cid *t*ransport), although, as indicated in Table 1.3, alternative names were used for the original non-human isoform clones. Functionally, the process for transport by EAAT1–3 is thought to involve extracellular binding and translocation of one amino acid, one proton and three sodium ions, with reorientation of the transporter to the extracellular face of the membrane being driven by the intracellular-to-extracelluar counter-transport of one potassium ion. In addition to the ion flux associated with EAAT1–3, EAAT4 and EAAT5 isoforms have a large inward chloride ion flux associated with their function, which may aid in the re-establishment of membrane potential by influencing cellular chloride permeability. The capacity for glutamate and aspartate uptake by EAAT4 and EAAT5 is less than those for EAAT1–3. Accordingly, it is thought that EAAT4 and

EAAT5 function as chloride channels that are activated by the sodium-dependent binding of anionic amino acids (Arriza *et al.*, 1997).

For the EAAT anionic family, the predicted protein sequences show structural features typical of membrane solute transporters, such as multiple membrane-spanning domains and glycosylation sites. Hydrophobicity analysis of EAAT family members predicts that the N-terminus will span the membrane six times. However, it is not clear whether the large hydrophobic C-terminal portion of the protein spans the membrane. In contrast, the protein sequences of most amino acid transporter families are predicted to span the extracellular membrane 10–12 times. Among mammals, the sequence identity of a given EAAT is typically >85%. In humans, across transporters, the five cloned EAATs share sequence identities of 36–46%. Compared with human EAATs, a recently cloned caterpillar EAAT isoform shares 37–42% sequence identity with human EAAT1–4 while salamander homologues of EAAT1, EAAT2 and EAAT5 share 87, 84 and 58% sequence identities, respectively.

EAAT1–4 are highly expressed in brain tissue, but with distinct patterns of distribution. In the brain, EAAT1 and EAAT2 represent glial-specific glutamate transporters, whereas EAAT3 and EAAT4 represent neuron-specific activities. Accordingly, EAAT1 and EAAT2 are involved in neurotransmission whereas EAAT3 and EAAT4 are thought to be responsible for more general metabolic functions of brain tissues. A reduction in the capacity to resorb glutamate from synaptic clefts has been associated with neuron degeneration in sporadic amyotrophic lateral sclerosis (Lou Gehrig's disease). Recent work has identified that this loss in glutamate transport capacity is due solely to reduced expression of EAAT2, resulting from the aberrant processing of EAAT2 mRNA (Lin *et al.*, 1998).

EAAT3 is the most widely distributed of the glutamate transporters outside of the brain. For example, in the rabbit, EAAT3 mRNA is expressed in the duodenum, jejunum, ileum, heart, liver, lung and placenta, but not the colon, lung or spleen. Therefore, EAAT3 is thought to be the primary EAAT isoform responsible for supplying anionic amino acids for general cellular metabolic processes. EAAT1 mRNA, however, is also fairly widely expressed outside of the brain, having been reported in heart, lung, skeletal muscle, placenta, and retinal Mueller and astrocyte cells. In contrast, EAAT2 and EAAT4 expression appears limited to brain and placenta tissues. EAAT5 has the most restricted pattern of the EAAT family, being expressed primarily in retinal tissue where it is thought to play a vital role in the retinal light response. Other expression of EAAT5 mRNA is restricted to liver and skeletal muscle tissue, at levels ~ 20-fold less than that of the retina (Arriza *et al.*, 1997).

Besides the brain, the one tissue that has been shown to express EAAT1–4 mRNA is the placenta. In the placenta, system X^-_{AG} activity is thought to be responsible for the absorption of maternal and fetal-derived glutamate (and aspartate), thereby providing trophoblasts with an

important source of oxidizable fuel in the form of glutamate, generated by fetal nitrogen assimilation from glutamine. Therefore, to the extent that the placenta can meet its demand for a readily oxidizable fuel by glutamate, the demand for maternal glucose for placental oxidation may be moderated. As illustrated in Fig. 1.1, transporters capable of system X^-_{AG} activity (EAAT1–3) have been identified on different membranes of the syncytial trophoblast of rat placenta (Matthews *et al.*, 1998a). The pattern of transporter expression changes, depending on the day of gestation. Accordingly, it is hypothesized that the increase in EAAT1 and EAAT3 content on the apical membrane, and the increase in EAAT3 and decrease in EAAT2 content on the basal membrane, provides an increased capacity to absorb glutamate (and aspartate) from the maternal and fetal circulations during the end of gestation. Additionally, the expression of EAAT1–3 protein by maternal decidual, giant and spongiotrophoblast cells was also altered with gestation. Overall, the expression of EAAT1–3 glutamate transport proteins in placental cells was altered in a manner

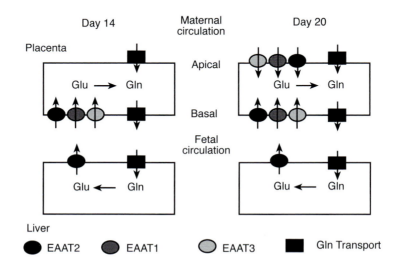

Fig. 1.1. Diagram illustrating the shift in transporter expression of EAAT1, EAAT2 and EAAT3 anionic amino acid transport proteins in the labyrinth apical and basal subdomains of gestation day 14 and 20 rat placentas. The model is based on the research of Matthews *et al.* (1998a) and is presented in terms of the maternal/fetal 'glutamine/glutamate cycle', as described in the text.

ASCT family of zwitterionic amino acid transporters

As noted above, Na[+]-dependent system ASC transports *a*lanine, *s*erine, *c*ysteine and other neutral α-amino acids. ASCT1 cDNA, originally cloned from human brain tissue, encodes system ASC-like activity and shares nearly 40% amino acid sequence identity with the anionic EAAT transporters. A second cDNA (ASCT2) has been cloned from mouse and human tissues that encodes system ASC-like activity. Human ASCT2 shares 61% identity with human ASCT1 and displays a broader pattern of substrate recognition than, but similar transport function to, ASCT1. The ASCT1 and ASCT2 cDNAs encode open reading frames of 532 and 541 amino acids, respectively. As with the EAAT family, hydrophobicity modelling of the ASCT transporter sequences predict six well-defined transmembrane sequences near the N-terminus of the protein and additional, less well-defined, hydrophobic stretches near the C-terminus. Although system ASC normally recognizes neutral amino acids, at pH ≤5.5, only glutamate and aspartate are substrates, not neutral amino acids. This pH-dependent recognition pattern is displayed by ASCT1 and ASCT2. The transport of anionic amino acids by ASCT1 and ASCT2 at low pH appears to be an example of similarities in structure/function that exist between the EAAT and ASCT families.

System ASC activity has been identified in nearly every mammalian tissue tested, and can account for the majority of uptake of several neutral amino acids in a number of cell types. For many years, it was thought that Na[+]-dependent system ASC functioned as a concentrative transporter. However, based on functional expression studies of ASCT1 in defolliculated *Xenopus laevis* oocytes, it is now thought that ASCT1-mediated system ASC activity is that of an obligatory exchanger system (Zerangue and Kavanaugh, 1996). As such, one extracellular amino acid would be exchanged for one intracellular transporter, resulting in no net accumulation of amino acids. Theoretically, however, because of potential differences in extracellular and intracellular binding affinities, the concentration of a given amino acid in the cytosol could be achieved at the expense of others being transported out of the cell. If system ASC is confirmed to be an obligatory exchanger in mammalian cell expression models, then system A, which has not been cloned, would remain as the only identified Na[+]-dependent transporter capable of concentrative neutral amino acid uptake in non-polarized cells.

ASCT1 mRNA is expressed highly in the brain, skeletal muscle and pancreas, moderately in the heart, and very weakly in liver, lung, placenta and kidney human tissues. The expression of ASCT2 mRNA appears limited to cells of the lung, skeletal muscle, kidney adipose, pancreas, placenta, testes and large intestine. The fact that ASCT1 and ASCT2 have not been reported in the small intestine, but that system ASC activity is high in intestinal tissue, suggests that other members of this family of neutral amino acid transporters have yet to be identified.

NBAT/4F2hc family of zwitterionic and cationic amino acid transporters

A new class of transport-related proteins has been identified in several animal species after induction of system b[o,+] (Na[+]-independent uptake of both zwitterionic (o) and cationic (+) amino acids) in oocytes following expression of size-fractionated kidney mRNA (Deves and Boyd, 1998). This chapter will refer to all cDNAs that encode system b[o,+] activity as NBAT (*neu*tral *b*asic *a*mino acid *t*ransport), even though cDNAs from several species were cloned and named independently (Table 1.3). NBAT is predicted to have 1–4 membrane-spanning domains, thereby differing from most solute transporters, which are predicted to possess 6–12 membrane-spanning domains. The NBAT proteins share 80–85% sequence identity and encode a protein of 683 amino acids with a non-glycosylated molecular mass of ∼ 78 kDa.

As noted, the expression of NBAT mRNA in oocytes results in increased system $b^{o,+}$ activity. Paradoxically, however, the expression of NBAT cDNA in mammalian cells has failed to result in increased system $b^{o,+}$ activity. Because of its unique predicted membrane topography, and because rat kidney NBAT appears to be associated with another protein of ∼ 50 kDa in size via disulphide bridging, it currently is thought that NBAT encodes a protein that activates an endogenous oocyte transporter, or that serves as an accessory subunit, rather than encoding a discrete transport protein.

System y^+L activity mediates the Na^+-independent absorption of cationic amino acids in a manner similar to system $b^{o,+}$, except that the transport of zwitterionic amino acids by system y^+L is Na^+-dependent and cystine is not a substrate. When expressed in oocytes, the human T-cell surface antigen 4F2hc (4F2 *heavy chain*) induces both cationic and zwitterionic amino acid high-affinity uptake in an system y^+L-like manner. Besides similar substrate recognitions, the 4F2hc and the NBAT proteins share significant (∼ 30%) sequence similarities and predicted membrane topographies. 4F2hc is an 85 kDa type II membrane glycoprotein that spans the membrane a single time and that forms a heterodimer functional unit with the 45 kDa non-glycosylated 4F2 light chain protein (Malandro and Kilberg, 1996). Implicit with its shared homology to 4F2hc, the system $b^{o,+}$/NBAT transport system may be composed of multiple proteins.

Because of their broad substrate specificity, the expression of NBAT and 4F2hc transport proteins/systems is considered to be important for rapid cellular growth. NBAT mRNA and protein are most highly expressed in the kidney and small intestine, but many other tissues express lower levels of NBAT mRNA. In the rat,

NBAT has been localized specifically to the epithelia of kidney proximal tubule and jejunal microvilli. Similarly, many polarized epithelial cells express 4F2hc mRNA and system y^+L activity. Based on the electroneutrality of transport across the basolateral membranes and consistent with its obligate exchanger function, it appears that system y^+L activity is localized to the basolateral membrane of polarized cells. In the apical membranes of enterocytes, systems $B^{o,+}$, y^+ and $b^{o,+}$ have all been measured, depending on diet, cell type and species differences. Accordingly, as a general model, the transport of cationic amino acids across polarized cells is proposed to occur by the transport of substrate across the apical membrane due to varying contributions by systems $B^{o,+}$, $b^{o,+}$ and/or y^+, followed by transfer across the basolateral membrane by system y^+L (Deves and Boyd, 1998). The expression on the apical membrane of multiple transporters with differing relative affinities for the same substrates ensures that the potential to absorb cationic substrates will be maximal at whatever concentration they are present.

PepT family of H^+/peptide co-transporters

PepT1 (*pep*tide *t*ransporter *1*; a 707 amino acid polypeptide for rabbit and a 708 amino acid polypeptide for human) cDNA encodes a low-affinity, high-capacity transporter that is predicted to contain one relatively large cytosolic domain and 12 α-helical membrane-spanning domains (Fei et al., 1994). PepT2 cDNA encodes a high-affinity, low-capacity transporter that is predicted to consist of 729 amino acids and possess 12 membrane-spanning domains (Leibach and Ganapathy, 1996). The amino acid sequences for human PepT1 and PepT2 share 50% identity, with the majority of the homology existing in the membrane-spanning regions.

The number of H^+ ions required for the intestinal apical membrane peptide transport system depends on the charge of the substrate; PepT1 displays H^+:substrate stoichiometries of 1:1, 2:1 and 1:1 for neutral, acidic and basic dipeptides (Steel *et al.*, 1997). Given that the enterocyte microenvironment of the apical membrane is maintained between pH 5.5 and 6.3, these findings suggest that PepT1 will bind preferentially to neutral and acidic dipeptides. In contrast, other expression studies indicate that the influence of pH on PepT1 and PepT2 function is to increase the velocity of transport, not the affinity of the transporter for its substrate (Brandsch *et al.*, 1997).

Rabbit PepT1 mRNA has been identified in the greatest quantity in epithelial cells of the small intestine, with lesser amounts in the liver and kidney tissue, and trace amounts in several brain tissues (Fei *et al.*, 1994). In contrast, the strongest expression of PepT2 is in the kidney, with weaker expression in brain, lung, liver, heart and spleen. The dual expression of PepT1 and PepT2 in the kidney is consistent with the biochemically defined high- and low-affinity peptide transport systems (Daniel *et al.*, 1992). Because the concentration of peptides is thought to increase from the proximal to distal nephron, future immunohistochemical research is expected to reveal that PepT2 (high-affinity, low-capacity) will be expressed primarily in the proximal nephron region, while PepT1 (low-affinity, high-capacity) will be expressed in the distal region of nephrons (Leibach and Ganapathy, 1996).

In the liver, the degree to which peptides are absorbed is controversial. Mediated uptake of carnosine and glycylsarcosine has been characterized in hamster liver slices (Matthews, 1991). However, the quantitative importance of hepatic peptide absorption is questioned by the observation that rat hepatocytes were incapable of absorbing dipeptides that are less resistant to hydrolysis than glycylsarcosine and carnosine (Lochs *et al.*, 1986). Instead, the absorption of peptide-bound amino acids occurs only after hydrolysis to their constituent amino acids. Therefore, the fact that the liver of rabbits contained mRNA for PepT1 (Fei *et al.*, 1994) and PepT2 (Boll *et al.*, 1996) suggests that species difference exists for tissue-specific peptide transporter expression. Alternatively, the expression of transporter protein may be limited to membranes other than the plasma membrane. In support of this hypothesis, low-affinity peptide transport activity has been demonstrated in the lysosomal membranes of rat hepatocytes using Gly-Gln (Thamotharan *et al.*, 1996). Also, the presence of PepT1 mRNA does not necessarily mean that PepT1 protein is expressed, or that the amount expressed is below detection. For example, even though EAAT4 mRNA is detectable in rat placenta, EAAT4 protein is not (Matthews *et al.*, 1998a). Finally, the expression of peptide transporters may be limited to a small subset of liver cells and/or in subcellular membranes, perhaps, in a manner analogous to the expression of system X^-_{AG} activity by only the pericentral hepatocytes, which constitute only ~ 7% of all hepatocytes (Kilberg and Haussinger, 1992). This controversy illustrates the point that even though molecular techniques can localize the expression of transporter mRNA and protein, biochemical assays are necessary to gauge the physiologic importance of their presence.

Unidentified transport proteins

Despite the tremendous success in the cloning and identification of many proteins responsible for the transport of amino acids and peptides, the proteins responsible for several physiologically important transport activities have not been cloned. Much of the cationic and zwitterionic amino acid transport across the apical membrane of polarized cells occurs by system $B^{o,+}$ activity. The eventual cloning of cDNAs that encode this activity, which is the only described Na^+-dependent activity capable of the transport of both cationic and neutral amino acids, should yield important insights into the teleologic development of amino acid transporters. System L activity, one of the first to be characterized, which transports long-chain, branched-chain and aromatic zwitterionic amino acids in an Na⁺-independent manner, also has not been cloned. Because system L is thought to be the primary mechanism for release of neutral amino acids from most mammalian cell types, understanding the molecular structure and patterns of regulation may yield important knowledge of how the transmembrane flux of amino acids is moderated to achieve intracellular amino acid homeostasis.

System N is the primary Na⁺-dependent transport activity for glutamine, asparagine and histidine in the liver. The heterogeneous absorption of anionic amino acids by the liver (system x^-_c, periportal hepatocytes; system X^-_{AG}, pericentral hepatocytes) is important to whole-animal nitrogen balance (Haussinger, 1990). Therefore, when combined with our ability to measure the expression of system X^-_{AG} proteins, the cloning of systems N and x^-_c will provide the ability to evaluate factors which affect the whole-body nitrogen homeostasis at the molecular level. Similarly, the elucidation of system A transport protein(s) and gene(s) will yield invaluable information as a model for the regulation of transporter expression. Normally, system A activity is low in most cells. However, in response to hormones, growth factors, cell division and/or substrate supply, system A activity increases from 2- to 50-fold. Accordingly, system A has been one of the most extensively biochemically characterized amino acid transport systems. Despite this fact, and the use of many imaginative protocols, including methodology successfully used for other transporters, the protein(s) responsible for system A activity has yet to be cloned. In terms of reported peptide transport activities, the protein(s) responsible for the putative basolateral membrane peptide transporter has yet to be identified. Once identified, two important questions to be answered using functional expression studies are what is the magnitude of the pH gradient required for transport and what regulates the capacity for peptide transport across the basolateral membrane.

Characterization of Gastrointestinal Tract Amino Acid and Peptide Transporters in Farm Animals

Chickens

It has been known for some time that the absorption of dietary amino acids across the chicken small intestine occurs by mediated processes, that neutral amino acids are transported more rapidly than cationic or anionic amino acids and that peptide absorption accounts for a substantial proportion of the total amount of amino acids absorbed (Duke, 1984). In a series of experiments designed to identify the transport system responsible for methionine and lysine uptake, the amino acid transport systems B, b⁰,⁺, y⁺ and L have been identified in the jejunal BBM of chicks (Torras-Llort et al., 1996; Soriano-Garcia et al., 1998). Methionine was transported by all four systems, whereas lysine uptake is reported to be by systems b⁰,⁺ and y⁺. In a subsequent trial, it was determined that feeding a lysine-enriched diet (68 g kg⁻¹ versus 48 g kg⁻¹) resulted in the increased activity of systems b⁰,⁺ and y⁺ (Torras-Llort et al., 1998). For system y⁺, only the velocity of transport was increased, indicating that the activity of resident system y⁺ transport protein increased and/or more transport proteins were present. In contrast, both the velocity and specificity of lysine transport by system b⁰,⁺ were increased. It is important to note from these studies that methionine was recognized by system y⁺ and that system L was not expressed in jejunal BBM. In other species, system y⁺ is reported to transport only cationic amino acids. Accordingly, the eventual molecular characterization of the complement of transport proteins expressed in chicken jejunum should either confirm this assignment, identify a new isoform of the CAT transporters (which may be unique to chickens) or demonstrate that methionine is actually transported by other Na⁺-independent transport systems that recognize cationic and neutral amino acids (such as system y⁺L/4F2hc). Additionally, once the genes for these transport proteins are identified, the study of how the feeding of elevated amounts of lysine in the diet ultimately caused an increase in transport system activity can be determined.

In terms of other transport systems in the chicken gastrointestinal tract, a high-affinity, Na^+-dependent anionic amino acid transport has been described, presumably corresponding to system X^-_{AG}-like activity (Wingrove and Kimmach, 1998). Also, the expression of H^+/peptide transporter activity has been reported in the BBM of the small intestine, caecum and rectum in chicks (Calonge *et al.*, 1990). Accordingly, with the noted exceptions for systems y^+ and L (above), it appears that the chicken intestinal tract expresses a complement of amino acid and peptide transporter activities that is similar to that of mammals. However, the molecular characterization of intestinal transporters in the chicken may increase our ability to manipulate the capacity for methionine and lysine transport, and, thereby, may optimize our ability to balance the supplementation of these limiting amino acids.

Pigs

In the pig, as with other monogastrics, the jejunum has the greatest capacity to absorb amino acids (Leibholz, 1998). As reviewed by Munck (1997), the BBM of the pig small intestine is known to express systems IMINO, B and probably x^-_c, but, unlike other monogastrics, not $B^{o,+}$. Consistent with this conclusion, measurements of amino acid fluxes across the small intestine suggest that transport systems capable of cationic amino acid transport in pig enterocytes are Na^+-independent in nature. As discussed previously (Matthews *et al.*, 1996c), the use of distal duodenal and proximal ileal cannulas in growing pigs resulted in the quantification of mutually inhibitable absorption of lysine and arginine. Additionally, the flux of lysine across isolated neonatal pig jejunal tissue sheets has been described as having

saturable (K_m = 200 μM) and non-saturable components. Because uptake was not measured in the absence of Na^+, mediated lysine uptake could have occurred by either systems $B^{o,+}$, y^+ and/or $b^{o,+}$. Lysine absorption in the presence of Na^+ by villi-tip enterocytes in the jejunal tissue of pigs (at approximately <1–28 days of age) has been shown to be non-concentrative, whereas alanine uptake in the presence of Na^+ was. Accordingly, lysine uptake could have occurred by systems y^+ and/or $b^{o,+}$, but not by $B^{o,+}$. Likewise, the non-concentrative component of alanine uptake was probably by system L and/or $b^{o,+}$. Consistent with the hypothesis that system $b^{o,+}$ is expressed by jejunal tissue, mRNA isolated from the jejunum of pigs encoded system $b^{o,+}$ activity when expressed in oocytes (Matthews *et al.*, 1996c). As with other monogastrics, the extracellular affinity for lysine was greater than that for leucine. Because system $B^{o,+}$ apparently is not expressed in the intestinal BBM of pigs, the observed Na^+-dependent concentrative alanine uptake may have been by systems A or ASC. Interestingly, however, neither of these transport systems have been shown to be expressed in intestinal BBM of other mammals (Table 1.1).

Clearly the complement of amino acid transporter activities expressed by the pig gastrointestinal tract has not been well defined. Additionally, reports of peptide transport systems are not known to this reviewer. Because the presence of leucine has been shown to stimulate both the influx and efflux of lysine across the basolateral membranes of enterocytes, ostensibly by the allosteric binding to system y^+ transporters (Deves and Boyd, 1998), and because system $b^{o,+}$ transport uptake of lysine is inhibitable by leucine (Matthews *et al.*, 1996c), the flux of lysine across pig jejunal enterocytes may be dependent on the luminal and serosal concentrations of leucine. If future research supports this hypothesis, then the determination of an optimal leucine:lysine dietary ratio may promote the more efficient feeding of lysine to pigs.

Sheep and cattle

*Intestinal absorption of amino acids
and peptides*

As with chickens and pigs, several characterized amino acid and peptide transport system activities have been identified in ruminants. Also, as in monogastrics, the duodenal, jejunal and ileal regions of the ruminant small intestine appear to have different abilities to absorb amino acids, with essential amino acids being absorbed preferentially over non-essential amino acids and absorption capacities unequally distributed throughout the length of the intestine. In contrast to pigs and other monogastrics, the ileal region of sheep and cattle has been identified as possessing the greatest potential for free amino acid absorption (Johns and Bergen, 1973; Phillips *et al.*, 1979; Guerino and Baumrucker, 1987). These reports also indicate that the relative contribution of transporter-mediated amino acid absorption to total amino acid absorption (versus that by non-mediated diffusion) will vary, depending on the concentration of luminal substrates. For peripheral tissues, which are exposed to much lower concentrations of amino acids, the contribution of mediated transport is expected to exceed that of non-mediated diffusion (Kilberg and Haussinger, 1992). For peptides, however, research with cultured cell lines indicates that a significant amount of non-mediated flux of peptides may occur across the plasma membranes of peripheral tissues (Oehlke *et al.*, 1997).

Although the specific transport systems in ruminants have not been characterized thoroughly, competitive uptake experiments performed using ileal mucosal strips isolated from beef and dairy cattle determined that methionine and lysine were absorbed by transport activities exhibiting system A, ASC, L and/or y^+ activities (Guerino and Baumrucker, 1987). The observations that alanine, glycine, leucine, lysine, phenylalanine and methionine mutually inhibited the uptake of each other across ileal BBM vesicles suggest that the bovine small intestine additionally expresses transporters capable of both neutral and cationic amino acid uptake (Moe *et al.*, 1987). However, because transport only was compared in the presence of Na^+, further delineation between the Na^+-dependent $B^{o,+}$ and Na^+-independent $b^{o,+}$ and y^+L transport systems cannot be determined. Additionally, the uptake of proline by system IMINO was indicated. Subsequently, the total uptake of methionine and lysine across ileal and jejunal BBM of steers was characterized as having active, facilitative and diffusional components (Wilson and Webb, 1990). At both 1.25 and 7.5 mM concentrations, a greater contribution to total uptake occurred by diffusion than by Na^+-dependent or Na^+-independent transport. It also was observed that ileal and jejunal tissue had lower affinities and higher capacities for methionine than for lysine.

Collectively, though limited, the above data suggest that the ruminant small intestine expresses a variety of amino acid transporter systems, similar to those reported for monogastrics. However, the membrane-specific localization has not been determined adequately. For example, on which membranes of enterocytes are systems A, ASC, L and/or y^+ activities expressed? If on the apical, then transporter expression in ruminants is dramatically different from that of monogastrics. As the bovine homologues of amino acid transporters are discovered, membrane-specific assignments of transporter expression can be made. To date, only EAAT1, EAAT2 and GLYT1 amino acid transporter homologues have been cloned from bovine-derived cell lines.

The expression of H^+-dependent peptide transport-like systems has been reported (preliminarily) in the intestinal epithelia of sheep and cattle. In one report, the observed K_m value of 0.005 mM for Gly–Pro uptake by sheep duodenal BBM is consistent with affinity constants typically reported for the high-affinity, low-capacity transporter (PepT2) (Backwell *et al.*, 1995). However, in a second report, velocities measured for peptide transport in both cattle and sheep proximal tissue are consistent with those reported for low-affinity, high-capacity peptide transport (PepT1) in monogastrics (Dyer *et al.*, 1996). Further research will be required to determine whether the dual expression of high- and low-affinity peptide transport systems is a unique property of ruminant intestinal epithelia, as compared with monogastrics.

Forestomach absorption of amino acids and peptides

The study of transport systems in fore-stomach tissues (rumen, reticulum and omasum) is complicated by the structure of their keratinized squamous epithelia. Starting proximal to the forestomach liquor, and ending adjacent to the basement membrane, the four strata of epithelial cells that make up these tissues have been classified as the basale, spinosum, granulosum and corneum. The number of cell layers that comprise the whole epithelium can range from eight to >30. Given the technical difficulties in performing kinetic characterization in such a complex tissue, and the classic hypothesis that the forestomach is responsible for little, if any, net absorption of amino acids, little research has been conducted to identify the capacity for forestomach absorption of amino acids or peptides. Consequently, mechanisms capable of α-amino nitrogen absorption in forestomach tissues are poorly characterized.

Given that pre-feeding levels of free amino acid concentrations in strained ruminal fluid of 0.12–1.5 mg dl^{-1} and post-feeding concentrations of 0.72–6 mg dl^{-1} have been reported in the rumen liquor of sheep fed common diets (as summarized by Matthews *et al.*, 1996a), it is likely that amino acid transporters would be of the high-affinity type. As discussed previously (Matthews and Webb, 1995), studies on measurement of the trans-epithelial passage of histidine (from 0.66 to 20 mM) across sheep ruminal epithelial sheets concluded that absorption was interpreted to mean that absorption was not saturatable. In retrospect, however, the fact that methionine, arginine and glycine inhibited histidine transfer indicates that

histidine transfer may have been at least partially mediated by transport proteins. Additional evidence that cationic amino acid absorption from forestomach liquor is mediated comes from the observation that the flux of lysine and arginine across ruminal tissue sheets is saturable from 0.3 to 30 mM. In omasal tissue, preliminary data from substrate competition trials in parabiotic chamber and oocyte expression models indicate that system b$^{o,+}$ is probably responsible for the absorption of cationic amino acids from across the omasal epithelium (Matthews *et al.*, 1996a). Because a lumen-to-blood Na$^+$ gradient does not typically exist, these competition profiles are consistent with the overlapping substrate recognition patterns of transporter systems y$^+$ or b$^{o,+}$.

From a teleological perspective, it seems reasonable to suggest that fore-stomach epithelial tissues may have evolved to express H$^+$/peptide co-transporters to absorb peptides from forestomach liquor. H$^+$ gradients of the magnitude used to demonstrate the presence of carrier-mediated dipeptide transport by intestinal and renal epithelial BBM vesicles and in cultured colon cells can develop between forestomach liquor and cells that comprise omasal and ruminal epithelia. Importantly, the Na$^+$/H$^+$ exchanger and Na$^+$/K$^+$ ATPase proteins, considered to be essential in re-establishing H$^+$ gradients in epithelial cells, are reported to exist and function in both ruminal and omasal epithelia. Finally, it is reasonable to expect pre-feeding concentrations of 1.5–5 mg dl^{-1} of peptide N and post-feeding concentrations of 10–27 mg dl^{-1} of peptide N in ruminal fluid of sheep and cattle (Matthews *et al.*, 1996a). Because omasal liquor amino acid and peptide N concentration values are unknown, it is not possible to predict the potential relative driving forces for amino acid absorption across the omasal epithelium. However, the absorption of water by omasal tissues would presumably result in the concentration of rumen liquor solutes, thereby potentially re-establishing (or generating greater) omasal liquor-to-blood concentration gradients and solvent drag forces that were present across ruminal epithelia, depending on the relative water and substrate absorption rates.

In a parabiotic study designed to evaluate the potential for forestomach epithelia to absorb dipeptides, the omasum demonstrated a markedly greater (approximately sixfold) ability to absorb carnosine and Met–Gly than did the rumen (Matthews and Webb, 1995). The expression of sheep omasal mRNA in oocytes (Matthews *et al.*, 1996b) resulted in H^+-dependent Gly-Sar uptake (K_m = 0.4 mM) that is consistent with PepT1 transport characteristics (Table 1.2). Additional work confirmed these findings and demonstrated that sheep omasal peptide transport protein(s) display differential affinities for di-, tri- and tetra-peptides (Pan *et al.*, 1997). As observed for PepT1 and PepT2 monogastric transporters (Daniel *et al.*, 1992), no relationship existed between the ability of these peptides to be transported and their molecular weight, hydrophobicity or net electrical charge.

The above data indicate that the ruminant gastrointestinal tract tissue of sheep and cattle possesses the capacity to absorb peptide-bound amino acids by peptide transport systems similar to those expressed by monogastric species. Unresolved questions regarding peptide absorption in ruminants include: (i) what the relative contribution of free versus peptide-bound amino acids is compared with the absorption of total amino acids across the gastrointestinal tract of ruminants; (ii) whether the forestomach epithelium is capable of absorbing nutritionally significant quantities of peptides; and (iii) whether specific dietary proteins and/or peptides can be supplied in a manner that increases total amino acid absorption.

Conclusions

The absorption of either free and peptide amino acids traditionally has been studied as separate events. Most of what is known regarding the structure, function and distribution of amino acid and peptide transport systems and proteins has been derived from the study of laboratory animal species and man. Information regarding the individual proteins responsible for the absorption of amino acids and peptides in farm animal species is limited. Amino acids typically are recognized by several transport systems, whereas most peptides apparently are transported by a single low-affinity, high-capacity and/or a high-affinity, low-capacity transporter. A variety of transporters in cells and cellular membranes provide a range of free and peptide-bound amino acid transport affinities and uptake capacities, thus promoting efficient absorption of these substrates, regardless of their extracellular concentration. In cells and membranes exposed to high substrate concentrations, the expression of low-affinity, high-capacity transporters is typical, whereas those normally exposed to low substrate concentrations often express high-affinity, low-capacity transporters. Some cells and membranes express both high- and low-affinity transporters.

The relative contribution of each transporter system/protein(s) to total amino acid nourishment of animals varies throughout the gastrointestinal and peripheral tissues, depending on substrate supply, cell type, tissue, species and/or the metabolic status of the animal. Accordingly, the ratio of free versus peptide-bound amino acid absorption will probably vary with production state. In the final analysis, however, it is the aggregate contribution of all these absorption phenomena, with their overlapping substrate affinities, that supplies the animal with its requisite amino acids. Therefore, the more we understand about how cells absorb amino acids, the greater our potential is to develop diets and feeding strategies that optimize protein synthesis and retention.

References

Adibi, S.A. (1997) Renal assimilation of oligopeptide: physiological mechanisms and metabolic importance. *American Journal of Physiology* 272, E723–E736.

Arriza, J.L., Eliasof, S., Kavanaugh, M.P. and Amara, S.G. (1997) Excitatory amino acid transporter 5, a retinal glutamate transporter coupled to a chloride conductance. *Proceedings of the National Academy of Sciences of the United States of America* 94, 4155–4160.

Backwell, C., Wilson, D. and Schweizer, A. (1995) Evidence for a glycyl-proline transport system in ovine enterocyte brush-border membrane vesicles. *Biochemical and Biophysical Research Communications* 215, 561–565.

Boll, M., Herget, M., Wagener, M., Weber, W.M., Markovich, D., Biber, J., Clayton, D.F., Murer, H. and Daniel, H. (1996) Expression cloning and functional characterization of the kidney cortex high-affinity proton-coupled peptide transporter. *Proceedings of the National Academy of Sciences of the United States of America* 93, 284–289.

Boyd, C.A.R. (1995) Intestinal oligopeptide transport. *Proceedings of the Nutrition Society* 54, 519–523.

Brandsch, M., Brandsch, C., Ganapathy, M.E., Chew, C.S., Ganapathy, V. and Leibach, F.H. (1997) Influence of proton and essential histidyl residues on the transport kinetics of the H^+/peptide cotransport systems in intestine (PEPT1) and kidney (PEPT2). *Biochimica et Biophysica Acta* 1324, 251–262.

Brandsch, M., Thunecke, F., Kuller, G., Schutkowski, M., Fischer, G. and Neubert, K. (1998) Evidence for the absolute conformational specificity of the intestinal H^+/peptide symporter, PEPT1. *Journal of Biological Chemistry* 273, 3861–3864.

Calonge, M.L., Ilundain, A. and Bolufer, J. (1990) Glycyl-L-sarcosine transport by ATP-depleted isolated enterocytes from chicks. *American Journal of Physiology* 259, G775–G780.

Christensen, H.N. (1984) Organic ion transport during seven decades. *Biochimica et Biophysica Acta* 779, 255–269.

Daniel, H., Morse, E.L. and Adibi, S.A. (1992) The high and low affinity transport systems for dipeptides in kidney brush border membrane respond differently to alterations in pH gradient and membrane potential. *Journal of Biological Chemistry* 266, 19917–19924.

Deves, R. and Boyd, C.A.R. (1998) Transporters for cationic amino acids in animal cells: discovery, structure, and function. *Physiology Reviews* 78, 487–545.

Duke, G.E. (1984) Avian digestion. In: Swenson, M.J. (ed.) *Dukes' Physiology of Domestic Animals*. Cornell University Press, Ithaca, Vol. 10, pp. 359–366.

Dyer, J., Allison, G., Scollan, N.D. and Shirazi-Beechey, S.P. (1996) Mechanism of peptide transport in ruminant intestinal brush-border membrane. *Biochemical Society Transactions* 24, 247S.

Fei, Y.-J., Kanai, Y., Nussberger, S., Ganapathy, V., Leibach, F.H., Romero, M.F., Singh, S.K., Boron, W.F. and Hediger, M.A. (1994) Expression cloning of a mammalian proton-coupled oligopeptide transporter. *Nature* 368, 563–566.

Ganapathy, V., Brandsch, M. and Leibach, F.H. (1994) Intestinal transport of amino acids and peptides. In: Johnson, L.R. (ed.) *Physiology of the Gastrointestinal Tract*, 3rd edn. Raven Press, New York, pp. 1773–1794.

Ganapathy, M.E., Huang, W., Ganapathy, V. and Leibach, F.H. (1998) Valacyclovir: a substrate for the intestinal and renal peptide transporters PEPT1 and PEPT2. *Biochemical and Biophysical Research Communications* 246, 470–475.

Gardner, M.L.G. (1994) Absorption of intact proteins and peptides. In: Johnson, L.R. (ed.) *Physiology of the Gastrointestinal Tract*, 3rd edn. Raven Press, New York, pp. 1795–1820.

Guerino, F. and Baumrucker, C.R. (1987) Identification of methionine and lysine transport systems in cattle small intestine. *Journal of Animal Science* 65, 630–640.

Haussinger, D. (1990) Nitrogen metabolism in liver: structural and functional organization and physiological relevance. *Biochemical Journal* 267, 281–290.

Johns, J.T. and Bergen, W.G. (1973) Studies on amino acid uptake by ovine small intestine. *Journal of Nutrition* 103, 1581–1586.

Kilberg, M.S. and Haussinger, D. (1992) *Mammalian Amino Acid Transport: Mechanisms and Control*. Plenum Press, New York.

Leibach, F.H. and Ganapathy, V. (1996) Peptide transporters in the intestine and the kidney. *Annual Review of Nutrition* 16, 99–119.

Leibholz, J. (1988) The utilization of free and protein-bound lysine. In: Friedman, M. (ed.) *The Utilization of Amino Acids*. CRC Press, Inc., Boca Raton, pp. 175–186.

Lin, C.L., Bristol, L.A., Jin, L., Dykes-Hoberg, M., Crawford, T., Clawson, L. and Rothstein, J.D. (1998) Aberrant RNA processing in a neurodegenerate disease: the cause for absent EAAT2, a glutamate transporter, in amyotrophic lateral sclerosis. *Neuron* 20, 589–602.

Lister, N., Bailey, P.D., Collier, I.D., Boyd, C.A.R. and Bronk, J.R. (1997) The influence of luminal pH on transport of neutral and charged dipeptides by rat small intestine, *in vitro*. *Biochimica et Biophysica Acta* 1324, 245–250.

Lochs, H., Morse, E.L. and Adibi, S.A. (1986) Mechanism of hepatic assimilation of dipeptides. *Journal of Biological Chemistry* 261, 14976–14981.

Mackenzie, B., Ahmed, A. and Rennie, M.J. (1992) Muscle amino acid metabolism and transport. In: Kilberg, M.S. and Haussinger, D. (eds) *Mammalian Amino Acid Transport*. Plenum Press, New York, pp. 195–231.

MacLeod, C.L., Finley, K.D. and Kekuda, D.K. (1994) y$^+$-type cationic amino acid transport: expression and regulation of the mCAT genes. *Journal of Experimental Biology* 196, 109–121.

Mailliard, M.E., Stevens, B.R. and Mann, G.E. (1995) Amino acid transport by small intestinal, hepatic, and pancreatic epithelia. *Gastroenterology* 108, 888–910.

Malandro, M.S. and Kilberg, M.S. (1996) Molecular biology of mammalian amino acid transporters. *Annual Review of Biochemistry* 65, 305–336.

Matthews, D.E. (1991) *Protein Absorption. Development and Present State of the Subject*. Wiley-Liss, New York.

Matthews, J.C. and Webb, K.E., Jr (1995) Absorption of L-carnosine, L-methionine, and L-methionyl-glycine by isolated sheep ruminal and omasal epithelial tissue. *Journal of Animal Science* 73, 3464–3475.

Matthews, J.C., Pan, Y.L., Wang, S., McCollum, M.Q. and Webb, K.E., Jr (1996a) Characterization of gastrointestinal amino acid and peptide transport proteins and the utilization of peptides as amino acid substrates by cultured cells (myogenic and mammary) and mammary tissue explants. In: Kornegay, E.T. (ed.) *Nutrient Management of Food Animals to Enhance and Protect the Environment*. CRC Press, Inc., Boca Raton, pp. 55–72.

Matthews, J.C., Wong, E.A., Bender, P.K., Bloomquist, J.R. and Webb, K.E., Jr (1996b) Demonstration and characterization of dipeptide transport system activity in sheep omasal epithelium by expression of mRNA in *Xenopus laevis* oocytes. *Journal of Animal Science* 74, 1720–1727.

Matthews, J.C., Wong, E.A., Bender, P.K. and Webb, K.E., Jr (1996c) Demonstration and characterization of the transport system capable of lysine and leucine absorption that is encoded in porcine jejunal epithelium by expression of mRNA in *Xenopus laevis* oocytes. *Journal of Animal Science* 74, 127–137.

Matthews, J.C., Beveridge, M.J., Malandro, M.S., Rothstein, J.D., Campbell-Thompson, M., Verlander, J., Kilberg, M.S. and Novak, D.A. (1998a) Activity and protein localization of multiple glutamate transporters in gestation day 14 vs. day 20 rat placenta. *American Journal of Physiology* 274, C603–C614.

Matthews, J.C., Beveridge, M.J., Malandro, M.S., Kilberg, M.S. and Novak, D.A. (1998b) Response of placental amino acid transport to gestational age and intrauterine growth retardation. *Proceedings of the Nutrition Society* 57, 257–263.

Moe, A.J., Pocius, P.A. and Polan, C.E. (1987) Transport of L-amino acids by brush border membrane vesicles from bovine small intestine. *Journal of Dairy Science* 70, 290–297.

Munck, L.K. (1997) Comparative aspects of chloride-dependent amino acid transport across the brush-border membrane. *Comparative Biochemistry and Physiology* 118A, 229–231.

Oehlke, J., Beyermann, M., Wiesner, B., Melzig, M., Berger, H., Krause, E. and Bienert, M. (1997) Evidence for extensive and non-specific translocation of oligopeptide across plasma membranes of mammalian cells. *Biochimica et Biophysica Acta* 1330, 50–60.

Pan, Y.X, Wong, E.A., Bloomquist, J.R. and Webb, K.E., Jr (1997) Poly(A)$^+$ RNA from sheep omasal epithelium induces expression of a peptide transport protein(s) in *Xenopus laevis* oocytes. *Journal of Animal Science* 75, 3323–3330.

Phillips, W.A., Webb, K.E., Jr and Fontenot, J.P. (1979) Characteristics of threonine, valine and methionine in the jejunum and ileum of sheep. *Journal of Animal Science* 48, 926–933.

Seal, C.J. and Parker, D.S. (1991) Isolation and characterization of low molecular weight peptides in steer, sheep and rat portal and peripheral blood. *Comparative and Biochemical Physiology* 99, 679–685.

Soriano-Garcia J.F., Torras-Llort, M., Ferrer, R. and Moreto, M. (1998) Multiple pathways for L-methionine transport in brush-border membrane vesicles from chicken jejunum. *Journal of Physiology* 509, 527–539.

Steel, A., Nussberger, S., Romero, M.F., Boron, W.F., Boyd, R.C.A. and Hediger, M.A. (1997) Stoichiometry and pH dependence of the rabbit proton-dependent oligopeptide transporter PepT1. *Journal of Physiology* 498, 563–569.

Thamotharan, M., Lombardo, Y.B., Bawani, S.Z. and Adibi, S.A. (1996) An active mechanism for completion of the final stage of protein degradation in the liver, lysosomal transport of dipeptides. *Journal of Biological Chemistry* 272, 11786–11790.

Thamotharan, M., Gomme, J., Zonno, V., Maffia, M., Storelli, C. and Ahearns, G.A. (1998) Electrogenic, proton-coupled, intestinal dipeptide transport in herbivorous and carnivorous teleosts. *American Journal of Physiology* 278, R939–R947.

Torras-Llort, M., Ferrer, R., Soriano-Garcia J.F. and Moreto, M. (1996) L-lysine transport in chicken jejunal brush border membrane vesicles. *Journal of Membrane Biology* 152, 183–193.

Torras-Llort, M., Soriano-Garcia, J.F., Ferrer, R. and Moreto, M. (1998) Effect of a lysine-enriched diet on L-lysine transport by the brush-border membrane of the chicken jejunum. *American Journal of Physiology* 274, R69–R75.

Webb, K.E., Jr and Matthews, J.C. (1998) Peptide absorption and its significance in ruminant protein metabolism. In: Grimbel, G. and Backwell, C. (eds) *Peptides in Mammalian Protein Metabolism: Tissue Utilization and Clinical Targeting*. Portland Press Ltd, London, pp. 1–10.

Wilson, J.W. and Webb, K.E., Jr (1990) Lysine and methionine transport by bovine jejunal and ileal brush border membrane vesicles. *Journal of Animal Science* 68, 504–514.

Wingrove, T.G. and Kimmach, G.A. (1998) High affinity L-aspartate transport in chick small intestine. *American Journal of Physiology* 252, C105–C114.

Zerangue, N. and Kavanaugh, M.P. (1996) ASCT-1 is a neutral amino acid exchanger with chloride channel activity. *Journal of Biological Chemistry* 271, 27991–27994.

Chapter 2

Measurement and Significance of Protein Turnover

J.A. Rathmacher

Metabolic Technologies Inc., Ames, Iowa, USA

Introduction

The accretion of body proteins is the net result of both the synthesis and breakdown of protein. The dynamic nature of protein metabolism has been known for 60 years thanks to the pioneering work of Schoenheimer and others (Schoenheimer *et al.*, 1939). Using stable isotopes of amino acids, they demonstrated that proteins continually were being broken down and resynthesized. In addition, they reported that different organs have different rates of protein synthesis. The dynamic process by which body proteins are continually synthesized and broken down is protein turnover.

Studies on the growth of body protein stores and the metabolism of protein have been a major area of research. For example, a major reason for this is the dramatic fact that up to 20–25% of the muscle protein can be broken down per day early in the life of humans and farm animals. This rate slows with age to 1–2% day^{-1} in adults. Rates of synthesis and breakdown are influenced not only by age, but by plane of nutrition, stress, disease, hormones, exercise and inactivity.

Nomenclature

The nomenclature employed in studying growth and protein metabolism is relatively straightforward, but it is a worthwhile exercise to define briefly the terms that will be used in this chapter.

- *Synthesis.* The conversion of amino acids into proteins by the protein synthetic apparatus in the cytoplasm in the cell.
- *Breakdown.* The proteolysis of polypeptides by different proteinases within both the cytoplasmic and lysosomal compartments of the cell. The terms breakdown and degradation are used interchangeably.
- *Growth.* The net accumulation of protein that occurs when the rate of synthesis is greater than the rate of breakdown. The term growth is often used interchangeably with accretion or net synthesis.
- *Wasting.* The loss of protein that occurs when the rate of breakdown is greater than the rate of synthesis.
- *Turnover.* A general term that involves both synthesis and breakdown. However,

it is sometimes used to represent breakdown. In this chapter, it will be used to describe protein metabolism, which includes both protein synthesis and protein breakdown.

- *Fractional synthesis and breakdown.* When quantitating protein synthesis and breakdown, one often expresses the rates as per cent per day. This allows one to compare different organs of different sizes or different muscles of different sizes.

Three intrinsic problems are associated with measuring protein synthesis and breakdown in body tissues. Details of these problems can be found reviewed elsewhere (Bier, 1989). The goal of this chapter will be to describe the methodology used to quantitate indirect whole-body protein turnover and direct measurement of tissue protein synthesis and breakdown.

One of the key problems in studying protein synthesis and degradation is that labelled (radio-labelled or stable isotopes) amino acids which are to measure their incorporation into protein, or conversely, release of amino acids from labelled proteins, and the true enrichment or specific activity of the amino acid or

metabolite are difficult to measure in an experiment. The labelled amino acid has various states in a cell, summarized in Fig. 2.1.

The amino acid can be transported into a free amino acid pool. Once in the cell, it can be transported back out, degraded to other metabolites (depending on the amino acid) or linked to a specific aminoacyl-tRNA. From the tRNA pool, it can be translated into protein by ribosomes (detailed below) and eventually degraded to free amino acids (mechanism described below).

Even though it is known that protein tissue accretion is influenced by both the synthesis and degradation of protein, protein synthesis and degradation are not always measured simultaneously. However, mechanisms controlling protein synthesis and degradation are distinct (Reeds, 1989) and, therefore, can be influenced independently. Often breakdown is ignored, especially when measuring direct tissue protein turnover. For example, very significant gains in muscle protein can be increased by decreasing protein breakdown, if protein synthesis remains the same. A 10% decrease in the fractional breakdown rate of muscle will result in a

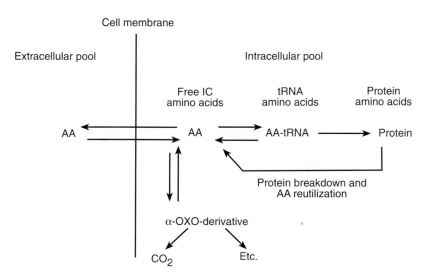

Fig. 2.1. Pathway of uptake, utilization and reutilization of amino acids for protein synthesis and breakdown.

23% increase in the protein accretion rate, whereas a 10% increase in the fractional synthesis rate will result in an 11% increase in the protein accretion rate. One could theorize even greater increases in growth if synthesis and degradation were both affected.

Protein synthesis and breakdown

It is evident that both synthesis and breakdown of proteins are necessary to evaluate the regulation of protein turnover. A better understanding of these processes is needed before we proceed. A brief overview of the mechanisms involved is presented.

Protein synthesis

Protein synthesis (translation) requires the coordination of >100 macromolecules working together. They include DNA, mRNA, tRNA, rRNA, activating enzymes and protein factors. Information encoded in DNA is transcribed into the RNA molecules, which are responsible for the synthesis of the individual protein. The formation of single-stranded mRNA occurs in the nucleus and is called transcription. The mRNA is transported to the cytosol, where it associates with ribosomes, and the translation of the mRNA sequence into an amino acid sequence occurs. There are three phases of protein synthesis: initiation, elongation and termination.

Initiation occurs when the mRNA and ribosome bind. The elongation cycle proceeds with aminoacyl-tRNA (tRNA molecules bound to specific amino acids) assembling on a specific codon on the mRNA. Many ribosomes can attach to a single mRNA and translate a protein. Synthesis is terminated when a stop codon is encountered. A newly synthesized protein may undergo post-translational modifications before it can become a functional protein. The protein synthetic process is probably regulated in two ways which can affect the rate of protein synthesis measured: the amount of RNA and the rate of translation to form protein.

Protein breakdown

Once a protein is synthesized, it is subject to breakdown. The mechanism of protein breakdown involves the hydrolysis of an intact protein to amino acids. Protein breakdown is selective, and specific proteins degrade within the cell at widely different rates. There are two general mechanisms involved in breakdown, lysosomal and non-lysosomal systems. The lysosomal system is characterized by the following: (i) it is located in lysosomes at pH 3–5 and includes the catheptic peptidases (cathepsins B, D, H and L); (ii) it is involved in degradation of endocytosed proteins; and (iii) it is involved in bulk degradation of some endogenous proteins. It is unclear how such a degradation system can produce different half-lives for different proteins.

A second system is the error-eliminating system which includes peptidases located in the cell cytoplasm. This system is specific for proteins containing errors of translation (abnormal), short-lived proteins, long-lived proteins and membrane proteins, and it requires ATP. This system is the ubiquitin–proteasome pathway reviewed by Mitch and Goldberg (1996). Proteins are degraded by this pathway when ubiquitin binds to the protein. It is accomplished by three enzymes: (i) the E1 enzyme activates ubiquitin in an ATP-requiring reaction; (ii) activated ubiquitin is transferred to E2 carrier protein; and (iii) this is transferred to the protein, catalysed by the E3 enzyme. This process is repeated to form a ubiquitin chain. The ubiquitin-conjugated proteins are recognized by the proteasome and degraded within the proteasome by multiple proteolytic sites. The peptides are released and degraded in the cytoplasm.

Another cytoplasmic system is the calpain system consisting of two iso-enzymes, μ- and m-calpain. This system is regulated by Ca^{2+}-binding, autoproteolytic modification, and its inhibitor, calpastatin (Emori *et al.*, 1987). It has been hypothesized that the calpain system is involved in the rate-limiting step of myofibrillar protein breakdown (Reeds, 1989). The calpains are candidates for the disassembly of the myofibril into filaments. The filament proteins are then broken down in the cytoplasm by other proteolytic enzymes.

The remainder of this chapter will deal with methodology used to measure protein synthesis and degradation. Discussion will be divided into two categories: (i) indirect and direct measurements of whole-body protein turnover; and (ii) measurement of tissue protein metabolism *in vivo*. Two methods to measure whole-body protein turnover include: the [^{15}N]glycine endproduct method; and the [$1-^{13}$C]leucine constant infusion method. Two methods commonly used to measure the synthetic rate of tissue protein directly are the 'constant infusion' and 'flooding dose' approaches, and these will be discussed in detail. In addition, the arterio-venous difference limb balance and tracee release method will be discussed. The traditional urinary 3-methylhistidine (3MH) endproduct method will be discussed and contrasted with a new compartmental tracer for measurement of muscle proteolysis for quantitating the 3MH end-product.

Indirect Measurement of Whole-body Protein Turnover

The subject of whole-body protein turnover has been reviewed extensively, and the following references are suggested reading Waterlow (1969); Waterlow *et al.* (1978); Waterlow (1981); Garlick and Fern (1985); Bier (1989); Nissen (1991); Wolfe (1992). Measurements of whole-body protein turnover have been based on either multicompartment or simple three-compartment models of protein metabolism. Multicompartmental models have an advantage because they produce information on compartments with distinct rates of turnover. If the mass of the compartments is known, the rates of synthesis and degradation can be determined. Many methods have been employed (Waterlow *et al.*, 1978), with some common assumptions and principles. It is difficult to validate these methods experimentally. Validation often involves

comparing different methods. If comparable data under similar circumstances are obtained, then a method would be considered valid. This is not always the case. If two different methods in the same animal give different conclusions, then one must be concerned about the conclusions drawn from each method.

Determination of whole-body protein turnover employs stochastic analysis. Stochastic analysis ignores all of the various pools and components of wholebody protein turnover, but focuses on the overall process. This technique uses either a single bolus or a continuous infusion technique. Samples are obtained with constant infusion once isotopic equilibrium is obtained. At isotopic equilibrium, the various pools become irrelevant in the stochastic model as sampling and infusion occur in a central pool.

Indirect methods of whole-body protein turnover determination are based on the concept of amino acid flux. Amino acid flux (Q) is the sum of all pathways of disposal of amino acids or is equal to the sum of all pathways of entry into the amino acid pool. For an essential amino acid, flux (Q) is Q = incorporation into protein(s) + irrevocable amino acid catabolism (E) + absorption from diet (D) + entry from protein catabolism (C) (Fig. 2.2). For a non-essential amino acid, *de novo* synthesis is based on the entry into the free amino acid pool.

There are some considerations that should be taken into consideration when performing such measurements of wholebody protein turnover: (i) infusion and sampling sites; (ii) amino acid absorption and catabolism; and (iii) choice of amino acid.

Constant infusion of [^{15}N]glycine (end-product method)

Rittenberg and colleagues were the first to use [^{15}N]glycine to measure whole-body protein turnover. They administered a single bolus of [^{15}N]glycine and measured the urinary ^{15}N decay curve for 3 days.

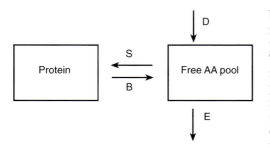

Fig. 2.2. Simple model of whole-body protein metabolism. S = protein synthesis; B = protein breakdown; D = dietary intake; E = nitrogen excretion.

They analysed the data using the modified three-compartment model depicted in Fig. 2.3.

Improvements were made to the model by Waterlow and colleagues (Picou and Taylor-Roberts, 1969; Waterlow *et al.*, 1978) by introducing the constant infusion steady-state approach. This approach reduces the number of samples and simplifies the mathematics required. The general concept is depicted in Fig. 2.4. There is a metabolic pool of N into which amino acids enter from the diet (I) and from the

breakdown (B) of body protein. N in the form of amino acids is synthesized into protein(s) or can be excreted into the urine. The [15N]glycine model is based on the following assumptions: (i) the metabolic pool of N remains constant during tracer infusions; (ii) [15N]glycine is not recycled; (iii) the three-pool model is correct; (iv) exogenous 15N is metabolized in a similar manner to endogenous and exogenous N; (v) synthesis and excretion are the major pathways of N disposal; and (vi) amino acids from breakdown and the diet are handled in the same way.

The method involves the administration of [15N]glycine (intravenously or orally) at a continuous rate until a plateau in the 15N enrichment is achieved. This usually takes 20–40 h. However, the time to reach plateau is greatly reduced with a primed constant infusion (Jeevanandam *et al.*, 1985). Urine samples are taken at the plateau. The enrichment of [15N]urea is then determined. At steady state (when the rate of amino acids entering the metabolic pool is equal to the rate at which they leave), the equation for the model is

$$Q = I + B = S + E. \qquad (2.1)$$

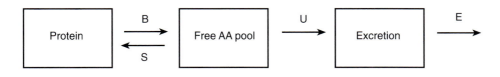

Fig. 2.3. Three-pool model of Rittenberg to describe protein metabolism. S = protein synthesis; B = protein breakdown; U = urea synthesis; E = nitrogen excretion.

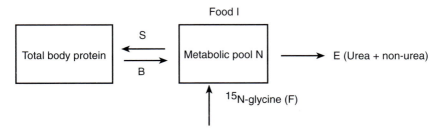

Fig. 2.4. Picou and Taylor-Roberts (1969) model of [15N]glycine protein metabolism. I = intake of dietary protein; F = infusion of [15N]glycine; B = protein breakdown; S = protein synthesis; E = excretion of both urinary urea and non-urea end-products.

The amino flux (Q) is equal to the infusion rate (F) divided by the enrichment of urea or ammonia (d), $Q = F \, d^{-1}$. Therefore, synthesis (S) = Q − E, where E is the total excretion and breakdown (B) = Q − I, where I is intake.

Constant infusion of [¹³C]leucine

The [¹³C]leucine method was developed based on common characteristics of the [¹⁵N]glycine method (Golden and Waterlow, 1977). The model is illustrated in Fig. 2.5. Leucine is an essential amino acid, therefore it is not produced *in vivo*. The first metabolite of leucine is α-ketoisocaproate (KIC). Leucine and KIC are interconvertable by a reversible transamination reaction. Both leucine and KIC have metabolic pools in plasma and inside the cell. Leucine enters the cell from protein breakdown and leaves through oxidative disposal (CO_2) and non-oxidative disposal (protein synthesis). These processes take place in all tissues and may exhibit different characteristics.

The difference between the leucine protein turnover model and the [¹⁵N]-glycine model are that the kinetics of the amino acid are measured directly. The difficulty with this model is the extrapolation of leucine kinetics to rates of protein breakdown and synthesis. For a further discussion, the advantages, limitations and difficulties associated with leucine metabolism can be found elsewhere (Waterlow *et al.*, 1978; Matthews and Bier, 1983; Bier, 1989). The original model proposed by Waterlow is illustrated in Fig. 2.6. Leucine was selected as the essential amino acid of choice because it is readily available cheaply in a pure form (L-leucine). In addition, when leucine is isotopically labelled as [1−¹³C]leucine or [1−¹⁴C]leucine, the label is completely removed as CO_2 (the first irreversible step). The model in Fig. 2.6 is resolved by infusing (constant) label leucine (L-[1−¹³C]leucine) into the blood stream until an isotopic steady state is reached in plasma. The measurements taken are the dilution of tracer by unlabelled leucine and the rate of labelled CO_2 excretion in the breath. The dilution of tracer defines the rate of appearance of leucine in plasma. The labelled CO_2 excretion divided by the leucine tracer infusion rate defines the oxidation rate (C). The breakdown rate (B) in the post-absorptive rate is equal to Q (leucine flux, leucine infusion/isotopic enrichment), and synthesis(s) is S = Q − C. In summary, neither Q or C protein are measured directly, and B and S are extrapolated from them. Other difficulties associated with this simple model are that the body does not have a single leucine pool or a single pool of protein entering and leaving it. In addition, the leucine tracer is infused into and sampled from blood, but leucine protein metabolism occurs within the cell. Leucine is transaminated (a reversible reaction) inside cells to KIC. The KIC may suffer one of three fates: it may be decarboxylated,

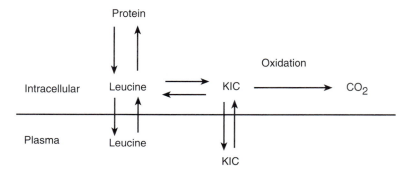

Fig. 2.5. Illustration of metabolism of leucine and α-ketoisotocaproate (KIC).

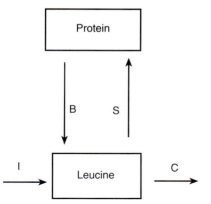

Fig. 2.6. Original model for leucine kinetics of an essential amino acid and its relationship to protein turnover. B = breakdown; S = synthesis (non-oxidative disposal); I = dietary intake; C = oxidation. Under steady-state conditions, leucine flux is Q = I + B = S + C. When I = O (post-absorptive), B = Q. Whole-body synthesis is calculated as S = Q − C.

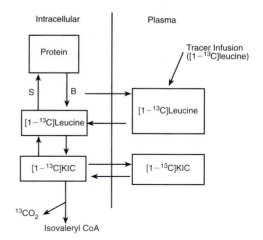

Fig. 2.7. The current model of whole-body synthesis of $[1-^{13}C]$leucine. The infused tracer reached an equilibrium with intracellular leucine and KIC. The use of plasma KIC enrichment allows for the calculation of the total intracellular rate of appearance and the correct calculation of leucine oxidation. Breakdown (B) = F/$[1-^{13}C]$KIC enrichment; oxidation (C) = $^{13}CO_2$/$[1-^{13}C]$KIC enrichment; synthesis (S) = B − C.

reaminated to leucine or it may leave the cell. Because KIC is only found in the cell from leucine transamination, plasma KIC reflects the intracellular KIC enrichment and can be used as an index of intracellular leucine tracer enrichment. This approach expands the single-pool model into a four-pool model. The calculations are made by substituting the leucine isotopic enrichment for the KIC enrichment (Fig. 2.7).

This approach is commonly called the 'reciprocal-pool' approach (measurement of the tracer in the metabolite opposite to the infused) (Schwenk *et al.*, 1985). There are still drawbacks that remain: (i) there are still multiple intracellular sites in the body, and it is not known what contribution they make to plasma KIC, and (ii) there are a variety of proteins in the body turning over at different rates.

Finally, Cobelli *et al.* (1991) designed a ten-compartment model, which involves simultaneously infusing dual tracers of leucine and KIC and measuring the resulting four enrichment curves in plasma and one in expired air. This model accounted for the complexity of the leucine system, but the authors failed to adopt a multi-tissue scheme for slow and fast kinetic events (liver as compared with muscle). These data demonstrated that there was no single intracellular pool for leucine and KIC. However, this model is mathematically difficult and is not solved easily. This model has not been used in an experimental design where protein metabolism is altered. Its value may be to test the structural errors of simpler but commonly used models.

Measurement of Tissue Protein Metabolism *in Vivo*

Currently, protein synthesis can be measured directly by two approaches (Garlick *et al.*, 1994; Rennie *et al.*, 1994), i.e. constant infusion or the 'flooding dose' of a labelled amino acid. The fractional rate of synthesis of a protein or mixture of proteins can be measured from an estimate of the change in incorporation of a labelled amino acid into protein over time in tissues.

Constant infusion

The primed constant infusion method was pioneered by Waterlow and Stephen (1966) and further developed extensively by Garlick (1969). This method aims to set up a steady state of labelling the amino acid in plasma and in the intracellular pools of the body. The method was developed to avoid the difficulty of measuring both the incorporation of the labelled amino acid into tissue protein and the time course of the enrichment of the tissue or plasma free amino acid compared with the rapid changes of both occurring after a single injection. In this method, a labelled amino acid tracer is given by a constant infusion (with and without a prime) at a rate sufficient to achieve an enrichment of 5–10% of the tracer amino acid. The infusion continues for 4–12 h depending on the tissue or protein of interest. The enrichment of the free amino acid remains constant for a substantial portion of the infusion period, thus the kinetics of the tissue protein labelling are simple and linear. At the end of the infusion, tissue samples are taken and rapidly frozen until they can be processed further. The enrichment of the precursor pool amino acid and the enrichment of the labelled amino acid in the isolated tissue or protein are determined.

The fractional synthetic rate (FSR) can be calculated by the following equation:

$$FSR = (E_1 - E_0)/[E_p \times (t_1 - t_0)] \times 100 \tag{2.2}$$

where $E_{0,1 \ldots 4}$ is the enrichment (tracer/tracee) of tracer amino acid in the tissue protein at different times and E_p is the average precursor enrichment during the same time period that the tissue protein is being labelled. The true value of the precursor enrichment is the tRNA molecule, but this is generally not a practical value to obtain. Many researchers using this method have adapted it by using L-[^{13}C]leucine as their tracer and measuring [^{13}C]KIC as the precursor enrichment.

An advantage of this method is that it is applicable to the measurement of proteins with a slow turnover. In addition, whole-body protein turnover may be measured at the same time so that a relationship between whole-body protein turnover and tissue protein synthesis may be determined. The method may be also suitable for arterio-venous sampling methods.

Flooding dose

The flooding dose technique was developed to overcome the limitations of the true precursor enrichment for the calculation of protein synthesis by the constant infusion method. Garlick and co-workers developed this method that was devised originally by Henshaw et al. (1971). The aim is to 'flood' the free amino acid pools, thereby eliminating the difference between the intracellular and extracellular (entire precursors pool) free amino acid enrichments. This is accomplished by administering the tracer with a large bolus of tracee. After the 'flooding dose', a biopsy of the tissue is taken and the enrichment determined. The FSR of tissue protein is determined using the following formula:

$$FSR = (e_{B+} - e_{Bo})/\int^+_0 e_A dt \tag{2.3}$$

where $e_{B+} - e_{Bo}$ is the increase in isotopic enrichment over time t and $\int^+_0 e_A dt$ is the area under the curve of the precursor enrichment versus time. The advantages of this method include: improved resolution of precursor enrichment; and shorter periods of measurement than constant infusion (10 min flood versus 6 h infusion in rat; 1–2 h flood versus 4–20 h infusion in humans). There are concerns that the flood dose itself may affect protein synthesis and degradation directly or change amino acid uptake. Also, the large dose of amino acids may cause a hormonal imbalance.

Arterio-venous difference

Although the measurement of the direct incorporation of isotope into protein is the preferred method to measure protein synthesis and degradation, it does have some disadvantages. The animal is often killed to collect samples or you must be able to take biopsies of the tissues, and the procedures themselves may alter protein turnover. Therefore, some researchers use an arterio-venous difference technique to define the net balances of amino acids. The balance of any amino acid within an organ or tissue is the result of the same processes that apply to the body as a whole, where amino acid net balance = input − amino acid catabolism = protein synthesis − proteolysis.

All of the components of the equation can be determined from the measurements of amino acid concentration, label uptake across a tissue, and blood flow. This method requires the constant infusion of a tracer amino acid. Both leucine (Pell *et al.*, 1986) and phenylalanine (Barrett *et al.*, 1987) tracers have been used, along with measurements of arterial and venous isotope enrichment, concentrations, metabolic output and blood flow. The technique measures the difference between total label uptake and irrevocable catabolism to protein synthesis, the difference between net uptake and irrevocable catabolism to protein deposition, and the difference between protein synthesis and deposition to degradation. Using phenylalanine metabolism of the hindlimb as an example,

$$
\begin{aligned}
&(E_A \times \text{conc}_A \times \text{blood flow}) \\
&- (E_V \times \text{conc}_V \times \text{blood flow}) \\
&= \text{total label uptake}
\end{aligned}
\tag{2.4}
$$

and

$$
\begin{aligned}
&(\text{conc}_A \times \text{blood flow}) \\
&- (\text{conc}_V \times \text{blood flow}) \\
&= \text{net amino acid balance}
\end{aligned}
\tag{2.5}
$$

where E_A and E_V are the isotopic enrichment of a phenylalanine tracer and conc_A and conc_V are the concentration of the tracee phenylalanine in arterial and venous blood, respectively. Based on Equations 2.4 and 2.5, protein synthesis = total label uptake $\div E_A$, and protein degradation = (total label uptake $\div E_A$) − net amino acid balance.

There are problems with this method. One is the definition of the isotopic enrich-

ment of protein synthesis and oxidative compartments. Another problem is the accurate measurement of amino acid concentrations and isotopic enrichments and, finally, the accurate measurement of blood flow. However, despite these problems, this method has great promise in large animals.

Indirect measurement of protein breakdown

The fractional breakdown rate of muscle protein can be estimated if the fractional accretion rate of muscle protein is known (fractional breakdown rate = fractional synthesis rate − fractional accretion rate, FBR = FSR − FAR) (Millward *et al.*, 1975). This approach to the study of protein degradation is somewhat unsatisfactory. The main problem with this method arises from the time scale of measurements. Synthesis is measured over a period of minutes or hours, while growth is integrated over the day and measured over a period of days or months; thus, estimation of protein synthesis will vary over the course of the day and before and after a meal. These changes in protein synthesis could, in turn, grossly over- or underestimate the degradation rate.

A more direct approach to measure muscle degradation is the 'tracee release method' (Zhang *et al.*, 1996). This approach involves infusing a labelled amino acid to an isotopic equilibrium and then observing the isotopic decay in arterial blood and the muscle intracellular pool. The FBR is calculated as the rate at which tracee dilutes the intracellular enrichment. This method can be combined with a tracer incorporation method in order to measure both the FSR and FBR in the same study.

Measurement of muscle protein breakdown: 3-methylhistidine metabolism

3-Methylhistidine: historical background
Tallen *et al.* (1954) were the first to identify 3MH as a component in urine in 1954, but they were not sure what the source of 3MH was. The metabolism of 3MH was first

investigated by Cowgill and Freeberg (1957) after injecting a radiotracer of 3MH into the bloodstream of rabbits, rats, chicks and frogs. The radioactivity was rapidly excreted in urine; recoveries ranging between 50 and 90% of the injected dose were observed. In 1967, 3MH was identified as a component of actin (Asatoor and Armstrong, 1967) and of myosin and actin (Johnson et al., 1967; Hardy et al., 1970). 3MH is present in the globular head of the myosin heavy chain (MHC) (Huszar and Elzinga, 1971) and is localized in the same area as the ATPase activity and actin-binding sites. However, there is no evidence that 3MH is involved in any of these functions. There is one mole of 3MH per mole of MHC in the myosin of fast-twitch, white fibres, but 3MH is absent in the myosin of the muscle of the fetus, cardiac muscle and slow-twitch, red muscle fibres (Huszar and Elzinga, 1971). Actin also contains this unique amino acid and it is located at residue 73 of the polypeptide chain. Unlike myosin, 3MH is found in all actin isoforms, including embryonic, smooth and cytoplasmic isoforms (Cass et al., 1983).

The methyl group is donated to 3MH by a post-translational event. It has been shown that S-adenosylmethionine was an effective methyl donor to histidine of the nascent polypeptide chains contained in actin and myosin (Reporter, 1969). Furthermore, when histidine was used as the source of labelled amino acid, the specific activities of histidine and 3MH were the same in muscle cultures.

Validation of 3-methylhistidine as an index of muscle protein breakdown

Before 3MH could be used as an index of myofibrillar protein breakdown, three assumptions had to be validated, as outlined by Young and Munro (1978): (i) it does not charge tRNA and is, therefore, not reutilized for protein synthesis; (ii) it is excreted quantitatively in the urine in an identifiable form; and (iii) the major portion of total body 3MH is present in skeletal muscle.

To show experimentally that 3MH was not reutilized for muscle protein synthesis,

3MH was demonstrated not to charge tRNA. This was accomplished using radio-labelled 3MH, demonstrating in vitro and in vivo that 3MH did not charge tRNA of the rat (Young et al., 1972). However, there was a high degree of incorporation of label achieved for histidine and leucine. As a marker of muscle protein breakdown, 3MH must be excreted quantitatively in the urine, i.e. once 3MH is released from actin and myosin of skeletal muscle it is not metabolized to any significant extent and is excreted in the urine. The common experimental protocol used to confirm quantitative recovery was to administer radiolabelled [^{14}C]3MH intravenously and measure the accumulative recovery in the urine. [^{14}C-methyl]N^t-methylhistidine was recovered quantitatively in the urine of rats after being administered either orally or intravenously. Ninety-three per cent of the tracer was recovered in the urine after the first 24 h, and 98–100% was recovered after 48 h. Only trace amounts were recovered in the faeces, and no $^{14}CO_2$ was recovered in the respired air. Similar recoveries were confirmed in humans (Long et al., 1975); 75% during the first 24 h and 95% in 48 h. In addition, quantitative recoveries were confirmed with rabbits (Harris et al., 1977), cattle (Harris and Milne, 1981b) and chickens (Jones et al., 1986). However, the tracer was not recovered quantitatively in the urine of sheep (Harris and Milne, 1980) or pigs (Harris and Milne, 1981a). More details will be given about domestic species in the following sections.

In rats, the radioactivity is distributed in two compounds, 3MH and N-acetyl-3MH. The N-acetyl form is the major form excreted by the rat (Young et al., 1972). The liver presumably is the site of acetylation in the rat. The analysis of 3MH from rat urine requires a hydrolysis step. Whereas 3MH is the major form excreted in humans and other species, the N-acetyl form has been detected in human urine (4.5%) (Long et al., 1975).

It has been debated whether urinary 3MH is primarily a product of skeletal muscle protein turnover or whether other tissues might contribute a significant amount to the daily production. Haverberg *et al.* (1975) showed that the mixed proteins in all of the organs sampled contained detectable levels of bound 3MH. However, when examining each organ as a whole, skeletal muscle contained the majority (98%) of the total amount. Nishizawa *et al.* (1977) concluded that the skin and intestine contributed up to 10% of the total body pool of 3MH. A study of humans with short-bowel syndrome indicated that skeletal muscle was the major source of urinary 3MH (Long *et al.*, 1988). In human patients with varying degrees of infection (Sjölin *et al.*, 1989), it was concluded that urinary 3MH was a valid marker of myofibrillar protein breakdown, because it was correlated with the release of 3MH from the leg. Furthermore, it was shown later in additional patients (Sjölin *et al.*, 1990) that there was a significant linear relationship between the leg effluxes of tyrosine, phenylalanine and 3MH and the resulting urinary excretion of 3MH. Therefore, urinary 3MH excretion is associated with net skeletal muscle protein breakdown. Our data using the 3MH kinetic model in portal vein cannulated swine (van den Hemel-Grooten *et al.*, 1997) suggest that 3MH production from the gastrointestinal tract is not increased in swine fed a protein-free diet. The FBR of the whole body in swine was 2.16 and 2.56 for controls and those fed a protein-free diet, respectively, and the percentage from the gastrointestinal tract was <6% for both treatments. In conclusion, based on previous studies, it is reasonable to assume that changes in 3MH production largely reflect muscle metabolism.

3-Methylhistidine metabolism in cattle
Cattle, like humans and rats, quantitatively excrete 3MH in urine. Harris and Milne (1981b) demonstrated that between 82 and 99% of a [^{14}C]3MH dose was recovered after 6 days in 21- to 98-month-old non-lactating cows, steers and a bull. Similarly, McCarthy *et al.* (1983) recovered 90% of the injected tracer dose after 120 h in two heifers. 3MH is excreted in the urine

unchanged, and occurs in muscle extracts both in the free form (4–10 nmol g^{-1} muscle) and as a perchloric acid-soluble, acid-labile form which account for 85% of the total non-protein-bound 3MH. This compound was later identified as balenine (Harris and Milne, 1987), a dipeptide composed of equal molar amounts of β-alanine and 3MH. Balenine was later identified in muscle extracts of sheep and pigs. There appears to be an age-related decline in the concentration of balenine in muscle, but this did not produce a measurable change in the recovery of radioactivity in urine. 3MH is present in whole blood of cattle at concentrations ranging from 2 to 6 nmol ml^{-1} blood.

The distribution of 3MH in organs has been determined for cattle (Holstein) (Nishizawa *et al.*, 1979). Skeletal muscle contained 93.4% of the total 3MH in the analysed cattle tissues. The concentration of 3MH was 3.5106 µmol of 3MH g^{-1} muscle protein or 0.587 µmol g^{-1} wet muscle in growing steers. This value is used commonly to calculate the protein-bound pool of muscle 3MH, when determining the fractional breakdown rate of skeletal muscle. Other values for the level of protein-bound 3MH in the muscle of cattle have been reported: 5.6 µmol g^{-1} protein and 1.8 µmol g^{-1} protein. This variability is of some concern because, in most studies, the amount of protein-bound 3MH is not determined.

3-Methylhistidine metabolism in sheep
Sheep are unlike cattle in that urinary 3MH is not a reliable index of muscle protein breakdown (Harris and Milne, 1980). After an intravenous dose of ^{14}C-labelled 3MH, only 25–50% of the label was recovered after 7 days. The recovery progressively increased with the age (4 weeks–7 years) of the animal, becoming almost quantitative in the older animals after 3 weeks. The incomplete recovery was not due to excretion in the faeces or elimination as expired gas, but was related to the presence of a muscle pool of non-protein-bound 3MH which was several times larger than the expected daily urinary excretion. The

concentration of free 3MH in muscle ranged from 17 to 120 nmol g^{-1} of muscle. This pool in newly synthesized muscle tissue was maintained by retention of some of the 3MH released by breakdown of muscle protein. Only a small proportion of the 3MH released from protein breakdown was available for excretion, and the proportion excreted in the urine increased with the age of the animal. Another non-protein-bound component of 3MH in muscle is the dipeptide, balenine (Harris and Milne, 1987), which comprises on average ~82% of the total non-protein-bound 3MH in muscle.

This percentage does not seem to change as the animal ages, and the same proportion was seen in cattle muscle. This dipeptide appeared to be synthesized in muscle from free 3MH and was not a terminal product of protein breakdown. The enzyme system responsible for the synthesis of the analogous peptides carnosine and anserine shows a broad specificity for histidine and histidine derivatives (Kalyankar and Meister, 1959). The occurrence of balenine in sheep muscle should be considered the norm rather than a rarity. Sheep also have a much higher concentration of 3MH in blood than cattle, with values ranging from 17 to 50 nmol ml^{-1} of whole blood. The acid-labile form is present in blood in a higher proportion than was observed in cattle, averaging 30% of the total non-protein-bound 3MH in sheep. The concentration of protein-bound 3MH in sheep was similar to that in cattle, with an average concentration from the *longissimus dorsi* and leg being 5.8 μmol g^{-1} protein. Buttery (1984) reported a value of 0.6 μmol g^{-1} muscle.

3-Methylhistidine metabolism in pigs

The pig is another species in which the recovery of radiolabelled 3MH is less than quantitative (Harris and Milne, 1981a). From five animals, <21% of the tracer dose was recovered after 7 days, after which the recovery was <0.3% day^{-1}. The incomplete recoveries of radiolabelled 3MH were associated with the presence of a large pool of

non-protein-bound 3MH in muscle, the concentration of which increased with age. The 3MH in the muscle pool was present as free 3MH, with values ranging from 4 to 8 nmol g^{-1} muscle, and as a dipeptide which constituted >90% of the total non-protein-bound 3MH. The contribution of the dipeptide, balenine (Harris and Milne, 1987), increased with age, reaching 99.8% in older animals, which was 2 μmol of the total non-protein-bound 3MH g^{-1} of muscle tissue at ~9 months of age. The concentration in blood was not as high as in sheep, but was comparable with that in cattle, with values in pigs ranging from 6 to 19 nmol ml^{-1} of blood.

In summary, urinary excretion of 3MH cannot be used as an index of myofibrillar protein breakdown in sheep and pigs, because 3MH is not excreted quantitatively in the urine. Sheep have elevated levels of 3MH in plasma and muscle, and a dipeptide of 3MH is also present at a high concentration. In pigs, the pool of non-protein-bound 3MH was maintained and increased in both established and newly synthesized tissue by retention of some of the 3MH released by muscle protein breakdown, only a proportion of which was available for excretion.

The traditional approach (Fig. 2.8) to quantitating 3MH production requires collecting total urinary output for 1–3 days. The fractional breakdown (day^{-1}) rate of muscle protein rate can be determined by total urinary 3MH excretion divided by the total body 3MH muscle pool: 3MH excretion day^{-1} ÷ total body 3MH muscle pool. An estimate of skeletal mass is often difficult to obtain. The rate of muscle protein breakdown can also be calculated as the rate of urinary 3MH excretion and its known concentration in muscle protein: 3MH excretion μmol kg^{-1} day^{-1} ÷ 3.63 μmol g^{-1} of muscle protein = B (g of protein kg^{-1} of BW day^{-1}). Another approach is to express the data on a urinary creatinine basis since urinary creatinine excretion is a satisfactory estimate of muscle protein.

The initial studies showing the inadequacy of 3MH as an index of muscle protein breakdown required the intravenous

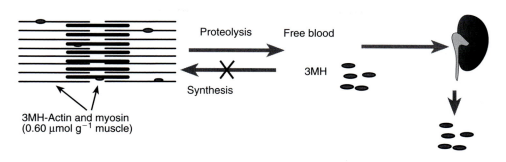

Fig. 2.8. Illustration of 3-methylhistidine (3MH) metabolism.

administration of a dose of labelled 3MH, but the decay curve of [^{14}C]3MH in plasma was not characterized. An alternative approach to quantitating urinary 3MH would be to describe the isotopic decay of a tracer of 3MH in plasma by a compartmental mathematical model. A compartmental model for swine or sheep must include a compartment for 3MH metabolism other than excretion into a urinary compartment. Swine not only have a large pool of free 3MH in muscle but also a large metabolic 'sink' of 3MH in the form of balenine. Likewise, sheep excrete ~15% of 3MH in the urine, with the remainder being retained in muscle as the dipeptide balenine. Hence a compartmental model describing the metabolism of 3MH in these two species must incorporate these metabolic differences as compared with humans, cattle, rats and rabbits.

Isotope model of 3MH kinetics

Urinary 3MH had been used in cattle and humans (Fig. 2.8) as an index of muscle protein breakdown but was invalid for use in swine and lambs. 3MH is produced in these species but is not excreted quantitatively in the urine. Previously, in validating urinary 3MH as an index of muscle proteolysis, researchers have injected [^{14}C]3MH intravenously and recovered the tracer in urine, but have never described its decay in plasma. 3MH is a histidine residue with one methyl group attached to the tau-nitrogen on the imidazole ring. To understand the metabolism of 3MH, we have used a deuterated molecule of 3MH, in which the three hydrogens of the methyl group have been replaced with three deuterium atoms, therefore the tracer is 3 mass units heavier than the natural occurring 3MH and can be detected by gas chromatography–mass spectrometry (Rathmacher *et al.*, 1992b). In constructing the three-compartment model, we kept in mind the known physiology of 3MH. It has been established that there are pools of 3MH in plasma, in other extracellular fluid pools, within muscle and in other tissues. The primary fate of 3MH in humans, cattle and dogs is into the urine (model exit from compartment 1), but in sheep and swine there is a balenine pool in muscle that accumulates over time (model exit from compartment 3).

The 3MH kinetic model was developed from the need to measure muscle proteolysis directly in growing lambs. However, the problem was that 3MH was a valid muscle protein turnover method in cattle and humans but invalid in sheep and swine. Model development proceeded by the strategy of developing the model first in sheep and swine and then validating the model in cattle and humans. Our basic experimental design involves the following: (i) an intravenous bolus dose of tracer (3-[methyl-^{2}H$_3$]methylhistidine); (ii) sampling (blood, urine and muscle tissue); (iii) 3MH isolation by ion-exchange chromatography; (iv) *t*-butyldimethylsilyl derivatization; (v) analysis by gas chromatography–mass spectrometry; and (vi) compartmental modelling using the SAAM/CONSAM program (Berman and Weiss, 1978; Boston *et al.*, 1981).

We have conducted a series of studies that propose that 3MH metabolism in humans (Rathmacher *et al.*, 1995), cattle (Rathmacher *et al.*, 1992a), dogs (Rathmacher *et al.*, 1993a), swine (Rathmacher *et al.*, 1996) and sheep (Rathmacher *et al.*, 1993c) can be defined from a single bolus infusion of a stable isotope, 3-[methyl-^{2}H$_3$]methylhistidine. Following the bolus dose of the stable isotope tracer, serial blood samples and/or urine were collected over 3–5 days. A minimum of three exponentials were required to describe the plasma decay curve adequately. The kinetic linear-time-invariant models of 3MH metabolism in the whole animal were constructed by using the SAAM/CONSAM modelling program. Three different configurations of a three-compartment model are described: (i) a simple three-compartment model for humans, cattle and dogs, in which plasma kinetics (3-[methyl-^{2}H$_3$]MH/3MH) are described by compartment 1 and which has one urinary exit from compartment 1; (ii) a plasma–urinary kinetic three-compartment model with two exits for sheep (a urinary exit out of compartment 1 and a balenine exit out of tissue compartment 3); and (iii) a plasma three-compartment model with an exit out of tissue compartment 3 in swine. The kinetic parameters reflect the differences in the known physiology of humans, cattle and dogs, compared with sheep and swine that do not quantitatively excrete 3MH into the urine. Steady-state model calculations define masses and fluxes of 3MH between the three compartments, and importantly the *de novo* production of 3MH. The *de novo* production of 3MH for humans, cattle, dogs, sheep and swine are 3.1, 6.0, 12.1, 10.3 and 7.2 μmol kg^{-1} day^{-1}, respectively.

The *de novo* production of 3MH as calculated by the compartmental model was not different when compared with 3MH production as calculated via traditional urinary collection. Additionally, the data suggest that steady-state compartment masses and mass transfer rates may be related to fat-free mass and muscle mass in humans and swine, respectively.

Species comparison of 3MH kinetics

Figures 2.9 and 2.10 and Tables 2.1 and 2.2 are a summary of the efforts to model 3MH metabolism using a three-compartment model in humans, cattle and dogs which quantitatively excrete 3MH in urine, as compared with sheep and swine which do not. Figure 2.10 is a comparison of model structures between the species. The diversity of models between humans, cattle and dogs, and sheep and swine reflects differences in known physiology. In each species, the tracer is injected into compartment 1 which, based on the size (volume and mass), is similar to plasma and extracellular water space. Compartment 1 was the sampling compartment and the compartment from which the steady-state calculations were initiated. All models for each species can be resolved by sampling only plasma. The exception is sheep, which, as shown in Fig. 2.10, required the sampling of both plasma and urine. However, the sheep model can be resolved from the plasma kinetics of 3MH if the rate of exit from compartment 1 is fixed. From the steady-state calculations, the *de novo* production of 3MH was obtained into compartment 3 for humans, cattle and dogs and into compartment 2 for sheep and swine. The *de novo* production of 3MH could be placed as an entry into compartment 2 and an identical rate calculated. The compartment identity of compartments 2 and 3 is intracellular pools of 3MH. The metabolic form of 3MH in these compartments may not be identical nor is the identity of compartments 2 or 3 for one species the same for another species (i.e. cattle versus sheep). The models also depict differences in the route by which 3MH exits the system. In humans, cattle and dogs, 3MH is excreted quantitatively in the urine as illustrated by the exit from compartment 1. This urinary exit has been confirmed by comparison of urinary excretion of 3MH and model calculated values (Fig. 2.11). Whereas sheep excrete only 15% of total

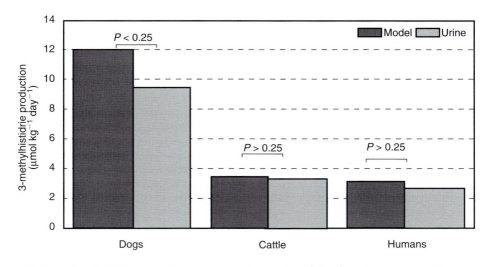

Fig. 2.9. Daily 3-methylhistidine production expressed as $\mu mol\ kg^{-1}\ day^{-1}$ for dogs, cattle and humans as calculated from urinary excretion and by a three-compartment model of 3-methylhistidine production. *There was no mean difference between urinary and model 3-methylhistidine production for cattle and humans, $P > 0.25$.

daily 3MH produced in the urine, swine excrete 1.5% day^{-1}. Therefore, accurate determination of 3MH production in sheep and swine requires an exit out of the system from compartment 3. This exit accounts for appreciable loss of 3MH into a balenine 'sink' which turns over slowly or not at all during the time frame of the study.

Representative plasma decay curves following a single dosing of 3-[methyl-$^2H_3$]methylhistidine tracer are illustrated in Fig. 2.9. In general, each species exhibited a similar exponential decay, characterized by rapid decay over the first 2–3 h, followed by a slower decay up to 12 h and a steady-state decay over the remainder of the study. The decays of the tracer are representative of the models used. Humans, cattle and dogs exhibit very similar decays, while sheep and swine are very different.

Table 2.1. Comparison of 3-methylhistidine kinetic parameters.

	Species				
Parameter	Cattle	Humans	Dogs	Swine	Sheep
Animals, n	39	4	5	20	40
Urinary 3MH loss, % of total	100	100	100	1	17
Fractional transfer rate, min^{-1a}					
$L_{2,1}$	0.18	0.08	0.11	0.23	0.21
$L_{1,2}$	0.06	0.06	0.06	0.09	0.08
$L_{3,2}$	0.003	0.009	0.006	0.014	0.007
$L_{2,3}$	0.002	0.002	0.008	0.006	0.005
$L_{0,3}$	NA	NA	NA	0.0009	0.0004
$L_{0,1}$	0.006	0.004	0.02	NA	0.0003

[a]Fractional transfer rate ($L_{i,j}$) from compartment j to i.
NA, not applicable.

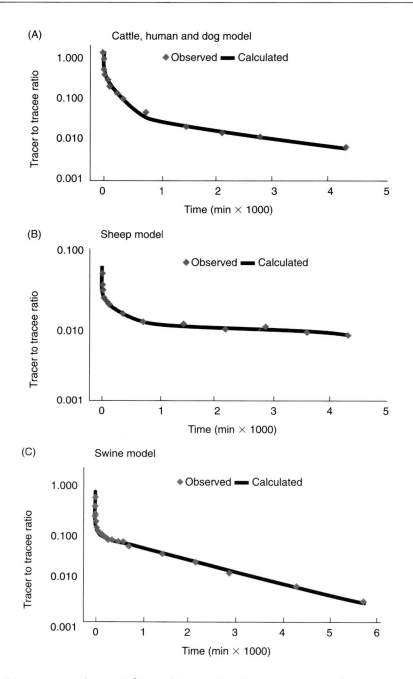

Fig. 2.10. Disappearance of tracer, 3-[^{2}H$_3$-methyl]methylhistidine, as the ratio of 3-[^{2}H$_3$-methyl]methylhistidine to 3-methylhistidine in plasma as described by a three-compartment model of 3-methylhistidine (see Fig. 2.11). Symbols (♦) represent observed data, and the line (■) represents best fit generated by the model.

Table 2.1 lists the model parameters and the fractional transfer rates ($L_{i,j}$ from compartment j to i). The fractional standard deviation of the parameters ranges from 5 to 50% and, in general, $L_{2,1}$, $L_{1,2}$ and $L_{0,1}$ or $L_{0,3}$ are solved with a higher precision than

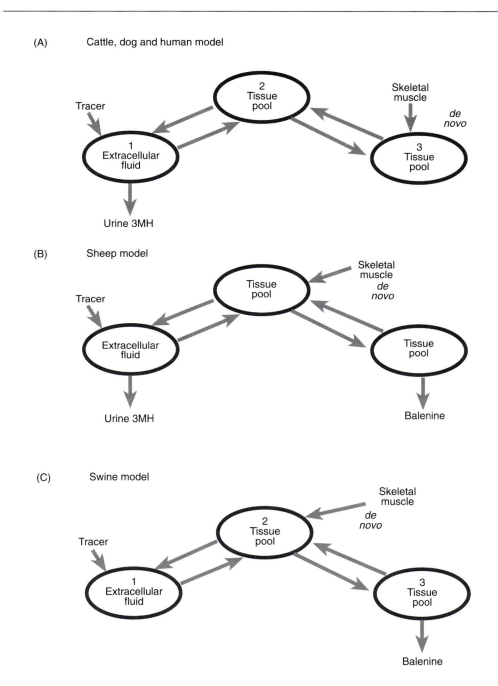

Fig. 2.11. Schematic of the three-compartment models used to analyse the kinetics of distribution, metabolism and *de novo* production of 3-methylhistidine (3MH). The tracer, 3-[^{2}H$_3$-methyl]methylhistidine (D$_3$-3MH), was injected into compartment 1. Sampling was performed from compartment 1. *De novo* production of 3MH and the exit from the system are dependent on the physiology of the species.

$L_{3,2}$ and $L_{2,3}$. Table 2.2 compares the compartment masses and mass transfer rates between compartments for each species. Also listed is the *de novo* production rate

Table 2.2. Steady-state compartment masses and mass transfer rates of a three-compartment model of 3-methylhistidine (3MH) metabolism.

Parameter	Human	Cattle	Swine	Sheep	Dogs
n	4	39	20	40	5
Plasma 3MH, μM	2.9	8.6	10.4	36.9	21.8
M_1, nmol kg^{-1a}	603	807	1,110	5,308	3,227
M_2, nmol kg^{-1}	912	2,291	2,857	12,483	7,973
M_3, nmol kg^{-1}	7,938	8,079	6,151	17,017	9,261
R_{21}, nmol kg^{-1} min^{-1b}	51	101	247	944	319
R_{12}, nmol kg^{-1} min^{-1}	53	105	247	946	329
R_{32}, nmol kg^{-1} min^{-1}	7.9	5.8	37	81	56
R_{23}, nmol kg^{-1} min^{-1}	9.6	9.9	32	77	56
R_{01}, nmol kg^{-1} min^{-1}	2.2	4.1	NA	1.4	9
R_{03}, nmol kg^{-1} min^{-1}	NA	NA	5.0	5.8	NA
3MH production[c], μmol kg^{-1} day^{-1}	3.1	6.0	7.2	10.3	12

[a]M_i = compartment mass I.
[b]R_{ij} = mass transfer rate from compartment j and i.
[c]3MH production was obtained from the model.

calculated by the model in Table 2.2. An important feature of these models is the description of 3MH metabolism within the body. The significance of mass transfer rates and compartment sizes is not fully understood. However, the model parameters and mass transfer rates may explain the failure of sheep and swine to excrete 3MH quantitatively in the urine (Rathmacher and Nissen, 1992). Three mechanisms may explain the failure of sheep and swine to excrete 3MH: (i) 3MH transport between the compartments limits the excretion of 3MH; (ii) 3MH is reabsorbed avidly by the kidney; and (iii) enzymatic conversion of 3MH to balenine is enhanced. In comparing the data from Tables 2.1 and 2.2, the low rate of 3MH excretion in sheep and swine is not due to impaired transfer of 3MH out of and between compartments. Cattle appear to have a slower exchange of 3MH between tissues despite near quantitative urinary excretion. The most likely reason for sequestering of 3MH in sheep and swine is that the kidneys are very efficient in conserving 3MH, which in turn increases the compartment size and plasma concentration, and through mass action could increase the synthesis of balenine.

The models described represent a framework and methodological approach describing steady-state 3MH kinetics in the whole animal and constitutes a working theory for testing by further experimentation using designs which alter muscle protein breakdown. The rate of 3MH production is an important tool in understanding the regulation of muscle protein degradation. The advantages of these models are that: (i) they do not necessitate quantitative urine collection (plasma model); (ii) they reduce error due to the frequency of plasma sampling versus the infrequency of urine collection in other models; (iii) they are more quantitative and measure the total production rate independently of the determination of free or conjugated forms; (iv) they give information about pool size and transfer rates; (v) they establish a relationship to muscle mass; (vi) they provide a method for direct measurement of muscle proteolysis in swine and sheep; and (vii) they do not require restraint of the animals for long periods.

Significance of Protein Turnover

Since isotopes were first used by Schoeheimer and his colleagues in 1940, many aspects of protein turnover have been described. The methods described in

Table 2.3. Tabulation of results from protein turnover studies in farm animals.

Model	Species	Response	Reference
3MH kinetic model	Swine	Myofibrillar proteolysis was increased by 27% in protein-deficient barrows; no direct relationship between myofibrillar proteolysis and *in vitro* proteinase activity	van den Hemel-Grooten *et al.* (1995)
3MH kinetic model	Swine	Myofibrillar proteolysis was not different from controls swine during the protein refeeding period	van den Hemel-Grooten *et al.* (1998)
3MH kinetic model	Cattle	There was a 20% decrease in 3MH production in the trenebolone acetate-implanted cattle, but when combined with an oestrogen implant the decrease was prevented	Rathmacher *et al.* (1993b)
3MH kinetic model	Dogs	In terms of post-surgical nutrition, meeting the protein requirement is critical in minimizing muscle protein catabolism, and hyper-supplementation of both energy and protein has little affect	Rathmacher *et al.* (1993a)
Urine 3MH	Cattle	FBR was increased in feed-restricted cattle	Jones *et al.* (1990)
Urine 3MH	Cattle	No effect on muscle protein breakdown	Hayden *et al.* (1992)
Arterio-venous Whole-body protein turnover–leucine	Sheep	Hepatic protein synthesis was maintained at the expense of muscle Muscle protein synthesis contributes to 50% of whole body protein synthesis	Pell *et al.* (1986)
Arterio-venous Whole-body protein turnover–leucine	Sheep	Whole-body and hind-limb protein synthesis is increased with food intake. Leucine oxidation increased with food intake	Harris *et al.* (1992)
[^{15}N]Glycine	Cattle	Whole-body protein synthesis and degradation increase when the limiting amino acid is given	Wessels *et al.* (1997)
[^{15}N]Glycine	Pigs	Increased protein accretion with lysine supplementation was due to a greater increase in protein synthesis	Salter *et al.* (1990)
Whole-body protein turnover–leucine	Cattle	Steroid-implanted steers had a greater increase in synthesis and reduced amino acid oxidation	Lobley *et al.* (1985)
Whole-body protein turnover–leucine/ constant infusion	Cattle	Bovine somatotropin increased the FSR in muscle and the small intestine	Eisemann *et al.* (1989)
Flooding dose	Sheep	The FSR was, in decreasing order, intestine, liver and muscle	Attaix *et al.* (1988)
Flooding dose	Sheep	Changes in nutrients at weaning enhance protein synthesis without any specific effect on small intestine site	Attaix *et al.* (1992)
Constant infusion	Swine	FSR was higher in ractopamine-fed pigs as compared with controls	Bergen *et al.* (1989)
Constant infusion	Swine	Testosterone levels had no effect on muscle growth or turnover	Skjaerlund *et al.* (1994)
Constant infusion/ flooding dose	Sheep	Protein synthesis increases with intake in muscle, skin and liver	Lobley *et al.* (1992)

this chapter have been used increasingly in farm animals to improve the production of muscle for meat and the relationship between whole-body protein turnover and muscle protein turnover. Table 2.3 summarizes some of these findings.

References

Asatoor, A.M. and Armstrong, M.D. (1967) 3-Methylhistidine, a component of actin. *Biochemical and Biophysical Research Communications* 26, 168–174.

Attaix, D., Aurousseau, E., Manghebati, A. and Arnal, M. (1988) Contribution of liver, skin and skeletal muscle to whole-body protein synthesis in the young lamb. *British Journal of Nutrition* 60, 77–84.

Attaix, D., Aurousseau, E., Rosolowska-Huszcz, D., Bayle, G. and Arnal, M. (1992) *In vivo* longitudinal variations in protein synthesis in developing ovine intestines. *American Journal of Physiology* 263, R1318–R1323

Barrett, E.J., Revkin, J.H., Young, L.H., Zaret, B.L., Jacob, R. and Gelfand, R.A. (1987) An isotopic method for measurement of muscle protein synthesis and degradation *in vivo*. *Biochemical Journal* 245, 223–228.

Bergen, W.G., Johnson, S.E., Skjaerlund, D.M., Babiker, A.S., Ames, N.K., Merkel, R.A. and Anderson, D.B. (1989) Muscle protein metabolism in finishing pigs fed ractopamine. *Journal of Animal Science* 67, 2255–2262.

Berman, M. and Weiss, M.F. (1978) *SAAM Manual, US Department of Health, Education and Welfare Publication No.(NIH) 78–180*. US Government Printing Office, Washington, DC.

Bier, D.M. (1989) Intrinsically difficult problems: the kinetics of body proteins and amino acids in man. *Diabetes/Metabolism* 5, 111–132.

Boston, R.C., Grief, P.C. and Berman, M. (1981) Conversational SAAM – an inter-reactive program for kinetic analysis of biological systems. *Comp. Programs in Biomedicine* 13, 111–119.

Buttery, P.J. (1984) Protein turnover and muscle metabolism in the ruminant. In: Gilchrist, F.M.C. and Mackie, R.I. (eds) *Herbivore Nutrition*. The Science Press, Craighell.

Cass, K.A., Clark, E.B. and Rubenstein, P.A. (1983) Is the onset of actin histidine methylation under developmental control in the chick embryo. *Archives of Biochemistry and Biophysics* 225, 731–739.

Cobelli, C., Saccomani, M.P., Tessari, P., Biolo, G., Luzi, L. and Matthews, D.E. (1991) Compartmental model of leucine kinetics in humans. *American Journal of Physiology* 261, E539–E550.

Cowgill, R.W. and Freeberg, B. (1957) The metabolism of methylhistidine compounds in animals. *Archives of Biochemistry and Biophysics* 71, 466–472.

Eisemann, J.H., Hammond, A.C. and Rumsey, T.S. (1989) Tissue protein synthesis and nucleic acid concentrations in steers treated with somatotropin. *British Journal of Nutrition* 62, 657–671.

Emori, Y., Kawasaki, H., Imajoh, S., Imahori, K. and Suzuki, K. (1987) Endogenous inhibitor for calcium-dependent cysteine protease contains four internal repeats that could be responsible for its multiple reactive sites. *Proceedings of the National Academy of Sciences of the United States of America* 84, 3590–3594.

Garlick, P.J. (1969) Turnover rate of muscle protein measured by constant intravenous infusion of ^{14}C-glycine. *Nature* 223, 61–62.

Garlick, P.J. and Fern, E.B. (1985) Whole-body protein turnover: theoretical considerations. In: *Substrate and Energy Metabolism*. John Libbey, London, pp. 7–15.

Garlick, P.J., McNurlan, M.A., Essen, P. and Wernerman, J. (1994) Measurement of tissue protein synthesis rates *in vivo*: a critical analysis of contrasting methods. *American Journal of Physiology* 29, E287–E297.

Golden, M.H.N. and Waterlow, J.C. (1977) Total protein synthesis in elderly people: a comparison of results with ^{15}N]glycine and ^{14}C]leucine. *Clinical Science, Molecular Medicine* 53, 277–288.

Hardy, M.F., Harris, C.I., Ferry, J.V. and Stone, D. (1970) Occurrence and formation of the N^t-methyllysines in myosin and the myofibrillar proteins. *Biochemical Journal* 120, 653–660.

Harris, C.I. and Milne, G. (1980) The urinary excretion of N^t-methyl histidine in sheep: an invalid index of muscle protein breakdown. *British Journal of Nutrition* 44, 129–140.

Harris, C.I. and Milne, G. (1981a) The inadequacy of urinary (*N*-tau)-methyl histidine excretion in the pig as a measure of muscle protein breakdown. *British Journal of Nutrition* 45, 423–429.

Harris, C.I. and Milne, G. (1981b) The urinary excretion of *N*-tau-methyl histidine by cattle: validation as an index of muscle protein breakdown. *British Journal of Nutrition* 45, 411–422.

Harris, C.I. and Milne, G. (1987) The identification of the *N*-methyl histidine-containing dipeptide, balenine, in muscle extracts from various mammals and the chicken. *Comparative Biochemistry and Physiology* 86B, 273–279.

Harris, C.I., Milne, G., Lobley, G.E. and Nicholas, G.A. (1977) 3-Methylhistidine as a measure of skeletal-muscle protein catabolism in the adult New Zealand white rabbit. *Biochemical Society Transactions* 5, 706–708.

Harris, P.M., Skene, P.A., Buchan, V., Milne, E., Calder, A.G., Anderson, S.E., Connell, A. and Lobley, G.E. (1992) Effect of food intake on hind-limb and whole-body protein metabolism in young growing sheep: chronic studies based on arterio-venous techniques [published erratum appears in *British Journal of Nutrition* 1992 Nov; 68(3): following 803]. *British Journal of Nutrition* 68, 389–407.

Haverberg, L.N., Omstedt, P.T., Munro, H.N. and Young, V.R. (1975) N^t-Methylhistidine content of mixed proteins in various rat tissues. *Biochemistry and Biophysiology Acta* 405, 67–71.

Hayden, J.M., Bergen, W.G. and Merkel, R.A. (1992) Skeletal muscle protein metabolism and serum growth hormone, insulin, and cortisol concentrations in growing steers implanted with estradiol-17 beta, trenbolone acetate, or estradiol-17 beta plus trenbolone acetate. *Journal of Animal Science* 70, 2109–2119.

Henshaw, E.C., Hirsch, C.A., Morton, B.E. and Hiatt, H.H. (1971) Control of protein synthesis in mammalian tissues through changes in ribosome activity. *Journal of Biological Chemistry* 246, 436–446.

Huszar, G. and Elzinga, M. (1971) Amino acid sequence around the single 3-methylhistidine residue in rabbit skeletal muscle. *Biochemistry* 10, 229–236.

Jeevanandam, M., Brennan, M.F., Horowitz, G.D., Rose, D., Mihranian, M.H., Daly, J. and Lowry, S.F. (1985) Tracer priming in human protein turnover studies with [^{15}N]glycine. *Biochemical Medicine* 34, 214–225.

Johnson, P., Harris, C.I. and Perry, S.V. (1967) 3-Methylhistidine in actin and other muscle proteins. *Biochemical Journal* 105, 361–370.

Jones, S.J., Aberle, E.D. and Judge, M.D. (1986) Estimation of the fractional breakdown rates of myofibrillar proteins in chickens from quantitation of 3-methylhistidine excretion. *Poultry Science* 65, 2142–2147.

Jones, S.J., Starkey, D.L., Calkins, C.R. and Crouse, J.D. (1990) Myofibrillar protein turnover in feed-restricted and realimented beef cattle. *Journal of Animal Science* 68, 2707–2715.

Kalyankar, G.D. and Meister, A. (1959) Enzymatic synthesis of carnosine and related beta-alanyl and gamma-aminobutryl peptides. *Journal of Biological Chemistry* 234, 3210–3218 (abstract).

Lobley, G.E., Connell, A., Mollison, G.S., Brewer, A., Harris, C.I., Buchan, V. and Galbraith, H. (1985) The effects of a combined implant of trenbolone acetate and oestradiol-17 beta on protein and energy metabolism in growing beef steers. *British Journal of Nutrition* 54, 681–694.

Lobley, G.E., Harris, P.M., Skene, P.A., Brown, D., Milne, E., Calder, A.G., Anderson, S.E., Garlick, P.J., Nevison, I. and Connell, A. (1992) Responses in tissue protein synthesis to sub- and supra-maintenance intake in young growing sheep: comparison of large-dose and continuous-infusion techniques. *British Journal of Nutrition* 68, 373–388.

Long, C.L., Haverberg, L.N., Young, V.R., Kinney, J.M., Munro, H.N. and Geiger, J.W. (1975) Metabolsim of 3-methylhistidine in man. *Metabolism* 24, 929–935.

Long, C.L., Dillard, D.R., Bodzin, J.H., Geiger, J.W. and Blakemore, W.S. (1988) Validity of 3-methyl-histidine excretion as an indicator of skeletal muscle protein breakdown in humans. *Metabolism* 37, 844–849.

Matthews, D.E. and Bier, D.M. (1983) Stable isotope methods for nutritional investigation. *Annual Review of Nutrition* 3, 309–339.

McCarthy, F.D., Bergen, W.G. and Hawkins, D.R. (1983) Muscle protein turnover in cattle of differing genetic backgrounds as measured by urinary *N*-tau-methylhistidine excretion. *Journal of Nutrition* 113, 2455–2463.

Millward, D.J., Garlick, P.J., Stewart, R.J.C., Nnanyelugo, D.O. and Waterlow, J.C. (1975) Skeletal-muscle growth and protein turnover. *Biochemical Journal* 150, 235–243.

Mitch, W.E. and Goldberg, A.L. (1996) Mechanisms of muscle wasting. The role of the ubiquitin–proteasome pathway. *New England Journal of Medicine* 335, 1897–1905.

Nishizawa, N., Noguchi, T. and Hareyama, S. (1977) Fractional flux rates of N^t-methylhistidine in skin and gastrointestine: the contribution of these tissues to urinary excretion of N^t-methylhistidine in the rat. *British Journal of Nutrition* 38, 149–151.

Nishizawa, N., Yoyoda, Y., Noguchi, T., Hareyama, S., Itabashi, H. and Funabiki, R. (1979) N-tau-methylhistidine content of organs and tissues of cattle and an attempt to estimate fractional catabolic and synthetic rates of myofibrillar proteins of skeletal muscle during growth by measuring urinary output of N-tau-methylhistidine. *British Journal of Nutrition* 42, 247–252.

Nissen, S. (1991) *Modern Methods in Protein Nutrition and Metabolism.* Academic Press, New York.

Pell, J.M., Caldarone, E.M. and Bergman, E.N. (1986) Leucine and alpha-ketoisocaproate metabolism and interconversions in fed and fasted sheep. *Metabolism* 35, 1005–1016.

Picou, D. and Taylor-Roberts, T. (1969) The measurement of total protein synthesis and catabolism and nitrogen turnover in infants in different nutritional states and receiving different amounts of dietary protein. *Clinical Science* 36, 283–296.

Rathmacher, J. and Nissen, S. (1992) Rate of 3-methylhistidine (3MH) exchange between tissues does not explain non-quantitative urinary excretion of 3MH in swine and sheep. *FASEB Journal* 6, A1965–A1965 (abstract).

Rathmacher, J.A., Link, G.A. and Nissen, S.L. (1992a) Technical note: The use of a compartmental model to estimate the *de novo* production rate of N^t-methylhistidine in cattle. *Journal of Animal Science* 70, 2104–2108.

Rathmacher, J.A., Link, G.A., Flakoll, P.J. and Nissen, S.L. (1992b) Gas chromatographic/mass spectrometric analysis of stable isotopes of 3-methylhistidine in biological fluids: application to plasma kinetics *in vivo*. *Biological Mass Spectrometry* 21, 560–566.

Rathmacher, J., Sperling, R., Coates, C. and Nissen, S. (1993a) A compartmental model to measure 3-methylhistidine production in dogs following surgery. *FASEB Journal* 7, A72–A72 (abstract).

Rathmacher, J., Trenkle, A. and Nissen, S. (1993b) The use of compartmental models of 3-methylhistidine flux to evaluate skeletal muscle protein turnover in implanted steers. *Journal of Animal Science* 71, 135–135 (abstract).

Rathmacher, J.A., Link, G. and Nissen, S. (1993c) Measurement of 3-methylhistidine production in lambs by using compartmental-kinetic analysis. *British Journal of Nutrition* 69, 743–755.

Rathmacher, J.A., Flakoll, P.J. and Nissen, S.L. (1995) A compartmental model of 3-methylhistidine metabolism in humans. *American Journal of Physiology* 296, E193–E198.

Rathmacher, J.A., Nissen, S.L., Paxton, R.E. and Anderson, D.B. (1996) Estimation of 3-methylhistidine production in pigs by compartmental analysis. *Journal of Animal Science* 74, 46–56.

Reeds, P.J. (1989) Regulation of protein turnover. In: Campion, D.R., Hausman, G.J. and Martin, R.J. (eds) *Animal Growth Regulation.* Plenum Press, New York, p. 183.

Rennie, M.J., Smith, K. and Watt, P.W. (1994) Measurement of human tissue protein synthesis: an optimal approach. *American Journal of Physiology* 266, 298–307.

Reporter, M. (1969) 3-Methylhistidine metabolism in proteins from cultured mammalian muscle cells. *Biochemistry* 8, 3489–3496.

Salter, D.N., Montgomery, A.I., Hudson, A., Quelch, D.B. and Elliott, R.J. (1990) Lysine requirements and whole-body protein turnover in growing pigs. *British Journal of Nutrition* 63, 503–513.

Schoenheimer, R., Rattner, S. and Rittenberg, D. (1939) Studies in protein metabolism. X. The metabolic activity of body proteins investigated with L(−) leucine containing two isotopes. *Journal of Biological Chemistry* 130, 703–732.

Schwenk, W.F., Beaufrere, B. and Haymond, M.W. (1985) Use of reciprocal pool specific activities to model leucine metabolism in humans. *American Journal of Physiology* 249, E646–E650.

Sjolin, J., Stjernström, H., Henneberg, S., Andersson, E., Martensson, J., Friman, G. and Larsson, J. (1989) Splanchnic and peripheral release of 3-methylhistidine in relation to its urinary excretion in human infection. *Metabolism* 38, 23–29.

Sjölin, J., Stjernström, H., Friman, G., Larsson, J. and Wahren, J. (1990) Total and net muscle protein breakdown in infection determined by amino acid effluxes. *American Journal of Physiology* 258, E856–E863.

Skjaerlund, D.M., Mulvaney, D.R., Bergen, W.G. and Merkel, R.A. (1994) Skeletal muscle growth and protein turnover in neonatal boars and barrows. *Journal of Animal Science* 72, 315–321.

Tallen, H., Stein, W.H. and Moore, S. (1954) 3-Methylhistidine, a new amino acid from human urine. *Journal of Biological Chemistry* 206, 825–834.

van den Hemel-Grooten, H.N.A., Koohmaraie, M., Yen, J.T., Arbona, J.R., Rathmacher, J.A., Nissen, S.L., Fiortto, M.L., Garssen, G.J. and Verstegen, M.W.A. (1995) Comparision between 3-methylhistidine production and proteinase activity as measures of skeletal muscle breakdown in protein-deficient growing barrows. *Journal of Animal Science* 73, 2272–2281.

van den Hemel-Grooten, H.N.A., Rathmacher, J.A., Garssen, G.J., Schreurs, V.V.A.M. and Verstegen, M.W.A. (1997) Contribution of gastrointestinal tract to whole-body 3-methylhistidine production in growing pigs. *Journal of Animal Physiology and Animal Nutrition* 77, 84–90.

van den Hemel-Grooten, H.N.A., Rathmacher, J.A., Garssen, G.J., Schreurs, V.V.A.M. and Verstegen, M.W.A. (1998) Whole body 3-methylhistidine production rate and proteinase activities in different skeletal muscles. *Livestock Production Science* 55, 145–156.

Waterlow, J.C. (1969) The assessment of protein nutrition and metabolism in the whole animal, with special reference to man. In: Munro, H. (ed.) *Mammalian Protein Metabolism*, Vol. III. Academic Press, New York, pp. 325–390.

Waterlow, J.C. (1981) ^{15}N end-product methods for the study of whole body protein turnover. *Proceedings of the Nutrition Society* 40, 317–320.

Waterlow, J.C. and Stephen, J.M. (1966) Adaptation of the rat to a low-protein diet: the effect of a reduced protein intake on the pattern of incorporation of L-[^{14}C]lysine. *British Journal of Nutrition* 20, 461–484.

Waterlow, J.C., Garlick, P.J. and Millward, D.J. (1978) *Protein Turnover in Mammalian Tissues and in the Whole Body*. Elsevier North-Holland, Amsterdam.

Wessels, R.H., Titgemeyer, E.C. and St Jean, G. (1997) Effect of amino acid supplementation on whole-body protein turnover in Holstein steers. *Journal of Animal Science* 75, 3066–3073.

Wolfe, R.R. (1992) *Radioactive and Stable Isotope Tracers in Biomedicine: Principles and Practice of Kinetic Analysis*. Wiley-Liss, New York.

Young, V.R. and Munro, H.N. (1978) N^t-Methylhistidine (3-methylhistidine) and muscle protein turnover: an overview. *Federation Proceedings* 37, 2291–2300.

Young, V.R., Alex, S.D., Baliga, B.S., Munro, H.N. and Muecke, W. (1972) Metabolism of administered 3-methylhistidine: lack of muscle transfer ribonucleic acid charging and quantitative excretion as 3-methylhistidine and its *N*-acetyl derivative. *Journal of Biological Chemistry* 217, 3592–3600.

Zhang, X.J., Chinkes, D.L., Sakurai, Y. and Wolfe, R.R. (1996) An isotopic method for measurement of muscle protein fractional breakdown rate *in vivo*. *American Journal of Physiology* 270, E759–E767.

Chapter 3

Inter-organ Amino Acid Flux

C.J. Seal and D.S. Parker[1]

Department of Biological and Nutritional Sciences, University of Newcastle,
Newcastle upon Tyne, UK
[1]Present address: Novus Europe s.a./n.v., Brussels, Belgium

Introduction

The integration of nitrogen metabolism in mammalian systems involves the complex interaction of several key processes which link together in a coordinated manner between, within and across individual tissues and organs. The principal role of these processes is the maintenance of finely tuned nitrogen cycles to meet the body's requirements for tissue mainten- ance, turnover and growth for any fixed level of dietary nitrogen intake. These processes include tissue protein turnover and degradation, salvage of the end- products of nitrogen metabolism, and the transport and redistribution of the end- products of nitrogen metabolism around the body. This chapter focuses on the role of amino acids in these processes and will consider transport of amino acids between tissues and organs in addition to flux across tissue beds. Quantitatively, muscle protein constitutes the largest pool of amino acids present in the body, in the form of protein and peptide-bound amino acids. The concentration of free amino acids in extracellular and intracellular compartments and blood is much smaller,

but nevertheless contributes the major route by which amino nitrogen is trans- ferred between metabolic compartments.

Transport of Amino Acids

Distribution between erythrocytes and plasma

Analysis of the distribution of individual amino acids between plasma and erythro- cytes (Table 3.1) shows that the concentra- tion of many amino acids is similar in both compartments and that there is generally good agreement between species in the relative distribution of individual amino acids. For some amino acids, notably aspartate, glutamate, glycine, histidine and lysine, the concentration of each amino acid in plasma is considerably less than that inside the red blood cell. Since Na^+-depen- dent concentrative uptake is not present in red blood cells (Young and Ellory, 1977), this indicates net production or synthesis of these amino acids within the erythro- cyte. In contrast, arginine and glutamine are more concentrated in plasma, suggest- ing catabolism of these amino acids in the

Table 3.1. Distribution of individual amino acids between plasma and erythrocytes.

Amino acid	Whole blood:plasma ratio					
	Elwyn (1966)[a] Dog	Felig *et al.* (1973) Humans	Aoki *et al.* (1976)[b] Humans	Koeln *et al.* (1993)[c] Calves	Heitmann and Bergman (1980) Sheep	Lobley *et al.* (1996)[a] Sheep
Histidine	2.21	ND	1.67	1.38	ND	2.55
Isoleucine	1.51	1.06	1.63	0.11	0.95	0.95
Leucine	1.54	1.03	1.65	0.20	1.11	1.48
Lysine	3.59	ND	1.59	0.44	1.13	2.75
Methionine	1.19	0.84	ND	0.56	ND	0.34
Phenylalanine	1.88	1.02	1.63	0.08	1.26	1.03
Threonine	1.59	1.23	1.73	0.40	1.20	1.16
Valine	1.42	1.06	1.64	0.11	0.99	1.02
Alanine	1.44	1.29	1.98	0.91	0.95	1.26
Arginine	4.08	ND	1.49	ND	0.72	ND
Aspartate	9.85	ND	ND	1.63	ND	4.24
Glutamate	4.11	ND	2.14	0.20	0.83	3.77
Glycine	ND	1.68	2.49	0.42	1.24	1.63
Proline	1.62	1.15	1.61	ND	ND	1.41
Serine	2.08	1.38	2.11	0.28	1.26	1.53
Tyrosine	3.34	1.13	1.80	0.34	1.19	1.17

[a]Erythrocyte:plasma ratio.
[b]Data from fasted humans.
[c]Data from fed calves.
ND, not determined.

red blood cell. The distribution of amino acids between the two blood compartments may vary across tissues. For example, it has been suggested that amino acids absorbed across the intestinal wall are transported to the liver in the plasma pool (Elwyn *et al.*, 1972; Houlier *et al.*, 1991; Lobley *et al.*, 1996) whereas erythrocytes may be more important in the transport of amino acids from the liver in non-ruminant species (Elwyn *et al.*, 1972). For ruminant animals, the data are conflicting; Houlier *et al.* (1991) have shown a similar differential distribution across the liver of cattle which has not been observed in studies with sheep (Lobley *et al.*, 1996).

The role of low-molecular weight peptides

The importance of low-molecular weight peptides in the transport of free amino acids (FAAs) is equivocal. Various analytical techniques have been employed to determine the concentration of peptide-bound amino acids (PBAAs) in plasma, and the results of these procedures indicate that the PBAA:FAA ratio in plasma varies between 0.4 and 3.6 depending on the species and the analytical technique used (Seal and Parker, 1997). There is considerable interest in the potential use of low-molecular weight peptides as nutritional substrates in parenteral nutrition (Stehle *et al.*, 1997) and there is convincing evidence that mixtures of peptides administered in this way can be hydrolysed and utilized by different tissues in several species (Albers *et al.*, 1988; Druml *et al.*, 1991; Stehle *et al.*, 1997). These studies suggest that hydrolysis of small synthetic peptides and utilization of the constituent amino acids can occur. It may be possible for PBAAs to be hydrolysed within specific tissues or organs, with the constituent amino acids then being available for intracellular use. The release of peptides back out of the cell during the process of intracellular protein turnover may also account for the apparent change in peptide composition observed across tissue beds (Seal and Parker, 1996). There is increasing evidence that dipeptides may be metabolized (hydrolysed) at different rates in different tissues (Druml *et al.*, 1997), which raises the intriguing possibility of targeting substrates to specific sites in the body. Recent research on the expression of peptide transporters suggests that these may be inducible under different dietary regimes (Walker and Hirst, 1997), again suggesting that these substrates may be important under different physiological situations. However, the contribution of these processes to overall α-amino N economy remains unresolved and will be a key area for future research.

Absorption of Amino Acids Across the Gastrointestinal Tract

The development of catheterization procedures for determining the composition of blood supplying and draining the gastrointestinal tissues, together with blood flow measurements and the use of isotopically labelled substrates, has substantially increased our understanding of the flux of amino acids across gut tissues (Seal and Reynolds, 1993). Where experiments have coupled these procedures with measurements of amino acid disappearance from the gut lumen, it is clear that fewer amino acids arrive in the portal vein than apparently disappear from digesta (Tagari and Bergman, 1978; MacRae and Reeds, 1980; Neutze *et al.*, 1990; MacRae *et al.*, 1996). Experiments with ruminant and non-ruminant animals have shown that amino acid flux across the portal-drained viscera is responsive to changes in diet and the supply of energy-yielding substrates within the gastrointestinal tissues (Seal *et al.*, 1992; Balcells *et al.*, 1995; Seal and Parker, 1996; van der Meulen *et al.*, 1997). These studies confirm that the net flux of amino acids is sensitive to many factors including metabolism of sequestered amino acids from the arterial supply. This latter process has been determined in sheep using a combination or arteriovenous difference procedures and isotopic

kinetic measurements (MacRae *et al.*, 1996). In this study, intravenous and intraluminal infusions of ^{13}C-labelled amino acids were used to apportion unidirectional fluxes from the arterial blood pool and from the gut lumen. The results of this experiment suggest that, whilst some essential amino acids are sequestered from the lumen, a much greater proportion comes from circulating blood supply to the tissue. Extraction of amino acids in this way reflects the high rates of protein turnover (relative to tissue mass) observed for gastrointestinal tissues (Lobley *et al.*, 1980). Stoll *et al.* (1998) also used ^{13}C-labelled amino acids from algal protein and showed in young pigs that first-pass splanchnic metabolism of enteral amino acids reflects intestinal rather than hepatic metabolism. In addition, they demonstrated that although this accounted for ~35% of dietary protein intake, the portal-drained viscera continued to utilize arterial amino acids, and amino acid catabolism accounted for ~80% of CO_2 production by the portal-drained viscera, predominantly through oxidation of glutamate and aspartate.

Net extraction of amino acids (i.e. a lower concentration of amino acids in portal blood compared with arterial blood supplying the tissues) across the gastrointestinal tissues is often observed, indicating that gastrointestinal tissue requirements for some amino acids cannot be met from luminal sources and must be derived from the arterial supply, especially in the fasted state. Glutamine, for example, is utilized readily by gut tissues for energy production (Windmeuller and Spaeth, 1980) and in the supply of amide nitrogen for purine and pyrimidine synthesis (Duée *et al.*, 1995). This intestinal utilization of glutamine is extensive. For example, in lambs, incorporation of [5–^{15}N]glutamine into intestinal proteins accounted for 73% of the gross flux of the amino acid across the small intestine (Gate *et al.*, 1997). In the pig, portal-drained visceral flux of glutamine is negative after feeding a wide range of diets (see van der Meulen and Jansman, 1997). The use of glutamine in enterocytes falls in growing pigs compared with neonatal pigs in which the amino acid is the preferred energy substrate compared with ATP and glucose. In ruminant animals, portal flux of glutamine is also negative, but the high concentration of the amino acid in herbage means that duodenal glutamine supply is much higher than in non-ruminant species. There is, however, considerable variability in portal glutamine flux across species and under different dietary regimes (Table 3.2). These data emphasize the sensitivity of the gut tissues not only to dietary amino acid supply but also to other luminal and arter-ial nutrients. In addition, different responses between ruminant species fed the same diets (see, for example, Prior et al., 1981) question the application of mean data in the development of mechanistic models of nutrient metabolism.

Net absorption of amino acids is strongly correlated with increasing protein intake in non-ruminants (Rérat et al., 1988) although the absorption coefficients of individual amino acids fall with increasing protein supply. These responses are different for non-essential and essential amino acids; increasing duodenal supply

Table 3.2. Effect of diet on net glutamine flux across portal-drained viscera of various species.

Species	Net flux[a]	Diet	Reference
Sheep	+ve	Cereal/straw	Balcells et al. (1995)
	−ve	Cereal/straw + i.v. glucose	
Sheep	−ve	Forage	Piccioli Capelli et al. (1997)
	+ve	Forage + i.v. glucose	
	++ve	Forage + intraduodenal glucose	
Sheep	−ve	High protein forage	Tagari and Bergman (1978)
	−−ve	Medium protein cereal by-products	
Sheep	+ve	Forage (hay based)	Prior et al. (1981)
	++ve	Concentrate	
Steers	+ve	Forage (hay based)	
	−ve	Concentrate	
Steers	+ve	Forage (lucerne)	Taniguchi et al. (1995)
	−ve	Forage + abomasal starch, intraruminal casein	
	−ve	Forage + intraruminal starch and casein	
Steers	−ve	Concentrate (maize based)	Guerino et al. (1991)
	+ve	Concentrate + postruminal casein (300 g day^{-1})	
Steers	+ve	Forage	Seal et al. (1992)
	−ve	Concentrate	
Steers	−ve	Forage	Seal and Parker (1996)
	+ve	Forage + intraruminal propionate	
Steers	−ve	Concentrate fed and starved	Koeln et al. (1993)
Dairy cows	+ve	Silage/concentrate 4 weeks post-partum	Reynolds et al. (1988)
	−ve	8 weeks post-partum	
Heifers	−ve	High concentrate	Harmon et al. (1988)
	−−ve	High concentrate + ionophores	
Pigs	−ve	Starch-based diets	van der Meulen et al. (1997)
Pigs	−ve	Pre-weaning	Wu et al. (1994)
	−ve	Maize-based diet	

[a]Negative values indicate net extraction and positive values net release of glutamine by portal-drained visceral tissues.

of the former is associated with increased portal flux not only of non-essential amino acids but also of ammonia, suggesting that gastrointestinal tissue metabolism (catabolism) of the amino acids is also increased (van der Meulen *et al.*, 1996). For ruminant animals, the effect of increasing nitrogen intake is more complex due to the moderating effect of the ruminal microflora in influencing the flow of protein (principally in the form of microbial protein) into the duodenum. Figure 3.1 shows that the relationship between net portal flux of amino acids and N intake is poor in comparison

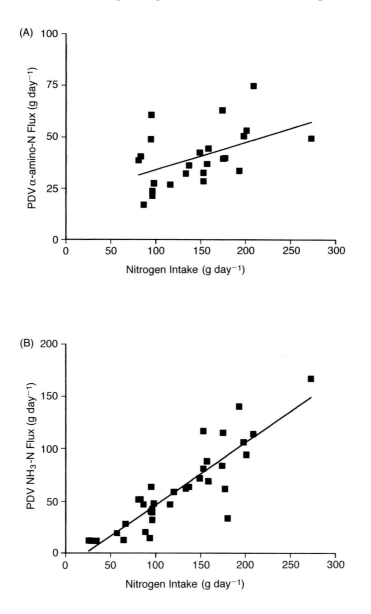

Fig. 3.1. Relationships between nitrogen intake, portal-drained visceral α-amino nitrogen flux (A: $y = 20.429 + 0.136x$, $R^2 = 0.235$) and portal-drained visceral NH_3N flux (B: $y = -12.96 + 0.594x$, $R^2 = 0.772$). From Seal and Reynolds (1993).

with the strong relationship between ammonia N flux and N intake (Seal and Reynolds, 1993). Metabolizable energy intake appears to be a better predictor of portal amino acid flux than protein intake (Reynolds *et al.*, 1994) since this is most closely linked to ruminally digestible organic matter, the principal determinant of microbial protein synthesis (Hoover and Stokes, 1991). Amino acid flux is also affected by the supply of glucose to the small intestine. In studies with pigs fed diets containing starches with differing rates of digestion, van der Meulen *et al.* (1997) showed that portal flux of amino acids was reduced when pea starch was fed compared with more rapidly digested maize starch. We have also shown that increasing glucose availability to the gastrointestinal tissues of sheep and steers, either by increasing ruminal propionate availability (Seal and Parker, 1996) or by infusion of glucose or starch into the small intestine (Seal *et al.*, 1994; Piccioli-Cappelli *et al.*, 1997), results in increased portal amino acid flux. The mechanism by which these responses are mediated is unclear but may be due to reduced catabolism of amino acids within gastrointestinal tissues, changes in transit of digesta in the gut lumen or, in the case of poorly digested starches in the small intestine, sequestration of protein within the digesta matrix.

The absorption of low-molecular weight peptides

There is increasing evidence that amino acids may be absorbed across intestinal tissues both as 'free' amino acids and 'bound' as low-molecular weight peptides (see Chapter 1), and studies in chronically catheterized steers have shown that the pattern of amino acids in the peptide fraction changes across both mesenteric- and portal-drained tissues (Seal and Parker, 1996). Experiments with sheep, in which labelled dipeptides have been infused into the rumen at rates calculated to maintain peptide concentrations seen post-feeding,

show that these dipeptides were absorbed intact into both the mesenteric and portal vein (Mesgaran, 1996). However, the concentrations recovered in blood were very small and were achieved using high infusion rates in order to elevate intra-ruminal peptide concentrations to levels which would not normally be maintained under physiological conditions. In contrast to these studies, Neutze *et al.* (1996) in lambs, and Dawson and Holdsworth (1962) in rats, were unable to show absorption of labelled peptides across the gut wall, suggesting that peptide material must be hydrolysed either at the cell wall, or within the cytosol before being transported across the basolateral membrane as free amino acids. Peptide transporters have been identified in tissues from different sites along the gastrointestinal tract in many non-ruminant and ruminant species (Walker and Hirst, 1997). These transporters show a wide substrate specificity, and the contribution of peptide transport to total amino acid flux across the gut wall remains an area of debate; at the time of writing, it is still generally considered that the great majority of amino acids are absorbed from the small intestine as free amino acids.

Trans-hepatic Flux of Amino Acids

Only a small proportion of the total amino acids absorbed from the small intestine into the hepatic portal vein reach the peripheral circulation in free form because substantial and variable amounts are removed by the liver (Lobley *et al.*, 1995, 1996). The proportion of individual amino acids which is removed is also species dependent (Wray-Cahen *et al.*, 1997). The balance of amino acids leaving the liver is important in influencing the subsequent availability of amino acids for extrahepatic use. For example, hepatic extraction of histidine (Wolff *et al.*, 1972) may leave insufficient amounts of this amino acid for milk synthesis. Data for hepatic extractions of individual amino acids in large animals are shown in Table 3.3. Such data are extremely variable and suffer from experimental problems in the accurate measurement of hepatic portal venous and arterial blood flow and corresponding amino acid concentrations, the venous-arterio concentration differences often being similar to levels of analytical precision. Absorbed amino acids have four potential fates in the liver (Wray-Cahen *et al.*, 1997): (i) retention in the free form as expanded intra- and extravascular fluid; (ii) conversion to specific nitrogenous metabolites (e.g. aromatic amino acids to neurotransmitters, glycine to hippurate, synthesis of small oligopeptides); (iii) oxidation to produce energy and non-nitrogenous intermediary metabolites; and (iv) incorporation into hepatic and export proteins. An additional fate of amino acids linked to catabolism of the carbon skeleton is their role as a method of detoxifying excess ammonia arriving at the liver (Parker *et al.*, 1995). For example, removal of amino acids by the liver is increased with increased portal absorption of ammonia N (Maltby *et al.*, 1991; Reynolds *et al.*, 1991). The mechanism for the increase in liver removal of amino acids under dietary conditions which

result in increased ammonia production is unclear; however, it has been suggested that this may be due to an increased requirement for amino acid N in transamination reactions to generate glutamate and aspartate required for urea biosynthesis (Reynolds, 1992). Under normal conditions, mitochondrial and cytosolic aspartate–glutamate transamination pools are in equilibrium (Cooper *et al.*, 1991), and the reversible action of glutamate dehydrogenase means that both N atoms in the urea molecule can arise from either NH_3 or amino acids (Meijer *et al.*, 1990). In contrast, under conditions of high urea flux, the mitochondrial supply of NH_3 may not be sufficient for both N moieties, inducing the obligatory use of amino acid N to maintain urea synthesis. Increased oxidation of alanine and reduced gluconeogenesis from this amino acid have been observed *in vitro* in hepatocytes isolated from sheep fed soluble nitrogen in the form of urea (Mutsvangwa *et al.*, 1996), and Lobley *et al.* (1995) showed that oxidation of [1–^{14}C]leucine was increased during infusions of NH_4Cl into the mesenteric vein. Studies *in vitro* with isolated

Table 3.3. Hepatic fractional extractions of absorbed amino acids from the plasma across the liver of sheep, pigs and cattle (reproduced with permission from Wray-Cahen *et al.*, 1997).

Amino acid	Wolff *et al.* (1972) Sheep	Rérat *et al.* (1992)[a] Pigs	Lobley *et al.* (1995)[b] Sheep	Lobley *et al.* (1996) Sheep	Wray-Cahen *et al.* (1997)[c] Cattle
Glycine	2.54	1.16	0.97	1.07	0.73
Alanine	1.39	0.86	0.69	1.14	0.54
Serine	1.13	0.63	0.97	0.75	0.37
Proline	0.91	0.53	0.47	0.96	0.47
Tyrosine	1.42	0.44	0.85	0.83	0.63
Arginine	2.53	0.48	0.73	0.72	0.70
Valine	0.58	0.48	0.43	0.47	0.25
Isoleucine	0.37	0.54	0.28	0.50	0.49
Leucine	0.36	0.50	0.56	0.34	0.30
Methionine	1.00	0.63	1.21	0.53	0.83
Phenylalanine	1.36	0.74	0.84	0.77	0.87
Lysine	0.81	0.50	0.64	0.57	0.31
Histidine	1.50	0.51	1.16	1.09	0.50
Threonine	1.05	0.62	0.44	0.85	0.49

[a]Mean value for peptide and free amino acid intraduodenal infusions.
[b]Values for blood only and mean of plus and minus exogenous ammonia infusion.
[c]Values during intramesenteric amino acid infusion corrected for basal level.

hepatocytes from fasted sheep using ^{15}N-labelled substrates have shown, however, that amino acid N is not essential for urea-genesis (Luo *et al.*, 1995). The mechanism for the interaction between NH_3 and amino acid deamination is not proven and requires further investigation.

Amino Acid Supply and Utilization by the Mammary Gland

Lactation imposes increased demands for protein synthesis, and the onset of lactation is accompanied by a shift in protein synthesis away from non-mammary tissues towards the mammary gland (Champredon *et al.*, 1990; Baracos *et al.*, 1991). This increase in protein synthesis is balanced by an increase in the supply of amino acids to the gland of between 20 and 40% (average across all amino acids, 25%; Bequette *et al.*, 1997). The major shift in protein metabolism during lactation is emphasized from studies in high-yielding dairy cows in which it was demonstrated that milk protein production may account for >80% of digestible protein intake (Clark *et al.*, 1978). The rate of milk production by the mammary gland is dependent on the combined influence of changes in blood flow and the concentration of specific nutrients in the blood. The fact that in some instances these may be inadequate to maintain maximal rates of milk synthesis has been demonstrated in several studies in which either peripheral intravenous or post-ruminal infusion of amino acids has resulted in increased milk protein output (Clark, 1975; Bequette and Backwell, 1997). Lysine and methionine are the first limiting amino acids for milk protein synthesis under normal conditions, and it is provision of these amino acids which may result in the observed increase in milk protein output in these studies. These data are not consistent, however, and many studies have shown either a small or no response to infusion of individual amino acids (see, for example, Mepham and Linzell, 1974; Metcalf *et al.*, 1991; Bequette *et al.*, 1996; Vanhatalo *et al.*, 1999; Varvikko *et al.*, 1999).

The control of nutrient supply, and in particular amino acid supply, to the mammary gland in non-ruminant animals is poorly understood in comparison with that in ruminant species, although it is recognized that the imbalances between the supply of individual amino acids to the gland and those found in milk in ruminants also exist in the pig (for a review, see Trottier, 1997). Measurements of milk output in non-ruminants is not easy, and this has been a major factor in limiting research in this area. However, there is considerable need for improved knowledge on the relationship between physiological and nutritional factors influencing lactational performance in non-ruminant farm animals in order to maximize performance and hence productivity.

The importance of low-molecular weight peptides in amino acid supply to the mammary gland

Several studies have demonstrated that on a net basis the extraction of non-essential amino acids by mammary tissue is insufficient to account for their output in milk protein. This suggests either the *de novo* synthesis of amino acids within the gland, or the utilization of the amino acid components of low-molecular weight peptides. There is no convincing evidence that synthesis of individual amino acids can account for this difference, since the exchange of C, N and S components between amino acids (for example, S from methionine and C from serine for cysteine synthesis) involves amino acids which may themselves become limiting or are already not extracted in adequate amounts in the free form. Backwell *et al.* (1996) used a dual-labelled tracer technique to demonstrate that the arterially infused peptides glycyl-phenylalanine and glycyl-leucine were used as substrates for casein synthesis in goats. In a further series of tracer studies, they have shown that naturally occurring low-molecular peptides can be used in milk protein synthesis and that there is some degree of substrate selectivity in this process (Backwell *et al.*, 1996; Bequette and Backwell, 1997).

Amino Acid Flux Across Muscle

The balance of the movement of individual amino acids across muscle tissue is determined by a number of competing pathways of metabolism. Skeletal muscle is the major protein store within the body, and in growing animals the rate of accretion is dependent upon amino acid supply, hormonal status and the relationship between synthetic and degradative pathways within the tissue-protein turnover. Small changes in the balance between these two latter processes can have a significant effect on rates of protein deposition and therefore production efficiency (Harris *et al.*, 1992; Sève and Ponter, 1997). Amino acid supply to, and flux from, muscle has been measured by a number of groups, and early work by Felig *et al.* (1973) established the presence of the glucose–alanine cycle in which alanine synthesized in muscle transfers amino groups to the liver and provides carbon for gluconeogenesis, thereby recycling glucose while disposing of the end-products of muscle amino acid degradation. This pathway, however, appears to be of minor importance in ruminant animals when compared with non-ruminants. The metabolism of the branched-chain amino acid (BCAA) leucine by muscle tissue also appears to differ between the two groups of animal species. In non-ruminants, skeletal muscle oxidizes a greater proportion of leucine derived from muscle protein degradation than in ruminants, and the transamination product α-ketoisocaproate (KIC) is re-aminated extensively in the liver. In the fasted ruminant, however, most of the leucine derived from muscle turnover is released, and in both gut and liver KIC and leucine contribute towards protein synthesis rather than acting as oxidative substrates (Pell *et al.*, 1986).

In addition to BCAAs, the role(s) of glutamine in the integration of nitrogen metabolism between tissues has also been an area of active research. It is the most abundant amino acid in the body, and muscle tissue appears to act as a source of supply for the requirements of gut and immune tissues during periods of metabolic stress. This efflux of glutamine has been demonstrated in both fed and fasted ruminants (McCormick and Webb, 1982), and in rats glutamine output from skeletal muscle increased as the plasma concentration decreased (Ardawi and Jamal, 1990). Given the putative roles of glutamine in energy metabolism and also in the provision of amino groups for nucleic acid synthesis in rapidly dividing cells (e.g. intestinal enterocytes and lymphocytes), it is apparent that amino group transfer from BCAAs in order to sustain glutamine output by muscle (Lobley, 1991) may represent a further integration of amino acid metabolism across the tissue.

As with other tissues, the form and complexity of amino acid supply to the muscle are still an area of debate. Arteriovenous studies by McCormick and Webb (1987) and Danilson *et al.* (1987) have suggested that peptides and serum proteins have the potential to contribute to amino acid flux to and from the tissue. Their studies also suggested that the nature of the diets fed to calves influenced the pattern of this flux. The hypothesis that hepatic protein output may provide a source of amino acids for peripheral tissues has been investigated (Connell *et al.*, 1997) in a study which measured changes in liver albumin synthesis in fed and fasted sheep. It was concluded that insufficient albumin was available to account for the shortfall in post-hepatic provision of free amino acids. A further evaluation of the potential role of a range of liver export proteins in the provision of a balanced supply of amino acids to meet the requirements for muscle protein accretion (Lobley and Milano, 1997), however, suggests that they could make an important contribution to the supply of histidine and phenylalanine. At present, the lack of specific methodology to investigate the fate(s) of plasma proteins across tissue beds is preventing further progress in this area.

Modelling Amino Acid Metabolism

Techniques for formulating feed for farm animals are based mainly on whole-animal studies, for the most part being designed to describe input and output situations developed to maximize productivity for given levels of financial expenditure (essentially equating to nutritive value of feed ingredients). The majority of early models of protein metabolism were simple in interpretation and were readily applicable to the feed industry. Early protein schemes were empirical models used to predict nitrogen requirements for growth and lactation (e.g. ARC, 1980; AFRC, 1984) and were based on the calculation of constants used to describe specific events in the gut and peripheral tissues. It is now recognized that these models are oversimplistic, and the reliance on average constants which do predict changes in response to perturbations in nutrient input is a major problem. Increased knowledge about metabolism in individual tissues has brought about a more integrated approach to modelling, incorporating a series of compartmentalized sub-models which are combined to provide a mechanistic integrated system which can still be applied in the feed industry (Hanigan et al., 1997). In order to describe amino acid requirements, these models adopt different approaches. The model described by Baldwin et al. (1987) introduced the concept of dynamic relationships integrated over time for three tissue types: lean body, adipose tissue and the viscera. This model treats amino acids as a single pool but allows competition between tissues for amino acids and different rates of tissue utilization. Gill et al. (1989) adopted a fully integrated approach which takes account of the effects of amino acid metabolism through ten tissue beds supplied from a single blood amino acid pool. The model does not include mammary metabolism and is necessarily complex using, as it does, data for ten different tissues. The Cornell net carbohydrate and protein system (CNCPS) includes sub-models of post-absorptive amino acid metabolism in which amino acid metabolism is split into discrete functions including needs for lactation, growth, urine and metabolic faecal losses, and scurf (O'Connor et al., 1993). The whole-animal and whole-tissue models described above are now supplemented by an increasing number of models in which intermediary metabolism of selected amino acids in some organs is added to the flux through the aggregated pool (Hanigan et al., 1997, 1998).

Conclusions

It is apparent that amino acid flux in blood represents the summation of a large number of processes in individual tissues. In farm livestock, the need to understand and quantify these processes is essential in order to optimize the use of dietary protein for animal production and minimize the impact of nitrogen loss from animal agriculture on the environment. The relationship between protein synthesis and degradation in individual tissues and the magnitude of the flux of amino acids between tissue beds and the plasma pool in the young growing lamb has been summarized (MacRae, 1993) and is shown in Fig. 3.2. These data provide a clear picture of the partition of amino acid metabolism between anabolic and catabolic processes in different tissues and the relationship between total protein synthesis (280 g day^{-1}) and protein accretion (39 g day^{-1}). In this respect, gut and skin represent ~50% of total protein synthesis on a daily basis but only contribute 10% towards protein accretion, whereas for muscle the values are 17.5 and 36%, respectively. The partition between these processes differentiates tissues in terms of their functions within the animal and often represents specific amino acid requirements; for example mucin production by the gut and export protein synthesis in the liver. Changes in the overall requirements of an individual tissue will inevitably have an effect on the balance of amino acid supply to others. In this respect, all tissues are 'competing' within the same amino acid pool, apart from the gut and liver both of which receive an exogenous supply of amino acids from the diet which supplements the

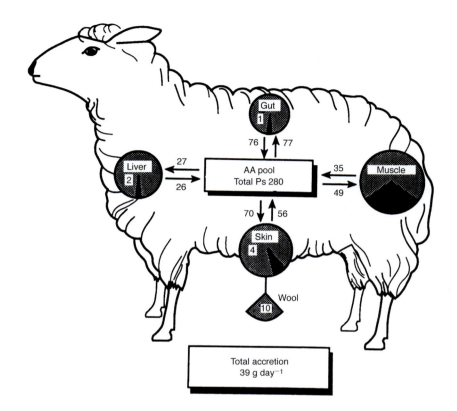

Fig. 3.2. Protein turnover rates (g day⁻¹) in different body components of young weaned lambs. Amino acid (AA) flux from the AA pool to a particular tissue represents protein synthesis, whereas flux into the AA pool represents protein degradation; Ps represents body protein synthesis. Reproduced with permission from MacRae (1993).

'endogenous' provision via arterial blood. In addition to tissue amino acid supply originating from the plasma pool, studies in muscle and mammary gland have identified the possible role of peptides in ensuring sufficient balance of amino acids for tissue synthetic requirements. This concept has been extended more recently to include plasma proteins, specifically the liver export proteins, as further 'currency' in the exchange between tissues. The relative importance of these different sources and the mechanisms involved in the control of amino acid flux to specific tissues are unknown. An understanding of these processes and the fundamental questions concerning regulation of the anabolic and catabolic fate of amino acids within tissues is essential if we are to improve our ability to formulate rations to meet the requirements of both ruminant and non-ruminant livestock.

References

Agricultural and Food Research Council (1984) *Report of the Agricultural Research Council Working Party on the Nutrient Requirements of Ruminants.* Commonwealth Agricultural Bureau, Farnham Common.

Agricultural Research Council (1980) *The Nutrient Requirements of Ruminant Livestock, Number 2 Ruminants.* Commonwealth Agricultural Bureau, Farnham Common.

Albers, S., Wernerman, J., Stehle, P., Vinnars, E. and Fürst, P. (1988) Availability of amino acids supplied by constant intravenous infusion of synthetic dipeptides in healthy man. *Clinical Science* 75, 463–468.

Ardawi, M.S.M. and Jamal, Y.S. (1990) Glutamine metabolism in skeletal muscle of glucocorticoid-treated rats. *Clinical Science* 79, 139–147.

Aoki, T.T., Brennan, M.F., Müller, W.A., Soeldner, J.S., Alpert, J.S., Saltz, S.B., Kaufmann, R.L., Tan, M.H. and Cahill, G.F. (1976) Amino acid levels across normal forearm muscle and splanchnic bed after a protein meal. *American Journal of Clinical Nutrition* 29, 340–350.

Backwell, F.R.C., Bequette, B.J., Wilson, D., Calder, A.G., Wray-Cahen, D., Metcalf, J.A., MacRae, J.C., Beever, D.E. and Lobley, G.E. (1996) Utilisation of dipeptides by the caprine mammary gland for milk protein synthesis. *American Journal of Physiology* 267, R1–R6.

Balcells, J., Seal, C.J. and Parker, D.S. (1995) Effect of intravenous glucose infusion on portal-drained visceral metabolism in sheep fed a cereal/straw-based diet. *Journal of Animal Science* 73, 2416–2155.

Baldwin, R.L., France, J. and Gill, M. (1987) Metabolism of the lactating cow. I. Animal elements of a mechanistic model. *Journal of Dairy Research* 54, 77–105.

Baracos, V.E., Brun-Bellut, J. and Marie, M. (1991) Tissue protein synthesis in lactating and dry goats. *British Journal of Nutrition* 66, 451–465.

Bequette, B.J. and Backwell, F.R.C. (1997) Amino acid supply and metabolism by the ruminant mammary gland. *Proceedings of the Nutrition Society* 56, 593–605.

Bequette, B.J., Metcalf, J.A., Wray-Cahen, D., Backwell, F.R.C., Sutton, J.D., Lomax, M.A., MacRae, J.C. and Lobley, G.E. (1996) Leucine and protein metabolism in the lactating cow mammary gland: responses to supplemental dietary crude protein intake. *Journal of Dairy Research* 63, 209–222.

Bequette, B.J., Backwell, F.R.C., Calder, A.G., Metcalf, J.A., Beever, D.E., MacRae, J.C. and Lobley, G.E. (1997) Application of a U-carbon-13-labelled tracer in lactating dairy goats for simultaneous measurements of the flux of amino acids in plasma and the partitioning of amino acids to the mammary gland. *Journal of Dairy Science* 80, 2842–2853.

Champredon, C., Debras, E., Mirand, P.P. and Arnal, M. (1990) Methionine flux and tissue protein synthesis in lactating dry goats. *Journal of Nutrition* 120, 1006–1015.

Clark, J.H. (1975) Lactational responses to postruminal administration of protein and amino acids. *Journal of Dairy Science* 58, 1178–1197.

Clark, J.H., Spires, H.R. and Davis, C.L. (1978) Uptake and metabolism of nitrogenous components by the lactating mammary gland. *Federation Proceedings* 37, 1233–1238.

Connell, A., Calder, A.G., Anderson, S.E. and Lobley, G.E. (1997) Hepatic protein synthesis in the sheep: effect of intake as monitored by stable-isotope-labelled glycine, leucine and phenylalanine. *British Journal of Nutrition* 77, 255–271.

Cooper, A.J.L., Nieves, E., Coleman, A.E., Filic-DeRicco, S. and Gelbard, A.S. (1991) Short-term metabolic fate of [^{13}N]ammonia in rat liver *in vivo*. *Journal of Biological Chemistry* 262, 1073–1080.

Danilson, D.A., Webb, K.E., Jr and Herbein, J.H. (1987) Transport and hindlimb exchange of peptide and serum protein amino acids in calves fed soy- or urea-based purified diets. *Journal of Animal Science* 64, 1852–1857.

Dawson, R. and Holdsworth, E.S. (1962) An investigation into protein digestion with ^{14}C-labelled protein. 1. The general pattern of ^{14}C incorporation into body tissues and fluids in the rat up to 3 h after feeding. *British Journal of Nutrition* 16, 13–26.

Druml, W., Lochs, H., Roth, E., Hübl, W., Balcke, P. and Lenz, K. (1991) Utilisation of tyrosine dipeptides and acetyltyrosine in normal and uremic humans. *American Journal of Physiology* 260, E280–E285.

Druml, W., Lochs, H. and Roth, E. (1997) Clearance of circulating dipeptides in humans. In: Grimble, G. and Backwell, F.R.C. (eds) *Peptides in Mammalian Protein Metabolism: Tissue Utilisation and Clinical Targeting*. Portland Press, London, pp. 55–68.

Duée, P.-H., Darcy-Vrillon, B., Blachier, F. and Morel, M.-T. (1995) Fuel selection of intestinal cells. *Proceedings of the Nutrition Society* 54, 83–94.

Elwyn, D.H. (1966) Distribution of amino acids between plasma and red cells in the dog. *Federation Proceedings* 25, 854–861.

Elwyn, D.H., Launder, W.J., Parikh, H.C. and Wise, E.M., Jr (1972) Roles of plasma and erythrocytes in inter-organ transport of amino acids in dogs. *American Journal of Physiology* 222, 1333–1342.

Felig, P., Wahren, J. and Räff, L. (1973) Evidence of inter-organ amino acid transport by blood cells in humans. *Proceedings of the National Academy of Sciences of the United States of America* 70, 1775–1779.

Gate, J.J., Parker, D.S. and Lobley, G.E. (1997) The incorporation of [5-^{15}N]glutamine into protein and nucleic acids in intestinal and other tissues in lambs. *Proceedings of the Nutrition Society* 56, 171A.

Gill, M., France, J., Summers, M., McBride, B.W. and Milligan, L.P. (1989) Mathematical integration of protein metabolism in growing lambs. *Journal of Nutrition* 119, 1269–1286.

Guerino, F., Huntington, G.B. and Erdman, R.A. (1991) The net portal and hepatic flux of metabolites and oxygen consumption in growing beef steers given postruminal casein. *Journal of Animal Science* 69, 387–395.

Hanigan, M.D., Dijkstra, J., Gerrits, W.J.J. and France, J. (1997) Modelling post-absorptive protein and amino acid metabolism in the ruminant. *Proceedings of the Nutrition Society* 56, 631–643.

Hanigan, M.D., France, J., Wray-Cahen, D., Beever, D.E., Lobley, G.E., Reutzel, L. and Smith, N.E. (1998) Alternative models for analyses of liver and mammary transorgan metabolite extraction data. *British Journal of Nutrition* 79, 63–78.

Harmon, D.L., Avery, T.B., Huntington, G.B. and Reynolds, P.J. (1988) Influence of ionophore addition to roughage and high-concentrate diets on portal blood flow and net nutrient flux in cattle. *Canadian Journal of Animal Science* 68, 419–429.

Harris, P.M., Skene, P.A., Buchan, V., Milne, E., Calder, A.G., Anderson, S.E., Connell, A. and Lobley, G.E. (1992) Effect of food intake on hind-limb and whole-body protein metabolism in young growing sheep: chronic studies based on arterio-venous techniques. *British Journal of Nutrition* 68, 389–407.

Heitmann, R.N. and Bergman, E.N. (1980) Transport of amino acids in whole blood and plasma of sheep. *American Journal of Physiology* 239, E242–E247.

Hoover, W.H. and Stokes, S.R. (1991) Balancing carbohydrates and proteins for optimal rumen microbial yield. *Journal of Dairy Science* 74, 3630–3644.

Houlier, M.L., Patureau-Mirand, P., Durand, D., Bauchart, D., Lefaivre, J. and Bayle, A. (1991) Transport of amino acids in blood and plasma across the splanchnic region of pre-ruminant calves. *Reproduction, Nutrition and Development* 31, 399–410.

Koeln, L.L., Schlagheck, T.G. and Webb, K.E., Jr (1993) Amino acid flux across the gastrointestinal tract and liver of calves. *Journal of Dairy Science* 76, 2275–2285.

Lobley, G.E. (1991) Some interactions between protein and 'energy' in ruminant metabolism. In: Eggum, B.O., Boisen, S., Børsting, C., Danfær, A. and Hvelplund, T. (eds) *Proceedings of the 6th International Symposium on Protein Metabolism and Nutrition.* National Institute of Animal Science, Foulum, pp. 66–79.

Lobley, G.E. and Milano, G.D. (1997) Regulation of hepatic nitrogen metabolism in ruminants. *Proceedings of the Nutrition Society* 56, 547–563.

Lobley, G.E., Milne, V., Lovie, J.M., Reeds, P.J. and Pennie, K. (1980) Whole body and tissue protein synthesis in cattle. *British Journal of Nutrition* 43, 491–502.

Lobley, G.E., Connell, A., Lomax, M.A., Brown, D.S., Milne, E., Calder, A.G. and Farningham, D.A.H. (1995) Hepatic detoxification of ammonia in the ovine liver, possible consequences of amino acid catabolism. *British Journal of Nutrition* 73, 667–685.

Lobley, G.E., Connell, A., Revell, D.K., Bequette, B.J., Brown, D.S. and Calder, A.G. (1996) Splanchnic-bed transfers of amino acids in sheep blood and plasma, as monitored through the use of a multiple U-^{13}C-labelled amino acid mixture. *British Journal of Nutrition* 75, 217–235.

Luo, Q.J., Maltby, S.A., Lobley, G.E., Calder, A.G. and Lomax, M.A. (1995) The effect of amino acids on the metabolic fate of ^{15}NH$_4$Cl in isolated sheep hepatocytes. *European Journal of Biochemistry* 228, 912–917.

MacRae, J.C. (1993) Metabolic consequences of intestinal parasitism. *Proceedings of the Nutrition Society* 52, 121–130.

MacRae, J.C. and Reeds, P.J. (1980) Prediction of protein deposition in ruminants. In: Buttery, P.J. and Lindsay, D.B. (eds) *Protein Deposition in Animals.* Butterworths, London, pp. 225–249.

MacRae, J.C., Bruce, L.A., Brown, D.S. and Calder, A.G. (1996) Amino acid use by the gastrointestinal tract of sheep given lucerne forage. *American Journal of Physiology* 273, G1158–G1165.

Maltby, S.A., Lomax, M.A., Beever, D.E. and Pippard, C.J. (1991) The effect of increased ammonia and amino acid supply on post-prandial portal-drained viscera and hepatic metabolism in growing steers fed maize silage. In: Wenk, C. and Boessinger, M. (eds) *Proceedings of the 12th Symposium on Energy Metabolism in Farm Animals. EAAP Publication No 58*. ETH-Zentrum, Zürich, Switzerland, pp. 20–23.

McCormick, M.E. and Webb, K.E., Jr (1982) Plasma free, erythrocyte free and plasma peptide amino acid exchange of calves in steady state and fasting metabolism. *Journal of Nutrition* 112, 276–282.

McCormick, M.E. and Webb, K.E., Jr (1987) Serum proteins as carriers of amino acids to and from the hindlimbs of fed and fasted calves. *Journal of Animal Science* 64, 586–593.

Meijer, A.J., Lamers, W.H. and Chamuleau, R.A.F.M. (1990) Nitrogen metabolism and ornithine cycle function. *Physiological Reviews* 70, 701–748.

Mepham, T.B. and Linzell, J.L. (1974) Hour to hour variations in amino acid arterio-venous difference across the lactating goat mammary gland. *Journal of Dairy Research* 41, 95–100.

Mesgaran, M.D. (1996) Ruminal accumulation and fate of low molecular weight peptides in sheep. PhD Thesis, The University of Newcastle, Newcastle upon Tyne, UK.

Metcalf, J.A., Sutton, J.D., Cockburn, J.E., Napper, D.J. and Beever, D.E. (1991) The influence of insulin and amino acid supply on amino acid uptake by the lactating mammary gland. *Journal of Dairy Science* 74, 3412–3420.

Mutsvangwa, T., Buchanan-Smith, J.G. and McBride, B.W. (1996) Interactions between ruminal degradable nitrogen intake and *in vitro* addition of substrates on patterns of amino acid metabolism in isolated ovine hepatocytes. *Journal of Nutrition* 126, 209–218.

Neutze, S.A., Oddy, V.H., Gooden, J.M., Forbes, W.A. and Warren, H.M. (1990) Portal uptake of amino acids by sheep given oaten chaff supplemented with rumen escape protein. *Proceedings of the Nutrition Society of Australia* 15, 145.

Neutze, S.A., Gooden, J.M. and Oddy, V.H. (1996) Uptake of labelled phenylalanine into different blood fractions in the portal vein and cranial mesenteric vein of lambs. *Journal of Agricultural Science, Cambridge* 126, 511–518.

O'Connor, J.D., Sniffen, C.J., Fox, D.G. and Chalupa, W. (1993) A net carbohydrate and protein system for evaluating cattle diets. IV. Predicting amino acid adequacy. *Journal of Animal Science* 71, 1298–1311.

Parker, D.S., Lomax, M.A., Seal, C.J. and Wilton, J.C. (1995) Metabolic implications of ammonia production in the ruminant. *Proceedings of the Nutrition Society* 54, 549–563.

Pell, J.M., Caldarone, E.M. and Bergman, E.N. (1986) Leucine and α-ketoisocaproate metabolism and interconversions in fed and fasted sheep. *Metabolism* 35, 1005–1016.

Piccioli Cappelli, F., Seal, C.J. and Parker, D.S. (1997) Glucose and [^{13}C]leucine metabolism by the portal-drained viscera of sheep fed on dried grass with acute intravenous and intraduodenal infusions of glucose. *British Journal of Nutrition* 78, 931–946.

Prior, R.L., Huntington, G.B. and Britton, R.A. (1981) Influence of diet on amino acid absorption in beef cattle and sheep. *Journal of Nutrition* 111, 2212–2222.

Rérat, A., Jung, J. and Kandé, J. (1988) Absorption kinetics of dietary hydrolysis products in conscious pigs given diets with different amounts of fish protein. 2. Individual amino acids. *British Journal of Nutrition* 60, 105–120.

Reynolds, C.K. (1992) Metabolism of nitrogenous compounds by ruminant liver. *Journal of Nutrition* 122, 850–854.

Reynolds, C.K., Huntington, G.B., Tyrell, H.F. and Reynolds, P.J. (1988) Net portal-drained visceral and hepatic metabolism of glucose, L-lactate, and nitrogenous compounds in lactating Holstein cows. *Journal of Dairy Science* 71, 1803–1812.

Reynolds, C.K., Tyrell, H.F. and Reynolds, P.J. (1991) The effect of diet forage-to-concentrate ratio and intake on energy metabolism in growing beef heifers: net nutrient metabolism by gut tissues. *Journal of Nutrition* 121, 1004–1015.

Reynolds, C.K., Harmon, D.L. and Cecava, M.J. (1994) Absorption and delivery of nutrients for milk protein synthesis by portal-drained viscera. *Journal of Dairy Science* 77, 2787–2808.

Seal, C.J. and Parker, D.S. (1996) Effect of intraruminal propionic acid infusion on metabolism of mesenteric- and portal-drained viscera in growing steers fed a forage diet. 2. Urea, ammonia, amino acids and peptides. *Journal of Animal Science* 74, 245–255.

Seal, C.J. and Parker, D.S. (1997) Methodological approaches for the quantification of peptide appearance across the gastrointestinal tract. In: Grimble, G. and Backwell, F.R.C. (eds) *Peptides in Mammalian Protein Metabolism: Tissue Utilisation and Clinical Targeting.* Portland Press, London, pp. 43–54.

Seal, C.J. and Reynolds, C.K. (1993) Nutritional implications of gastrointestinal and liver metabolism in ruminants. *Nutrition Research Reviews* 6, 185–208.

Seal, C.J., Parker, D.S. and Avery, P.J. (1992) The effect of forage and forage–concentrate diets on rumen fermentation and metabolism of nutrients by the mesenteric and portal drained viscera in growing steers. *British Journal of Nutrition* 67, 355–370.

Seal, C.J., Parker, D.S., MacRae, J.C. and Lobley, G.E. (1994) Effect of intraduodenal starch infusion on net portal absorption of amino acids in growing steers fed lucerne. *Animal Production* 58, 434A.

Sève, B. and Ponter, A.A. (1997) Nutrient-hormone signals relating to muscle protein turnover in pigs. *Proceedings of the Nutrition Society* 56, 565–580.

Stehle, P., Hertzog, B., Pogan, K. and Fürst, P. (1997) Intravenous dipeptide metabolism and the design of synthetic dipeptides for clinical nutrition. In: Grimble, G. and Backwell, F.R.C. (eds) *Peptides in Mammalian Protein Metabolism: Tissue Utilisation and Clinical Targeting.* Portland Press, London, pp. 103–118.

Stoll, B., Burrin, D.G., Jahoor, F., Henry, J., Yu, H. and Reeds, P.J. (1998) Dietary protein is the major source of energy for the portal-drained viscera of fed piglets. In: McCracken, K.J., Unsworth, E.F. and Wylie, A.R.G. (eds) *Energy Metabolism of Farm Animals. Proceedings of the 14th International Symposium on Energy Metabolism, Newcastle, County Down.* CAB International, Wallingford, pp. 23–26.

Tagari, H. and Bergman, E.N. (1978) Intestinal disappearance and portal blood appearance of amino acids in sheep. *Journal of Nutrition* 108, 790–803.

Taniguchi, K., Huntington, G.B. and Glenn, B.P. (1995) Net nutrient flux by visceral tissues of beef steers given abomasal and ruminal infusions of casein and starch. *Journal of Animal Science* 73, 236–249.

Trottier, N.L. (1997) Nutritional control of amino supply to the mammary gland during lactation in the pig. *Proceedings of the Nutrition Society* 56, 581–591.

van der Meulen, J. and Jansman, A.J.M. (1997) Nitrogen metabolism in gastrointestinal tissue of the pig. *Proceedings of the Nutrition Society* 56, 535–545.

van der Meulen, J., Lenis, N.P., Bakker, J.G.M., van Diepen, J.Th.M. and de Visser, H. (1996) Portal, hepatic, and splanchnic fluxes of amino acids, ammonia and urea in pigs after feeding a high and low protein diet. *Journal of Animal Science* 74 (Suppl. 1), 197A.

van der Meulen, J., Bakker, J.G.M., Smits, B. and de Visser, H. (1997) Effect of source of starch on net portal flux of glucose, lactate, volatile fatty acids and amino acids in the pig. *British Journal of Nutrition* 78, 533–544.

Vanhatalo, A., Huhtanen, P., Toivonen, V. and Varvikko, T. (1999) Response of dairy cows fed grass silage diets to abomasal infusions of histidine alone or in combinations with methionine and lysine. *Journal of Dairy Science* 82, 2674–2685.

Varvikko, T., Vanhatalo, A., Jalava, T. and Huhtanen, P. (1999) Lactation and metabolic responses to graded abomasal doses of methionine and lysine in cows fed grass silage diets. *Journal of Dairy Science* 82, 2659–2673.

Walker, D. and Hirst, B.H. (1997) Intestinal peptide transport and its regulation. *Nutrition Abstracts and Reviews (Series A)* 67, 802–808.

Windmueller, H.G. and Spaeth, A.E. (1980) Respiratory fuels and nitrogen metabolism *in vivo* in small intestine of fed rats. *Journal of Biological Chemistry* 255, 107–112.

Wolff, J.E., Bergman, E.N. and Williams, H.H. (1972) Net metabolism of plasma amino acids by liver and portal-drained viscera of fed sheep. *American Journal of Physiology* 223, 438–446.

Wray-Cahen, D., Metcalf, J.A., Backwell, F.R.C., Bequette, B., Brown, D.S., Sutton, J.D. and Lobley, G.E. (1997) Hepatic response to increased exogenous supply of plasma amino acids by infusion into the mesenteric vein of Holstein–Friesian cows in late gestation. *British Journal of Nutrition* 78, 913–930.

Wu, G., Borbolla, A.G. and Knabe, D.A. (1994) The uptake of glutamine and release of arginine, citrulline and proline by the small intestine of developing pigs. *Journal of Nutrition* 124, 2437–2444.

Young, J.D. and Ellory, J.C. (1977) Red cell amino acid transport. In: Ellory, J.C. and Lew, V.L. (eds) *Membrane Transport in Red Cells.* Academic Press, London, pp. 301–325.

Chapter 4

Phenethanolamine Repartitioning Agents

D.E. Moody, D.L. Hancock and D.B. Anderson
*Research and Development, Elanco Animal Health,
Greenfield, Indiana, USA*

Introduction

Phenethanolamine leanness-enhancing repartitioning agents have been studied in livestock species for nearly two decades. Work leading to the discovery of new compounds with repartitioning effects began at several pharmaceutical laboratories in the late 1970s. Patents were issued and initial reports were made in the mid-1980s (e.g. Asato *et al.*, 1984; Anderson *et al.*, 1987a; Convey *et al.*, 1987; Veenhuizen *et al.*, 1987). Since the mid-1980s, data have been generated to define the physiological effects and the parameters needed to optimize the response. One of these compounds manufactured by Hoechst Roussel Vet, zilpaterol, has been cleared for use and is being sold in South Africa and Mexico. Ractopamine, an Elanco Animal Health products, is cleared for use in swine in the US.

Several reviews of phenethanolamine repartitioning agent use in livestock have been published. Anderson *et al.* (1991) provide an extensive review with >360 citations, Moloney *et al.* (1991) provide a particularly complete summarization of the efficacy of various compounds, and Mersmann (1998) provides an updated review of mechanism of action. The objectives of this chapter are: (i) to summarize the effects of phenethanolamines on growth and carcass traits, including a review of factors that influence those effects; (ii) to describe the mode of action of phenethanolamines in livestock and explore topics currently under investigation that could contribute to a better understanding of their efficacy; (iii) to present safety information surrounding the use of phenethanolamines; and (iv) to discuss potential implications of the use of phenethanolamines in the livestock industry.

Effects of Phenethanolamines in Livestock

Compounds

The phenethanolamines are a general class of compounds that have been used successfully in human medicine for many years (Hoffman and Lefkowitz, 1996). More recently, the potential use of these compounds in improving the efficiency of livestock production has been evaluated (see reviews by Anderson *et al.*, 1991; Moloney *et al.*, 1991; Mersmann, 1998). The compounds most commonly studied include cimaterol, clenbuterol, L-644,969, ractopamine, salbutamol and zilpaterol (Fig. 4.1).

Summary of effects

Phenethanolamines are often referred to as repartitioning agents because of their ability to redirect nutrients away from adipose tissue and toward muscle (Ricks *et al.*, 1984). In general, the effects of phenethanolamines are: (i) increased rate of weight gain; (ii) improved feed utilization efficiency; (iii) increased leanness; and (iv) increased dressing percentage. Using ractopamine in swine as an example, a summary of the effects of phenethano-

lamines is presented in Fig. 4.2. Phenethanolamine efficacy has been demonstrated for lambs, broilers, turkeys, beef cattle and swine, although not all phenethanolamines are equally effective in all species (see Anderson *et al.*, 1991). Although comparisons across studies are difficult to make due to differences in compounds studied, dosage, duration and response parameters measured, a summarization of the available data on all phenethenolamines shows that cattle and sheep give substantially larger responses to phenethanolamines than swine, with the smallest response in chickens. Turkeys appear to be intermediate, although this represents data from only ractopamine (Wellenreiter, 1991; Mersmann, 1998; Fig. 4.3). The lower response in chickens may be due to intensive selection for growth rate in chickens, thus less potential for improvement; or perhaps due to species differences

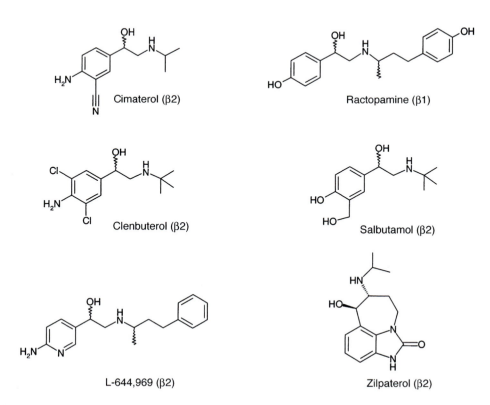

Fig. 4.1. Structure of several phenethanolamines evaluated as leanness enhancers in livestock. Current classifications of receptor subtype selectivity (β1- or β2-adrenergic receptor) are indicated.

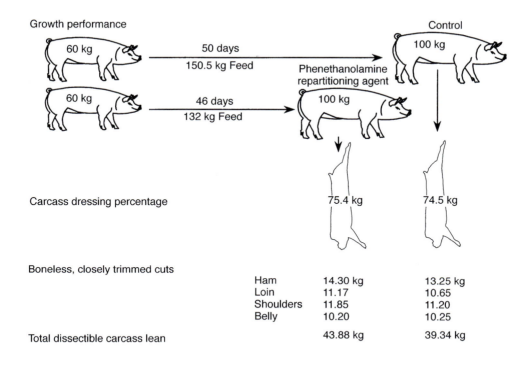

Fig. 4.2. Summary of the performance and carcass effects of ractopamine in swine. On average, pigs fed ractopamine from a body weight of 60 kg will reach 100 kg 4 days earlier and require 18.5 kg less feed compared with pigs without ractopamine treatment. The carcass of the 100 kg, ractopamine-fed pig will also have an improved dressing percentage (+0.9 kg hot carcass weight) and more dissectible carcass lean (+4.5 kg; adapted from Watkins *et al.*, 1990).

in β-adrenergic receptor selectivity and signalling pathways (Mersmann, 1998). In addition, stage of growth of the chicken at dosing relative to mammals may contribute to these species' differences in response.

There is also a substantial difference in response between phenethanolamines. The basis for the differences may lie in the specificity of a particular compound for adrenergic receptors (β1 versus β2 selectivity). For example, the β2-selective phenethanolamines clenbuterol, cimaterol and L-644,969 are particularly effective in sheep and cattle, but less effective in swine. The β1-selective phenethanolamine ractopamine is less effective in ruminants, particularly sheep (unpublished data not shown), but administration to swine has given consistent increases in both growth performance and carcass leanness as shown in Fig. 4.2.

Factors that influence response to phenethanolamines

Several factors including diet, dosage and duration of treatment, age, weight and genetics have been shown to influence the response to phenethanolamines (Table 4.1). It will be important to understand interactions of these factors with phenethanolamines if the use of phenethanolamines in the livestock industry is to be implemented successfully.

Diet
The interaction between dietary protein content and repartitioning agent treatment was first reported by Anderson *et al.* (1987b). In general, livestock fed phethanolamines require increased dietary protein to accommodate increased rates of lean deposition. In swine, dietary protein

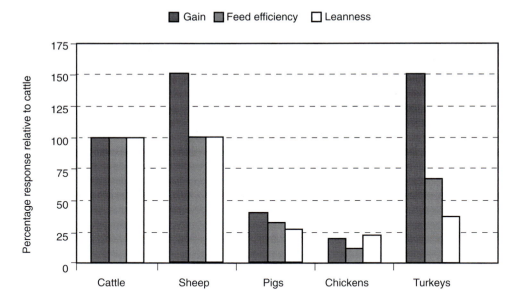

Fig. 4.3. Species differences in gain, feed efficiency and leanness with phenethanolamine administration. Values are relative differences compared with cattle. (Adapted from Mersmann, 1998; Wellenreiter, 1991.)

levels ≥167 g kg^{-1} were required to achieve a significant response to ractopamine (Dunshea *et al.*, 1993). Similarly, Mitchell *et al.* (1994) reported greater improvements in gain and carcass leanness in pigs that consumed an 180 relative to a 120 g kg^{-1} crude protein diet in combination with the phenethanolamine BRL47672, and Jones *et al.* (1988) concluded that rations containing 160–200 g kg^{-1} crude protein or lysine equivalent were needed in swine to optimize the growth performance response to ractopamine. However, in contrast to the protein levels needed for maximum gain, increased carcass leanness in ractopamine-fed pigs may be achieved at lower crude protein levels (Ji *et al.*, 1991; Jones *et al.*, 1992). In broilers, a linear response to dietary protein levels (220, 240 and 260 g of protein kg^{-1}) was observed in combination with clenbuterol treatment (Hamano *et al.*, 1998). These authors concluded that increased protein consumption is important to achieve maximal gains in body weight gain and protein to DNA ratio in clenbuterol-fed birds. Together, these studies indicate that increased dietary protein levels are essential to achieve the

maximum benefit of treatment with phenethanolamines in swine and poultry. Models can be used for estimating the specific level of dietary protein required based on anticipated rates of protein accretion (National Research Council, 1998).

Data describing the effect of protein on the response to phenethanolamines in ruminants are limited. However, Beermann *et al.* (1986) observed improved performance in cimaterol-treated sheep that were given supplemental by-pass protein. More work is needed in this area to confirm the interactions between phenethanolamines and nutrition in ruminants.

Duration of treatment
Phenethanolamines are often effective for a limited time period due in part to the desensitization or down-regulation of activated β-adrenergic receptors (see discussion in Mode of Action). The length of treatment before effects on weight gain begin to plateau varies for different compounds and species (see Table 4.2), but will probably limit the use of phenethanolamines to the final finishing phase in most cases. In ractopamine-treated swine,

Table 4.1. Factors that influence response to treatment with phenethanolamines (see text for references).

Factor	Requirement	Compounds studied	Species studied
Dietary protein	Greater response with higher dietary protein	Clenbuterol BRL47672 Ractopamine	Pigs, broilers, rats
Duration of treatment	Greater response during final finishing phase	Cimaterol Clenbuterol L-644,969 Ractopamine	Pigs, cattle, sheep
Dosage	Differential effect on growth and leanness	Ractopamine	Pigs
Age or weight	Greater response with older, heavier animals	Cimaterol Ractopamine	Pigs, cattle
Genetics	Effective in both fat and lean genetics	Cimaterol Ractopamine	Pigs, mice

average daily gain began to plateau after 3 weeks (Williams *et al.*, 1994), but benefits to carcass composition continued as ractopamine duration increased (Anderson *et al.*, 1987a; Williams *et al.*, 1994).

Dosage

There is a differential effect of dosage on the response of meat animals to phenethanolamines. As an example, when ractopamine is fed to swine, low dosages significantly improve weight gain and feed efficiency, and, to a lesser degree, carcass parameters. In contrast, higher dosages improve weight gain, feed efficiency and carcass parameters (Fig. 4.4). Weight gain is optimized at low dosages and is diminished at dosages >20 mg kg^{-1} due to reductions in feed intake. Alternately, leanness and dressing percentage continue to improve through the highest dosage tested

(30 mg kg^{-1}). These differential responses allow a selection of dose to optimize value under varying economic conditions (Fig. 4.4).

Age or weight

Typically, phenethanolamines are most efficacious when administered to older, heavier animals. Vestergaard *et al.* (1994) treated bulls with cimaterol for 90 days beginning at 162, 299 and 407 kg liveweight. The weight gain response to cimaterol increased from 10% for the 162 kg liveweight group to 25 and 22% at 299 and 407 kg, respectively, while the absolute difference in carcass gains were 18, 28 and 37 kg for the three weight groups, respectively. In pigs, cimaterol failed to effect growth or carcass traits in young growing animals (10–60 kg; Mersmann *et al.*, 1987), and ractopamine

Table 4.2. Phenethanolamines are effective for a relatively short period of time before response, measured as weight gain, reaches a plateau.

Drug	Species	Time (weeks) until response plateaus	Reference
Cimaterol	Sheep	3	O'Connor *et al.* (1991a)
L-644,969	Sheep	2	Pringle *et al.* (1993)
Clenbuterol	Cattle	5	Sillence *et al.* (1993)
Cimaterol	Cattle	10–16	Fiems *et al.* (1990)
Cimaterol	Cattle	8	Barash *et al.* (1994)
Ractopamine	Pigs	3	Williams *et al.* (1994)

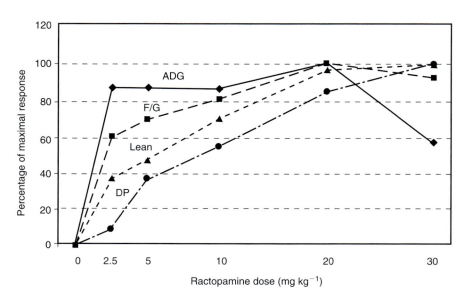

Fig. 4.4. Ractopamine dose–response relationship in swine. Beneficial effects on average daily gain (ADG) and feed efficiency (F/G) are achieved at lower dosages. However, higher doses are required to optimize the benefits on carcass leanness (Lean) and dressing percentage (DP). Data are adapted from Watkins *et al.* (1990).

had greater effects in heavier animals (Anderson *et al.*, 1988; Jones *et al.*, 1990). These results demonstrate that the greatest responses would be obtained from the use of phenethanolamines in heavier weight animals. This, along with limited duration of effectiveness, may direct the use of phenethanolamines to the final finishing phase of production systems.

Genetics

Phenethanolamines have been proven effective across a variety of genetic backgrounds. In particular, ractopamine has been shown to be equally effective in Landrace and Hampshire crossbred pigs (Mills *et al.*, 1990) and in Meishan, Meishan crossbred and US crossbred pigs (Yen *et al.*, 1991). Cimaterol also increased lean and decreased fat similarly in genetically lean and obese pigs (Yen *et al.*, 1990). A significant interaction between ractopamine and genotype was reported for lean growth rate, but not for growth performance or carcass merit, by Gu *et al.* (1991a,b). In this study, a greater response to ractopamine was observed in pigs from

leaner genotypes. Bark *et al.* (1992) also reported a significant interaction between genotype and ractopamine since ractopamine caused a greater increase in muscle accretion in pigs with a high genetic capacity for lean growth relative to a low genetic capacity. Finally, Eisen *et al.* (1988) reported a significant line × cimaterol interaction in mice. In this study, mice from lines selected for rapid 3–6 week post-weaning gain showed a greater response to cimaterol treatment than did mice from unselected control lines. Thus, it appears that phenethanolamines will be effective across divergent genetic backgrounds, but greater responses may be obtained from animals selected for superior genetic potential for lean tissue accretion.

Phenethanolamines and meat quality

The effects of phenethanolamine repartitioning agents on meat quality can be both positive and negative. For the purposes of this discussion, meat quality is defined as cooked meat palatability or those factors that are thought to influence meat palatability. These include cooked meat sensory panel tenderness, juiciness and flavour, as well as fresh meat quality factors such as colour, firmness, marbling and water-holding capacity of the muscle. When considering effects on meat quality, it must be remembered that reductions in carcass fat either through genetic selection or nutritional manipulation generally result in decreased tenderness and juiciness of the resulting edible meat (Wood and Warriss, 1992).

Tenderness

Phenethanolamines have the potential to reduce meat tenderness. These observed effects on meat quality appear to be dependent on dosage and the specific phenethanolamine under investigation, as well as the species of livestock studied (Merkel, 1988). An increase in the shear force required to cut through a standard cooked strip of muscle has been reported for phenethanolamines in poultry, cattle, sheep and pigs in response to specific phenethanolamines and experimental conditions (examples included in Table 4.3). Some effects of phenethanolamines on tenderness appear to be the result of decreased fat content, but some are clearly greater than that which would be expected for increased leanness alone. Early studies with β2-selective adrenergic receptor agonists in sheep and cattle gave significant reductions in tenderness. This reduced tenderness is thought to be related to an effect on the calpain protease system, and specifically to an increase in the level of calpastatin, an inhibitor of muscle protein degradation (Koohmaraie, 1992). It has been demonstrated that the mechanism of action of these β2-selective compounds is primarily through a reduction in the rate of muscle protein degradation *in vivo* (Reeds *et al.*, 1986; Bohorov *et al.*, 1987) and is therefore consistent with an increase in calpastatin.

A reasonable criterion for any phenethanolamine that is to be successfully developed for market is to affect

tenderness no more than expected from the direct effect of increasing leanness. The effects of ractopamine and zilpaterol on meat tenderness appear to be less severe than those of clenbuterol, cimaterol and L-644,969 in sheep and cattle. Although increases in shear force values have been reported in pigs fed ractopamine (Aalhus *et al.*, 1990; Uttaro *et al.*, 1993), other shear testing and taste panel studies detected no difference in meat tenderness due to ractopamine treatment (Merkel *et al.*, 1990; Stites *et al.*, 1994; Jeremiah *et al.*, 1994a,b). Zilpaterol also appears to have minimal effects on meat tenderness in cattle. Casey *et al.* (1997a) observed greater shear force values in steers treated with zilpaterol compared with controls, but shear force values for treated steers were not different from untreated steers with similar fat content. In another study, no significant effect of zilpaterol treatment on tenderness was observed (Casey *et al.*, 1997b). The increase in shear force values reported in animals treated with ractopamine and zilpaterol may be a reflection of differences in fatness of these animals. For example, Uttaro *et al.* (1993) found a greater difference in shear force value and leanness between gilts and barrows than between ractopamine-treated and control pigs. The minimal effect that ractopamine has on tenderness may also be related to its mechanism of action on muscle protein accretion. Ractopamine has been shown to increase muscle protein synthesis in swine, with no apparent decrease of protein degradation (Bergen *et al.*, 1989). It has also been shown that ractopamine has no effect on muscle calpastatin levels in swine (see Mode of Action, Skeletal Muscle). These apparent differences in mechanism may be related to the primary β1-adrenergic receptor selectivity of ractopamine compared with the β2-adrenergic receptor selectivity of clenbuterol, cimaterol and L-644,969. Therefore, tenderness effects of the phenethanolamines currently in use or under development (zilpaterol and ractopamine) appear to be similar to qualitative effects normally associated with leanness.

Table 4.3. References for the effects of phenethanolamines on meat quality.

Phenethanolamine	Cattle	Sheep	Pigs	Poultry
Cimaterol	Chikhou et al. (1993) Fabry et al. (1990) Fiems et al. (1990) Vestergaard et al. (1994)	Hanrahan (1988)	Jones et al. (1985) Walker et al. (1989) Yen et al. (1990)	Morgan et al. (1989) Gwartney et al. (1991)
Clenbuterol	Schiavetta et al. (1990)	Hamby et al. (1986)		
L-644,969	Wheeler and Koohmaraie (1992)	Pringle et al. (1993)		
Ractopamine	Schroeder et al. (1990)		Merkel et al. (1990) Aalhus et al. (1990) Uttaro et al. (1993) Stites et al. (1994) Jeremiah et al. (1994a,b)	
Salbutamol			Warriss et al. (1990)	
Zilpaterol	Casey et al. (1997a,b)			

Juiciness

Genetic selection for leanness results in a consistent decrease in cooked meat juiciness (Wood and Warris, 1992). A meat quality advantage of phenethanolamine repartitioning agents is that they improve leanness without reducing juiciness. This could be related to a lack of effect on marbling. Aalhus *et al.* (1990) showed reductions in both subcutaneous and intermuscular (seam) fat in swine fed ractopamine with no reduction of intramuscular fat. Merkel *et al.* (1990) and Anderson *et al.* (1988) showed a similar effect, although the phenomenon was time related. Short-term feeding of phenethanolamines results in a decrease in only subcutaneous and seam fat, while longer term treatment also affects marbling (Fig.

4.5). Therefore, longer term treatment with phenethanolamines may also result in reduced juiciness as seen with genetic selection for leanness. Short-term treatment with phenethanolamines at the end of the finishing period should allow improved leanness without affecting juiciness.

Additional meat quality traits

Merkel (1988) reported that phenethanolamine treatment has negligible effects on additional qualitative traits such as meat flavour, colour, firmness, marbling and water-holding capacity (WHC). More recent work has shown small, but consistent effects on colour (Uttaro *et al.*, 1993; Schroeder, personal communication, 1999) and WHC (Uttaro *et al.*, 1993). Ractopamine feeding results in a small, but consistent reduction

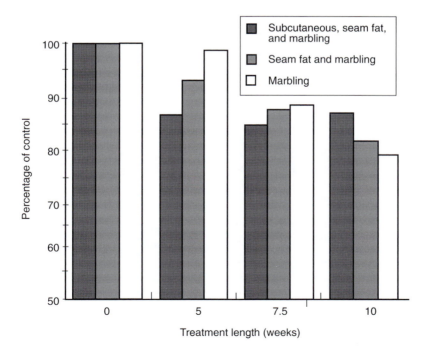

Fig. 4.5. Effect of length of ractopamine feeding on carcass fat content of finishing pigs. Ether extracts of subcutaneous + seam fat + marbling, seam fat + marbling, and marbling are shown as a percentage of the control for four treatment lengths. Marbling appears to be depleted more slowly than other fat depots. (Data adapted from Anderson *et al.*, 1988.)

in muscle colour score. Objective colour measurements of fresh loin and ham show significant reductions in 'a' value (redness) and 'b' value (yellowness) with no effect on 'L' value (lightness; Table 4.4). A reduction in the 'a' value suggests that the concentration of myoglobin may be reduced in pigs fed ractopamine. The reason is probably due to a shift in muscle fibre type in ractopamine-treated pigs, increasing the size and percentage of white fibres (Aalhus et al., 1992; Table 4.5). This shift is accompanied by an improvement in WHC (Uttaro et al., 1993; Table 4.6). This benefit was unexpected but may be related to greater functionality of muscle protein from muscle with high white fibre content (Parsons and Knight, 1990), translating to decreased cooking losses and increased processing yields (Uttaro et al., 1993; Table 4.6).

Fat composition

Variable and minor effects of ractopamine feeding on fatty acid profiles in swine have been reported (Engeseth et al., 1992; Perkins et al., 1992). A reduction in cholesterol content in muscle of pigs treated with ractopamine was reported by Perkins et al. (1992). These authors measured cholesterol content in longissimus dorsi muscles of 144 pigs representing two different trials. Two levels of ractopamine (10 or 20 mg kg^{-1}) were fed in each trial. Ractopamine treatment reduced cholesterol content in both trials, with an overall reduction of ~9%.

Table 4.4. Objective colour measurements of fresh pork loin and ham muscles (adapted from Uttaro et al., 1993).

	Ractopamine (mg kg^{-1})	
	0	20
Loin (longissimus dorsi)		
L value (lightness)	46.32	45.84
a value (redness)	7.59	6.48[a]
b value (yellowness)	3.14	2.42[b]
Ham (gluteus medius)		
L value (lightness)	44.37	43.47
a value (redness)	9.57	8.22[a]
b value (yellowness)	3.98	3.05[a]

[a]$P < 0.01$; [b]$P < 0.05$.

Table 4.5. Effect of ractopamine on myofibre distribution and diameter in swine (adapted from Aalhus et al., 1992).

	Ractopamine treatment (mg kg^{-1})	
	0	20
Number of animals	23	22
Red (%)	14.38	12.35
Intermediate (%)	12.86	10.39[a]
White (%)	72.81	77.26[b]
Red (μ^2)	2480	2564
Intermediate (μ^2)	1783	2216[b]
White (μ^2)	3467	4048[b]

[a]$P < 0.01$; [b]$P < 0.05$.

Engeseth et al. (1992) reported a similar trend, but with variable responses from limited numbers of pigs. A significant interaction affecting cholesterol content was identified between ractopamine treatment and sex by Uttaro et al. (1993). The feeding of ractopamine resulted in a 14% decrease in the cholesterol content of longissimus dorsi muscle of barrows, but did not affect cholesterol content of gilts. The difference between ractopamine-treated and control pigs without considering the sex interaction was 8.6%, which is similar to that reported by Perkins et al. (1992).

Mode of Action of Phenethanolamines

Adipose tissue

The effects of phenethanolamines on adipose tissue are facilitated by β-adrenergic

Table 4.6. Effect of ractopamine on quality characteristics of loin and ham in pigs (adapted from Uttaro et al., 1993).

	Ractopamine (mg kg^{-1})	
	0	20
Loin drip loss (%)	6.4	4.3
Loin cooking loss (%)	25.7	24.4[a]
Ham processing yield	96.4	99.5[b]
Bacon processing yield	95.5	97.1

[a]$P < 0.05$; [b]$P < 0.01$.

receptors. Activation of β-adrenergic receptors is coupled to Gs proteins and activation of adenyl cyclase, which converts adenosine triphosphate (ATP) to cyclic adenosine monophosphate (cAMP), an intracellular signalling molecule. The cAMP is thought to bind the regulatory subunit of protein kinase A to release its catalytic subunit. Regulation of intracellular enzymes is then accomplished through phosphorylation by protein kinase A (Fig. 4.6).

Activation of β-adrenergic receptors and the cAMP signalling pathway by phenethanolamines results in the activation of hormone-sensitive lipases and inactivation of lipogenic enzymes involved in *de novo* synthesis of fatty acids and triglycerides (Fain and Garcia-Sainz, 1983; Mersmann, 1987). Specific effects of phenethanolamines on adipose tissue have been studied in several species. For example, *in vivo* adiministration of ractopamine to swine enhances *in vitro* release of free fatty acids and depresses the

activity of lipogenic enzymes in adipose tissue (Merkel *et al.*, 1987). Ractopamine also depresses lipogenesis and triacylglycerol synthesis in the adipogenic cell line TA1 (Dickerson *et al.*, 1988), inhibits fat cell proliferation of stromalvascular cells obtained from rat inguinal fat pads (Jones *et al.*, 1987) and inhibits fat cell responsiveness to insulin (Williams *et al.*, 1987; Hausman *et al.*, 1989). Thus, phenethanolamines have the potential to increase the rate of lipolysis and decrease the rate of lipogenesis in adipose tissue via several mechanisms.

Skeletal muscle

The anabolic effects of phenethanolamines that result in muscle cell hypertrophy, muscle fibre type changes (Table 4.5) and increased lean mass (Beermann *et al.*, 1986; Maltin *et al.*, 1986; Kim *et al.*, 1987) are often attributed to activation of the β-adrenergic receptor pathway. However,

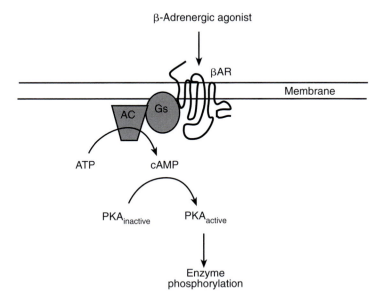

Fig. 4.6. Mechanism of signal transduction from β-adrenergic receptors (βAR). The β-adrenergic receptor is activated by an agonist and interacts with Gs proteins. The Gs proteins stimulate adenylyl cyclase (AC) to convert adenosine triphosphate (ATP) to cyclic adenosine monophosphate (cAMP) which acts as an intracellular signalling molecule. Increased levels of cAMP activate protein kinase A (PKA) to phosphorylate many enzymes and regulatory factors important in metabolic regulation (see text for references).

conclusive evidence linking activation of β-adrenergic receptors to the anabolic effects of phenethanolamines in livestock has yet to be presented. In rodents, antagonists of β-adrenergic receptors have been used in combination with agonists in efforts to block the anabolic effects of phenethanolamines. Reeds *et al.* (1988) used propranolol, a non-selective β1- and β2-antagonist, and atenolol, a β2-specific antagonist, in combination with clenbuterol in rats. The antagonists were administered orally at dosages 10–100 times greater than those of clenbuterol. The effects of clenbuterol on energy expenditure, cardiac growth and fat deposition were attenuated by the β-adrenergic receptor antagonists, but the effect of clenbuterol on muscle growth was not affected. Thus, these authors questioned whether the anabolic effects of clenbuterol were mediated by β-adrenergic receptor activation. The results of Reeds *et al.* (1988) were confirmed by MacLennan and Edwards (1989) when similar dosages of clenbuterol and propranolol were administered orally to rats. However, MacLennan and Edwards (1989) also administered propranolol by intraperitoneal injection, followed by subcutaneous injection of clenbuterol. Using this protocol, the ability of clenbuterol to induce muscle hypertrophy was blocked by propranolol, suggesting the involvement of β-adrenergic receptors. Likewise, Choo *et al.* (1992) showed that the anabolic effects of clenbuterol were inhibited by the β2-specific antagonist ICI-118,551, as well as by high dosages of propranolol administered orally. These authors also observed that when the anabolic effects of clenbuterol were inhibited by β-receptor antagonists, the lipolytic effects of clenbuterol were not affected. Thus, although the anabolic effects of clenbuterol were blocked by β-adrenergic receptor antagonists, they may not be facilitated by the same mechanisms that elicit changes in adipose tissue. It must also be recognized that these results represent the effects of specific agonists and antagonists in rats and have not been confirmed in livestock species to date.

Mechanisms responsible for the anabolic effects of phenethanolamines in livestock were investigated initially by measuring fractional protein synthesis and degradation rates *in vivo*. Individual studies reported increased, decreased and unchanged rates of protein synthesis and degradation following treatment with phenethanolamines (see Moloney *et al.*, 1991). The variability across studies is likely to be due in part to differences in the phenethanolamine used, its receptor specificity, the species studied, and the dose and duration of treatment. In general, results from these studies support the hypotheses that protein synthesis is enhanced and/or protein degradation is inhibited by treatment with the β2-agonists cimaterol, clenbuterol and L-644,969 (see Moloney *et al.*, 1991), whereas only protein synthesis is affected by the β1-agonist ractopamine (Bergen *et al.*, 1989).

Alternatives to measuring total protein synthesis or degradation are to measure total RNA produced in skeletal muscle, mRNA expression of specific genes or the activity of specific enzymes important in protein synthesis or degradation. Increased protein synthesis in response to phenethanolamines has been suggested based on increased total RNA and mRNA of α-actin in skeletal muscle of pigs treated with ractopamine (Bergen *et al.*, 1989; Helferich *et al.*, 1990) and sheep treated with L-644,969 (Koohmaraie *et al.*, 1991). Smith *et al.* (1989) reported an increase in the mRNA abundance of myosin in cattle treated with ractopamine, and Helferich *et al.* (1990) showed increased expression of additional unidentified muscle proteins by ractopamine-treated pigs based on the results of an *in vitro* translation assay.

Protein degradation rates have been predicted based on the expression and activity of proteolytic degradative enzymes. The calpains (μM and mM) are intracellular non-lysosomal calcium-dependent neutral proteases that contribute to protein degradation, and calpastatin is an endogenous inhibitor of the calpains. The calpain isoforms are named after their sensitivities to calcium required for activation. The μM calpain requires 3–50 μM calcium, and the mM calpain requires 400–800 μM calcium for one-half maximal activity (Goll *et al.*, 1998). Thus, μM calpain is the physiologically active isoform. For a review of the calpain system and skeletal muscle growth, including the effects of various phenethanolamines on the calpain system, see Goll *et al.* (1998). In general, there is good correlation between enzyme or inhibitor activity and mRNA expression (Bardsley *et al.*, 1992). An increase in calpastatin expression and activity combined with a decrease in μM calpain, suggesting a net decrease in protein degradation, has been observed in cattle treated with cimaterol (Parr *et al.*, 1992) and in sheep treated with L-644,969 (Kretchmar *et al.*, 1990; Koohmarie *et al.*, 1991; Pringle *et al.*, 1993). In contrast, Ji (1992) observed an increase in mM calpain activity in pigs treated with ractopamine, but detected no significant differences in μM calpain or calpastatin activity. Similarly, Bergen *et al.* (1989) reported increased activity of cathepsin L, but not of cathepsin B and H, nor the calcium-dependent proteases following ractopamine treatment in pigs. Consistent with the *in vivo* protein synthesis and degradation studies, this suggests that ractopamine does not affect protein degradation. One possible explanation for the conflicting results on muscle protein degradation in response to phenethanolamine treatment may relate to the differences in β-adrenergic receptor specificity of ractopamine (β1) compared with cimaterol and L-644,969 (β2). It may be postulated that activation of the β2-adrenergic receptor stimulates both an increase in protein synthesis and a decrease in protein degradation, while activation of the β1-adrenergic receptor affects only protein synthesis.

Protein synthesis and degradation in response to phenethanolamine treatment have also been evaluated *in vitro* using skeletal muscle cell cultures, but with varying results. Some authors concluded that phenethanolamines do not have a direct effect on cultured muscle cells, while others reported increased protein synthesis or increased protein synthesis combined with decreased degradation as direct responses to phenethanolamine treatment (see Mersmann, 1998). As with all *in vitro* studies, these results must be interpreted with caution as they do not represent the true muscle cell environment found *in vivo*. Bridge *et al.* (1998) suggested that some of the variation among *in vitro* studies may be attributed to differences in the densities and sub-populations of β-adrenergic receptors present in cultured muscle cells.

Endocrine effects

It has been suggested that the repartitioning effects of phenethanolamines may be due in part to opposing effects of phenethanolamines on insulin sensitivity in adipose tissue versus skeletal muscle (Anderson *et al.*, 1991). Decreased sensitivity to insulin in response to β-adrenergic agonists has been demonstrated in adipocytes from rats (Hausman *et al.*, 1989) and pigs (Liu and Mills, 1990), while increased sensitivity to insulin following prolonged treatment with β-adrenergic agonists has been observed from soleus muscle of rats (Budohoski *et al.*, 1987). However, adipocytes isolated from mice treated with clenbuterol did not differ from controls in sensitivity to insulin (Orcutt *et al.*, 1989), and insulin binding to mouse adipocytes following *in vivo* administration of ractopamine and clenbuterol was not significantly affected (Dubrovin *et al.*, 1990). Studies using the hyperinsulinaemic, euglycaemic clamp technique in cattle identified only a transient decrease in insulin sensitivity following clenbuterol administration (Sternbauer *et al.*, 1998), and no change in insulin sensitivity or responsiveness following ractopamine administration (Eisemann and Bristol, 1998). Therefore, the significance of changes in insulin sensitivity or responsiveness identified *in vitro* to the overall *in vivo* effects of phenethanolamines is unclear.

The effects of phenethanolamines on circulating hormones known to influence growth and metabolism have been measured in efforts to identify indirect mechanisms by which phenethanolamines may influence growth and body composition. In sheep administered cimaterol, increased growth hormone and T4, and decreased insulin-like growth factor 1 (IGF-1) concentrations were observed after 6 weeks of treatment (Beermann et al., 1987). In contrast, O'Connor et al. (1991b) observed no change in IGF-1 and decreased T4 concentrations after 3 weeks of cimaterol treatment in sheep. Young et al. (1995) also reported no significant change in IGF-1 concentration following chronic administration of clenbuterol in sheep. In cattle treated with cimaterol, Chikhou et al. (1991) reported an acute decrease in mean growth hormone concentration, followed by a chronic increase in growth hormone and decrease in IGF-1 concentrations. Also in steers treated with cimaterol, Dawson et al. (1993) identified no significant differences in mean concentrations of growth hormone or IGF-1. These authors also observed an absence of regular growth hormone secretion cycles in cattle treated with cimaterol, suggesting that cimaterol treatment may have disrupted the rhythm of growth hormone secretion. In broilers treated with clenbuterol, Buyse et al. (1991) reported no consistent effects on plasma thyroid hormone, growth hormone, IGF-1 or corticosterone concentrations.

In general, the effects of phenethanolamines on hormone concentrations have been insignificant or inconsistent across studies, indicating that these hormones are probably not important to the mechanism of action of phenethanolamines. Further evidence that the effects of phenethanolamines are not mediated through the growth hormone axis is provided by investigations of the effects of phenethanolamines and growth hormone administered in combination. Additive effects of growth hormone with clenbuterol in cattle (Maltin et al., 1990), salbutamol in pigs (Hansen et al., 1997) and ractopamine in pigs (Jones et al., 1989) were identified, suggesting that the growth-promoting effects of these compounds are mediated

by different mechanistic pathways. Additionally, it has been shown recently using direct hind-limb arterial infusion of steers that increased muscle protein accretion in response to cimaterol treatment is due to direct actions on the muscle, rather than indirect effects such as cardiovascular activity, endocrine status or splanchnic tissue metabolism (Byrem et al., 1998).

Blood flow

Increased blood flow has been demonstrated in cattle (Eisemann and Huntington, 1993; Byrem et al., 1998), sheep (Aurousseau et al., 1993) and pigs (Mersmann, 1989) in response to clenbuterol or cimaterol treatment. This response may enhance the effects of phenethanolamine treatment on skeletal muscle and adipose tissue by delivering increased amounts of substrate and energy source to skeletal muscle for protein synthesis, and by carrying non-esterified fatty acids away from adipose tissue to enhance lipid degradation (see Mersmann, 1998).

The β-adrenergic family of receptors

Although the effects of phenethanolamines on skeletal muscle have not yet been linked directly to activation of β-adrenergic receptors, the possibility that these receptors facilitate at least a portion of the anabolic effects of phenethanolamines cannot be eliminated. This, combined with the importance of β-adrenergic receptors in the regulation of lipid metabolism, make an understanding of the β-adrenergic family of receptors critical to discerning the mechanism of action of phenethanolamines in livestock.

Endogenous agonists of the β-adrenergic receptors include norepinephrine, a neurotransmitter produced by the sympathetic nervous system, and epinephrine, a circulating hormone produced by the adrenal medulla. The β-adrenergic receptors are members of the membrane-bound, G-protein-coupled receptor family that has a characteristic seven transmembrane domain structure (Fig. 4.7). To date, the presence of three unique receptors has been confirmed with the cloning of the β1-, β2- and β3-adrenergic receptor genes in several species (Table 4.7). Homology among the receptor subtypes is relatively low (30–50%), with conserved amino acids primarily restricted to the seven transmembrane domain segments and membrane-proximal regions of the intracellular loops (Fig. 4.7). Despite these differences among receptor subtypes, amino acid sequences of individual subtypes are highly conserved across species. For example, the β3-adrenergic receptor is 80–90% conserved across human, mouse, rat, canine and bovine amino acid sequences (see Table 4.7 for references).

The transmembrane domains of the β-adrenergic receptors have been implicated in receptor subtype-specific ligand binding. A series of β1–β2-adrenergic receptor chimeras was produced by Marullo *et al.* (1995) to study the role of the transmembrane domains in ligand binding. These authors concluded that receptor specificity is determined by unique interactions among agonists and several transmembrane domains. More recently, individual transmembrane domains of the β1- and β2-adrenergic receptors were exchanged to evaluate the role of each domain individually (Kikkawa *et al.*, 1998; Kurose *et al.*, 1998). Transmembrane domains 2 and 7 were implicated in affinity for the β2-adrenergic receptor, while transmembrane domain 2 was critical for β1-adrenergic receptor affinity.

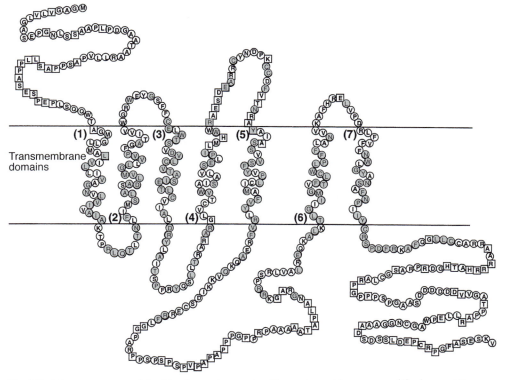

Fig. 4.7. Primary structure of the β1-adrenergic receptor. The amino acid sequence of the human β1-adrenergic receptor is represented by the one-letter code for amino acids. The polypeptide chain is arranged according to the model for rhodopsin. Shaded amino acids are conserved across the human β1-, β2- and β3-adrenergic receptors (31% of residues). Amino acids in circles are conserved across the β1-adrenergic receptor of humans, pigs and sheep (80% of residues; see Table 4.7 for references). Transmembrane domains are labelled in parentheses.

Table 4.7. The β1-, β2- and β3-adrenergic receptors have been cloned and sequenced in several species.

Species	Accession Number[a]		
	β1	β2	β3
Human	J03019	J02960	X72861
Monkey	X75540	L38905	U63592
Mouse	L10084	X15643	X72862
Rat	J05561	X17607	S73473
Cattle	AF188187	Z86037	X85961
Pigs	AF042454	AF000134	U55858 (fragment)
Sheep	AF072433	—	—
Dog	Huang et al. (1997)	Huang et al. (1997)	U92468
Turkey	[b]M14379	[c]U13977	—

[a]Accession numbers refer to the GenBank nucleotide database (www.ncbi.nlm.nih.gov).
[b]The sequence is named the avian β-adrenergic receptor and is not necessarily the β1-subtype homologue.
[c]The sequence is named the β4c-adrenergic receptor and is not necessarily the β2-homologue.

At least four of the seven transmembrane domains have been shown to be essential for binding to the β3-adrenergic receptor using computer modelling, site-directed mutagenesis and photoaffinity labelling (Strosberg, 1997). The second and third intracellular loops of the β2-adrenergic receptor are involved in signal transduction, and similar regions of the third intracellular loop are probably also involved in interactions that mediate signal transduction for the β3-adrenergic receptor (see Strosberg, 1997).

β1- and β2-adrenergic receptors

Phenethanolamines developed for use in livestock target the β1- and β2-adrenergic receptors. Agonists of these receptors have been used in humans for cardiac inotropic support, the treatment of asthma, and as uterine relaxants (Hoffman and Lefkowitz, 1996). Antagonists of the β-adrenergic receptors, or β-blockers, are used as treatment for high blood pressure, migraine, cardiac arrhythmias and myocardial infarction (Hoffman and Lefkowitz, 1996). In livestock, agonists of both the β1- and β2-receptors appear to act as repartitioning agents that shift energy away from adipose tissue and toward skeletal muscle.

The β1- and β2-adrenergic receptors are expressed in a variety of tissues. The rat heart and guinea pig trachea have been considered prototypical tissues for studying ligand binding to the β1- and β2-receptors, respectively. Most tissues contain a mixture of the β-adrenergic receptor subtypes with varying densities of each (Minneman et al., 1979). Expression of β-adrenergic receptors has been demonstrated in adipose and skeletal muscle tissues of livestock species, but the relative abundance of different β-adrenergic receptor subtypes has not been clearly defined (see Mersmann, 1998).

Classification of β-adrenergic receptor agonists

Classification of subtype selectivity of β-adrenergic receptor agonists is based on the ability of agonists and antagonists to stimulate or inhibit a particular physiological–pharmacological response, or to bind to the receptor (Mersmann, 1995). β-Adrenergic receptor ligands may be classified by their binding to human and rodent β-adrenergic receptors using stably transfected Chinese hamster ovary (CHO) cells that express a high copy number of one β-adrenergic receptor subtype. These cells may be used to investigate ligand binding as well as ligand activity (agonist or antagonist) by measuring cAMP accumulation. To date, the bovine β3-

adrenergic receptor (Pietri-Rouxel *et al.*, 1995) and porcine β1- and β2-adrenergic receptors (Mills, personal communication) have been expressed in CHO cells. However, the current classification of ligands tested in livestock is based on data obtained from rodent or human receptors.

Response to specific β-adrenergic receptor ligands varies across species, presenting a significant limitation to the extrapolation of data from one species to another (Pietri-Rouxel *et al.*, 1995). For example, bupranolol acts as an antagonist in both humans and rodents, but as a partial agonist at bovine β3-receptors, while propranolol is an antagonist at the rodent β3-receptor but a partial agonist at the human and bovine homologues of this receptor (see Strosberg, 1997). These findings demonstrate the need to characterize β-adrenergic receptor ligand activity in the species of interest.

The receptor subtype selectivity of phenethanolamines used in livestock has been evaluated only with regard to the β1- and β2-adrenergic receptors. Salbutamol, clenbuterol and cimaterol were all developed as β2-selective bronchodilators (Brittain *et al.*, 1976; Asato *et al.*, 1984; Engelhardt, 1984). Studies in human heart (Hall *et al.*, 1989) and guinea pig trachea (O'Donnell and Wanstall, 1978; Colbert *et al.*, 1991) with salbutamol and in rat jugular vein with clenbuterol (Cohen *et al.*, 1982) have confirmed this β2-receptor selectivity. The β-adrenergic receptor profile of ractopamine-HCl was determined in isolated smooth and cardiac muscle tissues of rat and guinea pig (Colbert *et al.*, 1991). Ractopamine possessed a 100-fold higher affinity than salbutamol at the β1-adrenergic receptor but only one-tenth the affinity of salbutamol at the β2-adrenergic receptor. The selectivity of ractopamine for the β1- and β2-adrenergic receptor subtypes was evaluated by competition binding analysis with crude membrane preparations from C6 rat glioma cells (Smith *et al.*, 1990) and by nuclear magnetic resonance (NMR) evaluation of the β-adrenergic receptor peptide binding (Schmidt *et al.*, 1993). Ractopamine possessed higher binding affinity for crude membranes prepared from rat heart (β1) than from rat lung (β2). Thus, ractopamine has been shown to be selective for the β1-adrenergic receptor, in contrast to other phenethanolamine repartitioning agents that are β2-selective.

Receptor desensitization and down-regulation
Many membrane-bound receptors, including β1- and β2-adrenergic receptors, undergo decreased sensitivity to agonists following prolonged exposure. This may occur by uncoupling of the receptors from Gs proteins (desensitization), as well as by receptor sequestration and internalization (down-regulation; see Benovic *et al.*, 1988; Barnes, 1995).

Desensitization of receptors occurs through phosphorylation (Fig. 4.8). Phosphorylation of β1- and β2-adrenergic receptors occurs in the C-terminal region by the activity of a family of serine-threonine kinases known as G-protein-coupled receptor kinases (GRKs; Benovic *et al.*, 1986; Inglese *et al.*, 1993). The β-adrenergic receptor kinase (βARK) is one member of the GRK family. Phosphorylation in the C-terminal region facilitates the binding of arrestin proteins that uncouple the interactions between receptor and Gs proteins, resulting in receptor desensitization (Pippig *et al.*, 1993). Desensitization of β-adrenergic receptors by members of the GRK family has been demonstrated for the β1- (Freedman *et al.*, 1995) and β2- (Inglese *et al.*, 1993) receptors, but not for the β3-adrenergic receptor (Liggett and Raymond, 1993). The β3-adrenergic receptor lacks phosphorylation sites in its C-terminal region which may make it resistant to GRK-mediated desensitization.

Down-regulation of receptors, resulting in decreased numbers of receptors on the cell membrane, also decreases responsiveness to receptor agonists (Benovic *et al.*, 1988). Spurlock *et al.* (1994) studied the effect of ractopamine on β-adrenergic receptor density in skeletal muscle and adipose tissue of pigs. These authors reported decreased receptor density in adipose, but not skeletal muscle tissue, in response to

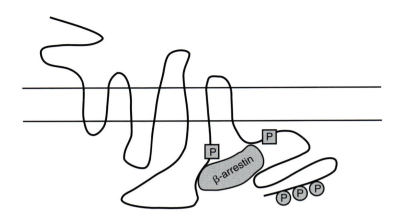

Fig. 4.8. Phosphorylation of β-adrenergic receptors. The β1- and β2-adrenergic receptors are phosphorylated on the carboxy tail by G-protein receptor kinases (GRK; phosphorylation sites shown by circles) and on the third intracellular loop by protein kinase A (phosphorylation sites shown by squares). Phosphorylation by GRK results in increased binding of β-arrestin. Binding of β-arrestin leads to uncoupling and internalization of the receptor, resulting in desensitization. (Adapted from Barnes, 1995.)

ractopamine. This result may indicate that ractopamine-induced down-regulation differs between tissues. Likewise, Smith (1989) observed no down-regulation of skeletal muscle β-adrenergic receptors in cattle or swine fed ractopamine, although cimaterol did down-regulate skeletal muscle β-adrenergic receptors in swine. These data are consistent with the *in vivo* accretion data of Dunshea *et al.* (1993) showing that pigs fed ractopamine had significantly increased protein accretion rates but only slightly decreased fat accretion rates (Table 4.8). This differential response may be a reflection of differences in receptor down-regulation or desensitization between tissues, or due to the involvement of additional receptors.

Potential involvement of other receptors in phenethanolamine mechanism of action

Pathways or receptors in addition to β1- and β2-adrenergic receptors that elicit responses to phenethanolamines have not yet been identified in livestock. However, the β3-adrenergic receptor, atypical β-adrenergic receptors that currently are unidentified, interactions among β-receptors or between β-receptors and other physiological pathways, and receptors that do not belong to the β-adrenergic receptor family are possible candidates. Currently, the β3-adrenergic receptor is being investigated for its role in energy expenditure and lipid metabolism; several authors have suggested the presence of additional, or atypical, β-

Table 4.8. Effect of ractopamine on empty body protein and fat accretion of finishing swine. Data are combined for barrows, boars and gilts that were fed ractopamine beginning at 60 kg and ending at 90 kg body weight (adapted from Dunshea *et al.*, 1993).

	Ractopamine		
	0	20	% change
Net protein accretion (g day^{-1})	144	188[a]	30
Net fat accretion (g day^{-1})	442	414	−6

[a]$P < 0.001$.

adrenergic receptors; and complex inter-actions involving the β-adrenergic recep-tors are being investigated using transgenic and knock-out mice that over- or underex-press, respectively, specific β-adrenergic receptors. Although much of this data is from rodent studies and species differences in the pharmacology of β-receptors are known to exist, insights may prove valu-able to a thorough understanding of the mechanism of action of phenethano-lamines in livestock.

β3-Adrenergic receptor

The β3-adrenergic receptor is the pre-dominant adrenergic receptor in rodent brown and white adipose tissue (Giacobino, 1995), and its effects have been described in greatest detail in these tissues. Important functions of β3-adrenergic receptor activation include the stimulation of energy expenditure and lipolysis, and administration of selective β3-agonists leads to weight loss and resistance to diet-induced obesity in rodents (Himms-Hagen et al., 1994; Collins et al., 1997). Selective agonists of the β3-adrenergic receptor currently are being investigated as potential anti-obesity agents for humans (for reviews, see Yen, 1995; Arch and Wilson, 1996; Strosberg, 1997) and dogs (Sasaki et al., 1998), but there are no reports to date of studies using selective β3-adrenergic receptor agonists in livestock species.

In rodents, the weight-reducing effects of β3-adrenergic receptor agonists may be due largely to increased energy expendi-ture occurring through the stimulation of brown adipose tissue (BAT) activity. Increased energy expenditure in BAT is accomplished in part by increased expres-sion of the BAT-specific uncoupling protein 1 (UCP1). UCP1 is located in the mitochondrial membrane and facilitates the transport of protons across a concentra-tion gradient without the capture of energy as ATP, thereby allowing energy to be dissipated as heat. Additional proteins with sequence homology to UCP1 have been identified in tissues other than BAT, including UCP2 which is expressed in many tissues (Fleury et al., 1997; Gimeno

et al., 1997) and UCP3 expressed primarily in skeletal muscle and adipose tissue (Boss et al., 1997). Changes in expression of UCP2 and UCP3 mRNA in brown and white adipose tissue, and in skeletal muscle of rodents have been reported in response to β3-agonists (Emilsson et al., 1998; Savontaus et al., 1998; Yoshitomi et al., 1998). Additionally, ectopic expression of UCP1 and the appearance of brown adipocytes in white adipose tissue follow-ing treatment with β3-agonists has been described in rodents (Cousin et al., 1992; Collins et al., 1997), humans (Garruti and Ricquier, 1992) and dogs (Champigny et al., 1991; Sasaki et al., 1998). Thus, β3-agonists may influence energy expenditure and body composition of mammals with-out clearly defined BAT depots through the regulation of uncoupling protein expres-sion in several tissues and recruitment of brown adipocytes in white adipose tissue.

Atypical receptors

Several authors have suggested that addi-tional, or 'atypical', β-adrenergic receptors exist. However, a 'β4'-adrenergic receptor has not yet been cloned. Galitzky et al. (1997) evaluated lipolytic effects of CGP12177, a non-conventional partial β3-agonist that acts as an antagonist of β1- and β2-adrenergic receptors, in rat and human fat cells. These authors suggested that lipolysis was stimulated through a novel β-adrenergic receptor that is distinct from the β3-receptor. In rat adipose cells, this novel receptor appeared to coexist with and regulate lipolysis in combination with the β3-adrenergic receptor, whereas the novel receptor appeared to mediate all of the lipolytic effects of the non-conventional β3-agonist in human adipose cells. Evidence of an 'atypical' binding site was also found in bovine skeletal muscle and adipose tissues using radioligand binding and second messenger adenyl cyclase assays (Sillence and Matthews, 1994). The clearest evidence for the existence of additional β-adrenergic receptors has come from experimentation using mice that do not express the β3-adrenergic receptor (β3 knock-out mice; Kaumann et al., 1998).

The cardiostimulant effects and receptor affinity of CGP12177 that are observed in wild-type mice were also observed in the β3 knock-out mice, suggesting that a cardiac β-adrenergic receptor that is distinct from β1-, β2- and β3-adrenergic receptors was present.

Manipulation of β-adrenergic receptor genes
Several techniques currently are used to alter expression of specific genes *in vivo* (see Roher and Kobilka, 1998). Mouse models have been developed to study the effects of increased β1-adrenergic receptor expression in adipose tissue (Soloveva *et al.*, 1997), inhibition of β3-adrenergic receptor expression (Susulic *et al.*, 1995; Revelli *et al.*, 1997) and replacement of the murine β3-adrenergic receptor gene with the human gene and regulatory elements (Ito *et al.*, 1998). Several interesting insights regarding the effects and interactions of β-adrenergic receptor agonists can be gained from these experiments. However, these studies must be interpreted with care because of differences between the mouse model and livestock species, and because of the unusual physiological environment created by genetic manipulation.

It has been proposed that the β3-receptor is a primary regulator of lipolysis because of its abundance relative to β1- and β2-receptors in rodent adipose tissue. However, significant reductions in the percentage of white adipose tissue and adipocyte cell size were reported in mice with increased expression of β1-adrenergic receptors in white adipose tissue, indicating that β1 also has the ability to stimulate lipolysis (Soloveva *et al.*, 1997). Furthermore, although two β3 knock-out models demonstrated increased adiposity, the increase was not as great as would be expected if a primary stimulator of lipolysis were removed (Susulic *et al.*, 1995; Revelli *et al.*, 1997). One possible explanation for the lack of obesity in these mice is the stimulation of lipolysis by adrenergic receptors other than β3. The mice described by Susulic *et al.* (1995) had increased mRNA expression of the β1-receptor, particularly in BAT. Therefore, the results

from the β1 transgenic and β3 knock-out models indicate that the control of lipolysis may depend more on the total population of β-adrenergic receptors than on the presence of specific receptor subtypes.

The same mouse models also demonstrate a potential difference in responsiveness of β3-adrenergic receptors between males and females. Susulic *et al.* (1995) reported a greater increase in adiposity in female compared with male β3 knock-out mice, indicating that females were more sensitive than males to changes in β3-adrenergic receptor activation. Soloveva *et al.* (1997) observed a greater decrease in adiposity of male compared with female mice that overexpressed β1-adrenergic receptors. This may be attributed to a more potent regulation of fat accretion by β3-adrenergic receptors in females compared with males, which would make additional lipolytic effects mediated by overexpression of the β1-adrenergic receptor more apparent in males than in females.

The mice described by Ito *et al.* (1998) are a very intriguing model that were generated by transgenic introduction of the human β3-adrenergic receptor gene and promoter region into β3 knock-out mice, resulting in mice that express human but not murine β3-receptors. Human β3-receptors were expressed in BAT of transgenic mice, but little or no expression was observed in white adipose tissue. This is different from the normal expression pattern of the rodent β3-receptor, which is abundant in both brown and white adipose tissues. These mice demonstrate the importance of species-related differences in the regulation of expression and function of β-adrenergic receptors and will be valuable for further investigations of the human β3-receptor.

Summary

The repartitioning effects of phenethanolamines in livestock occur through a combination of increased protein synthesis and lipolysis, and decreased protein degradation and lipogenesis to varying degrees depending on the specific phenethanolamine. The lipolytic and lipogenic effects of phenethanolamines on adipose tissue are facilitated by activation of β-adrenergic receptors and may be transient due to receptor desensitization or down-regulation. β-Adrenergic receptors may also be involved in the muscle protein accretion effects of phenethanolamines, but definitive data showing this mechanism of action in livestock remain elusive. Phenethanolamines studied in livestock activate β1- and β2-adrenergic receptors, but classification of receptor subtype specificity has been based primarily on data from rodent and human receptors. It has become increasingly evident that species differences exist in the pharmacology of β-adrenergic receptors and that a full understanding of phenethanolamine binding and activation will only occur when evaluated in the species of interest. Further research is needed to better define the relationship of β1- and β2-adrenergic receptors, as well as other receptors and pathways, to the anabolic effects of phenethanolamines in livestock.

Safety and Residue Issues

Detailed safety and residue testing is required on any repartitioning agent that is developed for use in meat animals. These tests are directed toward human food safety, safety to the environment and safety to the animals of intended use (target animal safety). For example, effective doses of ractopamine were reported to have negligible to undetectable residue levels in swine (Dalidowicz *et al.*, 1992; see Anderson *et al.*, 1993), and zilpaterol residues in cattle were well below the threshold that posed any human health risk (Zilmax Technical Manual, 1998). Extensive reviews of safety and residue data by regulatory agencies will ensure that phenethanolamines are cleared for use only if all safety questions have been answered to the satisfaction of the Food and Drug Administration (FDA) and other regulatory agencies.

The phenethanolamine clenbuterol was the subject of considerable negative publicity in the early 1990s when its illegal use and indiscriminate misuse was linked to cases of acute food poisoning (Martinez-Navarro, 1990; Pulce *et al.*, 1991; Salleras *et al.*, 1995) and illegal show-ring use. People in France (Pulce *et al.*, 1991) and Spain (Salleras *et al.*, 1995) who suffered from food poisoning after consumption of contaminated liver from livestock fed clenbuterol reported symptoms of tachycardia, tremor, headache and dizziness. At the 1995 EU Scientific Conference on Growth Promotion in Meat Production (Brussels), it was concluded that large-scale application of pharmacologically potent agents for growth-promoting purposes should not be recommended because of the potential for misuse leading to adverse health effects in humans. In March 1996, the EU banned the use of β-adrenergic receptor agonists (Directive 96/22/EC), and national monitoring programmes have been put in place to eliminate their illegal misuse (see Kuiper *et al.*, 1998).

In the USA, the illegal use of clenbuterol has been limited primarily to show animals. Reports of illegal use of clenbuterol to increase muscle and reduce fat mass, combined with the association between clenbuterol residue and food poisoning, led to the development of sensitive assays for the detection of clenbuterol and other β-adrenergic receptor agonist residues (see Mitchell and Dunnavan, 1998). The identification of clenbuterol residues and subsequent disqualification of champion steers, lambs and barrows at the Tulsa State Fair and National Western Stock Show led to an increased awareness of the illegal use of clenbuterol. Since that time, several convictions have been made for illegal distribution of clenbuterol (Mitchell and Dunnavan, 1998). Clearly, the misuse of clenbuterol needs to be closely monitored and eliminated. However, other phenethanolamines have the potential to improve the efficiency of livestock production without adverse effects on human health.

Structural diversity among phenethanolamines and differences in their oral potencies provide ample opportunity for other β-adrenergic receptor agonists to be safely developed for use in livestock (Smith, 1998). Clenbuterol and other phenethanolamines have been developed for use in humans for bronchodilation and tocolytic purposes, and extreme differences in oral dosage are required to achieve therapeutic effects. For example, a total dose of only 10 µg of clenbuterol is an effective bronchodilator while an oral dose of 10,000 µg preceded by intravenous infusion is required for effectiveness from ritodrine (see Smith, 1998). Because of these large differences in minimum dosage needed to observe effects in humans, it is reasonable to expect that the maximum dosage with no observable effects (NOEL) in humans differs greatly among phenethanolamines. Therefore, the problems that arose from the illegal treatment of animals with clenbuterol are not representative of the appropriate use of all phenethanolamines.

Industry Applications

Phenethanolamines will probably be administered as a feed additive during the final phase of finishing. Because phenethanolamines are short acting and efficacious over limited time periods, their use may be limited to intensive production systems. Currently, the only phenethanolamines available for use as repartitioning agents are zilpaterol (Zilmax®), which is manufactured by Hoechst Roussel and currently is on the market in Mexico and South Africa, and ractopamine, an Elanco Animal Health product that is cleared for use in swine in the US.

Additionally, a novel approach to activate the β-adrenergic receptors is being investigated by researchers in Australia (Sillence, 1996; Hill et al., 1998). The long-term objective of these researchers is the development of a vaccine to stimulate the production of antibodies that will interact with the β2-adrenergic receptor and mimic the anabolic effects of β-agonist drugs. Using this approach, one or two doses of the vaccine could be administered to stimulate the production of antibodies, allowing the system to be used in non-intensive systems and grazing animals (see Sillence, 1996). Although the efficacy of this approach remains to be demonstrated in vivo, the successful production of rabbit antibodies with functional activity at the bovine β2-adrenergic receptor in vitro has been described (Hill et al., 1998).

The development of phenethanolamines initially was targeted to decrease fatness so producers could provide more efficiently the leaner meat products demanded by consumers. Since the initial work with phenethanolamines was completed, genetic selection has resulted in leaner animals, particularly in swine (PIC Technical Update, 1993). The use of phenethanolamines may allow slaughter at heavier weights and maintenance of the same level of leanness as with current slaughter weights. Increased lean produced per day in a grow-out facility will remain important to the producer. Additionally, the repartitioning effects of phenethanolamines may be useful as a management tool to increase lean muscle and decrease fatness in lines of animals selected for criteria other than carcass composition, such as reproductive efficiency, improved meat quality or increased longevity. Such a strategy would enable selection pressure to be applied to traits that would result in livestock that are better able to reproduce and raise offspring in an efficient manner.

The development and use of phenethanolamine repartitioning agents has the potential to impact all aspects of the meat and livestock industries (Fig. 4.9). Producers will be able to raise livestock more efficiently, meat packers will have higher yielding carcasses, and meat processors will have the opportunity to develop new low-fat meat products more efficiently. In addition, consumers will benefit from products with reduced cholesterol (Perkins et al., 1992) and reduced calories. Finally, the use of phenethanolamine repartitioning agents will provide environmental benefits. Less

**Segment of
meat industry**

**Benefit of phenethanolamine
repartitioning agent**

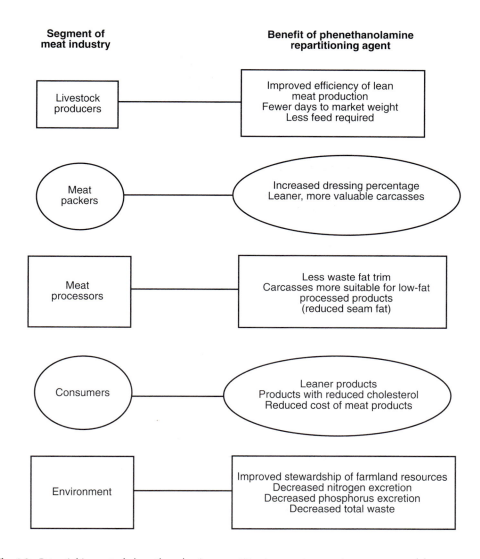

Livestock
producers

Improved efficiency of lean
meat production
Fewer days to market weight
Less feed required

Meat
packers

Increased dressing percentage
Leaner, more valuable carcasses

Meat
processors

Less waste fat trim
Carcasses more suitable for low-fat
processed products
(reduced seam fat)

Consumers

Leaner products
Products with reduced cholesterol
Reduced cost of meat products

Environment

Improved stewardship of farmland resources
Decreased nitrogen excretion
Decreased phosphorus excretion
Decreased total waste

Fig. 4.9. Potential impact of phenethanolamine repartitioning agents on various segments of the meat industry. (Adapted from Anderson *et al.*, 1991.)

land will be required to produce the feed-stuffs needed for the meat that is consumed, and the greater nitrogen retention in the animal for lean tissue growth will result in less nitrogen excreted as waste and less total volume of waste. Phenethanolamine reparti-tioning agents that are demonstrated to be safe and efficacious will provide the meat industry with a powerful tool to aid in the production of health-conscious meat products.

Acknowledgements

The authors express their appreciation to Drs Charles K. Smith II, Bruce Martin, D. Jay Jones, Emerson Potter, Thomas Jeffers, Aubrey Schroeder, Marlene Cohen, Gail Williams and Ron Schoner for their review of this manuscript, and to Ms Marcia Draper for assistance with manuscript preparations.

References

Aalhus, J.L., Jones, S.D.M., Schaefer, A.L., Tong, A.K.W., Robertson, W.M., Merrill, J.K. and Murray, A.C. (1990) The effect of ractopamine on performance, carcass composition and meat quality of finishing pigs. *Canadian Journal of Animal Science* 70, 943–952.

Aalhus, J.L., Schaefer, A.L., Murray, A.C. and Jones, S.D.M. (1992) The effect of ractopamine on myofibre distribution and morphology and their relation to meat quality in swine. *Meat Science* 31, 397–409.

Anderson, D.B., Veenhuizen, E.L., Waitt, W.P., Paxton, R.E. and Mowrey, D.H. (1987a) Effect of ractopamine on nitrogen retention, growth performance and carcass composition of finisher pigs. *Journal of Animal Science* 65 (Suppl. 1), 130–131.

Anderson, D.B., Veenhuizen, E.L., Waitt, W.P., Paxton, R.E. and Young, S.S. (1987b) The effect of dietary protein on nitrogen metabolism, growth performance and carcass composition of finishing pigs fed ractopamine. *Federation Proceedings* 46, 1021.

Anderson, D.B., Veenhuizen, E.L., Waitt, W.P., Paxton, R.E. and Mowrey, D.H. (1988) The effect of starting weight on growth performance and carcass composition of finishing pigs fed ractopamine. *Journal of Animal Science* 66 (Suppl. 1), 279–280.

Anderson, D.B., Veenhuizen, E.L., Schroeder, A.L., Jones, D.J. and Hancock, D.L. (1991) The use of phenethanolamines to reduce fat and increase leanness in meat animals. In: Haberstroh, C. and Morris, C.E. (eds) *Proceedings of Symposium on Fat and Cholesterol Reduced Foods – Advances in Applied Biotechnology Series*. Portfolio Publishing Company, New Orleans, pp. 43–73.

Anderson, D.B., Veenhuizen, E.L., Smith, C.K., Dalidowicz, J.E., Donoho, A.L., Williams, G.D., Jones, D.J., Schroeder, A.L., Turbert, M.P. and Guneratne, R.J. (1993) Ractopamine hydrochloride: a unique PLE (phenethanolamine lean enhancer) for swine. In: Ingkaninum, P. and Poomvises, P. (eds) *Prodeedings of the 11th WAVFH Symposium*. Bangkok, Thailand, The Thai Veterinary Medical Association Under the Royal Patronage, pp. 96–102.

Arch, J.R. and Wilson, S. (1996) Prospects for beta 3-adrenoceptor agonists in the treatment of obesity and diabetes. *International Journal of Obesity and Related Metabolic Disorders* 20, 191–199.

Asato, G., Baker, P.K., Bass, R.T., Bentley, T.J., Chari, S., Dalrymple, R.H., France, D.J., Gingher, P.E., Lences, B.L., Pascavage, J.J., Pensack, J.M. and Ricks, C.A. (1984) Repartitioning agents, 5-[1-hydroxy-2(isopropylamino)ethyl]-anthranilonitrile and related phenethanolamines; agents for promoting growth, increasing muscle accretion and reducing fat deposition in meat-producing animals. *Agricultural and Biological Chemistry* 48, 2883–2888.

Aurousseau, B., Connell, A., Revell, D.K., Rocha, H.J. and Lobley, G.E. (1993) Hind-limb protein metabolism in growing sheep; effects of acute and chronic infusion of clenbuterol by close arterial and systemic routes. *Comparative Biochemistry and Physiology. C: Comparative Pharmacology and Toxicology* 106, 529–535.

Barash, H., Peri, I., Gertler, A. and Bruckental, I. (1994) Effects of energy allowance and cimaterol feeding during the heifer rearing period on growth, puberty and milk production. *Animal Production* 59, 359.

Bardsley, R.G., Allcock, S.M.J., Dawson, J.M., Dumelow, N.W., Higgins, J.A., Lasslett, Y.V., Lockley, A.K., Parr, T. and Buttery, P.J. (1992) Effect of beta-agonists on expression of calpain and calpastatin activity in skeletal muscle. *Biochimie* 74, 267–273.

Bark, L.J., Stahly, T.S., Cromwell, G.L. and Miyat, J. (1992) Influence of genetic capacity for lean tissue growth on rate and efficiency of tissue accretion in pigs fed ractopamine. *Journal of Animal Science* 70, 3391–3400.

Barnes, P.J. (1995) Beta-adrenergic receptors and their regulation. *American Journal of Respiratory and Critical Care Medicine* 152, 838–860.

Beermann, D.H., Hogue, D.E., Fishell, V.K., Dalrymple, R.H. and Ricks, C.A. (1986) Effects of cimaterol and fishmeal on performance, carcass characteristics and skeletal muscle growth in lambs. *Journal of Animal Science* 62, 370–380.

Beermann, D.H., Butler, W.R., Hogue, D.E., Fishell, V.K., Dalrymple, R.H., Ricks, C.A. and Scanes, C.G. (1987) Cimaterol-induced muscle hypertrophy and altered endocrine status in lambs. *Journal of Animal Science* 65, 1514–1524.

Benovic, J.L., Strasser, R.H., Caron, M.G. and Lefkowitz, R.J. (1986) β-Adrenergic receptor kinase: identification of a novel protein kinase that phosphorylates the agonist-occupied form of the receptor. *Proceedings of the National Academy of Sciences of the United States of America* 83, 2797–2801.

Benovic, J.L., Bouvier, M., Caron, M.G. and Lefkowitz, R.J. (1988) Regulation of adenylyl cyclase-coupled β-adrenergic receptors. *Annual Review of Cell Biology* 4, 405–428.

Bergen, W.G., Johnson, S.E., Skjaerlund, D.M., Babiker, A.S., Ames, N.K., Merkel, R.A. and Anderson, D.B. (1989) Muscle protein metabolism in finishing pigs fed ractopamine. *Journal of Animal Science* 67, 2255–2262.

Bohorov, O., Buttery, P.J., Correia, J.H.R.D. and Soar, J.B. (1987) The effect of the β2-adrenergic agonist clenbuterol or implantation with oestradiol plus trenbolone acetate on protein metabolism in wether lambs. *British Journal of Nutrition* 57, 99–107.

Boss, O., Samec, S., Paoloni-Giacobino, A., Rossier, C., Dulloo, A., Seydoux, J., Muzzin, P. and Giacobino, J.P. (1997) Uncoupling protein-3, a new member of the mitochondrial carrier family with tissue-specific expression. *FEBS Letters* 408, 39–42.

Bridge, K.Y., Smith, C.K. II, and Young, R.B. (1998) Beta-adrenergic receptor gene expression in bovine skeletal muscle cells in culture. *Journal of Animal Science* 76, 2382–2391.

Brittain, R.T., Dean, C.M. and Jack, D. (1976) Sympathomimetic bronchodilator drugs. *Pharmacology and Therapeutics* 2, 423–462.

Budohoski, L., Challiss, R.A.J., Dubaniewicz, A., Kaciuba-Uscilko, H., Leighton, B., Lozeman, F.J., Nazar, K., Newsholme, E.A. and Porta, S. (1987) Effects of prolonged elevation of plasma adrenaline concentration *in vivo* on insulin-sensitivity in soleus muscle of the rat. *Biochemical Journal* 244, 655–660.

Buyse, J., Decuypere, E., Huyghebaert, G. and Herremans, M. (1991) The effect of clenbuterol supplementation on growth performance and on plasma hormone and metabolite levels of broilers. *Poultry Science* 70, 993–1002.

Byrem, T.M., Beermann, D.H. and Robinson, T.F. (1998) The beta-agonist cimaterol directly enhances chronic protein accretion in skeletal muscle. *Journal of Animal Science* 76, 988–998.

Casey, N.H., Montgomery, T.H. and Scheltons, M.L. (1997a) The effect of zilpaterol on feedlot performance, carcass quality, USDA carcass grades and meat quality. In: Bass, J. (ed.) *43rd International Congress of Meat Science and Technology*. Auckland, New Zealand, Congress Organizing Committee, p. C-6.

Casey, N.H., Webb, E.C. and Maritz, J.L. (1997b) Effect of zilpaterol and its withdrawal on carcass and meat quality of young steers. In: Bass, J. (ed.) *43rd International Congress of Meat Science and Technology*. Auckland, New Zealand, Congress Organizing Committee, p. C-7.

Champigny, O., Ricquier, D., Blondel, O., Mayers, R.M., Briscoe, M.G. and Holloway, B.R. (1991) Beta 3-adrenergic receptor stimulation restores message and expression of brown-fat mitochondrial uncoupling protein in adult dogs. *Proceedings of the National Academy of Sciences of the United States of America* 88, 10774–10777.

Chikhou, F., Moloney, A.P., Austin, F.H., Roche, J.F. and Enright, W.J. (1991) Effects of cimaterol administration on plasma concentrations of various hormones and metabolites in Friesian steers. *Domestic Animal Endocrinology* 8, 471–480.

Chikhou, F.H., Moloney, A.P., Allen, P., Joseph, R., Tarrant, P., Quirke, J., Austin, F. and Roche, J. (1993) Long-term effects of cimaterol in friesian steers. II: Carcass composition and meat quality. *Journal of Animal Science* 71, 914–922.

Choo, J.J., Horan, M.A., Little, R.A. and Rothwell, N.J. (1992) Anabolic effects of clenbuterol on skeletal muscle are mediated by β2-adrenoceptor activation. *American Journal of Physiology* 263, E50–E56.

Cohen, M.L., Wiley, K.S. and Bemis, K.G. (1982) Analysis of beta-1 and beta-2 adrenoceptor interactions of the partial agonist, clenbuterol (NAB365), in the rat jugular vein and atria. *Naunyn-Schmiedeberg's Archives of Pharmacology* 320, 145–151.

Colbert, W.E., Williams, P.D. and Williams, G.D. (1991) β-Adrenoceptor profile of ractopamine HCl in isolated smooth and cardicac muscle tissues of rat and guinea-pig. *Journal of Pharmacy and Pharmacology* 43, 844–847.

Collins, S., Daniel, K.W., Petro, A.E. and Surwit, R.S. (1997) Strain-specific response to beta 3-adrenergic receptor agonist treatment of diet-induced obesity in mice. *Endocrinology* 138, 405–413.

Convey, E.M., Rickes, E., Yang, Y.T., McElligot, M.A. and Olson, G. (1987) Effects of the beta-adrenergic agonist L-644,969 on growth performance, carcass merit and meat quality. *Reciprocal Meat Conference Proceedings* 40, 47–55.

Cousin, B., Cinti, S., Morroni, M., Raimbault, S., Ricquier, D., Penicaud, L. and Casteilla, L. (1992) Occurrence of brown adipocytes in rat white adipose tissue: molecular and morphological characterization. *Journal of Cell Science* 103, 931–942.

Dalidowicz, J.E., Thomson, T.D. and Babbitt, G.E. (1992) Ractopamine hydrochloride, a phenethanolamine repartitioning agent, metabolism and tissue residues. In: Hutson, D.H., Hawkins, D.R., Paulson, G.D. and Struble, C.B. (eds) *ACS Symposium Series 503*. American Chemistry Society, New York, pp. 234–243.

Dawson, J.M., Craigon, J., Buttery, P.J. and Beever, D.E. (1993) Influence of diet and beta-agonist administration on plasma concentrations of growth hormone and insulin-like growth factor-1 in steers. *British Journal of Nutrition* 70, 93–102.

Dickerson, P.S., Merkel, R.A. and Bergen, W.G. (1988) The time related effect of continual ractopamine treatment on lipogenesis and triacylglycerol synthesis in the adipogenic cell line TAl. *Journal of Animal Science* 66 (Suppl. 1), 250–251.

Dubrovin, L.C., Liu, C.Y. and Mills, S.E. (1990) Insulin binding to mouse adipocytes exposed to clenbuterol and ractopamine *in vitro* and *in vivo*. *Domestic Animal Endocrinology* 7, 103–109.

Dunshea, F.R., King, R.H. and Campbell, R.G. (1993) Interrelationships between dietary protein and ractopamine on protein and lipid deposition in finishing gilts. *Journal of Animal Science* 71, 2931–2941.

Eisemann, J.H. and Bristol, D.G. (1998) Change in insulin sensitivity or responsiveness is not a major component of the mechanism of action of ractopamine in beef steers. *Journal of Nutrition* 128, 505–511.

Eisemann, J.H. and Huntington, G.B. (1993) Effects of dietary clenbuterol on net flux across the portal-drained viscera, liver and hindquarters of steers (*Bos taurus*). *Comparative Biochemistry and Physiology. C: Comparative Pharmacology and Toxicology* 104, 401–406.

Eisen, E.J., Croom, W.J., Jr and Helton, S.W. (1988) Differential response to the beta-adrenergic agonist cimaterol in mice selected for rapid gain and unselected controls. *Journal of Animal Science* 66, 361–371.

Emilsson, V., Summers, R.J., Hamilton, S., Liu, Y.L. and Cawthorne, M.A. (1998) The effects of the beta3-adrenoceptor agonist BRL 35135 on UCP isoform mRNA expression. *Biochemical and Biophysical Research Communications* 252, 450–454.

Engelhardt, G. (1984) Structure–activity relationships in further series of amino-halogen substituted phenyl-aminoethanols. *Drug Research* 34, 1625–1632.

Engeseth, N.J., Lee, K.O., Bergen, W.G., Helferich, W.G., Knudson, B.K. and Merkel, R.A. (1992) Fatty acid profiles of lipid depots and cholesterol concentration in muscle tissue of finishing pigs fed ractopamine. *Journal of Food Science* 57, 1060–1062.

Fabry, J., Deroanne, C., Buts, B., Demeyer, D. and Sommer, M. (1990) Effect of cimaterol on carcass and meat characteristics in cull cows. *Journal of Animal Science* 68 (Suppl. 1), 332.

Fain, J.N. and Garcia-Sainz, J.A. (1983) Adrenergic regulation of adipocyte metabolism. *Journal of Lipid Research* 24, 945–966.

Fiems, L.O., Buts, B., Bouchque, C.V., Demeyer, D.I. and Cottyn, B.G. (1990) Effect of a β-agonist on meat quality and myofibrillar protein fragmentation in bulls. *Meat Science* 27, 29–39.

Fleury, C., Neverova, M., Collins, S., Raimbault, S., Champigny, O., Levi-Meyrueis, C., Bouillaud, F., Seldin, M.F., Surwit, R.S., Ricquier, D. and Warden, C.H. (1997) Uncoupling protein-2, a novel gene linked to obesity and hyperinsulinemia. *Nature Genetics* 15, 269–272.

Freedman, N.J., Liggett, S.B., Drachman, D.E., Pei, G., Caron, M.G. and Lefkowitz, R.J. (1995) Phosphorylation and desensitization of the human beta 1-adrenergic receptor. Involvement of G protein-coupled receptor kinases and cAMP-dependent protein kinase. *Journal of Biological Chemistry* 270, 17953–17961.

Galitzky, J., Langin, D., Verwaerde, P., Montastruc, J.L., Lafontan, M. and Berlan, M. (1997) Lipolytic effects of conventional beta 3-adrenoceptor agonists and of CGP 12,177 in rat and human fat cells: preliminary pharmacological evidence for a putative beta 4-adrenoceptor. *British Journal of Pharmacology* 122, 1244–1250.

Garruti, G. and Ricquier, D. (1992) Analysis of uncoupling protein and its mRNA in adipose tissue deposits of adult humans. *International Journal of Obesity and Related Metabolic Disorders* 16, 383–390.

Giacobino, J.P. (1995) Beta 3-adrenoceptor: an update. *European Journal of Endocrinology* 132, 377–385.

Gimeno, R.E., Dembski, M., Weng, X., Deng, N., Shyjan, A.W., Gimeno, C.J., Iris, F., Ellis, S.J., Woolf, E.A. and Tartaglia, L.A. (1997) Cloning and characterization of an uncoupling protein homolog: a potential molecular mediator of human thermogenesis. *Diabetes* 46, 900–906.

Goll, D.E., Thompson, V.F., Taylor, R.G. and Ouali, A. (1998) The calpain system and skeletal muscle growth. *Canadian Journal of Animal Science* 78, 503–512.

Gu, Y., Schinckel, A.P., Forrest, J.C., Kuel, C.H. and Watkins, L.E. (1991a) Effects of ractopamine, genotype and growth phase on finishing performance and carcass value in swine. I. Growth performance and carcass merit. *Journal of Animal Science* 69, 2685–2693.

Gu, Y., Schinckel, A.P., Forrest, J.C., Kuei, C.H. and Watkins, L.E. (1991b) Effects of ractopamine, genotype and growth phase on finishing performance and carcass value in swine. II. Estimation of lean growth rate and lean feed efficiency. *Journal of Animal Science* 69, 2694–2702.

Gwartney, B.L., Calkins, C.R. and Jones, S.J. (1991) The effect of cimaterol and its withdrawal on carcass composition and meat tenderness of broiler chickens. *Journal of Animal Science* 69, 1551–1558.

Hall, J.A., Petch, M.C. and Brown, M.J. (1989) Intracoronary injections of salbutamol demonstrate the presence of functional β2-adrenoceptors in the human heart. *Circulation Research* 65, 546–553.

Hamano, Y., Kume, K., Yamazaki, S., Kobayashi, S. and Terashima, Y. (1998) Combined effects of clenbuterol and various concentrations of protein on performance of broiler chickens. *British Poultry Science* 39, 117–122.

Hamby, P.L., Stouffer, J.R. and Smith, S.B. (1986) Muscle metabolism and real-time ultrasound measurement of muscle and subcutaneous adipose tissue growth in lambs fed diets containing a beta-agonist. *Journal of Animal Science* 63, 1410–1417.

Hanrahan, J.P. (1988) Influence of cimaterol on growth and carcass composition of sheep. In: Quirke, J.F. and Schmid, H. (eds) *Control and Regulation of Animal Growth, Proceedings of the EAAP Seminar.* Center for Agricultural Publishing and Documentation, The Netherlands, pp. 149–160.

Hansen, J.A., Yen, J.T., Klindt, J., Nelssen, J.L. and Goodband, R.D. (1997) Effects of somatotropin and salbutamol in three genotypes of finishing barrows: blood hormones and metabolites and muscle characteristics. *Journal of Animal Science* 75, 1810–1821.

Hausman, D.B., Martin, R.J., Veenhuizen, E.L. and Anderson, D.B. (1989) Effect of ractopamine on insulin sensitivity and response of isolated rat adipocytes. *Journal of Animal Science* 67, 1455–1464.

Helferich, W.G., Jump, D.B., Anderson, D.B., Skjaerlund, D.M., Merkel, R.A. and Bergen, W.G. (1990) Skeletal muscle alpha-actin synthesis is increased pretranslationally in pigs fed the phenethanolamine ractopamine. *Endocrinology* 126, 3096–3100.

Hill, R.A., Hoey, A.J. and Sillence, M.N. (1998) Functional activity of antibodies at the bovine beta2-adrenoceptor. *Journal of Animal Science* 76, 1651–1661.

Himms-Hagen, J., Cui, J., Danforth, E., Jr, Taatjes, D., Lang, S.S., Waters, B.L. and Claus, T.H. (1994) Effect of CL-316,243, a thermogenic beta 3-agonist, on energy balance and brown and white adipose tissues in rats. *American Journal of Physiology* 266, R1371–R1382.

Hoffman, B.B. and Lefkowitz, R.J. (1996) Catecholamines, sympathomimetic drugs, and adrenergic receptor antagonists. In: Hardman, J.G. and Limbird, L.E. (eds) *Goodman and Gilman's: The Pharmacological Basis of Therapeutics.* McGraw-Hill, New York, pp. 100–248.

Huang, R.R., Rapoport, D., Schaeffer, M.T., Cascieri, M.A. and Fong, T.M. (1997) Molecular cloning of the dog beta 1 and beta 2 adrenergic receptors. *Journal of Receptor and Signal Transduction Research* 17, 599–607.

Inglese, J., Freedman, N.J., Koch, W.J. and Lefkowitz, R.J. (1993) Structure and mechanism of the G protein-coupled receptor kinases. *Journal of Biological Chemistry* 268, 23735–23738.

Ito, M., Grujic, D., Abel, E.D., Vidal-Puig, A., Susulic, V.S., Lawitts, J., Harper, M.E., Himms-Hagen, J., Strosberg, A.D. and Lowell, B.B. (1998) Mice expressing human but not murine beta3-adrenergic receptors under the control of human gene regulatory elements. *Diabetes* 47, 1464–1471.

Jeremiah, L.E., Ball, R.O., Merrill, J.K., Dick, P., Stobbs, L., Gibson, L.L. and Uttaro, B. (1994a) Effects of feed treatment and gender on the flavor and texture profiles of cured and uncured pork cuts. I. Ractopamine treatment and dietary protein level. *Meat Science* 37, 1–20.

Jeremiah, L.E., Merrill, J.K., Stobbs, L., Gibson, L.L. and Gibson, R. (1994b) Effects of feed treatment and gender on the flavor and texture profiles of cured and uncured pork cuts. II. Ractopamine treatment and dietary protein source. *Meat Science* 37, 21–35.

Ji, S. (1992) Mode of action of beta-adrenergic agonists on muscle protein metabolism. PhD Thesis, Purdue University, West Lafayette, Indiana.

Ji, S., Hancock, D.L., Paxton, R.E. and Anderson, D.B. (1991) The effects of dietary protein on the responses of ractopamine on nitrogen metabolism of finishing pigs. *Journal of Animal Science* 69 (Suppl. 1), 329–330.

Jones, D.D., Hausman, G., Neal, M., Anderson, D.B., Veenhuizen, E.L. and Martin, R.J. (1987) A phenethanolamine (ractopamine) alters preadipocyte proliferation and differentiation in primary culture. *Federation Proceedings* 46, 1178.

Jones, D.J., Waitt, W.P., Mowery, D.H. and Anderson, D.B. (1988) Effect of ractopamine hydrochloride on the growth performance and carcass composition of finisher pigs fed corn–soy diets with 5% added fat. *Journal of Animal Science* 66 (Suppl. 1), 324.

Jones, D.J., Anderson, D.B., Waitt, W.P., Wagner, J.F. and Mowrey, D.H. (1989) Effect of ractopamine hydrochloride (RAC) and pituitary derived porcine somatotropin (pPST) alone and in combination on swine growth and carcass parameters. *Journal of Animal Science* 67 (Suppl. 1), 221.

Jones, D.J., Waitt, W.P., Mowery, D.H., Anderson, D.B., Veenhuizen, E.L. and Mckeith, F.K. (1990) Effect of ractopamine hydrochloride on growth performance and carcass composition of finisher pigs slaughtered at 107 and 125 kg. *Journal of Animal Science* 68 (Suppl. 1), 360.

Jones, D.J., Waitt, W.P., Mowery, D.H., Veenhuizen, E.L. and Anderson, D.B. (1992) Performance responses to ractopamine with a 0 or 5 day withdrawal when fed in 16 or 13% crude protein diets to barrows and gilts. *Journal of Animal Science* 70 (Suppl. 1), 241.

Jones, R.W., Easter, R.A., McKeith, F.K., Dalrymple, R.H., Maddock, H.M. and Bechtel, P.J. (1985) Effect of the β-adrenergic agonist cimaterol (CL 263, 780) on the growth and carcass characteristics of finishing swine. *Journal of Animal Science* 61, 905–913.

Kaumann, A.J., Preitner, F., Sarsero, D., Molenaar, P., Revelli, J.P. and Giacobino, J.P. (1998) (−)-CGP 12177 causes cardiostimulation and binds to cardiac putative beta 4-adrenoceptors in both wild-type and beta 3-adrenoceptor knockout mice. *Molecular Pharmacology* 53, 670–675.

Kikkawa, H., Isogaya, M., Nagao, T. and Kurose, H. (1998) The role of the seventh transmembrane region in high affinity binding of a beta 2-selective agonist TA-2005. *Molecular Pharmacology* 53, 128–134.

Kim, Y.S., Lee, Y.B. and Dalrymple, R.H. (1987) Effect of the repartitioning agent cimaterol on growth, carcass and skeletal muscle characteristics in lambs. *Journal of Animal Science* 65, 1392–1399.

Koohmaraie, M. (1992) The role of Ca(2+)-dependent proteases (calpains) in post mortem proteolysis and meat tenderness. *Biochimie* 74, 2239–2245.

Koohmaraie, M., Shackelford, S.D., Muggli-Cockett, N.E. and Stone, R.T. (1991) Effect of the beta-adrenergic agonist L644,969 on muscle growth, endogenous proteinase activities and post-mortem proteolysis in wether lambs. *Journal of Animal Science* 69, 4823–4835.

Kretchmar, D.H., Hathaway, M.R., Epley, R.J. and Dayton, W.R. (1990) Alterations in postmortem degradation of myofibrillar proteins in muscle of lambs fed a beta-adrenergic agonist. *Journal of Animal Science* 68, 1760–1772.

Kuiper, H.A., Noordam, M.Y., van Dooren-Flipsen, M.M., Schilt, R. and Roos, A.H. (1998) Illegal use of beta-adrenergic agonists, European Community. *Journal of Animal Science* 76, 195–207.

Kurose, H., Isogaya, M., Kikkawa, H. and Nagao, T. (1998) Domains of beta1 and beta2 adrenergic receptors to bind subtype selective agonists. *Life Sciences* 62, 1513–1517.

Liggett, S.B. and Raymond, J.R. (1993) Pharmacology and molecular biology of adrenergic receptors. *Baillieres Clinical Endocrinology and Metabolism* 7, 279–306.

Liu, C.Y. and Mills, S.E. (1990) Decreased insulin binding to porcine adipocytes *in vitro* by beta-adrenergic agonists. *Journal of Animal Science* 68, 1603–1608.

MacLennan, P.A. and Edwards, R.H.T. (1989) Effects of clenbuterol and propranolol on muscle mass. *Biochemical Journal* 264, 573–579.

Maltin, C.A., Delday, M.I. and Reeds, P.J. (1986) The effect of a growth promoting drug, clenbuterol, on fibre frequency and area in hind limb muscles from young male rats. *Bioscience Reports* 6, 293–299.

Maltin, C.A., Delday, M.I., Hay, S.M., Innes, G.M. and Williams, P.E. (1990) Effects of bovine pituitary growth hormone alone or in combination with the beta-agonist clenbuterol on muscle growth and composition in veal calves. *British Journal of Nutrition* 63, 535–545.

Martinez-Navarro, J.F. (1990) Food poisoning related to consumption of illicit beta-agonist in liver. *Lancet* 336, 1311.

Marullo, S., Nantel, F., Strosberg, A.D. and Bouvier, M. (1995) Variability in the regulation of beta-adrenoceptor subtypes. *Biochemical Society Transactions* 23, 126–129.

Merkel, R.A. (1988) Is meat quality affected by the use of repartitioning agents? *Reciprocal Meat Conference Proceedings* 41, 101–111.

Merkel, R.A., Dickerson, P., Johnson, S., Burkett, R., Burnett, R., Schroeder, A., Bergen, W. and Anderson, D. (1987) The effect of ractopamine on lipid metabolism in pigs. *Federation Proceedings* 46, 1177.

Merkel, R.A., Burkett, R.J., Babiker, A.S., Schroeder, A.L., Bergen, W.G., Anderson, D.B. and Veenhuizen, E.L. (1988) Qualitative properties and carcass composition of pigs fed ractopamine. In: Chandler, C.S. and Thornton, R.F. (eds) *Proceedings of the 34th International Congress of Meat Science and Technology*. Congress Organizing Committee, Brisbane, Australia, pp. 605–606.

Merkel, R.A., Babiker, A.S., Schroeder, A.L., Burnett, R.J. and Bergen, W.G. (1990) The effect of ractopamine on qualitative properties of porcine longissimus muscle. *Journal of Animal Science* 68 (Suppl. 1), 336.

Mersmann, H.J. (1987) Acute metabolic effects of adrenergic agents in swine. *American Journal of Physiology* 252, E85–E95.

Mersmann, H.J. (1989) Acute changes in blood flow in pigs infused with beta-adrenergic agonists. *Journal of Animal Science* 67, 2913–2920.

Mersmann, H.J. (1995) Species variation in mechanisms for modulation of growth by beta-adrenergic receptors. *Journal of Nutrition* 125, 1777S–1782S.

Mersmann, H.J. (1998) Overview of the effects of beta-adrenergic receptor agonists on animal growth including mechanisms of action. *Journal of Animal Science* 76, 160–172.

Mersmann, H.J., Hu, C.Y., Pond, W.G., Rule, D.C., Novakofski, J.E. and Smith, S.B. (1987) Growth and adipose tissue metabolism in young pigs fed cimaterol with adequate or low dietary protein. *Journal of Animal Science* 64, 1384–1394.

Mills, S.E., Liu, C.Y., Gu, Y. and Schinckel, A.P. (1990) Effects of ractopamine on adipose tissue metabolism and insulin binding in finishing hogs. Interaction with genotype and slaughter weight. *Domestic Animal Endocrinology* 7, 251–263.

Minneman, K.P., Hedberg, A. and Molinoff, P.B. (1979) Comparison of beta adrenergic receptor subtypes in mammalian tissues. *Journal of Pharmacology and Experimental Therapeutics* 221, 502–508.

Mitchell, A.D., Steele, N.C., Solomon, M.B., Alila, H.W., Lindsey, T.O. and Cracknell, V. (1994) Influence of dietary background on the response of pigs to the beta-adrenergic agonist BRL 47672. *Journal of Animal Science* 72, 1516–1521.

Mitchell, G.A. and Dunnavan, G. (1998) Illegal use of beta-adrenergic agonists in the United States. *Journal of Animal Science* 76, 208–211.

Moloney, A., Allen, P., Joseph, R. and Tarrant, V. (1991) Influence of beta-adrenergic agonists and similar compounds on growth. In: Pearson, A.M. and Dutson, T.R. (eds) *Growth Regulation in Farm Animals*. Elsevier, New York, pp. 455–513.

Morgan, J.B., Jones, S.J. and Calkins C.R. (1989) Muscle protein-turnover and tenderness in broiler-chickens fed cimaterol. *Journal of Animal Science* 67, 2646–2654.

National Research Council (1998) *Nutrient Requirements of Swine*, 10th edition. National Academy Press, Washington, DC.

O'Connor, R.M., Butler, W.R., Hogue, D.E. and Beermann, D.H. (1991a) Temporal pattern of skeletal muscle changes in lambs fed cimaterol. *Domestic Animal Endocrinology* 8, 549–554.

O'Connor, R.M., Butler, W.R. Finnerty, K.D., Hogue, D.E. and Beermann, D.H. (1991b) Acute and chronic hormone and metabolite changes in lambs fed the beta-agonist, cimaterol. *Domestic Animal Endocrinology* 8, 537–548.

O'Donnell, S.R. and Wanstall, J.C. (1978) Evidence that the efficacy (intrinsic activity) of fenoterol is higher than that of salbutamol on beta-adrenoceptors in guinea-pig trachea. *European Journal of Pharmacology* 47, 333–340.

Orcutt, A.L., Cline, T.R. and Mills, S.E. (1989) Influence of the β2-adrenergic agonist clenbuterol on insulin-stimulated lipogenesis in mouse adipocytes. *Domestic Animal Endocrinology* 6, 59–69.

Parr, T., Bardsley, R.G., Gilmour, R.S. and Buttery, P.J. (1992) Changes in calpain and calpastatin mRNA induced by beta-adrenergic stimulation of bovine skeletal muscle. *European Journal of Biochemistry* 208, 333–339.

Parsons, N. and Knight, P. (1990) Origin of variable extraction of myosin from myofibrils treated with salt and pyrophosphate. *Journal of the Science of Food and Agriculture* 51, 71–90.

Perkins, E.G., McKeith, F.K., Jones, D.J., Mowrey, D.H., Hill, S.E., Novakofski, J. and O'Connor, P.L. (1992) Fatty acid and cholesterol changes in pork longissimus muscle and fat due to ractopamine. *Journal of Food Science* 57, 1266–1268.

PIC Technical Update (1993) Estimates of genetic trend. In: *Genetics 1.1–93*. The Pig Improvement Company, Inc., Franklin, Kentucky.

Pietri-Rouxel, F., Lenzen, G., Kapoor, A., Drumare, M.F., Archimbault, P., Strosberg, A.D. and Manning, B.S. (1995) Molecular cloning and pharmacological characterization of the bovine beta 3-adrenergic receptor. *European Journal of Biochemistry* 230, 350–358.

Pippig, S., Andexinger, S., Daniel, K., Puzicha, M., Caron, M.G., Lefkowitz, R.J. and Lohse, M.J. (1993) Overexpression of beta-arrestin and beta-adrenergic receptor kinase augment desensitization of beta 2-adrenergic receptors. *Journal of Biological Chemistry* 268, 3201–3208.

Pringle, T.D., Calkins, C.R., Koohmaraie, M. and Jones, S.J. (1993) Effects over time of feeding β-adrenergic agonist to wether lambs on animal performance, muscle growth, endogenous muscle proteinase activities and meat tenderness. *Journal of Animal Science* 71, 636–644.

Pulce, C., Lamaison, D., Keck, G., Bostvironnois, C., Nicolas, J. and Descotes, J. (1991) Collective human food poisonings by clenbuterol residues in veal liver. *Veterinary and Human Toxicology* 33, 480–481.

Reeds, P.J., Hay, S.M., Dorwood, P.M. and Palmer, R.M. (1986) Stimulation of muscle growth by clenbuterol: lack of effect on muscle protein biosynthesis. *British Journal of Nutrition* 56, 249–258.

Reeds, P.J., Hay, S.M., Dorward, P.M. and Palmer, R.M. (1988) The effect of β-agonists and antagonists on muscle growth and body composition of young rats (*Rattus* sp.). *Comparative Biochemistry and Physiology* 89C, 337–341.

Revelli, J.P., Preitner, F., Samec, S., Muniesa, P., Kuehne, F., Boss, O., Vassalli, J.D., Dulloo, A., Seydoux, J., Giacobino, J.P., Huarte, J. and Ody, C. (1997) Targeted gene disruption reveals a leptin-independent role for the mouse beta3-adrenoceptor in the regulation of body composition. *Journal of Clinical Investigation* 100, 1098–1106.

Ricks, C.A., Baker, P.K. and Dalrymple, R.H. (1984) Use of repartitioning agents to improve performance and body composition of meat animals. *Reciprocal Meat Conference Proceedings* 37, 5–11.

Rohrer, D.K. and Kobilka, B.K. (1998) G protein-coupled receptors, functional and mechanistic insights through altered gene expression. *Physiology Reviews* 78, 35–52.

Salleras, L., Dominguez, A., Mata, E., Taberner, J.L., Moro, I. and Salva, P. (1995) Epidemiologic study of an outbreak of clenbuterol poisoning in Catalonia, Spain. *Public Health Report* 110, 338–342.

Sasaki, N., Uchida, E., Niiyama, M., Yoshida, T. and Saito, M. (1998) Anti-obesity effects of selective agonists to the beta 3-adrenergic receptor in dogs. II. Recruitment of thermogenic brown adipocytes and reduction of adiposity after chronic treatment with a beta 3-adrenergic agonist. *Journal of Veterinary Medical Science* 60, 465–469.

Savontaus, E., Rouru, J., Boss, O., Huupponen, R. and Koulu, M. (1998) Differential regulation of uncoupling proteins by chronic treatments with beta 3-adrenergic agonist BRL 35135 and metformin in obese fa/fa Zucker rats. *Biochemical and Biophysical Research Communications* 246, 899–904.

Schiavetta, A.M., Miller, M.F., Lunt, D.K., Davis, S.K. and Smith, S.B. (1990) Adipose tissue cellularity and muscle growth in young steers fed the β-adrenergic agonist clenbuterol for 50 days and after 78 days of withdrawal. *Journal of Animal Science* 68, 3614–3623.

Schmidt, W.F., Waters, R.M., Mitchell, A.D., Warthen, J.D., Jr, Honigbert, I.L. and Van Halbeek, H. (1993) Association of beta-agonists with corresponding beta 2- and beta 1-adrenergic pentapeptide sequences. *International Journal of Peptides and Protein Research* 41, 467–475.

Schroeder, A.L., Koohmaraie, M., Burnett, R., Merkel, R.A. and Anderson, D.B. (1990) Calcium-dependent protease activity, collagen content and electrical stimulation on meat tenderness in steers fed ractopamine (RAC). *Journal of Animal Science* 68 (Suppl. 1), 282.

Sillence, M.N. (1996) Evaluation of new technologies for the improvement of nitrogen utilization in ruminants. In: Kornegay, E.T. (ed.) *Nutrient Management of Food Animals to Enhance and Protect the Environment*. CRC Press, Boca Raton, pp. 105–133.

Sillence, M.N. and Matthews, M.L. (1994) Classical and atypical binding sites for β-adrenoceptor ligands and activation of adenylyl cyclase in bovine skeletal muscle and adipose tissue membranes. *British Journal of Pharmacology* 111, 866–872.

Sillence, M.N., Hunter, R.A., Pegg, G.G., Brown, L., Matthews, M.L., Magner, T., Sleeman, M. and Lindsay, D.B. (1993) Growth, nitrogen metabolism and cardiac responses to clenbuterol and ketoclenbuterol in rats and underfed cattle. *Journal of Animal Science* 71, 2942–2951.

Smith, C.K., II (1989) Affinity of phenethanolamines for skeletal muscle β-adrenoceptors and influence on receptor downregulation. *Journal of Animal Science* 67 (Suppl. 1), 190–191.

Smith, C.K., II, Lee, D.E. and Coutinho, L.L. (1990) Quantitative analysis of the selectivity of ractopamine for β-adrenergic receptor subtypes. *Journal of Animal Science* 68 (Suppl. 1), 284.

Smith, D.J. (1998) The pharmacokinetics, metabolism and tissue residues of beta-adrenergic agonists in livestock. *Journal of Animal Science* 76, 173–194.

Smith, S.B., Garcia, D.K., Davis, S.K. and Anderson, D.B. (1989) Elevation of a specific mRNA in longissimus muscle of steers fed ractopamine. *Journal of Animal Science* 67, 3495–3502.

Soloveva, V., Graves, R.A., Rasenick, M.M., Spiegelman, B.M. and Ross, S.R. (1997) Transgenic mice overexpressing the beta 1-adrenergic receptor in adipose tissue are resistant to obesity. *Molecular Endocrinology* 11, 27–38.

Spurlock, M.E., Cusumano, J.C., Ji, S.Q., Anderson, D.B., Smith, C.K., II, Hancock, D.L. and Mills, S.E. (1994) The effect of ractopamine on beta-adrenoceptors density and affinity in porcine adipose and skeletal muscle tissue. *Journal of Animal Science* 72, 75–80.

Sternbauer, K., Luthman, J., Hanni, A. and Jacobsson, S.O. (1998) Clenbuterol-induced insulin resistance in calves measured by hyperinsulinemic, euglycemic clamp technique. *Acta Veterinaria Scandinavica* 39, 281–289.

Stites, C.R., McKeith, F.K., Singh, S.D., Bechtel, P.J., Mowrey, D.H. and Jones, D.J. (1994) Palatability and visual characteristics of hams and loin chops from swine treated with ractopamine hydrochloride. *Journal of Muscle Foods* 5, 367–376.

Strosberg, A.D. (1997) Structure and function of the beta 3-adrenergic receptor. *Annual Review of Pharmacology and Toxicology* 37, 421–450.

Susulic, V.S., Frederich, R.C., Lawitts, J., Tozzo, E., Kahn, B.B., Harper, M.E., Himms-Hagen, J., Flier, J.S. and Lowell, B.B. (1995) Targeted disruption of the beta 3-adrenergic receptor gene. *Journal of Biological Chemistry* 270, 29483–29492.

Uttaro, B.E., Ball, R.O., Dick, P., Rae, W., Vessie, G. and Jeremiah, L.E. (1993) Effect of ractopamine and sex on growth, carcass characteristics, processing yield and meat quality characteristics of crossbred swine. *Journal of Animal Science* 71, 2439–2449.

Veenhuizen, E.L., Schmiegel, K.K., Waitt, W.P. and Anderson, D.B. (1987) Lipolytic growth, feed efficiency and carcass responses to phenethanolamines in swine. *Journal of Animal Science* 65 (Suppl. 1), 130.

Vestergaard, M., Sejrsen, K. and Klastrup, S. (1994) Growth, composition and eating quality of longissimus dorsi from young bulls fed the beta-agonist cimaterol at consecutive developmental stages. *Meat Science* 38, 55–66.

Walker, W.R., Johnson, D.D., Brendemuhl, J.H., Dalrymple, R.H. and Combs, G.E. (1989) Evaluation of cimaterol for finishing swine including a drug withdrawal period. *Journal of Animal Science* 67, 168–176.

Warriss, P.D., Kestin, S.C., Rolph, T.P. and Brown, S.N. (1990) The effects of the beta-adrenergic agonist salbutamol on meat quality in pigs. *Journal of Animal Science* 68, 128–136.

Watkins, L.E., Jones, D.J., Mowrey, D.H., Anderson, D.B. and Veenhuizen, E.L. (1990) The effect of various levels of ractopamine hydrochloride on the performance and carcass characteristics of finishing swine. *Journal of Animal Science* 68, 3588–3595.

Wellenreiter, R.H. (1991) Beta-adrenergic agonists for poultry. *Critical Reviews in Poultry Biology* 3, 229–237.

Wheeler, T.L. and Koohmaraie, M. (1992) Effects of the beta-adrenergic agonist L644,969 on muscle protein turnover, endogenous proteinase activities and meat tenderness in steers. *Journal of Animal Science* 70, 3035–3043.

Williams, A.C., Brunjes, P.M., Martin, R.J., Veenhuizen, E.L. and Anderson, D.B. (1987) Influence of feeding ractopamine to finishing swine on the *in vitro* responsiveness of adipose tissue to ractopamine and insulin. *Journal of Animal Science* 65 (Suppl. 1), 249–250.

Williams, N.H., Cline, T.R., Schinckel, A.P. and Jones, D.J. (1994) The impact of ractopamine, energy intake and dietary fat on finisher pig growth performance and carcass merit. *Journal of Animal Science* 72, 3152–3162.

Wood, J.D. and Warriss, P.D. (1992) The influence of the manipulation of carcass composition on meat quality. In: Boorman, K.N., Buttery, P.J. and Lindsay, D.B. (eds) *The Control of Fat and Lean Deposition*. Butterworth-Heinemann Ltd, Oxford, pp. 331–353.

Yen, J.T., Mersmann, H.J., Nienaber, J.A., Hill, D.A. and Pond, W.G. (1990) Responses to cimaterol in genetically obese and lean pigs. *Journal of Animal Science* 68, 2698–2706.

Yen, J.T., Nienaber, J.A., Klindt, J. and Crouse, J.D. (1991) Effect of ractopamine on growth, carcass, and fasting heat production of U.S. contemporary crossbred and Chinese-Meishan pure- and crossbred pigs. *Journal of Animal Science* 69, 4810–4822.

Yen, T.T. (1995) Beta-agonists as antiobesity, antidiabetic and nutrient partitioning agents. *Obesity Research* 3, 531S–536S.

Yoshitomi, H., Yamazaki, K., Abe, S. and Tanaka, I. (1998) Differential regulation of mouse uncoupling proteins among brown adipose tissue, white adipose tissue and skeletal muscle in chronic beta 3 adrenergic receptor agonist treatment. *Biochemical and Biophysical Research Communications* 253, 85–91.

Young, O.A., Watkins, S., Oldham, J.M. and Bass, J.J. (1995) The role of insulin-like growth factor I in clenbuterol-stimulated growth in growing lambs. *Journal of Animal Science* 73, 3069–3077.

Zilmax® Technical Brochure (1998) Hoechst Roussel Vet., GmbH, Rheingaustrasse 190, D-65203 Wiesbaden, Germany.

Chapter 5
Lipid Metabolism

J.K. Drackley

*Department of Animal Sciences, University of Illinois,
Urbana, Illinois, USA*

Introduction

Traditionally, the study of lipid absorption and metabolism in farm animals has centred on the role of dietary lipids in provision of dietary energy and in processes of fat deposition in meat, milk and eggs. Interest in these areas remains intense because of the importance of fat deposition in determining the efficiency and, hence, profitability, of meat and milk production. The content and composition of fat in animal products has become increasingly important to consumer perceptions of the healthfulness of meat and milk. Although a normal part of animal growth or milk synthesis, fat synthesis decreases the efficiency of conversion of feed nutrients into lean meat or low-fat milk products that consumers desire. Furthermore, metabolism of lipids in the liver is an integral component of animal production and is a key factor in development of metabolic disorders such as ketosis and fatty liver. Consequently, this chapter will focus primarily on aspects of digestion, absorption and transport of dietary lipids, lipid synthesis, lipid mobilization and lipid metabolism in the liver.

In addition to the primary and well-studied roles of lipids as energy substrates, however, many new roles of lipids as biological mediators and second messengers in processes of signal transduction have been discovered in recent years. An overview of these functions will also be presented.

Digestion, Absorption and Transport of Dietary Lipids

Digestion and absorption of lipids in non-ruminants

Lipids consumed by non-ruminant animals are predominantly triacylglycerols (triglycerides), with the exception of herbivorous animals such as horses and rabbits that may consume considerable amounts of galactolipids from vegetative material. Proteolytic activity in the stomach helps to release lipids from feed matrices, and the acid conditions and churning activity caused by gastric motility serve to disperse the lipids into a coarse emulsion. Lipase activity is present in the stomach, which may arise from enzymes synthesized and secreted by the salivary glands (salivary lipase) as well as by the fundic region of the stomach (Gargouri *et al.*, 1989). Salivary lipase possesses significant hydrolytic activity at pH 3.5, near that of the stomach. Gastric lipase is present at higher activities in neonatal animals and has higher hydrolytic activity toward milk triacylglycerols than does pancreatic lipase (Jensen *et al.*, 1997). Gastric lipase attacks primarily short- and medium-chain fatty acid linkages on the sn-3 position of triacylglycerol, such as those prevalent in milk of ruminants and swine.

Bile is essential for further lipid digestion and absorption in the small intestine (Brindley, 1984). The primary components of bile necessary for lipid digestion are the bile salts and phospholipids. Bile salts, which are responsible for emulsification of lipid droplets, are synthesized from cholesterol in hepatocytes of the liver. The bile salts are conjugated by the liver with the amino acids taurine or glycine, which increases the water solubility and decreases the cellular toxicity of the bile salts. Pigs conjugate bile salts to both taurine and glycine, whereas poultry only produce taurine conjugates (Freeman, 1984). The structure of the bile salts is such that it provides a flat molecule, with one side being polar and hydrophilic and the other non-polar and hydrophobic. Thus, the bile salts lie at the water–lipid interface and do not penetrate deeply into either surface. Bile salts in bile are present in cylindrical structures termed bile micelles (Brindley, 1984). The presence of bile imparts detergent-like effects on dietary lipids, causing lipid droplets to be subdivided into smaller and smaller droplets.

Pancreatic secretions into the small intestine are also critical for lipid digestion and absorption. Dispersion of lipid by bile salts enables attachment of the pancreatic polypeptide colipase, which attracts pancreatic lipase and enables it to interact at the surface of the lipid droplet (Brindley, 1984). Although the pancreatic lipase itself has no specific requirement for bile salts, the increased surface area created by the action of bile salts greatly increases the rate of pancreatic lipase-catalysed triacylglycerol hydrolysis. Pancreatic lipase specifically attacks the sn-1 and sn-3 linkages of triacylglycerols, resulting in formation of 2-monoacylglycerols and free fatty acids. Phospholipases, particularly of the A_1 and A_2 types, are secreted in pancreatic juice and convert the phospholipid lecithin (phosphatidylcholine) to lysolecithin (lysophosphatidylcholine).

Absorption of lipids is dependent on the formation of mixed micelles and on continued movement of lipids from oil droplets in the intestinal lumen into the mixed micelles. In the presence of bile salts, the fatty acids and monoacylglycerols produced by pancreatic lipase action spontaneously aggregate into mixed micelles. Lysolecithin produced from biliary and dietary phospholipids plays a key role in formation and stabilization of micelles. In particular, lysolecithin is highly efficient at solubilizing highly non-polar lipids such as stearic acid (18:0) into mixed micelles (Brindley, 1984). Formation of mixed micelles is necessary to move the non-polar lipids across the unstirred water layer present at the surface of the intestinal microvillus membranes; this unstirred water layer is thought to be the main barrier to lipid absorption (Brindley, 1984). Fatty acids and monoacylglycerols can enter the intestinal cells by simple diffusion into the lipid membrane, although the presence of transmembrane carrier proteins has been postulated (Glatz *et al.*, 1997).

Absorption of fatty lipids into intestinal epithelial cells is an energy-independent process that is facilitated by maintenance of a concentration gradient into the cells. Several putative fatty acid translocase proteins have been identified in tissues, but their role and mechanism of action have not been resolved (Glatz *et al.*, 1997). After fatty acids are absorbed into cells, they become bound to low-molecular weight (12–15 kDa) binding proteins (Glatz *et al.*, 1997). These binding proteins aid in fatty acid absorption, prevent accumulation of potentially toxic free fatty acids and may direct fatty acids to the appropriate intracellular sites for metabolism.

Most absorption of fatty acids and monoacylglycerols takes place in the jejunum in mammals. In fowl, some fatty acid absorption has been demonstrated in both the duodenum and the ileum. The extensive degree of antiperistaltic or reflux activity in the avian intestinal tract may contribute to this more diffuse location of lipid absorption (Freeman, 1984). Bile salts are not absorbed until they reach the terminal ileum, but instead cycle back to the intestinal lumen to participate in further micelle formation. The bile salts are absorbed efficiently in the ileum by an active transport process and are returned to the liver (enterohepatic circulation) to be reincorporated into bile. In both pigs and fowl, this active recycling means that the quantity of bile salts that must be synthe- sized by the liver is quite low (Freeman, 1984). Small quantities of bile salts are not reabsorbed but enter the large intestine, where they are converted into products known as 'secondary bile salts' by anaerobic gut bacteria. Loss of this quantity of bile salts in the faeces is the only route for cholesterol excretion from the body.

Fatty acids are activated for further metabolism within intestinal epithelial cells by esterification to coenzyme A (CoA), a process that consumes two high- energy phosphate bonds from ATP. In non- ruminants, the acyl-CoA molecules largely are re-esterified to triacylglycerols by the monoacylglycerol pathway, in which acyl- CoA molecules are added sequentially to 2-monoacylglycerols absorbed from the intestinal lumen. A smaller quantity of triacylglycerol is formed by the α-glycerol- phosphate pathway. Absorbed lysolecithin is re-acylated in intestinal cells to form lecithin. Cholesterol is actively synthesized from acetyl-CoA in intestinal cells of most farm animal species. Some of the cholesterol is esterified with a long-chain fatty acyl-CoA by acyl-CoA–cholesterol acyltransferase (ACAT) to form cholesterol esters.

Delivery of triacylglycerol from the intestine to other organs of the body requires that these highly non-polar lipids are packaged into a form that is stable in aqueous environments. To do so, the non- polar lipids (triacylglycerol, cholesterol esters, fat-soluble vitamins) are surrounded by amphipathic compounds such as free cholesterol, phospholipids and specific proteins called apoproteins (Hussain *et al.*, 1996). The major apoproteins synthesized by intestinal cells of most species are apo- B48, apo-AI and apo-AIV. The resulting particles, called chylomicrons, are quite large in mammalian species (50–500 nm) and contain by weight 85–95% triacyl- glycerol, 4–9% phospholipids, ~1% free cholesterol, ~0.5% esterified cholesterol and ~0.6% protein (Brindley, 1984). The size, but not number, of the chylomicrons increases in proportion to larger dietary intakes of lipid. Chylomicrons are secreted from the intestinal cells and enter the lacteals of the lymphatic system, which then drains into the venous blood at the thoracic duct. Fatty acids of less than 14 carbons are not actively esterified by intestinal enzymes, and instead are absorbed directly into the portal vein as free fatty acids.

In fowl, the intestinally synthesized lipoprotein particles are classified as very low-density lipoproteins (VLDLs), and are much lower in triacylglycerol content than mammalian chylomicrons or even VLDLs from pigs or humans (Freeman, 1984). The lymphatic system is poorly developed in fowl, and consequently the VLDL are absorbed directly into the portal vein.

Fatty acid digestibility is high in non- ruminants, with values often >80% in pigs and poultry and >90% in pre-ruminant calves (Doreau and Chilliard, 1997). Intestinal fatty acid digestibility decreases with increasing chain length and increases with increasing unsaturation. Absorption of saturated fatty acids is greater when they are in the *sn*-2 position of triacylglycerols, because they are absorbed as the 2-mono- acylglycerol after pancreatic lipase action. Fatty acid digestibility increases somewhat with age in both pigs and poultry; fat digestibility in young chicks in particular is quite poor because of the limited pro- duction of bile salts (Doreau and Chilliard, 1997).

Digestion and absorption of lipids in ruminants

Ruminant and non-ruminant animals differ with respect to strategies for lipid digestion, primarily because of the nature of the dietary lipids and the microbial processes within the rumen (Moore and Christie, 1984). In forage-fed ruminants, dietary lipids consist primarily of galactolipids and other glycolipids that are rich in linolenic acid (18:3). Cereal grains and other concentrate ingredients contribute triacylglycerols that are high in linoleic acid (18:2). Oilseeds and animal fats contribute triacylglycerols. A variety of commercial fat products are available, including calcium soaps of long-chain fatty acids, saturated or protected triacylglycerols, or mostly saturated free fatty acids. Phospholipids are smaller components of both grains and forages.

Bacteria and protozoa in the rumen hydrolyse complex lipids (glycerides) into their constituent long-chain fatty acids, sugars, organic bases (choline, ethanolamine, serine) and glycerol. Thus, the rumen is the primary site of complex lipid hydrolysis, rather than the small intestine as in non-ruminants and pre-ruminants. The glycerol and sugars are fermented rapidly to volatile fatty acids (mainly acetic, propionic and butyric).

Unsaturated fatty acids are hydrogenated extensively to saturated fatty acids (stearic, 18:0 and palmitic, 16:0) by ruminal bacteria and protozoa. The process of hydrogenation, which only occurs on free fatty acids, requires a mixed population of microbial species (Doreau and Chilliard, 1997). The biohydrogenation of linoleic acid occurs through the sequence of reactions shown in Fig. 5.1. The first isomerization reaction converts the *cis*-9, *cis*-12 linoleic acid to the *cis*-9, *trans*-11 form, known as conjugated linoleic acid (CLA). Most of the CLA that is produced in the rumen is hydrogenated to *trans*-11

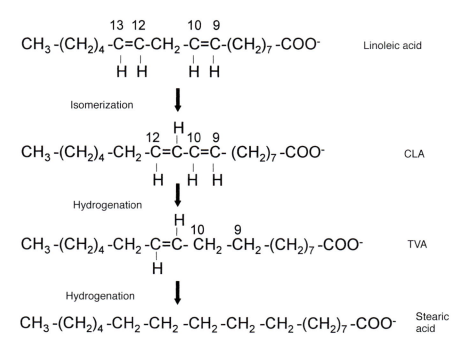

Fig. 5.1. General pathway for ruminal microbial hydrogenation of linoleic acid (*cis*-9, *cis*-12 18:2) through conjugated linoleic acid (CLA; *cis*-9, *trans*-11 18:2) and *trans*-vaccenic acid (TVA; *trans*-11 18:1) to stearic acid (18:0).

octadecenoic acid (vaccenic acid), which subsequently is hydrogenated to stearic acid. However, small amounts of *trans* isomers and CLA escape hydrogenation and are absorbed from the small intestine. These isomers are incorporated into milk and meat, which explains their relatively high content in ruminant products.

Eight positional isomers of CLA are possible, but the predominant product in the rumen is the *cis*-9, *trans*-11 isomer. Research has demonstrated that this compound has widespread effects in a number of biological systems, including inhibition of carcinogenesis, decreased body fat accumulation, modulation of the immune system and prevention of atherosclerotic lesions (Belury, 1995). Factors that increase the accumulation of CLA in the rumen and its subsequent absorption into milk and meat currently are the subject of intense research effort.

Rumen microorganisms also synthesize fatty acids, most of which are incorporated into cell membrane phospholipids. Bacteria synthesize odd-chain fatty acids containing 15–17 carbons, as well as branched-chain fatty acids, which also are relatively unique to ruminant fats (Doreau and Chilliard, 1997). As a consequence of the unique actions of the rumen microbes, ~85% of the lipids entering the small intestine of ruminants are free fatty acids, which are predominantly saturated and adsorbed to the surface of small feed particles. At the prevailing pH in the rumen, most of the fatty acids are present as salts of sodium, potassium or calcium. The remaining 15% of lipids reaching the duodenum consist mostly of bacterial phospholipids.

Pancreatic juice and bile enter the duodenum through the common bile duct and are essential for lipid digestion and absorption in the small intestine. Ruminants secrete more taurine-conjugated bile salts than glycine-conjugated bile salts because the former are more soluble at the low pH found in the ruminant small intestine (Moore and Christie, 1984). Bile salts are essential to dissociate fatty acids adsorbed to feed particles and enable micelle formation. Phospholipase A_2 secreted in pancreatic juice becomes active in the upper jejunum where the pH is more favourable and hydrolyses fatty acids from the *sn*-2 position of phospholipids. The major phospholipid in the intestine is phosphatidylcholine (lecithin), which enters in bile, pancreatic juice and digesta from the abomasum. The resultant product of phospholipase-catalysed hydrolysis is lysophosphatidylcholine (lysolecithin), which is an excellent detergent for formation of mixed micelles from the highly saturated fatty acids in the ruminant small intestine.

Bile salts and lysolecithin promote micelle formation from free fatty acids. The mixed micelle associates with the brush border of the intestinal epithelium and facilitates transfer of the hydrophobic fatty acids across the unstirred water layer at the surface of the brush border membranes. Fatty acids and lysolecithin then diffuse across intestinal cell membranes into the cells. The bile salts are not absorbed in the jejunum, but continue to form micelles. Most bile salts are absorbed in the ileum and are returned to the liver to be reincorporated into bile.

Within the small intestinal cells, fatty acids are re-esterified to glycerol-3-phosphate to form triacylglycerols. The glycerol-3-phosphate is formed from blood glucose via glycolysis. Pre-ruminants consuming milk triacylglycerol function like non-ruminants and absorb large amounts of 2-monoacylglycerol that can be re-esterified to form triacylglycerol. Along with apolipoproteins (B48, AI and AIV), cholesterol and phospholipids, the triacylglycerols are packaged into lipoprotein particles that are secreted from the cells and enter the lacteals to be carried into the lymph and reach the peripheral circulation. These particles are analogous to chylomicrons in non-ruminants but are classified more correctly as VLDLs because of their small size in functioning ruminants. This is a factor of the highly saturated nature of the triacylglycerols, the low dietary fat content of ruminant diets and the constant flow of digesta into the intestine as compared with the episodic nature of digesta entry in meal-feeding non-ruminants. Recent evidence also indicates that some triacylglycerol-rich lipoproteins may be secreted into the portal vein of calves and functioning ruminants (Bauchart, 1993).

Fatty acid digestibility in ruminants is usually lower and more variable than that in non-ruminants (Doreau and Chilliard, 1997). Intestinal digestibility does not differ appreciably between 16- and 18-carbon fatty acids (average of 79 and 77%, respectively), and is slightly greater for unsaturated than saturated fatty acids (77, 85 and 83% for 18:0, 18:1 and 18:2, respectively; Doreau and Chilliard, 1997).

Lipid transport: lipoprotein metabolism

With the exception of free fatty acids, which circulate bound to serum albumin, lipids circulate as components of large lipoprotein particles. Lipoproteins generally are classified according to their buoyant density, which is determined by the relative proportions of lipids and proteins. The largest lipoproteins are the chylomicrons, followed by VLDLs. These are also the least dense materials because they carry large lipid loads with relatively small protein contents. High-density lipoproteins (HDLs) are the smallest particles and the most dense, having higher amounts of protein and less lipid. Low-density lipoproteins (LDLs) have densities between those of HDLs and VLDLs.

Intestinally derived lipoproteins rich in triacylglycerols (chylomicrons, VLDL) function to deliver dietary long-chain fatty acids to peripheral tissues (Fig. 5.2). The liver also secretes VLDLs as a way to package endogenous triacylglycerols for transport in plasma. Following secretion from intestinal cells or liver, these triacylglycerol-rich lipoproteins acquire apo-CII from circulating HDLs (Hussain et al., 1996). Apo-CII is an activator of the enzyme lipoprotein lipase (LPL), which is responsible for clearance of plasma triacylglycerol (Braun and Severson, 1992). LPL is present in most tissues and is found in high activities in

adipose tissue, lactating mammary gland, heart and skeletal muscle. Synthesis of LPL occurs in the parenchymal cells of the tissue; the LPL is secreted from the cells and translocated to the interior surfaces of capillaries perfusing the tissue. There, the highly glycosylated LPL is anchored to the vascular surface of the endothelial cells by interactions with heparin sulphate proteoglycans on the cell surface (Braun and Severson, 1992).

As chylomicrons and VLDLs move through the capillary beds, they become trapped by LPL through interactions of the carbohydrate moieties of apo-B and LPL. Binding is facilitated by the presence of apo-CII in the triacylglycerol-rich lipoproteins. Triacylglycerol hydrolysis occurs rapidly, with release of free fatty acids and monoacylglycerols. The fatty acids can diffuse into the cells or exit the tissue in the venous blood. Although LPL is a product of a single gene in all tissues, its transcription is regulated differently in different tissues through the presence of tissue-specific cis-acting elements (Braun and Severson, 1992). For example, LPL activity is higher in adipose tissue during mid-gestation, and is high in mammary gland during lactation. In cows, adipose LPL increases markedly during mid- to late lactation to restore energy reserves (McNamara, 1991). During fasting, the activity of LPL decreases in adipose tissue and increases in the heart. Thus, LPL may help to direct dietary fatty acids to appropriate tissues depending on the nutritional state of the animal, which in turn is signalled by insulin and other hormones.

After triacylglycerol hydrolysis, the lipoprotein particles remaining are termed remnants (from chylomicrons) and intermediate-density lipoproteins (IDLs; from VLDLs). Continued triacylglycerol hydrolysis by LPL and, in some species, hepatic lipase, eventually decreases the size of the particles so that they can be removed by the liver. Remnants and IDLs are actively removed by the liver in most species via interaction with the apo-B,E receptors (Hussain et al., 1996). Other portions of IDLs are converted to LDLs, which are end-products of the intravascular metabolism of VLDLs. The LDLs, which are rich in cholesterol esters and phospholipids, are taken up by receptors in the skeleton, intestine, liver, adrenals and corpus luteum (Fig. 5.2).

The HDLs are synthesized and secreted by the liver and small intestine as small discoidal particles consisting of a phospholipid bilayer containing only apo-A and free cholesterol (Fielding and Fielding, 1995). The particles become spherical as cholesterol esters are formed via the lecithin–cholesterol acyltransferase (LCAT)

reaction (Fig. 5.2). This enzyme, synthesized in liver and secreted into plasma, binds to the discoidal HDLs and catalyses the transfer of a fatty acid (usually linoleic acid) from the *sn*-2 position of lecithin (phosphatidylcholine) to free cholesterol, forming cholesterol esters and lysolecithin. The non-polar cholesterol esters move into the interior of the particle, causing it to become spherical and to enlarge as more cholesterol ester is formed. Lysolecithin is transferred to albumin in plasma. The HDLs acquire excess surface components (phospholipids, apo-C, apo-E) from VLDLs

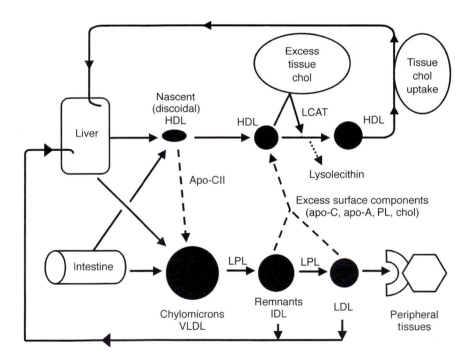

Fig. 5.2. Schematic diagram of lipoprotein metabolism in farm animals. Chylomicrons or very low-density lipoproteins (VLDLs) secreted from the intestine or liver acquire apoprotein CII (apo-CII) from newly secreted (nascent) high-density lipoproteins (HDLs). Triacylglycerols in chylomicrons or VLDLs are hydrolysed by lipoprotein lipase (LPL) in peripheral tissues, which is activated by apo-CII and allows fatty acid uptake by tissues. The remaining particles (remnants or intermediate-density lipoproteins, IDLs) are cleared by the liver or undergo further triacylglycerol hydrolysis to produce low-density lipoproteins (LDLs). Excess surface components (phospholipids, PLs; apoproteins C and A; free cholesterol, chol) are transferred to HDLs. LDLs are degraded in the liver or after receptor-mediated uptake in peripheral tissues. HDLs take up excess cholesterol (chol) from peripheral tissues and convert it to cholesterol esters by the action of lecithin cholesterol acyltransferase (LCAT); lysolecithin is released into plasma, and cholesterol esters enter the core of HDLs. HDLs can deliver cholesterol to tissues or return it to the liver for conversion to bile salts. In some species, cholesterol esters may be transferred from HDLs to LDLs by cholesterol ester transfer protein.

or chylomicrons as these particles are metabolized by LPL in peripheral tissues.

These metabolic functions of HDLs result in these particles carrying out a cycle known as reverse cholesterol transport, in which HDLs pick up excess free cholesterol from tissues and convert it to cholesterol ester (Fielding and Fielding, 1995). The HDL particles thus enlarge and grow less dense as their content of cholesterol esters increases. The HDLs then transfer cholesterol esters to the liver for conversion into bile acids (the only route for excretion of cholesterol from the body), and the now smaller HDLs can return to repeat the cycle (Fig. 5.2). Clearance of HDL particles occurs in liver and bone.

The basic scheme of lipoprotein metabolism as just discussed exhibits many species variations (Hollanders et al., 1986). Pigs have high concentrations of LDLs, similarly to humans, and are often used as models of human lipoprotein metabolism. In horses and ruminants, HDLs are the predominant lipoproteins and serve to deliver cholesterol to steroidogenic tissues (liver, ovary, adrenals, testis) and to a variety of tissues for membrane synthesis. Many of the functions that LDLs play in transport of cholesterol esters in humans and rabbits are replaced by HDLs in ruminants and horses. In ruminants, there is considerable overlap in the density range of LDLs and HDLs, which makes separation by traditional ultracentrifugal methods difficult (Bauchart, 1993).

Lipid Synthesis and Mobilization

Lipid synthesis

Lipogenesis

Lipogenesis (lipid synthesis) refers in the strictest sense to synthesis of fatty acids and not to the esterification of those fatty acids to glycerides. Adipose tissue is the main site of lipogenesis in non-lactating cattle, sheep, goats, pigs, dogs and cats (Beitz and Nizzi, 1997). In poultry, similarly to humans, the liver is the major site of lipogenesis, while in rodents (rats and mice) both liver and adipose tissue are important lipogenic sites. The mammary gland of lactating farm animals actively synthesizes fatty acids.

De novo lipogenesis occurs in the cytosol and is a sequential cyclical process in which acetyl (2-carbon) units are added successively to a 'primer' or initial starting molecule, usually acetyl-CoA but also 3-hydroxybutyrate in the lactating mammary gland of ruminants. The source of the acetyl units is acetyl-CoA, derived either from glucose through glycolysis in non-ruminants or pre-ruminants, or from acetate via rumen fermentation of dietary carbohydrates in ruminants. In functioning ruminants, glucose is not used for fatty acid synthesis, which serves to spare glucose for other essential functions.

The nature of the mechanism that minimizes lipogenic use of glucose by ruminants remains unclear. Since the discovery that activities of ATP-citrate lyase and NADP-malate dehydrogenase were lower in bovine adipose tissue than in liver and adipose tissue of rats (Hanson and Ballard, 1967), it was believed that these enzymes limited lipogenic use of glucose by ruminants. However, subsequent research showed that lactate was used by bovine adipose tissue (Whitehurst et al., 1978) and mammary gland (Forsberg et al., 1985) at rates similar to those of acetate. Lactate, after being converted to pyruvate, is metabolized similarly to pyruvate produced from glycolysis. Consequently, lactate also requires the enzymes ATP-citrate lyase and NADP-malate dehydrogenase in order to be converted to fatty acids. The activity of ATP-citrate lyase in bovine adipose tissue and mammary gland, albeit lower than that in rat tissues, is still sufficient to allow the observed rates of lactate conversion to fatty acids (Forsberg et al., 1985). Moreover, ATP-citrate lyase activity is at least equal to that of acetyl-CoA carboxylase, the rate-limiting step in fatty acid synthesis (Beitz and Nizzi, 1997). Probably the most likely explanation for the low rate of incorporation of glucose into fatty acids in ruminant adipose tissue and mammary gland is the limited flux of glucose carbon past the triose phosphate stage in glycolysis (Forsberg *et al.*, 1985), because of the high demand for glycerol-3-phosphate for triacylglycerol synthesis, and the active metabolism of glucose in the pentose phosphate pathway to produce NADPH.

The rate-limiting step in fatty acid synthesis is catalysed by the enzyme acetyl-CoA carboxylase (Hillgartner *et al.*, 1995). This enzyme converts acetyl-CoA to malonyl-CoA, which is the actual 'donor' of acetyl units in the elongation process. Two forms of the enzyme, termed α and β, are found in animals (Kim, 1997). The α-form is the enzyme found in lipogenic tissues that regulates the rate of fatty acid synthesis. The β-form is found in non-lipogenic tissues and is associated with control of mitochondrial fatty acid oxidation (discussed later). The α-form of the enzyme is subject to several levels of metabolic regulation from signals of nutrient status. Insulin, released when dietary energy is plentiful, activates the enzyme and so promotes fat storage. Increased concentrations of citrate and isocitrate, which also would signal increased substrate availability for storage as fat, activate the reaction. In contrast, glucagon and the catecholamines inhibit its activity via cyclic AMP (cAMP)-dependent phosphorylation. In this way, fat synthesis is inhibited during times when mobilization of energy stores is required. Increased concentrations of fatty acyl-CoA in the cytosol inhibit the reaction, a form of negative feedback. In addition to short-term changes in enzyme activity caused by these hormones and metabolites, the abundance of the enzyme protein is also regulated. Starvation decreases the amounts of both the mRNA and the protein, while refeeding after a fast causes a large increase in transcription and translation of mRNA for acetyl-CoA carboxylase (Hillgartner *et al.*, 1995).

The fatty acid synthase enzyme complex consists of two multifunctional polypeptide chains, each containing seven distinct enzyme activities necessary to elongate a growing fatty acid (Smith, 1994).

The two polypeptide chains are arranged head-to-tail, resulting in two separate sites for synthesis of fatty acids; thus each enzyme complex can assemble two fatty acids simultaneously. The activity of the enzyme complex is not limiting to the overall rate of fatty acid synthesis. The overall reaction for synthesis of one molecule of palmitic acid is:

$$\text{Acetyl-CoA} + 7 \text{ malonyl-CoA} + 14 \text{ NADPH} + 14 \text{ H}^+ \rightarrow \text{palmitic acid} + 7 \text{ CO}_2 + 8 \text{ CoA} + 14 \text{ NADP}^+ + 6 \text{ H}_2\text{O} \tag{5.1}$$

In non-ruminants the hydrogen donor, NADPH, is generated through metabolism of glucose in the pentose phosphate pathway and in the malic enzyme reaction. In ruminants, cytosolic isocitrate dehydrogenase can generate over one-half of the NADPH needed through metabolism of acetate (Beitz and Nizzi, 1997). The remainder of the NADPH in ruminants is derived from glucose metabolism in the pentose phosphate pathway. The presence of glucose enhances fatty acid synthesis in ruminants, probably through enhanced production of NADPH. Regulation of fatty acid synthase is largely through intracellular concentrations of dietary or synthesized fatty acids, which decrease its activity (Smith, 1994). High-fat diets decrease the intracellular concentration of fatty acid synthase, whereas refeeding after a fast increases its concentration. High concentrations of insulin increase the abundance of fatty acid synthase, whereas growth hormone, glucagon and glucocorticoids decrease its abundance (Hillgartner *et al.*, 1995).

Lipogenesis generally increases as animals age, although changes are depot-specific and may be modulated by diet (Smith, 1995). Thus, lipogenesis in internal adipose depots such as perirenal fat is more active earlier in the growth stage, and less active as the animal reaches physiological maturity. Somatotropin treatment of pigs and cattle leads to decreased lipogenesis, primarily by decreasing the sensitivity of adipose cells to the actions of insulin (Etherton and Bauman, 1998).

Other acyl-CoA molecules such as propionyl-CoA can be used as primers by the fatty acid synthase complex. In this case, odd-carbon numbered fatty acids will be produced, most commonly of 15 or 17 carbon length. In addition, methylmalonyl-CoA can replace malonyl-CoA in the elongation reactions, resulting in branched-chain (methyl-branched) fatty acids. In most lipogenic tissues, these fatty acids are only minor products, but in sebaceous (skin) glands of some species the production of methyl-branched fatty acids may be substantial (Smith, 1994). In ruminants, higher concentrations of odd-chain and branched-chain fatty acids are found in milk and adipose tissue because of the greater synthesis of these fatty acids by rumen bacteria.

In adipose tissue, the predominant product of the lipogenic pathway is palmitic acid. In the mammary gland of lactating animals, however, large quantities of fatty acids <16 carbons in length are synthesized. This is due to the action of specific chain-terminating mechanisms, which differ between ruminants and non-ruminants. In ruminants, the fatty acid synthase complex allows the release of short- and medium-chain fatty acyl-CoA esters, which are incorporated rapidly into milk fat. In non-ruminants, a specific enzyme, thioesterase II, is responsible for hydrolysing the thioester bond of the 8–14 carbon acyl chain, thus releasing the medium-chain fatty acids (Smith, 1994).

Elongation and desaturation

The end-product of the *de novo* lipogenic pathway in animal tissues is usually palmitic acid, yet this fatty acid constitutes only 20–30% of total fatty acids in adipose tissue lipids (Rule *et al.*, 1995). Considerable amounts of stearic (18:0) and oleic (18:1) acids are present in adipose tissue lipids, and may arise either from intestinally derived triacylglycerol-rich lipoproteins or by conversion from palmitic acid in adipose tissue. Elongation of palmitic acid (16:0) to stearic acid occurs by the action of fatty acid elongase, found in the microsomal fraction (endoplasmic

reticulum) of adipocytes. Malonyl-CoA is the source of the additional two carbons. Fatty acid elongase is found in much larger activities in bovine adipose tissue than in mammary gland, liver, muscle or intestinal mucosa (Smith, 1995).

The concentration of stearic acid in tissue lipids is regulated by the presence of stearoyl-CoA desaturase (Δ9 desaturase), which converts stearic acid to oleic acid. This microsomal enzyme is a mixed function oxidase that inserts a double bond nine carbons from the methyl end of the fatty acid. Considerable activity of stearoyl-CoA desaturase is found in mammary gland, muscle and duodenal muscosa, but little activity is found in bovine liver (Smith, 1995). The primary function of the enzyme seems to be to regulate lipid fluidity by preventing excessive accumulation of the very high-melting stearic acid.

Glycerolipid synthesis

Few free (non-esterified) fatty acids are found in the animal body; rather, most fatty acids are found esterified to glycerol as glycerolipids such as triacylglycerols and phospholipids. In adipose tissue and the lactating mammary gland, most fatty acids are esterified to form triacylglycerols as a non-toxic form of energy storage or for transfer to the young, respectively. In liver and other tissues, most fatty acids are esterified to form phospholipids as components of intracellular and plasma membranes. The liver actively synthesizes triacylglycerols when presented with high concentrations of non-esterified fatty acids from the blood.

The enzymes necessary for glycerolipid biosynthesis are found in the microsomal fraction of cells. The general pathways of esterification of fatty acids are shown in Fig. 5.3. Acyl chains from acyl-CoA are transferred consecutively to glycerol-3-phosphate produced via glycolysis. Production of diacylglycerol (diglyceride) from phosphatidate by phosphatidate phosphohydrolase and subsequent production of triacylglycerol from diacylglycerol by diacylglycerol acyltransferase may be regulatory steps for triacylglycerol synthesis, but these enzymes have not been well characterized in farm animals. Esterification of fatty acids in adipose tissue increases with increasing energy intake in meat animals (Rule, 1995) and is lower in times of dietary energy deficit, such as during early lactation in dairy cows (McNamara, 1991).

Fatty acid composition of milk, muscle and body fat

A variety of fatty acids are found in complex lipids of animal tissues. These fatty acids range primarily from 14 to 20 carbons in length, with varying degrees of unsaturation. Characteristic profiles of fatty acids are found in individual tissues and among species of animals. Sample profiles of muscle and adipose tissue of beef cattle, sheep and pigs are shown in Table 5.1. Adipose tissue lipids from ruminants generally are more highly saturated than lipids from non-ruminants such as pigs because of ruminal biohydrogenation of dietary

unsaturated fatty acids. Experimental post-ruminal infusions of unsaturated oils and feeding formaldehyde-protected oils to sheep and cattle results in increasing unsaturation of adipose tissue lipids (Rule *et al.*, 1995). In pigs and chickens, increasing amounts of dietary fat will result in adipose tissue lipids reflecting the fatty acid composition of the dietary fat. Body fat generally becomes softer in these species with supplementation of fats and oils, because the relative amounts of *de novo* synthesized palmitic acid decrease and those of 18-carbon unsaturated fatty acids increase (Rule *et al.*, 1995).

Bovine milk fat contains considerable amounts of fatty acids shorter than 14 carbons that are synthesized within the mammary gland (Table 5.2). The fatty acid composition of milk fat can be altered markedly by supplementation of the diet with fat (Palmquist *et al.*, 1993). Dietary long-chain fatty acids suppress *de novo* synthesis of short- and medium-chain fatty

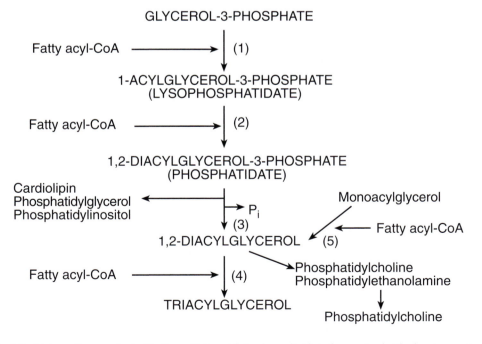

Fig. 5.3. Major pathways of esterification of fatty acids to glycerolipids in farm animals. The key enzymes involved are: (1) glycerophosphate acyltransferase; (2) lysophosphatidate acyltransferase; (3) phosphatidate phosphohydrolase; (4) diacylglycerol acyltransferase; and (5) monoacylglycerol acyltransferase. P_i, inorganic phosphate. Adapted from Rule (1995).

Table 5.1. Typical profiles of major fatty acids found in lipids from subcutaneous adipose tissue or longissimus muscle from cattle, sheep and pigs (g kg^{-1}). (Adapted from Rule *et al.*, 1995.)

Fatty acid	Cattle	Sheep	Pigs
Adipose tissue			
14:0	40	40	10
16:0	280	260	240
18:0	110	160	130
18:1	430	410	440
18:2	30	30	120
Muscle			
14:0	40	30	10
16:0	270	250	250
18:0	130	110	110
18:1	380	460	490
18:2	80	60	70

Table 5.2. Fatty acid composition of milk fat from cows fed a basal low-fat diet or the basal diet supplemented with tallow. (Adapted from Palmquist *et al.*, 1993.)

Fatty acid	Diet (g kg^{-1} of methyl esters)	
	Basal	Basal + tallow
4:0	33	35
6:0	27	23[a]
8:0	18	13[a]
10:0	40	26[a]
12:0	46	29[a]
14:0	130	103[a]
14:1	15	13
15:0	13	10[a]
16:0	299	284
16:1	17	18
17:0	6	8[a]
18:0	90	104
18:1	172	233[a]
18:2	22	16[a]
18:3	6	9[a]

[a]Different from basal diet, $P < 0.05$.

acids in the mammary gland. Unprotected fats lead to only slight increases in polyunsaturated fatty acids in milk fat, but may lead to appreciable increases in oleic acid because of intestinal and mammary desaturation of stearic acid produced by ruminal biohydrogenation of dietary unsaturated fatty acids (Table 5.2). The bovine mammary gland readily incorporates unsaturated fatty acids presented to it (LaCount *et al.*, 1994). Producing milk with more monounsaturated and polyunsaturated fatty acids depends on the development of practical strategies to protect dietary unsaturated fatty acids from hydrogenation by rumen microbes. Currently, formaldehyde treatment of protein–fat mixtures is the best methodology for rumen protection (Doreau and Chilliard, 1997), but regulatory approval may limit its application in many countries.

Lipolysis

Mobilization of fatty acids from adipose tissue triacylglycerols (lipolysis) occurs during times of negative energy balance or in response to stresses. The reaction proceeds by the sequential release of fatty acids from the glycerol backbone. The fatty acids released increase the size of the intracellular free fatty acid pool and, in the absence of stimuli to re-esterify those fatty acids, they diffuse from the cell into the blood. The free fatty acids are adsorbed quickly to binding domains on serum albumin, and circulate to various tissues as a fatty acid–albumin complex. Physiological states characterized by high rates of lipolysis, such as early lactation in dairy cows and sows (McNamara, 1991), often are also characterized by relatively lower concentrations of albumin in the blood. Hence, the ratio of free fatty acids to albumin in blood increases, which favours greater uptake of the free fatty acids by tissues of the body because more fatty acids occupy lower affinity binding sites on the albumin molecule. Furthermore, the increased ratio of fatty acids to albumin increases the size of the tissue free fatty acid pool, which in turn increases re-esterification of fatty acids in adipose tissue and thus provides feedback regulation on lipolysis (Metz and van den Bergh, 1977).

The initial step in lipolysis is catalysed by hormone-sensitive triacylglycerol lipase. This enzyme is activated by binding of hormones that stimulate formation of cAMP by adenyl cyclase. In mammals, the primary agonists for this reaction are the catecholamines, such as epinephrine and norepinephrine. In poultry, glucagon is the major lipolytic hormone. Binding of these hormones to cell surface receptors causes activation of adenyl cyclase, depending on the balance between activation of the stimulatory guanine nucleotide-binding protein (G_s protein) and activation of the inhibitory G_i protein (Lafontan and Langin, 1995). Receptor types vary among tissues and species in the relative activation of these two G proteins. Agonists that activate β-adrenergic receptors cause activation of G_s. Activation of G_s activates adenyl cyclase, which increases the concentration of cAMP in the cell. In turn, cAMP activates protein kinase A, which phosphorylates the regulatory subunit of hormone-sensitive lipase. The activated hormone-sensitive lipase then catalyses lipolysis of triacylglycerol.

Inhibition of lipolysis depends on a greater activation of G_i proteins, which inhibit adenyl cyclase and increase the activity of phosphodiesterase, the enzyme that degrades cAMP. Agonists that bind to α-adrenergic receptors activate G_i and thus suppress lipolysis (Lafontan and Langin, 1995). Factors such as insulin, adenosine and the E series of prostaglandins are associated with decreased activity of hormone-sensitive lipolysis. Treatment of animals with somatotropin results in an indirect stimulation of lipolysis by increasing the sensitivity of adipose tissue to the effects of the catecholamines. Somatotropin causes this increased sensitivity by diminishing the ability of the G_i proteins to inhibit adenyl cyclase. Thus, suppression of the inhibitory controls of lipolysis allows higher rates of lipolysis to occur during treatment with somatotropin.

Another factor controlling the relative degree of lipolysis is the degree to which fatty acids are re-esterified to form triacylglycerols before they can diffuse out of the cells. Insulin stimulates uptake of glucose and glycolysis, increasing the supply of glycerol-3-phosphate available for esterification. Insulin also stimulates the activity of the esterification pathway. Control of lipolysis is interwoven tightly with regulation of lipogenesis, so that the overall function of adipose tissue to accrete or release energy stores is coordinated according to the physiological needs of the animal.

Metabolism of Lipids in the Liver

Oxidation and ketogenesis

The liver takes up free fatty acids from blood in proportion to their concentration. Within the hepatocytes (liver cells), long-chain fatty acids of 14 carbons or more are activated by acyl-CoA synthetases found in the microsomes and outer mitochondrial membrane. Acyl-CoA may either enter the mitochondria for oxidation or be esterified within the endoplasmic reticulum (microsomes). Under conditions of increased fatty acid uptake, the liver often produces large amounts of the ketone bodies, acetoacetate and β-hydroxybutyrate, in the process known as ketogenesis. The two main factors regulating the degree to which fatty acids are oxidized by the liver are the supply of fatty acids to the liver via lipolysis and the partitioning within hepatocytes between mitochondrial oxidation and microsomal esterification.

No acyl-CoA synthetase enzymes that can activate fatty acids with 14 carbons or more are present within the mitochondrial matrix (McGarry *et al.*, 1989). Therefore, entry of these long-chain fatty acids into the mitochondria is regulated effectively by the activity of the enzyme carnitine palmitoyltransferase I (CPT-I). This enzyme is an integral membrane protein of the outer mitochondrial membrane, and catalyses the formation of fatty acyl-carnitine from fatty acyl-CoA and free L-carnitine. The acyl-carnitine molecules are then transported across the mitochondrial membrane by a specific carrier protein, and are reconverted to acyl-CoA within the mitochondrial matrix by the action of CPT-II, a peripheral protein of the inner mitochondrial membrane. Short- and medium-chain fatty acids (12 carbons or less) pass through the mitochondrial membrane and are activated by acyl-CoA synthetases found within the mitochondrial matrix. Consequently, oxidation of these fatty acids is not controlled by CPT-I.

The activity of CPT-I is inhibited by interaction with malonyl-CoA, the product of the first committed step of lipogenesis catalysed by acetyl-CoA carboxylase. Insulin stimulates the activity of acetyl-CoA carboxylase. Conditions of negative energy balance as signalled by lower ratios of insulin to glucagon thus result in decreased concentrations of malonyl-CoA and increased rates of fatty acid oxidation. Furthermore, in rats, the sensitivity of CPT-I to malonyl-CoA is decreased during times of low insulin or insulin resistance, which decreases the ability of the low concentrations of malonyl-CoA to inhibit acyl-carnitine formation and thereby further increases the rate of fatty acid oxidation (Zammit, 1996).

Classical studies (reviewed by McGarry et al., 1989) that delineated the control of CPT-I by malonyl-CoA in rats described this mechanism as a means of preventing simultaneous oxidation and synthesis of fatty acids within the liver cell, a potential futile cycle. However, in cattle, sheep and swine, rates of lipogenesis are very low in liver, which obviates the need for such a control mechanism. Nevertheless, production of malonyl-CoA by acetyl-CoA carboxylase does occur in bovine, ovine and swine liver (Brindle et al., 1985), probably as a control mechanism for oxidation rather than as a quantitatively important site of fatty acid synthesis. Likewise, skeletal muscle and heart muscle are also non-lipogenic tissues that use fatty acids as energy sources. Both heart and skeletal muscle of rats contain a high activity of acetyl-CoA carboxylase of the β-isoform (Kim, 1997). Physiological situations that lead to low insulin to glucagon ratios and decreased activity of acetyl-CoA carboxylase in these tissues result in increased rates of fatty acid oxidation. Whether the acetyl-CoA carboxylase present in the liver of ruminants and swine is similar to the β-isoform of rats has not been determined.

Intramitochondrial oxidation of fatty acyl-CoA occurs through the β-oxidation pathway, resulting in formation of acetyl-CoA. During this process, electrons are transferred to FAD and NAD$^+$ to form the reduced forms of these coenzymes, which in turn can donate electrons to the electron transport chain to drive ATP synthesis. The acetyl-CoA can be oxidized completely to carbon dioxide in the tricarboxylic acid (TCA) cycle. Alternately, acetyl-CoA can be diverted to formation of ketone bodies. Ketogenesis is enhanced in times of increased fatty acid mobilization and uptake by the liver, when low ratios of insulin to glucagon cause activation of CPT-I that allows extensive uptake of fatty acids into mitochondria (Zammit, 1990). Conversion of acetyl-CoA to ketone bodies rather than complete oxidation in the TCA cycle results in formation of less ATP per mole of fatty acid oxidized. For example, complete oxidation of palmitate in the TCA cycle, followed by oxidative phosphorylation in the electron transport chain, yields 129 ATP per molecule of palmitate. In contrast, β-oxidation of palmitate with acetyl-CoA converted to ketone bodies generates only 27 ATP per molecule of palmitate. Because the production of ATP must match its utilization for energy-requiring reactions in the liver, ketogenesis allows the liver to metabolize about five times more fatty acid for the same ATP yield. Conversion of fatty acids into water-soluble fuels may be an important strategy to allow the animal to cope with extensive mobilization of fatty acids during energy deficit.

In addition to control at the levels of fatty acid supply and CPT-I, ketogenesis is controlled by the activity of the key regulatory enzyme, 3-hydroxy-3-methylglutaryl-CoA (HMG-CoA) synthase. This enzyme is controlled both through increased transcription and translation during prolonged energy deficit and by inactivation through succinylation (Emery et al., 1992). Increased flux of metabolites such as pyruvate, propionic acid or glucogenic amino acids into the TCA cycle, resulting from greater feed intake and improved energy balance, results in increased pool size of succinyl-CoA, an intermediate of the TCA cycle. The succinyl-CoA is used to add a succinyl group to a regulatory sub-unit of HMG-CoA synthase, which inactivates the enzyme.

In ruminants, CPT-I also is highly sensitive to inhibition by methylmalonyl-CoA (Brindle *et al.*, 1985), which is an intermediate in the conversion of propionate to succinyl-CoA in the process of gluconeogenesis. This may constitute an additional adaptation of ruminants to link the supply of energy-yielding compounds from the diet with the need for hepatic fatty acid oxidation. Furthermore, the ability to distinguish between glucogenic molecules originating primarily through ruminal fermentation of dietary carbo-hydrates (propionate) and those originating from catabolism of endogenous amino acids (e.g. pyruvate) has been proposed as a unique adaptation of regulation of fatty acid oxidation in ruminants during energy deficit situations (Zammit, 1990).

Accelerated ketogenesis in response to low blood glucose from insufficient dietary energy intake may occur in both lactating cows and pregnant ewes. The increased ketogenesis is probably a factor of increased mobilization of free fatty acids from adipose tissue, increased uptake of fatty acids by the liver, increased activity of CPT-I, decreased sensitivity of CPT-I to malonyl-CoA and increased activity of HMG-CoA synthase.

Ketogenesis has been shown to occur at lower rates in swine than in many other species (Odle *et al.*, 1995; Adams *et al.*, 1997). This may be due to limitations both in the ability of swine to form acylcarnitines for transport into the mitochondria (Odle *et al.*, 1995) and in the activity of HMG-CoA synthase (Adams *et al.*, 1997). Limitations are particularly pronounced in neonates, with some developmental increase in oxida-tive capacity observed with advancing age in pigs (Adams *et al.*, 1997; Yu *et al.*, 1997).

Peroxisomal metabolism

An alternate pathway for β-oxidation in liver is found in peroxisomes, which are subcellular organelles present in most tissues (Singh, 1997). The peroxisomal pathway for β-oxidation functions similarly to the mitochondrial pathway, with notable exceptions. First, the first dehydrogenase step of mitochondrial β-oxidation is replaced with an oxidase step (acyl-CoA oxidase) in the peroxisome, resulting in formation of hydrogen peroxide rather than reduced NAD^+. Second, peroxisomes do not contain an electron transport chain. As a result of these factors, peroxisomal β-oxidation results in capture of less energy as ATP than does mitochondrial β-oxidation. Another unique aspect of the peroxisomal pathway is that two enzymic activities of the β-oxidation pathway (enoyl-CoA hydratase and 3-hydroxyacyl-CoA dehydrogenase) are performed by a single multifunctional protein, called the bifunctional protein.

Peroxisomal β-oxidation is active with very long-chain fatty acids (20 carbons or more) that are relatively poor substrates for mitochondrial β-oxidation. Because peroxisomal β-oxidation enzymes are induced in rats by situations leading to increased supply of fatty acids in the liver, such as high dietary fat, starvation and diabetes, the peroxisomal β-oxidation path-way has been discussed as an 'overflow' pathway to help cope with increased flux of fatty acids (Singh, 1997).

Recent investigations in dairy cows (Grum *et al.*, 1994), sheep (Hansen *et al.*, 1995) and pigs (Yu *et al.*, 1997) have shown that the livers of these farm animals possess relatively high peroxisomal β-oxidation activity. In neonatal pigs, peroxisomal β-oxidation increases rapidly after birth in response to milk intake and may be an adaptive mechanism to aid in oxidation of long-chain fatty acids from milk in the face of relatively low capacity for mitochondrial fatty acid oxidation (Yu *et al.*, 1997). In dairy cows, peroxisomal β-oxidation is not induced by dietary fat during lactation or by starvation (Grum *et al.*, 1994), but increases in response to dietary fat and nutrient restriction during the periparturient period. Subsequent to the increased peroxisomal β-oxidation prepartum, less triacylglycerol accumulates in the liver at the time of calving (Grum *et al.*, 1996). This may be an adaptation to allow increased metabolism of fatty acids during their extensive mobilization.

During the last decade, research has identified specific nuclear receptors that are activated by fatty acids and chemicals that cause peroxisomal proliferation in rodents. These receptors, called peroxisome proliferator-activated receptors (PPARs), in turn bind to specific peroxisome proliferator response elements (PPREs) located in the regulatory region of a number of genes whose products are associated with lipid metabolism (Schoonjans *et al.*, 1996). These include long-chain acyl-CoA synthetase; the peroxisomal enzymes acyl-CoA oxidase and bifunctional protein; the mitochondrial enzymes CPT-I, medium-chain acyl-CoA dehydrogenase and HMG-CoA synthase; and the microsomal cytochrome P450 enzymes CYP4A1 and CYP4A6, which catalyse ω-oxidation. Furthermore, the liver fatty acid-binding protein gene contains a PPRE. In rats, the gluconeogenic enzymes phosphoenolpyruvate carboxykinase and malic enzyme also contain PPREs in their regulatory regions. Although limited research has been conducted with farm animals to date, it is attractive to speculate that the PPARs represent a molecular mechanism that would function to coordinate the activity of the metabolic machinery necessary for fatty acid metabolism with the supply of fatty acids to tissues.

Esterification and export

Esterification is believed to 'compete' with oxidation for acyl-CoA in the liver of farm animals. The pathways for esterification of acyl-CoA to glycerolipids in liver are similar to those discussed earlier for adipose tissue. In rodents, the activities of phosphatidate phosphohydrolase and diacylglycerol acyltransferase appear to be increased in times of high insulin; little is known about regulation of these enzymes in farm animals. In dairy cows, hepatic

capacity for esterification of fatty acids is increased around calving (Grum *et al.*, 1996), which may contribute to the propensity of dairy cows to develop fatty livers around the time of calving. The enzymes glycerophosphate acyltransferase, diacylglycerol acyltransferase and phosphatidate phosphohydrolase (Fig. 5.3) are potential regulatory sites for accumulation of triacylglycerol in the liver, but data supporting their role are inconclusive.

The general mechanisms for synthesis and secretion of VLDLs from liver are well known (Bauchart, 1993). Apoprotein B is the key component whose rate of synthesis in the rough endoplasmic reticulum is believed to control the overall rate of VLDL production. Lipid components that are synthesized in the smooth endoplasmic reticulum are added to apoprotein B as it moves to the junction of the two compartments. After being carried to the Golgi apparatus in transport vesicles, the apoproteins are glycosylated. Secretory vesicles bud off the Golgi membrane and migrate to the sinusoidal membrane of the hepatocyte. The vesicles fuse with the membrane and release the VLDLs into blood in the space of Disse.

Ruminants and swine do not export triacylglycerol from the liver as VLDLs as efficiently as do poultry or laboratory rodents. In particular, ruminants have a very low rate of VLDL export compared with rats, despite similar rates of esterification of fatty acids to triacylglycerols (Kleppe *et al.*, 1988). Where the limitation in VLDL synthesis or secretion resides is unknown (Bauchart, 1993). Based on available evidence, it appears that the rate of synthesis or assembly of VLDLs is more likely to be limiting than is the secretory process *per se*. Possible limitations include a low rate of synthesis or a high rate of degradation of apoprotein B, or deficient synthesis of phosphatidylcholine or cholesterol.

The rate of export of triacylglycerol from the liver corresponds in general to the relative rate of *de novo* fatty acid synthesis among species, with species such as cattle and pigs that do not synthesize fatty acids in the liver also having the lowest rates of triacylglycerol export (Pullen *et al.*, 1990). On the other hand, poultry and fish actively synthesize fatty acids in the liver and secrete VLDLs at very high rates. Rates of VLDL export are intermediate for species that have lipogenesis in both liver and adipose tissue, such as rats and rabbits. In rats, the origin of the fatty acids incorporated into triacylglycerol can affect the rate of VLDL export. Dietary conditions that promote lipogenesis in liver also stimulate VLDL output. In contrast, high fat diets or conditions that promote mobilization of fatty acids from adipose tissue decrease the rate of VLDL synthesis but promote formation of a separate pool of storage triacylglycerol (Wiggins and Gibbons, 1996). Because the latter condition (uptake by the liver of fatty acids mobilized from adipose tissue) is similar to that usually encountered in ruminants, similar factors may govern the rate of VLDL synthesis in ruminants (Bauchart, 1993).

Consequently, conditions in ruminants that promote extensive body fat mobilization usually result in accumulation of triacylglycerol within the liver, potentially resulting in fatty liver. Problems with fatty liver in dairy cows are more likely in over-fattened cows, possibly as a result of high insulin and its effects on fatty acid esterification in the liver, and increased insulin resistance in peripheral tissues such as adipose tissue. The mechanism of clearance of accumulated triacylglycerol has not been determined definitively. No hormone-sensitive lipase is present in the liver of farm animals. In rats, the stored lipid droplets do not contribute appreciably to synthesis of VLDLs (Wiggins and Gibbons, 1996). Rather, it appears that the lipid droplet must be degraded by lysosomal acid lipases to free fatty acids, which then can be metabolized by the liver (Cadórniga-Valiño *et al.*, 1997).

Metabolism of Essential Fatty Acids

Animals can synthesize fatty acids with double bonds no closer than nine carbons from the methyl end of the fatty acyl chain. For example, stearic acid (18:0) can be desaturated to oleic acid (18:1) by desaturase enzymes in liver, adipose tissue, intestinal mucosa and mammary gland. The convention for nomenclature of the position of double bonds within the fatty acyl chain refers to the carbon number starting from the methyl carbon end of the fatty acid, with the methyl carbon referred to as the 'ω-carbon'. Thus, oleic acid is referred to in shorthand notation as 18:1 ω-9, because the double bond occurs at the ninth carbon from the methyl end. Alternate nomenclature refers to this as the 'n-9' or 'Δ9' position. Likewise, the enzyme activity responsible for conversion of stearic to oleic acid is usually referred to as Δ9-desaturase.

Polyunsaturated fatty acids with double bonds nearer to the end of the chain are required for normal formation of cell membranes and synthesis of other key regulatory molecules such as prostaglandins (Sardesai, 1992). These fatty acids fall into two groups, the ω-6 series and ω-3 series. Because animal tissues are unable to synthesize fatty acids with double bonds in the ω-6 or ω-3 positions, such fatty acids must be supplied in the diet. In most species, the parent compounds of these families, linoleic acid (18:2 ω-6) and linolenic acid (18:3 ω-3), respectively, are the only fatty acids that are required from dietary sources. Consequently, these are referred to as dietary essential fatty acids. These fatty acids can be elongated and desaturated to produce longer chain fatty acids that are more highly unsaturated. For example, linoleic acid can be converted to arachidonic acid (20:4 ω-6) beginning with Δ6-desaturation, followed by elongation and Δ5-desaturation (Fig. 5.4). However, because the position of the final double bond in the chain is always fixed from the methyl end, linoleic acid cannot be converted to eicosapentaenoic acid (20:5 ω-3) or docosahexaenoic acid (22:6 ω-3). Cats and some other carnivores have very limited activities of the Δ6-desaturase enzyme, and thus require dietary arachidonic acid as well as linoleic and linolenic acid.

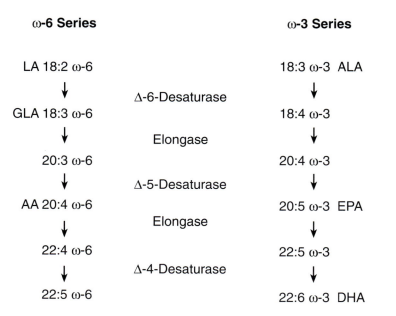

Fig. 5.4. Metabolism of essential fatty acids of the ω-6 (linoleic) and ω-3 (linolenic) series. LA, linoleic acid; GLA, γ-linolenic acid; AA, arachidonic acid; ALA, α-linolenic acid; EPA, eicosapentaenoic acid; DHA, docosahexaenoic acid.

The enzymes for elongation and desaturation are found in the microsomal fraction of cells. The distribution of enzyme activity varies among organs of animals, with the greatest activity in the liver and the adrenal glands and only limited activity in tissues such as the heart, kidneys and brain (Bézard *et al.*, 1994).

One function of the essential unsaturated fatty acids is in maintaining the appropriate fluidity of cell membranes (Sardesai, 1992). Because unsaturated fatty acids have lower melting points than saturated fatty acids, their presence in membranes makes the membranes more fluid. Changes in the fluidity of cell membranes can affect the degree to which integral membrane proteins such as receptors are assembled into and diffuse laterally in the membrane. Such changes can also affect the activity of membrane-associated enzymes, change the expression and function of receptors and alter the transport of molecules across the membrane.

While the biochemical basis of the requirement for linoleic acid and its metabolites in animal metabolism has been relatively well understood for some time, functions of the ω-3 family of fatty acids have been harder to delineate (Sardesai, 1992). Docosahexaenoic acid is a component of lipids in the grey matter of the cerebral cortex of the brain and of the photoreceptor membranes of the rod outer segment of the retina. As a result, deprivation of linolenic acid in pregnant female rats leads to impairments in cognitive function, learning and vision in the rat pups. Thus, the presence of adequate linolenic acid during fetal and neonatal development is critical.

Arachidonic acid in cell membrane phospholipids can be released in response to various signals that activate phospholipase activity. Arachidonic acid can then become a substrate for conversion to the eicosanoids of the so-called series 2 type (prostaglandin E_2, thromboxane A_2, 12-hydroxyeicosatetraenoic acid and leukotriene B_4), which have strong pro-inflammatory and pro-aggregatory actions. In contrast, the series 3 products produced from eicosapentaenoic acid released from cell membrane phospholipids (prostaglandin E_3, thromboxane A_3 and leukotriene B_5) have anti- or weakly inflammatory effects and only weak aggregation-promoting effects. Because linoleic and linolenic acid compete for the same pathways of elongation and desaturation, an increased supply of one will decrease the elongation–desaturation products of the other that are incorporated into membrane phospholipids (Sardesai, 1992). In this way, the fatty acid composition of cell membranes can be altered by the type of dietary fat. Interest has grown in whether sources of ω-3 fatty acids such as fish oil could be used to confer advantages to animals by increasing eicosapentaenoic acid and decreasing arachidonic acid in cell membranes, thereby decreasing the influence of the series 2 eicosanoid products. Numerous questions remain about the effectiveness of such approaches, and to date few conclusive data are available.

Several fundamental questions remain about the metabolism of essential fatty acids in farm animal species. One of these is how these fatty acids are transferred *in utero* to the fetus, given the complex nature of the placenta in ruminants and pigs. A second issue is how ruminants are able to obtain sufficient essential fatty acids in the face of extensive rumen microbial hydrogenation of dietary unsaturated fatty acids (Noble, 1984). A small, and evidently at least marginally sufficient, amount of the essential fatty acids escapes hydrogenation in the rumen and is absorbed. Nearly all of the linoleic (and presumably linolenic) acid that reaches the small intestine is incorporated into phospholipids (through reacylation of lysophosphatidic acid) and cholesterol esters (via the ACAT reaction). These lipids have a very slow turnover in the body, so that the essential fatty acids are retained for their critical functions (Noble, 1984). Very few essential fatty acids normally are incorporated into the triacylglycerol fraction, which has a very rapid turnover in the body. However, if protected unsaturated lipids are fed or the

rumen is by-passed experimentally to allow absorption of large amounts of unsaturated fatty acids, essential fatty acids can be incorporated into lymph triacylglycerols, which will then be transferred to tissues and milk (LaCount *et al.*, 1994). An additional factor in conservation of essential fatty acids by ruminants is that they oxidize linoleic acid less efficiently than other more abundant fatty acids such as oleic, and less efficiently than do non-ruminants (Reid and Husbands, 1985).

Role of Lipids in Cell Signalling and Signal Transduction

Cells within and among tissues of animals must communicate with one another to ensure coordinated growth, differentiation, metabolism and apoptosis (regulated cell death). A variety of endocrine (hormonal), paracrine and autocrine factors communicate such information to the surface of neighbouring or distant cells. During the last two decades, research has exploded on the ways in which receptor-borne messages are translated into intracellular function. These processes, which are referred to as signal transduction mechanisms, have profound effects on both normal growth and carcinogenesis (Eyster, 1998). One of the most exciting current areas of research in lipid metabolism relates to the role of lipids as signalling compounds.

Recent evidence has shown that various polyunsaturated fatty acids can serve directly as second messengers or modulators of enzymes. Polyunsaturated fatty acids play a key role in regulating expression of genes for lipid-metabolizing or lipogenic enzymes in both lipogenic and non-lipogenic tissues (Sessler and Ntambi, 1998). Other lipids, such as platelet-activating factor and the eicosanoids, have regulatory effects on the inflammatory response. Platelet-activating factor is a type of ether-linked lipid called a plasmalogen.

The first discovery of the involvement of phospholipids was of the agonist-induced hydrolysis of phosphatidylinositol 4,5-bisphosphate by phospholipase C to produce inositol-1,4,5-trisphosphate and diacylglycerols. In turn, the diacylglycerols and the calcium mobilized by inositol trisphosphate activate protein kinase C, which has many diverse effects on cellular growth and metabolism. Many hormones and growth factors activate isoforms of phospholipase C, including epinephrine and norepinephrine, serotonin, thromboxane A_2, histamine, cholecystokinin, epidermal growth factor, nerve growth factor and platelet-derived growth factor (Exton, 1997).

During the last decade, phosphatidyl-choline also has been found to participate in cell signalling mechanisms, through agonists that stimulate phospholipase D activation. The products of this reaction are choline and phosphatidic acid, which may in itself serve as a signalling mechanism as well as being converted rapidly to diacylglycerol by phosphatidate phosphohydrolase. Phosphatidic acid also may be converted by a specific phospholipase A_2 to form lysophosphatidic acid, which is recognized as an important intercellular messenger, particularly in stimulating growth. As discussed earlier, hydrolysis of arachidonic acid from phosphatidylcholine by phospholipase A_2 leads to formation of the eicosanoids.

Recently, a new pathway of cell signalling has been discovered that works through sphingomyelin (Exton, 1997). Activation of sphingomyelinase by agonists such as tumour necrosis factor-α, interferon-γ and 1,25-dihydroxycholecalciferol causes hydrolysis of sphingomyelin to produce ceramide and phosphocholine. Ceramide is a potent intracellular signalling factor that has widespread effects on cellular growth, differentiation and viability. Furthermore, ceramide can be converted by removal of its fatty acyl group to sphingosine, which is an inhibitor of protein kinase C. Sphingosine in turn can be phosphorylated to form sphingosine-1-phosphate, which

has different cell signalling properties. Progress in this exciting area is extremely rapid (Eyster, 1998) and it is likely that additional information on these pathways in farm animals will be forthcoming.

Future Perspectives

Although much is known about the basic pathways of lipid metabolism and their regulation in farm animals, the processes of lipid accretion and lipid secretion in milk will continue to assume great importance in future research. This prominence is stimulated by the tremendous impact that lipid synthesis has on the efficiency, or inefficiency, of meat and milk production. In turn, this directly affects profitability of livestock enterprises. Lipid metabolism also plays a key role in development of metabolic disorders such as fatty liver, ketosis and pregnancy toxaemia, which continue to plague livestock producers. Supplemental fats are now standard components of diets fed to high-producing dairy cows, and are common in both swine and beef diets. Continued efforts to enhance the digestibility and utilization of dietary fatty acids will improve the energetic efficiency of milk and meat production.

Increased understanding of lipid metabolism should lead to practical approaches to enhance the productivity and health of farm animals. Various biotechnological approaches to manipulate the process of growth or milk production, such as somatotropin, target key aspects of lipid synthesis. Development of transgenic livestock may be able to exploit desirable pathways or overcome limitations in others to alter lipid metabolism. Finally, unravelling the roles and metabolism of the lipid-derived cell signalling mechanisms will have a huge impact on understanding the cellular processes of growth in farm animals, as well as on the cellular mechanisms underlying homeostatic actions of circulating hormones and growth factors.

References

Adams, S.H., Alho, C.S., Asins, G., Hegardt, F. and Marrero, P.F. (1997) Gene expression of mitochondrial 3-hydroxy-3-methylglutaryl-CoA synthase in a poorly ketogenic mammal: effect of starvation during the neonatal period of the piglet. *Biochemical Journal* 324, 65–73.

Bauchart, D. (1993) Lipid absorption and transport in ruminants. *Journal of Dairy Science* 76, 3864–3881.

Beitz, D.C. and Nizzi, C.P. (1997) Lipogenesis and lipolysis in bovine adipose tissue. In: Onodera, R., Itabashi, H., Ushida, K., Yano, H. and Sasaki, Y. (eds) *Rumen Microbes and Digestive Physiology in Ruminants*. Japan Science Society Press, Tokyo/S. Karger, Basel, pp. 133–143.

Belury, M.A. (1995) Conjugated dienoic linoleate: a polyunsaturated fatty acid with unique chemoprotective properties. *Nutrition Reviews* 53, 83–89.

Bézard, J., Blond, J.P., Bernard, A. and Clouet, P. (1994) The metabolism and availability of essential fatty acids in animal and human tissues. *Reproduction, Nutrition, Development* 34, 539–568.

Brindle, N.P.J., Zammit, V.A. and Pogson, C.I. (1985) Regulation of carnitine palmitoyltransferase activity by malonyl-CoA in mitochondria from sheep liver, a tissue with a low capacity for fatty acid synthesis. *Biochemical Journal* 232, 177–182.

Brindley, D.N. (1984) Digestion, absorption and transport of fats: general principles. In: Wiseman, J. (ed.) *Fats in Animal Nutrition*. Butterworths, London, pp. 85–103.

Braun, J.E.A. and Severson, D.L. (1992) Regulation of the synthesis, processing, and translocation of lipoprotein lipase. *Biochemical Journal* 287, 337–347.

Cadórniga-Valiño, C., Grummer, R.R., Armentano, L.E., Donkin, S.S. and Bertics, S.J. (1997) Effects of fatty acids and hormones on fatty acid metabolism and gluconeogenesis in bovine hepatocytes. *Journal of Dairy Science* 80, 646–656.

Doreau, M. and Chilliard, Y. (1997) Digestion and metabolism of dietary fat in farm animals. *British Journal of Nutrition* 78 (Suppl. 1), S15–S35.

Emery, R.S., Liesman, J.S. and Herdt, T.H. (1992) Metabolism of long chain fatty acids by ruminant liver. *Journal of Nutrition* 122, 832–837.

Etherton, T.D. and Bauman, D.E. (1998) Biology of somatotropin in growth and lactation of domestic animals. *Physiological Reviews* 78, 745–761.

Exton, J.H. (1997) Cell signaling through guanine-nucleotide-binding regulatory proteins (G proteins) and phospholipases. *European Journal of Biochemistry* 243, 10–20.

Eyster, K.M. (1998) Introduction to signal transduction: a primer for untangling the web of intracellular messengers. *Biochemical Pharmacology* 55, 1927–1938.

Fielding, C.J. and Fielding, P.E. (1995) Molecular physiology of reverse cholesterol transport. *Journal of Lipid Research* 36, 211–228.

Forsberg, N.E., Baldwin, R.L. and Smith, N.E. (1985) Roles of lactate and its interactions with acetate in maintenance and biosynthesis in bovine mammary tissue. *Journal of Dairy Science* 68, 2550–2556.

Freeman, C.P. (1984) The digestion, absorption and transport of fats – non-ruminants. In: Wiseman, J. (ed.) *Fats in Animal Nutrition*. Butterworths, London, pp. 105–122.

Gargouri, Y., Moreau, H. and Verger, R. (1989) Gastric lipases: biochemical and physiological studies. *Biochimica et Biophysica Acta* 1006, 255–271.

Glatz, J.F.C., van Nieuwenhoven, F.A., Luiken, J.J.F.P., Schaap, F.G. and van der Vusse, G.J. (1997) Role of membrane-associated and cytoplasmic fatty acid-binding proteins in cellular fatty acid metabolism. *Prostaglandins, Leukotrienes and Essential Fatty Acids* 57, 373–378.

Grum, D.E., Hansen, L.R. and Drackley, J.K. (1994) Peroxisomal β-oxidation of fatty acids in bovine and rat liver. *Comparative Biochemistry and Physiology* 109B, 281–292.

Grum, D.E., Drackley, J.K., Younker, R.S., LaCount, D.W. and Veenhuizen, J.J. (1996) Nutrition during the dry period and hepatic lipid metabolism of periparturient dairy cows. *Journal of Dairy Science* 79, 1850–1864.

Hansen, L.R., Drackley, J.K., Berger, L.L., Grum, D.E., Cremin, J.D., Jr, Lin, X. and Odle, J. (1995) Prenatal androgenization of lambs: II. Metabolism in adipose tissue and liver. *Journal of Animal Science* 73, 1701–1712.

Hanson, R.W. and Ballard, F.J. (1967) The relative significance of acetate and glucose as precursors for lipid synthesis in liver and adipose tissue from ruminants. *Biochemical Journal* 105, 529–536.

Hillgartner, F.B., Salati, L.M. and Goodridge, A.G. (1995) Physiological and molecular mechanisms involved in nutritional regulation of fatty acid synthesis. *Physiological Reviews* 75, 47–76.

Hollanders, B., Mougin, A., N'Diaye, F., Hentz, E., Aude, X. and Girard, A. (1986) Comparison of the lipoprotein profiles obtained from rat, bovine, horse, dog, rabbit and pig serum by a new two-step ultracentrifugal gradient procedure. *Comparative Biochemistry and Physiology* 84B, 83–89.

Hussain, M.M., Kancha, R.K., Zhou, Z., Luchoomun, J., Zu, H. and Bakillah, A. (1996) Chylomicron assembly and catabolism: role of apolipoproteins and receptors. *Biochimica et Biophysica Acta* 1300, 151–170.

Jensen, M.S., Jensen, S.K. and Jakobsen, K. (1997) Development of digestive enzymes in pigs with emphasis on lipolytic activity in the stomach and pancreas. *Journal of Animal Science* 75, 437–445.

Kim, K.-H. (1997) Regulation of mammalian acetyl-coenzyme a carboxylase. *Annual Review of Nutrition* 17, 77–99.

Kleppe, B.B., Aiello, R.J., Grummer, R.R. and Armentano, L.E. (1988) Triglyceride accumulation and very low density lipoprotein secretion by rat and goat hepatocytes *in vitro*. *Journal of Dairy Science* 71, 1813–1822.

LaCount, D.W., Drackley, J.K., Laesch, S.O. and Clark, J.H. (1994) Secretion of oleic acid in milk fat in response to abomasal infusions of canola or high-oleic sunflower fatty acids. *Journal of Dairy Science* 77, 1372–1385.

Lafontan, M. and Langin, D. (1995) Cellular aspects of fuel mobilization and selection in white adipocytes. *Proceedings of the Nutrition Society* 54, 49–63.

McGarry, J.D., Woeltje, K.F., Kuwajima, M. and Foster, D.W. (1989) Regulation of ketogenesis and the renaissance of carnitine palmitoyltransferase. *Diabetes/Metabolism Reviews* 5, 271–284.

McNamara, J.P. (1991) Regulation of adipose tissue metabolism in support of lactation. *Journal of Dairy Science* 74, 706–719.

Metz, S.H.M. and van den Bergh, S.G. (1977) Regulation of fat mobilization in adipose tissue of dairy cows in the period around parturition. *Netherlands Journal of Agricultural Science* 25, 198–211.

Moore, J.H. and Christie, W.W. (1984) Digestion, absorption and transport of fats in ruminant animals. In: Wiseman, J. (ed.) *Fats in Animal Nutrition*. Butterworths, London, pp. 123–149.

Noble, R.C. (1984) Essential fatty acids in the ruminant. In: Wiseman, J. (ed.) *Fats in Animal Nutrition*. Butterworths, London, pp. 185–200.

Odle, J., Lin, X., van Kempen, T.A.T.G., Drackley, J.K. and Adams, S.H. (1995) Carnitine palmitoyl-transferase modulation of hepatic fatty acid metabolism and radio-HPLC evidence for low ketogenesis in neonatal pigs. *Journal of Nutrition* 125, 2541–2549.

Palmquist, D.L., Beaulieu, A.D. and Barbano, D.M. (1993) Feed and animal factors influencing milk fat composition. *Journal of Dairy Science* 76, 1753–1771.

Pullen, D.L., Liesman, J.S. and Emery, R.S. (1990) A species comparison of liver slice synthesis and secretion of triacylglycerol from nonesterified fatty acids in media. *Journal of Animal Science* 68, 1395–1399.

Reid, J.C.W. and Husbands, D.R. (1985) Oxidative metabolism of long-chain fatty acids in mitochondria from sheep and rat liver. Evidence that sheep conserve linoleate by limiting its oxidation. *Biochemical Journal* 225, 233–237.

Rule, D.C. (1995) Adipose tissue glycerolipid biosynthesis. In: Smith, S.B. and Smith, D.R. (eds) *The Biology of Fat in Meat Animals*. American Society of Animal Science, Champaign, Illinois, pp. 129–143.

Rule, D.C., Smith, S.B. and Romans, J.R. (1995) Fatty acid composition of muscle and adipose tissue of meat animals. In: Smith, S.B. and Smith, D.R. (eds) *The Biology of Fat in Meat Animals*. American Society of Animal Science, Champaign, Illinois, pp. 144–165.

Sardesai, V.M. (1992) Nutritional role of polyunsaturated fatty acids. *Journal of Nutritional Biochemistry* 3, 154–166.

Schoonjans, K., Staels, B. and Auwerx, J. (1996) The peroxisome proliferator activated receptors (PPARs) and their effects on lipid metabolism and adipocyte differentiation. *Biochimica et Biophysica Acta* 1302, 93–109.

Sessler, A.M. and Ntambi, J.M. (1998) Polyunsaturated fatty acid regulation of gene expression. *Journal of Nutrition* 128, 923–926.

Singh, I. (1997) Biochemistry of peroxisomes in health and disease. *Molecular and Cellular Biochemistry* 167, 1–29.

Smith, S. (1994) The animal fatty acid synthase: one gene, one polypeptide, seven enzymes. *FASEB Journal* 8, 1248–1259.

Smith, S.B. (1995) Substrate utilization in ruminant adipose tissue. In: Smith, S.B. and Smith, D.R. (eds) *The Biology of Fat in Meat Animals*. American Society of Animal Science, Champaign, Illinois, pp. 166–188.

Whitehurst, G.B., Beitz, D.C., Pothoven, M.A., Ellison, W.R. and Crump, M.H. (1978) Lactate as a precursor of fatty acids in bovine adipose tissue. *Journal of Nutrition* 108, 1806–1811.

Wiggins, D. and Gibbons, G.F. (1996) Origin of hepatic very-low-density lipoprotein triacylglycerol: the contribution of cellular phospholipid. *Biochemical Journal* 320, 673–679.

Yu, X.X., Drackley, J.K. and Odle, J. (1997) Rates of mitochondrial and peroxisomal β-oxidation of palmitate change during postnatal development and food deprivation in liver, kidney, and heart of pigs. *Journal of Nutrition* 127, 1814–1821.

Zammit, V.A. (1990) Ketogenesis in the liver of ruminants – adaptations to a challenge. *Journal of Agricultural Science (Cambridge)* 115, 155–162.

Zammit, V.A. (1996) The role of insulin in hepatic fatty acid partitioning: emerging concepts. *Biochemical Journal* 314, 1–14.

Chapter 6

Glucose Availability and Associated Metabolism

R.W. Russell and S.A. Gahr

Division of Animal and Veterinary Sciences, West Virginia University, Morgantown, West Virginia, USA

Introduction

Glucose is the sugar that is central to carbohydrate metabolism in all vertebrates. It is the carbohydrate that circulates throughout the body via blood plasma and/or cells, the concentration of which is tightly controlled. Failure of control in either direction has dire physiological consequences, e.g. coma, energy 'spillage', dehydration and vascular damage. Although the scheme of metabolism is constant throughout nature, the strategies of procuring and metabolizing carbohydrates vary markedly, even among farm animals.

Classification of animals by feeding types yields three categories: (i) herbivores, consumers of plants; (ii) carnivores, consumers of animals; and (iii) omnivores, consumers of both plants and animals. The majority of farm animals are herbivores, e.g. cattle, sheep, goats, rabbits, horses and catfish; or omnivores, e.g. swine and poultry. Carnivores have not been prominent farm animals, although fur-bearing animals are predominantly carnivores. The increase in aquaculture has also increased the number of farm animal carnivores, e.g. trout, salmonoids and alligators.

Aquaculture has also challenged traditional animal scientists to expand their understanding of metabolism to include that of carnivores and poikilotherms, cold-blooded animals.

There are three major routes by which animals procure glucose.

1. Direct enzymatic digestion and absorption of dietary carbohydrates. Non-glucose dietary carbohydrates that are absorbed are processed to glucose before passage from the liver such that extrahepatic metabolism of carbohydrate is restricted to glucose metabolism.
2. Fermentation of dietary carbohydrates by enteric microbial ecosystems. Glucose is synthesized by the host, primarily from end-products of the microbial ecosystem. Typically, fermentation chambers are located near the beginning or end of the alimentary canal, or both.
3. Direct enzymatic digestion of dietary or enteric microbial protein with absorption of peptides and amino acids. Selected amino acids from the absorbed peptides and amino acids then become substrate for gluconeogenesis, the synthesis of glucose from non-carbohydrate precursors.

The various farm animals use different routes or combination of routes to obtain blood glucose. Even within a species, the route of obtaining glucose may vary with physiological state or husbandry system. Poultry, growing swine and newborn ruminants typically will use primarily route 1. Functional ruminants will use route 2. Horses and grazing, mature swine will use a combination of routes 1 and 2. Carnivores will use primarily route 3.

Different routes of obtaining glucose are also related to different types of dietary carbohydrates. Some carbohydrates are present in the diet in an absorbable form, but most require at least some digestion for conversion to an absorbable form. Some carbohydrates can be digested only with microbial assistance. Carbohydrates of this sort are of minimal nutritional value to animals that rely on route 1 for obtaining blood glucose.

Classification of Dietary Carbohydrate

There are four major categories in classification of carbohydrates by dietary form (see Van Soest, 1994): free; intracellular; cell wall carbohydrates; and chitin (Table 6.1). From the standpoint of the plant or animal forming the food, free and intracellular carbohydrates can be considered together as non-structural carbohydrates. Cell wall carbohydrates would only be found in plant tissue and often are referred to as structural carbohydrates. Free carbohydrates are those carbohydrates that are not associated with the cellular structure of the food. They are in an absorbable form or require minimal digestion for absorption. Generally these are minor components of the diet, but there are important exceptions. Lactose in milk is included in this category and is the sole dietary carbohydrate for many newborn animals. Trehalose is a non-reducing disaccharide of glucose found in the haemolymph of insects and is a readily available form of dietary carbohydrate of insect-eating animals. Fructose in honey is another example in a natural food.

Table 6.1. Classification of carbohydrate by dietary form.

I. Free – not associated with the cellular structure of food
  A. Lactose – milk
  B. Fructose – honey
  C. Trehalose – haemolymph
II. Intracellular – inside the cell
  A. Soluble – dissolved in the cytosol of cell
  B. Storage polysaccharide
    a. Starches
      1. Amylose, $\alpha1$–4 glucose polymer
      2. Amylopectin $\alpha1$–4 and $\alpha1$–6 glucose polymer
      3. Glycogen, $\alpha1$–4 and $\alpha1$–6 glucose polymer
    b. Fructans
      1. Levans, $\beta2$–6 fructose polymer
      2. Inulins, $\beta2$–1 fructose polymer
III. Cell wall
  A. Cellulose, $\beta1$–4 glucose polymer
  B. Hemicellulose, $\beta1$–4 xylose polymer
  C. Pectin, $\alpha1$–4 galacturonic acid
  D. Gums, $\beta1$–4 and $\beta1$–3 polymers of various sugars
  E. Lignin, phenylpropenoid polymers (not carbohydrate)
IV. Chitin, $\beta1$–4 N-acetylglucosamine polymer
  A. Exoskeleton
  B. Cell wall

Intracellular carbohydrate is divided into two subcategories: soluble and storage polysaccharide. Soluble intracellular carbohydrate includes those carbohydrates that are soluble in the cytoplasm of cells. Most common feed ingredients contain <5% soluble sugars (Webster and Hoover, 1998), but some ingredients contain much more. Citrus pulp contains ~300 g kg^{-1}, and soybean meal and hays harvested in an early vegetative stage contain ~100 g kg^{-1} of the dry matter (DM) as free sugars. Maize plants harvested for silage are rich in soluble sugars but these sugars serve as substrates for fermentation and very few remain after ensiling. Care must be taken in interpretation of these data because some analyses may include fructans in the soluble sugars.

Storage polysaccharides are also divided into two major subcategories: starches and fructans. Starches include glycogen, also referred to as animal starch, and various mixtures of amylose and amylopectin. Amylose is a linear polymer of glucose linked by α1–4 glycosidic bonds. There are typically 1000–2000 glucose monomers per molecule of amylose. Amylopectin also is a polymer made solely of glucose. It differs from amylose because it is branched and it is larger. The general structure of amylopectin resembles that of a tree. There is a single trunk with a reducing end (free carbon 1 hydroxyl) elongated with other glucose monomers attached by α1–4 glycosidic bonds. From this single trunk, branch points are formed by α1–6 glycosidic bonds. The branches are elongated by glucose monomers linked by α1–4 glycosidic bonds. On average, there are branch points every 20–25 glucose residues. There may be up to 200,000 glucose monomers per molecule of amylopectin. Glycogen is similar to amylopectin but is more branched. Glycogen contains a branch point approximately every 10–12 glucose residues. There is no reducing end on glycogen. The 'trunk' of glycogen is anchored on a specific glycoprotein, glycogenin.

Starches make up ~700 g kg^{-1} of the DM of cereal grains, and ~300 g kg^{-1} of the DM of fruits, roots and tubers, and are the principal storage polysaccharide of tropical grasses. Starches, therefore, are a principal constituent of the diet of many farm animals, and at least potentially are digestible by enzymes produced by animals. The properties of the starch are determined primarily by the proportions of amylose and amylopectin in the starch, the degree of crystallinity of the starch and the degree of interaction of starch and protein. This is obvious to the baker who will select different types of flour (starch) depending on whether he is making bread, pastries or pizza crust. Digestion is also influenced by the type of starch. Starches may be rapidly and completely digested, slowly but completely digested, partially digested or resistant to digestion. Knowledge of these properties and how the properties can be altered by processing is important in formulating diets.

Fructans are a second group of intracellular storage polysaccharides. Fructans are polymers of fructose attached by β2–6 (levans) or β2–1 (inulins) to each other and to a sucrose primer. Fructans, therefore, have no reducing end. There are ~30 fructose monomers in a molecule of fructan. The fructans are the principal storage polysaccharide of temperate grasses. Levans are typical of grasses and are more soluble than inulins. Fructans are soluble in water and are digested rapidly by enteric microorganisms but are not digested by digestive enzymes produced by animals. The glycosidic linkages of fructans are hydrolysed easily by acid. This, along with their water solubility, may include fructans in the intracellular soluble carbohydrate category.

Cell wall carbohydrates are also referred to as structural carbohydrates. There are four major types of carbohydrates in this group: cellulose; hemicellulose; pectins; and gums. All of the carbohydrates in this group require microbial enzymes for digestion. Cellulose is a linear polymer of glucose linked by β1–4 glycosidic bonds. Cellulose is the most abundant organic compound on earth. There are ~10,000 glucose monomers per molecule of cellulose. The β1–4 linkages of cellulose versus the α1–4 linkages of amylose cause marked differences in the properties of the two polymers. Cellulose has a flat, straight structure. This allows cellulose molecules to align tightly together in straight, parallel rows to provide structural rigidity. Despite the rather simple chemical definition of cellulose, the nutritional characteristics of cellulose vary from indigestible to completely digestible by enteric microbes independently of a host. Cellulose interacts with other cell wall components such as hemicellulose, lignin, pectin, cutin and minerals to various extents. The extent and nature of the interactions alter the nutritional characteristics of the cellulose.

Hemicellulose is more heterogeneous than cellulose, with the overall composition of hemicellulose differing from one plant species to another. Generally, the base polymer is xylose linked by β1–4 glycosidic bonds. The degree of branching varies from nearly linear to highly branched. The branches usually are polymers of arabinose or uronic acid, but both types of branches will not be present on the same molecule of hemicellulose. The interactions of hemicellulose and lignin are numerous and varied. Exposure of hemicellulose to gastric digestion improves its digestibility by enteric microorganisms.

Pectin is a water-soluble polymer composed primarily of galacturonic acid linked by $\alpha1–4$ glycosidic bonds. Pectin serves as a 'cement' that holds the various components of the cell wall together. The carboxyl moieties of galacturonic acid are cross-linked by Ca^{2+}. Phosphates in the lumen of the alimentary canal chelate the Ca^{2+} and solubilize the pectin. Enteric microorganisms rapidly ferment pectin, but the $\alpha1–4$ bonds are not a substrate for amylases. Galactose, being a C4-epimer of glucose, makes the C4-hydroxy of pectin axial rather than equatorial as in glucose. Thus the $\alpha1–4$ galactosidic bond is similar in character to a $\beta1–4$ glucosidic bond. Pectin, however, is not a flat molecule like cellulose but tends to coil like amylose. Interspersed in the galacturonic chains are rhamnose moieties inserted with $\alpha1–4$ and 2–4 rhamnosyl galacturonate linkages. The vicinal linkages with rhamnose cause sharp bends in the pectin polymer.

Various gums are found in the cell wall of the seeds of many plants. The gums are polymers of various sugars linked $\beta1–4$ with $\beta1–3$ branch points. The branching prevents these molecules from packing together, rendering them as open structures that are soluble in water or form viscous gels in water. The gums are indigestible by mammalian enzymes but are fermented readily by enteric microorganisms.

Another important component of the cell wall is lignin. Lignin is not a carbohydrate and is, for the most part, indigestible, but lignin does affect the digestion of cell wall carbohydrates. Lignin is an extremely variable structure made primarily of polymers of phenylprope(a)noid monomers. Phenylpropenoid compounds are strong electron sinks that polymerize by free-radical condensation. Lignin influences digestion by encrustation of potentially digestible cell wall carbohydrates. Lignins can also complex with digestive enzymes or glycoprotein substrate to inhibit digestion.

Chitin is the second most abundant organic compound on earth. Chitin forms the cell walls of lower plants and the exoskeleton of arthropods. Chitin is a linear polymer of N-acetyl-glucosamine linked by $\beta1–4$ glycosidic bonds. Chitinase, the hydrolytic enzyme for chitin, is found in a wide variety of animals as well as being produced by enteric microflora (Stevens and Hume, 1995).

Procurement of Carbon

Direct absorbers

Direct digestion and absorption of dietary carbohydrate is the most efficient method of obtaining carbohydrate if large quantities of substrate are available in the diet (Table 6.2). Swine and poultry are the major groups of farm animals that rely predominantly, but not solely, on the direct digestion and absorption of dietary carbohydrates. Rabbits and grain-fed fish would also be included in this category. This group contains wide diversity in the structure of the alimentary canal.

Swine

We will begin with a discussion of swine because the structure of the alimentary canal in swine most closely resembles that of humans. The natural diet of swine consists primarily of starch foods such as roots, tubers and nuts that are harvested by rooting with their rigid snout (Ensminger, 1991) and chewed thoroughly prior to swallowing. Grains are the source of starch for the Western swine industry, although swine are still used as a part of the 'garbage disposal' system in China and developing countries. While being chewed, ingesta is insalivated with a mixture of mucus and

Table 6.2. Summary of carbohydrate digestion in direct absorbers.

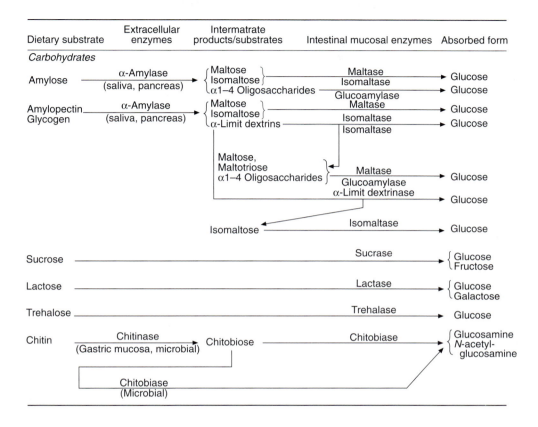

Dietary substrate	Extracellular enzymes	Intermatrate products/substrates	Intestinal mucosal enzymes	Absorbed form
Carbohydrates				
Amylose	α-Amylase (saliva, pancreas)	Maltose, Isomaltose, α1–4 Oligosaccharides	Maltase Isomaltase / Glucoamylase	Glucose, Glucose
Amylopectin, Glycogen	α-Amylase (saliva, pancreas)	Maltose, Isomaltose, α-Limit dextrins	Maltase Isomaltase Isomaltase	Glucose, Glucose
		Maltose, Maltotriose α1–4 Oligosaccharides	Maltase Glucoamylase α-Limit dextrinase	Glucose, Glucose
		Isomaltose	Isomaltase	Glucose
Sucrose			Sucrase	{ Glucose Fructose
Lactose			Lactase	{ Glucose Galactose
Trehalose			Trehalase	Glucose
Chitin	Chitinase (Gastric mucosa, microbial)	Chitobiose	Chitobiase	{ Glucosamine N-acetyl-glucosamine
	Chitobiase (Microbial)			

serous saliva containing α-amylase from the parotid salivary glands. Swine, like most farm species, do not have an abundant supply of salivary amylase (Vonk and Western, 1984). The ingesta is formed into a bolus by the tongue and swallowed.

The importance of salivary amylase in those species that posses it is poorly defined and probably under-appreciated. Typically, it is assumed that salivary amylase is inactivated rapidly by the acid environment in the stomach. It requires a measurable time for boli entering the stomach to be disrupted by the churning action of the stomach and, hence, stomach acid slowly penetrates the boli. In humans consuming a starchy meal, 40% of the starch is digested in the stomach (Vonk and Western, 1984). Salivary amylase activity eventually is overpowered by pancreatic amylase in terms of starch digestion *per se.*

The extent of salivary amylase activity expressed in the stomach, however, would be expected to affect the viscosity of digesta in animals consuming starchy feeds. Viscosity is a factor in rates of passage and digestion. Thus salivary amylase could affect practical factors as the glycaemic index and feed intake.

There are no other carbohydrases added to the ingesta until the digesta enters the small intestine. Thus the acidic material entering the small intestine from the stomach will contain native starch, dextrins resulting from partial digestion of starch and other saccharides contained in the feeds, e.g. sucrose, lactose, mannose, fructose, glucose, trehalose, chitin and cellulose. The carbohydrates must be digested to their monosaccharide units for absorption.

Continued processing of the carbohydrates requires interaction of the digesta with gut tissues. The presence of acid in the duodenum sensitizes the mucosa to release the hormone, secretin. Secretin stimulates the exocrine pancreas to secrete approximately isotonic bicarbonate solution into the lumen of the intestine. A pH-neutral environment is essential to maintain the activity of the digestive enzymes present in the intestinal tract and to allow the fragile surface necessary for absorption. Peptides generated by gastric digestion of dietary proteins or lipids are necessary in the digesta to stimulate the intestinal mucosa to release the hormone, cholecystokinin (CCK). CCK stimulates the exocrine pancreas to release digestive enzymes, some in the form of zymogens, into the lumen of the intestine. The pancreatic secretions are carried to the intestine via the pancreatic duct and common bile duct. CCK also causes relaxation of the sphincter of Oddi, an area of increased tonation where the common bile duct enters the duodenum, and which prevents backflux of intestinal contents into the liver and pancreas.

Pancreatic amylase enters the intestinal lumen in an active form where it mixes with the digesta and continues catalysing hydrolysis of the α1–4 glycosidic bonds in starch and dextrins in a random manner as initiated by salivary amylase. The end-products of starch digestion by amylase are maltose (disaccharide of glucose with α1–4 linkage), maltotriose (trisaccharide of glucose with α1–4 linkage) and α-limit dextrins. The α-limit dextrins have various structures. They contain the α1–6 linkage of the branch points of amylopectin. The number of glucose units before and after the branch point and the length of the branch vary. α-Amylase does not hydrolyse the glucose unit immediately before or until two glucose units after branch points (Newsholme and Leech, 1989). The minimum size, therefore, of α-limit dextrin is five glucose units, but the average size is eight glucose units. No free glucose is released by α-amylase-catalysed hydrolysis of starch (Alpers, 1987).

Completion of starch digestion is catalysed by saccharidases attached to the brush border of the small intestine. There is some disagreement as to the relative importance of the saccharidases (Gray et al., 1979; Taraval et al., 1983; Rodriguez et al., 1984), but for swine it appears that α-limit dextrinase is most active in hydrolysing oligosaccharides. Limit dextrins are hydrolysed to multiple units of glucose and isomaltose (disaccharide of glucose linked by a α1–6 bond). The isomaltose then is hydrolysed to glucose by isomaltase, although isomaltase could cleave the α1–6 bond first, generating substrate for maltase and glucoamylase. Maltose and maltotriose are hydrolysed to glucose by maltase. Longer α1–4 oligosaccharides are hydrolysed one glucose unit at a time from the non-reducing end by glucoamylase.

Dietary disaccharides are hydrolysed by brush border disaccharidases. Sucrose, plentiful in fruits and cell solubles, is hydrolysed by sucrase to fructose and glucose. Sucrose should not be included in the diet of neonatal pigs and most other animals because sucrase activity is not expressed in most young animals (Kidder and Manners, 1980). Lactose, the sugar found in milk, is hydrolysed to galactose and glucose by lactase. Trehalose, plentiful in algae and fungi and the main circulating carbohydrate of insects, is hydrolysed to glucose by trehalase.

The pH optimum for these enzymes is ~6.0. Intestinal pH is maintained near neutral by the secretin–pancreas system described above. The K_m of the enzymes for sugars range from ~1 to 20 mM (Alpers, 1987). The difference in K_ms for α-limit dextrins between isomaltase and α-limit dextrinase may explain some of the controversy concerning their importance. The difference is about an order of magnitude, so isomaltase activity may appear more important when α-limit dextrin is plentiful and α-limit dextrinase more important when substrate is less plentiful.

With the exception of lactase in mature animals and sucrase in young animals, the capacity for digestion exceeds the capacity for absorption. After a meal containing disaccharides, monosaccharides accumulate in the intestinal lumen (Alpers,

1987). The activities of the intestinal saccharidases vary along the length of both the intestine (Vonk and Western, 1984) and the villus (Alpers, 1987). There are a number of factors that affect enzyme activity along the length of the villus. Cells differentiate as they migrate from the crypt to the villus tip and change their pattern of proteins synthesized. Different enzymes also have different half-lives on the brush border. This is due primarily to pancreatic proteases hydrolysing the glycoprotein anchors of the disaccharidases and releasing them into the lumen. In some species, including swine, the activities of some membrane saccharidases such as sucrase and maltase are modified differentially, but lactase activity is rather constant (Karasov and Hume, 1997). The distinction between luminal and membrane digestion becomes blurred. Membrane enzymes are released into the lumen by proteases and cell sloughing; in contrast, pancreatic amylase adheres, to some extent, to the enterocyte membrane (Alpers, 1987).

In the scheme of digestion of dietary carbohydrates, most of the absorbable monosaccharides are generated on the surface of the absorptive enterocytes. Logically, this would enhance the efficiency of absorption (Ugolev, 1968), but this logic is questioned (Alpers, 1987). Glucose is the major monosaccharide available for absorption from most practical diets. It is believed that glucose is absorbed by both transcellular and paracellular routes. The paracellular route, however, is dependent on the transcellular route.

The major transcellular route is the Na^+-dependent co-transport system (SGLT1). There are several reviews on the mechanism of SGLT1 (Semenza *et al.*, 1984; Hopfer, 1987; Baly and Horuk, 1988; Widdas, 1988; Wright, 1993). Na^+ is the primary solute transported. Glucose is a co-solute. In the absence of Na^+, glucose cannot be transported. Under *in vitro* conditions, other cations may substitute for Na^+ although less effectively, but Na^+ is virtually the sole binding cation *in vivo*. The preponderance of data suggest a single SGLT1 in the intestine with a 2:1

Na^+:glucose stoichiometric ratio. There is some support, however, for two Na^+-dependent transporters in the intestine with different affinities for glucose and 1:1 and 2:1 or even 3:1 Na^+:glucose stoichiometric ratios, more similar to renal proximal tubule glucose transporters.

Apical membrane events of the SGLT1 transport system appear to follow an ordered mechanism. The first Na^+ binds to a luminal portion of the SGLT1 protein referred to as the gate. The gate has a valence of -1 or -2. Binding of the first Na^+ causes the gate to extend and expose the binding site for glucose to the luminal contents. Binding of Na^+ also decreases the K_m for glucose. Glucose binds, followed by binding of a second Na^+, causing the gate to be neutralized or changed to a positive charge. The gate snaps back, translocating the binding sites to the cytosolic surface of the enterocyte. The intracellular concentration of Na^+ is much lower than the extracellular concentration and therefore Na^+ dissociates from SGLT1. Dissociation of Na^+ increases the K_m for glucose and the glucose dissociates. The second Na^+ dissociates, returning a negative valence to the 'gate'. The electrical gradient of the cell membrane (inside negative) slowly returns the 'gate' of SGLT1 to the luminal surface. Return of protein with empty binding sites from the interior to the exterior of the apical membrane is the rate-limiting step.

The affinity of SGLT1 for Na^+ is dependent on the electrical potential of the membrane. At 0 and -150 mV, the K_m for Na^+ is 50 and 5 mM Na^+, respectively. Under physiological conditions, the electrical potential is estimated to be approximately -120 mV. Luminal, intracellular and extracellular concentrations of Na^+ typically are 150, 10 and 150 mM Na^+, respectively (Guyton, 1971; Ferraris *et al.*, 1990). Likewise, the affinity of SGLT1 for glucose is dependent on Na^+ concentration. At 2 and 100 mM Na^+, the K_m for glucose is >10 and <0.1 mM glucose, respectively. The luminal and intracellular concentrations of glucose vary and are difficult to measure. Both increase during the absorptive state. The intracellular concentration increases from <0.4 mM in the non-absorptive state to several mM during the absorptive state. The range in concentration will be even more for luminal glucose concentration, conservatively estimated from 0.2 to ~50 mM (Ferraris *et al.*, 1990). Glucose concentration in the unstirred layer can be estimated only with uncertainty, and may exceed several hundred mM (Pappenheimer, 1993). Measurements of K_ms were made for luminal substrates. Assuming the K_ms are similar on the cytosolic surface, SGLT1 will be loaded with substrate on the luminal surface and substrates unloaded on the cytosolic surface. A summary diagram is provided in Fig. 6.1.

The SGLT1 system for glucose transport is active, requiring expenditure of ATP. The events on the apical membrane that bring glucose into the enterocyte do not involve direct hydrolysis of ATP. Na^+ is the primary solute and is transported down an electrochemical gradient requiring no energy. The secondary solute, glucose, can be carried up a concentration gradient with no immediate expenditure of ATP. Energy must be used, however, to maintain the electrochemical gradient for Na^+. The Na^+ gradient is maintained by the Na^+/K^+-exchange ATPase pump on the basolateral membrane of the enterocytes. Exchange of intracellular Na^+ for extracellular K^+ requires hydrolysis of an ATP. Inhibition of the exchange pump quickly stops active absorption of glucose.

A second means for transepithelial transport of sugars is the GLUT5 transporter protein. GLUT5 catalyses insulin-independent facilitated diffusion of monosaccharides across the apical membrane of enterocytes. Carbohydrate-facilitated diffusion transporters, GLUT1–GLUT5, have been reviewed (Baly and Horuk, 1988; Widdas, 1988; Birnbaum, 1992; Elsas and Longo, 1992; Pessin and Bell, 1992; Thorens, 1992, 1993; Bird *et al.*, 1996; Olson and Pessin, 1996). Despite the name GLUT5, glucose is not transported by GLUT5. GLUT5 is the major route of uptake for fructose, and fructose uptake is not inhibited by the presence of glucose. The transporter is present on the apical membrane of enterocytes from approxi-

mately mid-villus to the tip. Other sugars not actively transported, such as ribose, mannose, arabinose, glucosamine, *N*-acetylglucosamine and xylose, are probably transported by GLUT5. Galactose shares SGLT1 with glucose.

Transport of glucose across the basolateral membrane of the enterocyte is an important component of the paracellular route of glucose absorption. Thus, basolateral glucose transport will be presented before discussing paracellular absorption. GLUT2 is the transporter that catalyses transport of glucose across the basolateral membrane. The process is insulin-independent facilitated diffusion. GLUT2 is expressed on the basolateral membranes of mature enterocytes, i.e. from the sides of the villi to the tip but not at the base or in the crypts. GLUT2 is characterized by a high K_m and high V_{max}. The intestinal GLUT2 displays slight asymmetry with regard to transport kinetics. The K_m for glucose efflux is 23 mM glucose, approximately half that of the K_m of influx (48 mM glucose); favouring glucose efflux from the enterocyte. Transport asymmetry is not unique. GLUT1, the erythrocyte glucose transporter, has a difference between efflux and influx K_ms of approximately an order of magnitude, favouring influx. The GLUT2 expressed in hepatocytes and pancreatic islet cells is symmetrical. GLUT2 transports glucose, galactose and fructose, the major sugars absorbed by a transcellular route. Other absorbed sugars are probably transported by GLUT2.

Accumulation of solutes of active transport (Na^+, glucose, amino acids) stimulates paracellular absorption (for reviews, see Madara, 1988; Pappenheimer, 1993; Ballard *et al.*, 1995; Pappenheimer, 1998). Paracellular transport cannot occur in the absence of active transport. Thus active transport provides most of the driving force for paracellular transport. What is clear is that during the rapid absorptive state *in vivo*, the SGLT1 system is saturated. The mechanisms for the connections are not determined fully and the hypothesis itself is not accepted universally (Ferraris *et al.*, 1990; Fine *et al.*, 1993). It appears that absorbed solutes

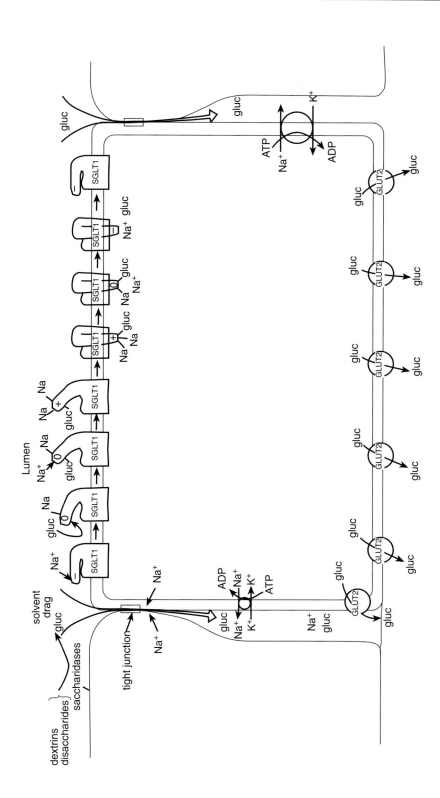

Fig. 6.1. Absorption of glucose through the small intestine.

establish a standing osmotic gradient in the epithelial interstitium that increases water transport from the lumen to the interstitium. There is no debate on this part of the hypothesis. What is not established is the proportion of water entering the interstitium by transcellular versus paracellular routes. The Pappenheimer hypothesis suggests that the intracellular Na^+ induced by active transport triggers a contraction of the cytoskeleton that causes a rearrangement of the tight junction proteins and making the junction more porous. This is a point of contention, but has good support. Cytochalasin D, which also stimulates con-traction of the cytoskeleton of enterocytes, increases tight-junction permeability to an extent similar to that observed concomitant with active glucose absorption. In large animals, the proportion of glucose absorbed via the paracellular route may be much greater than carrier-mediated absorption. It cannot be construed, however, that the para-cellular route is more important because the paracellular route will not operate in the absence of an active transport system.

Generally, most of the α-linked glucose polymers, lactose and sucrose (except in neonates) are digested and absorbed during the transit time of the digesta through the small intestine. Starches that are resistant to the digestive process are not common in feedstuffs fed to swine. Digestion-resistant starches are those that form crystalline starch granules. Sorghum harvested as high moisture, then dried and fed without further processing, contains some resistant starch. The quantity of resistant starch in legume seed is significant. The resistant starch and fibre (fructans and cell wall carbohydrates) will pass into the caecum and large intestine to provide substrate for the enteric microorganisms. Fermentation by the microorganisms does not provide an important source of energy for growing and finishing swine, but hindgut fermentation can provide a substantial energy source for the breeding herd. Independently of the magnitude of energy supply to the host, hindgut fermentation is an important process. Details of hindgut fermentation will be discussed in a subsequent section.

Poultry

Much of the previous discussion on swine is also applicable to poultry, but there are important differences in poultry (Duke, 1986a,b). The beak replaces the lips and teeth. Feed is consumed, one peck at a time; hence there is very little residence time per peck in the oral cavity. Lacking a soft palate, poultry raise their heads to swallow in order to prevent ingesta from filling the nasal cavity. Dry, non-pelleted feeds often are moistened prior to ingesting with saliva or water carried in the beak and dumped on the feed. This practice causes practical problems in maintaining feed intake and freshness of the feed. Most poultry feeds are pelleted. Pellets more closely resembling the natural diet of seeds, insects, worms, berries and carrion are easier for the birds to ingest and the pellets are not moistened before ingestion.

The lumen of the oesophagus is very large relative to the size of the animal in order to accommodate the lack of physical breakdown of ingesta in the oral cavity. The oesophagus is divided into three distinct sections: the pre-crop oesophagus; the crop; and the post-crop oesophagus. The crop is a distensible pouch in the oesophagus that stores the ingesta during meals. Between meals, the crop meters ingesta to the post-crop oesophagus and gastric digestion. Salivary and oesophageal secretions, mostly mucus, are added to the ingesta during its retention in the crop. The saliva of poultry lacks amylase, although that of some wild birds, e.g. sparrows, contains amylase. Amylase is present in the crop contents of poultry. The sources are primarily bacteria ingested with the feed and the feed itself. As much as 25% of the ingested starch may be converted to sugars in the crop, and ~10% of the starch disappears during storage in the crop. Disappearance is due to microbial fermentation and absorption of glucose through the crop wall.

As material is metered from the crop through the post-crop oesophagus, it traverses the proventriculus. The proventriculus is the secretory portion of the stomach releasing HCl, pepsinogen, intrinsic factor and chitinase. Chitinase activity in poultry is much less than in insectivorous birds, but adequate to hydrolyse approximately one-third of purified shrimp chitin added to normal diets (Vonk and Western, 1984). Its lumen is approximately the same size as the oesophagus. The ingesta is mixed thoroughly with gastric secretions in the ventriculus (gizzard). The ventriculus is the site where both physical and chemical digestion is initiated as a major effort. Each batch of digesta entering the ventriculus is churned into a pulpy consistency by muscular contractions.

The digesta passes into the small intestine and is processed similarly to what was discussed for swine. Poultry, however, lack lactase. No chitinobiase is found in either the small intestine or the pancreas. The function of chitinase, therefore, is mainly to solubilize chitin in order to enhance digestion of other nutrients in the feedstuff, rather than to obtain energy from chitin itself. Relative to body size, the length of the small intestine is short. There is some question of the completeness of starch digestion and absorption in the small intestine. The proximal caeca has SGLT1 activity similar to that expressed in mid-small intestine (Planas *et al.*, 1986; Vinardell *et al.*, 1986). The extent of glucose absorption from the caeca in commercial production systems is unknown.

Other

Hindgut fermenters and carnivores will also process digesta similarly to direct absorbers. They too are direct absorbers but have alternative routes for obtaining a substantial portion of their carbohydrate carbon. Very strict carnivores have a reduced capacity for digesting carbohydrate, and excess carbohydrate in their diet may impede their ability to digest protein.

Fermenters

Pre-gastric fermentation

Ruminant animals rely on pre-gastric fermentation for initial processing of ingesta. Ruminants actually harvest nutrients to supply a complex microbial ecosystem inhabiting their forestomach. The ruminant obtains its nutrients from the wastes and effluent from the fermentation. There are ~20–25 billion bacteria and 200,000–2 million protozoa ml^{-1} of ruminal fluids. The population of fungi is more variable and the role of fungi defined less accurately. The rumen of an adult dairy cow has a capacity of ~210 l. The number of microorganisms inhabiting the rumen of a single cow exceeds the world's human population by 1 million-fold! The fundamentals of this complex system were established by the classic work of Hungate (1966), and this has been updated recently (Hobson and Stewart, 1997). More general reviews are available (Church, 1988; Van Soest, 1994).

To ruminate means to chew again, hence the name ruminant. The process of rumination is essential for efficient metabolism of fibrous feeds. Ruminants are meal-feeding animals, eating twice per day each morning and evening. The ruminal ecosystem is most efficient if fermentation is continuous at a constant rate. Microorganisms do not have the ability to store nutrients during times of abundance for use when nutrients are limited; they grow by dividing and their metabolism is most efficient during the exponential growth phase. Cycling of nutrient availability causes surges in microbial growth followed by periods of maintenance metabolism with little cell division. Rumination converts the meal-feeding habits of the ruminants into a continuous feeding regimen for the microorganisms. Ruminants consume large quantities of coarse feeds rapidly. As the feeds are ingested, not all of the material is available immediately as a substrate for the microorganisms. The waxy cuticle on the surface of plants impedes microbial digestion. The microorganisms attack the broken ends and places where there are nicks in the cuticle. The nearly continual process of rumination continues to provide 'new substrate' to the microorganisms long after the meal has been consumed. The digestion by microorganisms causes loci of structural weakness in the plant material that are fractured by the mixing contractions of the rumen (Ulyatt *et al.*, 1986). Rumination is also a potent stimulus for salivation. The continual addition of saliva to the fermentation helps neutralize acids generated by fermentation. This is important because acid inhibits fermentation.

The feeds consumed by ruminants to be digested by the microbial ecosystem are physically much larger than the microorganisms themselves. The microorganisms, therefore, must solubilize the feeds by secreting enzymes to digest the feed chemically into soluble components. There are many different enzymes manufactured intracellularly by the microorganisms for excretion into the ruminal environment in various forms. These enzymes include cellulases, hemicellulases, pectinases, amylases, proteases and lipases. There are multiple enzymes within each class that act concurrently in hydrolysing the substrate into a soluble, absorbable form. The enzymes may be released altruistically into the environment of the microorganism, i.e. whatever effect the released enzyme has in making soluble substrate available to the microorganisms by catalysing hydrolysis of substrate, the soluble products of hydrolysis are available to any microorganism in the area. The released enzyme may remain attached to the exterior surface of the secreting microorganism similarly to the brush border enzymes described previously. As the microorganism comes in contact with substrate, the solubilized products are generated in very close proximity to the cell that manufactured the enzyme. Many microorganisms attach themselves to the 'surface' (keep in mind this is an inner surface of the substrate to which the microorganism gained access via a nick in the outer surface, i.e. the substrates are digested from the inside to the outside) of the substrate by means of a glycoprotein matrix between the cell wall of the substrate and the cell wall of the microorganism. This is the predominant mode of digestion (Cheng *et al.*, 1991). Enzymes are secreted into the space enclosed by the glycoprotein matrix. As substrate is solubilized, the products are captured by the glycoprotein matrix, making these nutrients available only to the microorganism that secreted the enzyme. Some microorganisms secrete enzymes that hydrolyse the structural components of plant material but do not use the solubilized products as an energy substrate. Like the chitinase activity in poultry, this hydrolysis is necessary to gain access to more desirable substrate. The solubilized structural components, however, are used as substrate by other species of microorganisms.

Not all microorganisms have the same complement of enzymes in the same proportions. Ruminal microorganisms can be organized into 11 groups by substrate and product preferences (Yokoyama and Johnson, 1988), though there is considerable overlap of species among the substrate/product-grouping scheme.

1. Cellulolytic, e.g. *Bacteroides succinogens*, *Ruminococcus flavefaciens*, *Ruminococcus albus* and *Butyrivibrio fibrisolvens*.
2. Hemicellulolytic, e.g. *Butyrivibrio fibrisolvens*, *Bacteroides ruminicola* and *Ruminococcus* sp.
3. Pectinolytic, e.g. *Butyrivibrio fibrisolvens*, *Bacteroides ruminicola*, *Lachnospira multiparus*, *Succinivibrio dextrinosolvens*, *Treponema bryantii* and *Streptococcus bovis*.
4. Amylolytic, e.g. *Bacteroides amylophilus*, *Streptococcus bovis*, *Succinimonas amylolytica* and *Bacteroides ruminicola*.
5. Ureolytic, e.g. *Succinivibrio dextrinosolvens*, *Selenomonas* sp., *Bacteroides ruminicola*, *Ruminococcus bromii*, *Butyrivibrio* sp. and *Treponema* sp.
6. Methanogens, e.g. *Methanobrevibacter ruminantium*, *Methanobacterium formicicum* and *Methanomicrobium mobile*.
7. Sugar-utilizing, e.g. *Treponema bryantii*, *Lactobacillus vitulinus* and *Lactobacillus ruminus*.
8. Acid-utilizing, e.g. *Megasphera elsdenii* and *Selenomonas ruminantium*.
9. Proteolytic, e.g. *Bacteroides amylophilus*, *Bacteroides ruminicola*, *Butyrivibrio fibrisolvens* and *Streptococcus bovis*.
10. Ammonia-producing, e.g. *Bacteroides ruminicola*, *Megasphera elsdenii* and *Selenomonas ruminantium*.

11. Lipolytic, e.g. *Anaerovigrio lipolytica*, *Butyrivibrio fibrisolvens*, *Treponema bryantii*, *Eubacterium* sp., *Fusocillus* sp. and *Micrococcus* sp.

After solubilizing substrates, the soluble nutrients are transported across the plasma membrane of the microbial cell. The major soluble substrates derived from dietary carbohydrates are glucose, cellobiose, xylose and galacturonic acid. The soluble carbohydrates enter microbial cells via an ATP-driven active transport system similar to that described previously or via a phosphoenolpyruvate (PEP)-dependent phosphotransferase system (PTS) (Fig. 6.2) (Konings *et al.*, 1986; Erni, 1992). High-energy phosphate is transferred from PEP in glycolysis through a series of phospho-protein intermediates to a sugar being transported across the plasma membrane. The first two proteins, EI and HPr, are cytosolic and are intermediates common to all sugars being transported. The other two protein intermediates are sugar-specific, EIII^{sugarx} and EII^{sugarx}. EIII may be either cytosolic or membrane-bound. The dephosphorylated form of EIII (dephosphorylated because sugar x is being transported rapidly from the medium into the cell) binds to ATP-driven permeases in the cell membrane inhibiting them. The EIII~P form (which accumulates when sugar x is unavailable in the medium) activates adenylate cyclase to generate cAMP to turn on synthesis of other sugar transport proteins. EII is a transmembrane protein that binds sugar x on the outside surface of the membrane, phosphorylates the sugar, and releases the phosphorylated sugar into the cytosol of the cell. Coupling transport with phosphorylation conserves ATP. If the sugar is cellobiose, even more ATP savings are realized. The PTS will release cellobiose phosphate (on C-6 of the reducing sugar) on the interior of the cell. Phosphorylysis then will yield glucose-6-phosphate and a glucose-1-phosphate.

The ATP-dependent systems usually are symport transporters, with the specific sugars being the co-solute as in SGLT1. The primary solute is a proton or Na$^+$. As with SGLT1, both solutes must bind on the exterior prior to protein conformational change in order to bring the solutes to the interior. The K_ms of solutes when the binding sites are on the interior of the membrane are high, causing release of the solutes and preventing transport to the exterior. The primary solute is pumped out of the cell at the expense of ATP.

The Embden–Meyerhof–Parnas glycolytic pathway is the basis for metabolism of the phosphorylated sugars under anaerobic conditions (Fig. 6.3) to pyruvate. Pentoses, dietary and derived from decarboxylation of galacturonic acid of pectins, enter glycolysis via the pentose phosphate shunt. An alternative route of metabolism of pentoses is the pentose phosphate phospho-ketolase reaction. In this reaction, ribulose-5-phosphate (an intermediate of the pentose phosphate shunt) is phosphorylated (cleavage of a carbon–carbon bond by addition of phosphate) to glyceraldehyde-3-phosphate (an intermediate in glycolysis) and acetyl-phosphate. With this exception noted, virtually all carbon entering the ruminal anaerobic fermentation is converted to pyruvate. In conversion of 1 mol of hexose to pyruvate there are 2–5 mol of ATP generated by substrate-level phosphorylation, depending on the transport system used in getting the carbohydrate into the cells, and 2 mol of reducing power generated (NAD$^+$→NADH,H$^+$). The NADH,H$^+$ must be oxidized for glycolysis to continue. Thus reactions that produce NADH,H$^+$ must be balanced with reactions that consume NADH,H$^+$.

The secondary degradation of pyruvate in ruminal fermentation differs from that of mammalian glycolysis. Lactate, although an intermediate in ruminal fermentation, is not an end-product of a normal, healthy fermentation. The major end-products of a normal fermentation are acetate, propionate, butyrate, CO$_2$ and CH$_4$. A typical molar ratio of acetate:propionate:butyrate is 66:20:14. Balancing this molar production ratio of volatile fatty acids (VFAs) for redox potential (Wolin, 1960), the molar ratio for major end-products is 34:10:8:30:18, for acetate, propionate, butyrate, CO$_2$ and CH$_4$, respectively. Expressing these values as

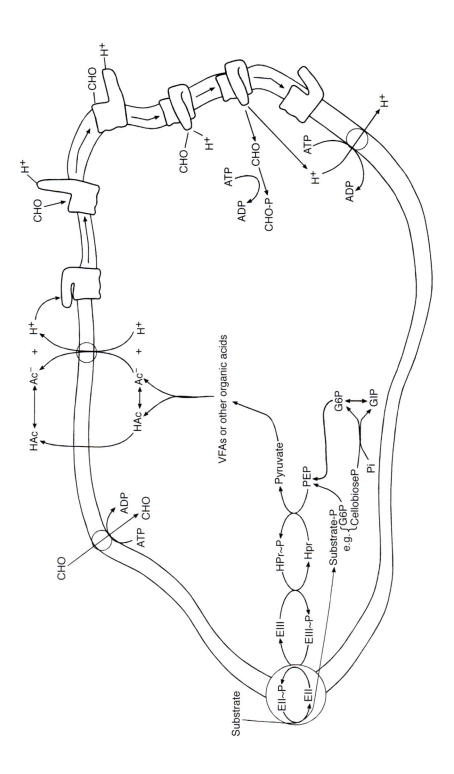

Fig. 6.2. Absorption of carbohydrates by enteric microorganisms.

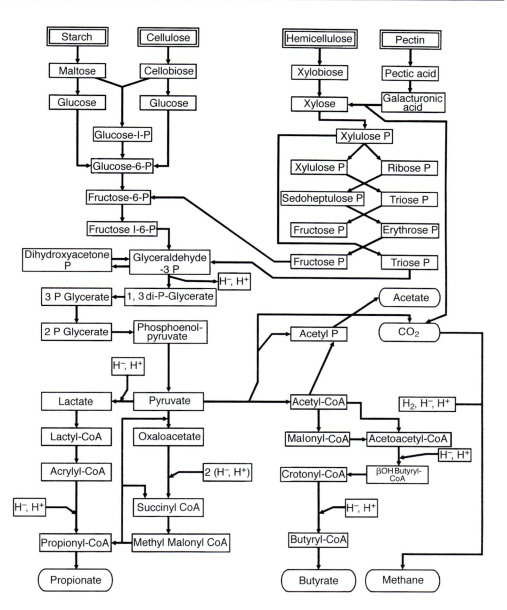

Fig. 6.3. Summary of ruminal fermentation (modified from Czerkawski, 1986).

percentage carbon fermented yields 38, 17, 17, 17 and 11%. Management practices such as diet and meal frequency influence these ratios: grains increase propionate and decrease methane, forages increase acetate and methane. The important thing to remember is that the production of end-products is linked such that, overall, there must be a redox balance. Feeding forages versus concentrates causes divergent ecological changes in the ruminal eco-system. Both are stable, although grain feeding taken to extreme may collapse, but are not compatible.

To see how the end-products are linked, we shall examine how each is produced. They all start from pyruvate and in the production of pyruvate there is a redox imbalance. The redox could be balanced by reducing pyruvate to lactate as occurs in mammalian metabolism. This works chemically, but such metabolism eliminates many places where microorganisms can gain production of ATP. Keep in mind that due to management errors, the ruminal ecosystem may switch to generating lactate as its major end-product. When this happens, the ruminant is likely to be dead within hours.

In the production of acetate, pyruvate is first oxidatively decarboxylated to yield CO_2, a reducing equivalent, and acetyl-CoA. Formate also could be released instead of CO_2, but the reducing equivalent eventually would be generated as the formate was oxidized to CO_2. Transesterification of acetyl-CoA yields acetyl-phosphate and CoA. A phosphotransferase catalyses formation of acetate and ATP from acetyl-phosphate and ADP. The production of acetate from pyruvate produces one unit each of CO_2, ATP and reducing power per acetate.

Butyrate is produced by the condensation of two units of acetyl-CoA forming CoA and acetoacetyl-CoA and consuming an ATP. The acetoacetyl-CoA is reduced to β-hydroxybutyryl-CoA followed by dehydration to crotonyl-CoA. Crotonyl-CoA serves as a terminal electron acceptor of an electron transport chain coupled to phosphorylation of ADP (Fig. 6.4). The electron transport chain transfers reducing power from NADH,H$^+$/FADH$_2$ and reduces crotonyl-CoA to butyryl-CoA. The energy of the butyryl-CoA thioester is captured in the form of ATP via transesterification and phosphotransferase, similarly to that described for the acetate pathway. The production of butyrate from acetyl-CoA produces an ATP and consumes two units of reducing power per unit of butyrate formed.

Propionate is produced by two pathways, the randomizing and acrylate pathways. The randomizing pathway predominates, producing 90–95% of the propionate when ruminants are fed forage-based diets and 60–70% of the propionate when fed mixed diets. The acrylate pathway predominates in grain-fed ruminants, accounting for 70–90% of the propionate produced after a meal of grain. The acrylate pathway is more tolerant of the acid conditions induced by grain feeding (more rapid production of acid coupled with reduced stimulus for rumination and therefore less buffer from saliva) with increases in propionate and decreases in methane production.

The randomizing pathway is initiated by a carboxytransphosphorylase reaction in which PEP reacts with CO_2 and P$_i$ forming oxaloacetate (OAA) and PP$_i$. This may or may not be equivalent to expenditure of an ATP, depending on the efficiency of coupling, because phosphofructokinase in propionate-producing bacteria can use PP$_i$ as the phosphate donor in forming fructose-1,6-bisphosphate. The OAA is reduced to malate, consuming a unit of reducing power. The malate is dehydrated to fumarate. Fumarate, like crotonyl-CoA, is the terminal electron acceptor in an electron transport chain, resulting in the reduction of fumarate to succinate and production of ATP. Initially, the succinate is converted to succinyl-CoA by a thiokinase, consuming an ATP. Once succinyl-CoA is formed, the pathway becomes autocatalytic, eliminating the need for the thiokinase and carboxytransphosphorylase reactions. These reactions are necessary only for priming the pathway. The succinyl-CoA is mutated to methylmalonyl-CoA by a vitamin B$_{12}$-catalysed reaction. Methylmalonyl-CoA is epimerized from the (R) to the (S) stereoisomer. The next reactions, catalysed by a biotin-containing transcarboxylase, are central to the randomizing pathway. Methylmalonyl-CoA donates a CO_2, forming carboxybiotin on the enzyme and propionyl-CoA. The carboxybiotin form of the enzyme reacts with pyruvate, carboxylating pyruvate to OAA and reforming the uncarboxylated enzyme. Thus the initial CO_2 of the transcarboxyphosphorylase becomes catalytic, and pyruvate rather than PEP is the subsequent source of propionate carbon. Conversion of PEP to pyruvate captures energy in the form of ATP when the transcarboxyphosphorylase is eliminated. The

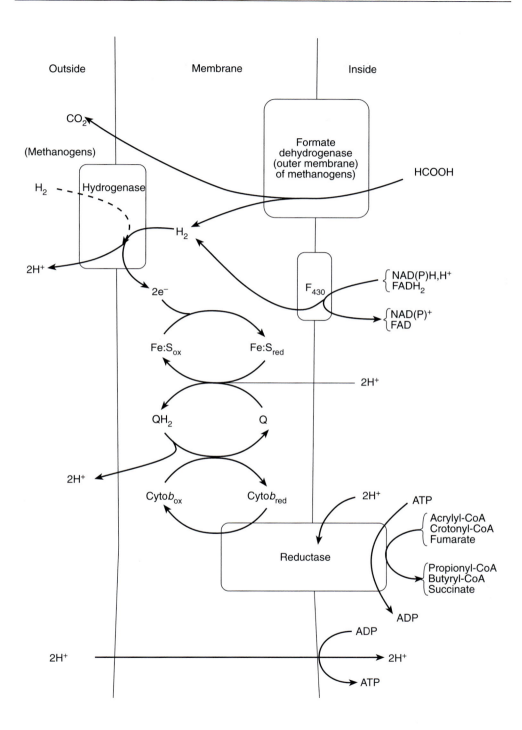

Fig. 6.4. Representation of anaerobic electron transport systems (putative). Not all components are found in all microorganisms nor are all components observed in ruminal microorganisms included. Based on Erfle *et al.* (1986).

propionyl-CoA formed in the transcarboxy-lase reaction undergoes transesterification with succinate yielding succinyl-CoA and propionate. The transesterification reaction eliminates the thiokinase reaction. Once primed, the randomizing pathway produces an ATP and consumes two NADH,H[+] per propionate produced.

The acrylate pathway converts pyruvate to propionate and acetate in a coordinated and stoichiometric manner. Pyruvate is reduced to lactate, consuming a reducing equivalent. The lactate is energized to lactyl-CoA by a transesterifica-tion reaction with acetyl-CoA. The acetyl-CoA generation was discussed in the acetate section. The lactyl-CoA is phos-phorylated using acetyl-phosphate as the donor. The phosphate is a much better leaving group than a hydroxyl, and sets up the next reaction which is phosphate elimination. In effect, the phosphoryla-tion/phosphate elimination dehydrates lactyl-CoA to acrylyl-CoA. Acrylyl-CoA is a terminal electron acceptor of an electron transport chain, and an ATP is generated as acrylyl-CoA is reduced to propionyl-CoA. The propionyl-CoA is transesterified with acetate yielding propionate and acetyl-CoA. Overall, two pyruvates are converted to a propionate, a CO_2 and an acetate while generating an ATP and consuming an NADH,H[+]. Considering the pathway with-out the contribution of pyruvate to acetate, there are two units of reducing power consumed per propionate produced and no change in ATP.

Production of CO_2, in effect, was described concurrently with the pathways of VFA production. Glycolysis and produc-tion of acetate generate reducing power, and production of propionate and butyrate consumes reducing power. Acetate is the dominant end-product of ruminal fermentation. The VFA ratios normally encountered produce more reducing power than is consumed by VFA production alone. Species that generate excess reduc-ing power balance the excess by using a proton as a terminal electron acceptor, which in combination with a hydride ion generates H_2 gas. This system can only be

effective if there is a means of consuming the H_2. The methanogens use H_2 to reduce CO_2 to methane. The methanogenic path-way is a series of oxidation–reduction reac-tions of a series of electron transport chains that ultimately use CO_2 or its reduction products as terminal electron acceptors. ATP is generated concurrently with electron transport. A branch from the methanogenic pathway also fixes carbon for anabolic processes (Fig. 6.5). In addi-tion to fumarate, crotonyl-CoA, acrylyl-CoA, H^+ and CO_2, other compounds that serve as significant terminal electron acceptors are SO_4 and NO_3. Methanogens generate virtually all of the ATP from electron transport-coupled phosphoryla-tion, but there is a wide range in non-methanogenic species, e.g. B. succinogens, 50%; B. ruminicola, 33%; B. fibrisolvens, 25%, and S. bovis, ~0%.

The summary in Fig. 6.3 represents the whole of the ruminal ecosystem and not the metabolism of individual species. There is interspecies metabolite transfer. End-products of the metabolism of one species are used as substrates for meta-bolism of another species. The inter-species hydrogen transfer to methanogens may prove to be quite interesting. There are indications that methanogens physic-ally attach themselves to the cells of larger microorganisms. Typically, the metabolic characteristics expressed by micro-organisms in monoculture are quite different from those in mixed culture. This effect is very dramatic in ruminal micro-organisms grown in the absence of methanogens. Although methanogens may be politically incorrect, they are vital to the ruminal ecology. Methane produced by ruminants worldwide is significant (~12% of total world production) but must be kept in context. Ruminants produce the same amount of methane as rice fields. Methane production from landfills is half that from ruminants. The major generator of methane is natural wetlands (42%) (Crutzen, 1995).

Organic acid end-products of meta-bolism of individual microbes (VFAs and metabolic intermediates for interspecies

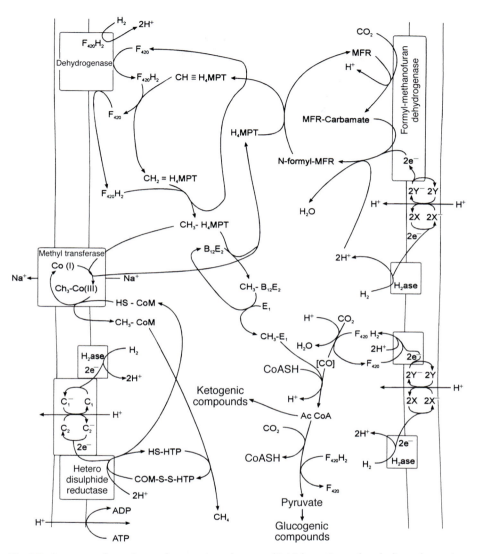

Fig. 6.5. Summary of putative methanogenic pathway and initial reactions of anabolic pathways in ruminal methanogens. Composited from Muller *et al.* (1993), Simpson and Whitman (1993) and Thauer *et al.* (1993).

metabolite transfer) must exit the cell into the fluid environment of the rumen. Exit is by diffusion and by permeases (Fig. 6.2).

Most of the VFAs, the waste products of the fermentation, are removed from the fermentation by absorption through the rumen epithelium. Not all details of the absorption process are understood but the process has been reviewed recently (Gabel, 1995; Rechkemmer *et al.*, 1995; von

Engelhardt, 1995). It had been thought previously that the major route of absorption was by passive diffusion of the undissociated acids through the epithelium. The absorption rate is influenced by luminal pH and chain length of the acids in the direction consistent with passive diffusion, but the magnitude of influence is very small relative to differences in absorption rates observed at different concentrations of VFAs. A schematic diagram

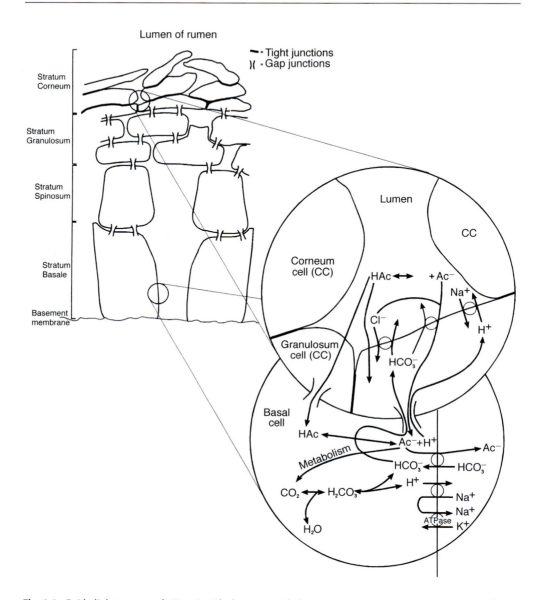

Fig. 6.6. Epithelial transport of VFAs. Stratified rumen epithelium shown (anatomy based on Steven and Marshall, 1970). Caecal and colonic epithelia are only one cell thick.

garnered from the cited references is presented in Fig. 6.6. Although passive diffusion of the undissociated acid does occur, uptake of the anion predominates. Anion uptake is coupled with exchange of intracellular bicarbonate with luminal anion. The VFA anions compete with chloride directly on the same exchange permease, or the competition is indirect for the same pool of intracellular bicarbonate and the presence of a separate luminal chloride/intracellular bicarbonate exchanger. The anions of VFAs are weaker bases than bicarbonate and the exchange acidifies the cytosol of the epithelial cell. Na⁺/H⁺ exchangers in both the apical and basolateral membranes diminish the change in cytosolic pH. The apical exchanger enhances Na⁺

uptake that is extruded on the basolateral membrane by the Na^+/K^+ ATPase. The stoichiometry has not been determined. The acetate anion is a significant source of energy for the epithelial cells and is a source of CO_2 for intracellular bicarbonate. Transport of the anions across the basolateral membranes is less certain, but intracellular anion/basolateral extracellular bicarbonate exchange is likely.

The strategy of ruminants is to retain materials in the rumen for extensive fermentation. The mechanisms causing this are not defined clearly (Mathison *et al.*, 1995). Physical characteristics of the feed have an influence, but are not the only factor. There is a 'threshold' size for particulate passage through the reticulo-omasal orifice. The rate at which feeds break into particles smaller than the threshold is important, but many particles less than threshold size are retained in the rumen. Particulates to be passed into the omasum appear to concentrate in the honeycomb pattern of epithelia folds in the reticulum and migrate toward the orifice during reticular contractions. Liquid passage rate and omasal 'fill' influence the rate at which these particulates are transferred into the omasum. Generally, slowly digested feeds remain in the rumen longer than rapidly digested feeds, but there are exceptions. Very fibrous feeds with minimal available protein, i.e. straw, may be digested and passed from the rumen so slowly that they reduce nutrient intake below requirements. On the other hand, extremely nutritious forage, i.e. spring pasture, which is digested rapidly, may pass from the rumen too rapidly for significant digestion. As a consequence, animal performance declines. The decline in performance can be avoided by providing a small amount of coarse roughage to slow the rate of passage. Although many farmers have known this for generations, scientists are beginning to understand the reasons. Grains, which are digested rapidly, have a relatively long retention time because they are less stimulatory of rumen motility than forages, and the rapid generation of fermentation acids is inhibitory to motility.

The relationship between a ruminant and its ruminal microbial ecosystem is symbiotic. The ruminant provides substrate, a warm anaerobic space (with some assistance by facultative anaerobes attached to the rumen epithelium), buffers to help maintain a desirable pH and systems for removal of microbial wastes (eructation to eliminate CO_2 and methane; passage to eliminate undigestable residue; absorption to eliminate VFAs and ammonia). The VFAs are a waste product of microbial metabolism, but are an important fuel for ruminants, providing 60–80% of total energy. The microorganisms also are an important source of protein for the ruminant, providing up to 2.5 kg of microbial protein per day to the ruminant (lactating dairy cow; Clark *et al.*, 1992) as the microorganisms pass from the stomach to be digested by the ruminant. Much of the microbial protein is derived from non-protein N from the feed and metabolic waste N from the ruminant's metabolism. Microorganisms have the ability to synthesize B vitamins and with rare exception do so to the extent that there is no need to supplement the ruminant's diet with B vitamins.

There are costs associated with this relationship. Generally, ~25% of the energy of the carbohydrates fermented is lost, i.e. the VFAs retain ~75% of the energy. Most (90% or more) of the carbohydrate carbon that becomes available for metabolism by the ruminant is in the form of VFAs, thus very little glucose is available for absorption and the microorganisms ferment carbohydrates that potentially would be available to the ruminant directly (starches) as well as or rather than the structural carbohydrates that are unavailable directly. Ruminants, therefore, are very dependent on gluconeogenesis for maintaining blood glucose concentrations. Of the VFAs, only propionate is a major source of carbon for gluconeogenesis. Conversion of propionate to glucose also costs metabolic energy (4 ATP mol^{-1} glucose). Combining the costs of fermentation and gluconeogenesis (ignoring the costs of the futile cycle embedded in the gluconeogenic pathway from propionate), complete oxidation of glucose yields only 65% of the energy that would have been available if the dietary carbohydrates were digested and metabolized directly.

This may appear to be a high price. Most carbohydrates that ruminants eat during their lifetime, however, are totally unavailable by the direct route. The microbial ecosystem gives ruminants the advantage of being able to thrive on feeds that would not sustain other animals, including humans. There is lots of good news in this good news/bad news story. Of the solar energy captured by the earth's biomass, only 5% potentially is available for human food directly, leaving lots of feed for ruminants.

Attempts to improve the efficiency of ruminant metabolism by providing a post-ruminal source of starch have been unsuccessful. Unlike the case in direct absorbers, starch entering the small intestine of ruminants does not disappear rapidly. Typically, only half the starch that enters the duodenum disappears during transit through the small intestine (Owens et al., 1986; for discussion see Hill et al., 1991). Huntington (1997) concluded that enzymatic capacity, both luminal and membrane, is the limiting factor in disappearance of starch. Another factor to consider is that after weaning, ruminants stop expressing SGLT1 (Shirazi-Beechey et al., 1995). Expression of SGLT1 has been induced in adult ruminants by infusing the intestine with 30 mM glucose for 4 days. It has not been determined whether practical conditions can generate the combination of starch supply and intestinal enzymatic activity necessary to achieve the threshold concentration of free glucose for induction of SGLT1. There is a wide range of individual variability, making it probable that rapid changes could be made by genetic selection. Intestinal starch disappearance ranged from 10 to 93% in beef steers (Harmon, 1992) and intestinal glucose absorption ranged from 10 to 100% in dairy steers (Russell and Schmidt, 1984; and unpublished).

Hindgut fermentation

Fermentation in the hindgut is similar to that described for the ruminal ecosystem in most species incorporating the process into their digestive strategy. Most species use hindgut fermentation, at least to some extent. Even in species, such as humans, where the fermentation is an insignificant source of energy, the VFAs produced are important in maintaining a healthy intestinal epithelium (Cummings et al., 1995). Fermentation is combined with direct absorption, but the host animal has the first access to available substrate. Feed consumed by the animal is processed initially as described for direct absorbers. Much of the starches and non-structural carbohydrates is digested and absorbed prior to exposure to fermentation. Absorption of VFAs differs slightly from that described for the rumen, with variations depending on the location in the hindgut (von Engelhardt, 1995).

Ruminants expose digesta to hindgut fermentation as well as to pre-gastric fermentation. Most of the hindgut fermentation in ruminants occurs in the caecum. The caecum is a blind pouch at the junction of the small and large intestine and functions like a small rumen with a steady flow of material in and out. Hindgut fermentation in ruminants provides <10% of the VFAs relative to ruminal production (Bergman, 1990).

Equids and swine are colon fermenters; most of the fermentation occurs in the colon. The caecum, although quite large, operates functionally as an extension of the proximal colon. In these animals, the large, distinct haustrations of the colon retain the digesta for fermentation. There is good mixing of material within each haustration but minimum mixing of contents among the haustrations. From a functional viewpoint, this is analogous to many small, 'closed' (exchange of material only with epithelium) rumens in series passing down the tract. A distinct and important difference between colonic and ruminal fermentation is that acetogenesis largely replaces methanogenesis in colonic fermentation (Miller, 1995). For a comprehensive review of acetogenesis see Drake (1994). The acetogenic and methanogenic pathways are parallel, differing primarily in substrate specificity. Replacing methanogenesis with acetogenesis in the rumen would increase carbohydrate energy retained as VFAs from 75% to ~95%. A worthy project for industrious students.

Colonic fermentation has advantages over ruminal fermentation when feeds are either of very high quality or very low quality, if available in abundance. The advantage when fed high-quality feeds is obvious. The host has first access to the feed, and non-structural carbohydrates can be digested and absorbed directly by the host without fermentation losses. The hindgut microorganisms then provide additional energy to the host by digesting structural carbohydrates. When there is an abundance of poor-quality feeds, colonic fermenters perform better than ruminants. Colonic fermenters adapt to poor-quality feeds by increasing the transit rate through the tract. Digestibility decreases but nutrient availability increases by increasing intake. The ruminant strategy of maximizing digestibility becomes a liability because passage rate slows, filling the rumen with undigestible material, which limits intake.

Poultry are caecal fermenters. The process in poultry differs from that in ruminants. The caeca are filled by antiperistaltic flow. The contents of the caeca ferment, followed by emptying of the caeca. Thus in poultry, it is a 'batch' process rather than a continuous flow process as in ruminants. Because poultry feeds are digested very well in the small intestine and urine mixes with the digesta, we hypothesized that caecal microorganisms would have an abundance of available nitrogen relative to energy. Supplementing the hindgut microorganisms with an energy source in the form of lactose fed to young turkeys (poultry lack lactase) increased weight gains by 50% relative to control turkeys (Russell, 1999, unpublished).

Coprophagic strategy

Rabbits are hindgut, caecal fermenters and are the only wanted farm animals (rats in the granary do not count) with a coprophagic feeding strategy. Their digestive strategy differs markedly from that of other farm animals. Like poultry, the caecal fermentation is a 'batch-type' fermentation, but differs in function. Excellent reviews of rabbit physiology and nutrition are available (Cheeke, 1987; McNitt *et al.*, 1996). The initial ingesta is chewed to a very fine consistency in the mouth. Upon swallowing, the digesta is processed as described for direct absorbers. A significant difference is that the digesta is acidified to ~pH 1.5 in the stomach. This is 5- to 10-fold more acidic than that of most animals. The consequence is that there are very few species of microorganisms that survive these conditions to eventually inhabit the hindgut. As a result, the ecology in the hindgut is much more fragile.

Rabbits are paradoxical. They require fibre in their diet but, contrary to popular belief, they are poor digesters of fibre. Fibre is essential to maintain motility in the hindgut. As digesta enters the caecum, the particulates are separated from the solubles. Solubles are retained in the caecum for fermentation and the large particulates are propelled down the tract, with solubles and small particulates captured in the haustrations, and pushed toward the caecum by antiperistalsis. The large particulates are evacuated from the tract as 'hard' or 'day' faeces. These faeces are not recycled. The solubles and small particulates are retained in the caecum for fermentation. Excretion of the hard faeces precedes excretion of the 'soft' or 'night' faeces, called caecotrophs. Approximately 8 h after feeding, the caecal contents become coated with mucus. The mucus-coated caecal contents (caecotrophs) are evacuated via the anus directly into the mouth and swallowed. The caecotrophs remain in the stomach for up to 12 h where a lactate-producing fermentation occurs until the acid stomach fluids penetrate the caecotrophs. The fermentation in the caecum is similar to that described for the rumen. In rabbits, the VFA ratio is still dominated by acetate, but butyrate generally is increased and propionate decreased.

Feeds such as maize that can provide a source of readily fermentable carbohydrate to the caecum without a supply of fibre to maintain motility can have devastating effects on rabbits. Rapid fermentation increases the acidity of the caecum which inhibits motility. Reduced motility allows the fermentation to continue in the caecum, producing more acids. The acids cause irritation and damage to the epithelium, allowing a large influx of tissue water into the lumen. A severe and potentially lethal diarrhoea ensues. This is an important practical problem. Nearly 20% of all rabbits born alive in commercial rabbit production die as a result of this type of situation. A second paradox of rabbit physiology is that constipation induces diarrhoea. The constipation can be initiated by many factors: lack of water, inadequate fibre, resistant starch in the diet, genetics, stress and antibiotics.

Carnivores

Carnivores have not been a significant farm animal raised for human food. Until recently, commercial production of carnivores was restricted to fur-bearing animals. Recently there has been increased interest in raising fish, some of which are carnivores, alligators, and in some parts of the world, dogs. Of these species, only some fish and alligators are true carnivores. The less strict carnivores can obtain 30–50% of their glucose need by the process described for direct absorbers. Strict carnivores have very little carbohydrate in their diet and lack the capacity for significant digestion of carbohydrate. Carnivores are direct absorbers, but not of carbohydrates.

Protein must provide the carbon for gluconeogenesis necessary to supply blood glucose. Dietary protein is processed analogously to carbohydrates as described

for direct absorbers. The enzymes, substrates and products differ. Luminal proteases are secreted as inactive zymogens that are activated by specific cleavage. There also are several brush border peptidases. Active transporters similar to SGLT1 absorb free amino acids. Many amino acids are absorbed in the form of short peptides. The mechanisms for peptide transport are less well defined. Paracellular transport is also probable.

The dietary protein hydrolysis products that are absorbed are carried to the liver by the hepatic portal vein. The mechanisms that determine which and how many amino acids are used as precursors of glucose synthesis, surprisingly, have not been determined. It has been observed that carnivores clear excesses of dietary non-essential amino acids more rapidly than dietary essential amino acids (Coulson and Hernandez, 1983).

This does not do justice to carnivores, but there appears to be very little known about where their glucose carbon comes from specifically. The area of fish nutrition is fascinating, with much diversity in their anatomy and feeding habits. Fish warrant a separate chapter on their own.

Concluding Comments

The purpose of this chapter was to trace the routes of carbon from the diet to glucose available to farm animals. It is important for students to see beyond this context to the overall challenge to agricultural scientists. Examination of the human population curve reveals that we as a society must produce as much food for human consumption during the next 40 years as we have produced since the beginning of time. The driving force for all of agriculture is solar radiation that must be captured and converted to food for humans. Of the biomass captured by photosynthesis, most of which is carbohydrate, 95% is unavailable as a direct source of food for humans. Animals can convert much of this non-food biomass into high-quality food.

References

Alpers, D.H. (1987) Digestion and absorption of carbohydrates and proteins. In: Johnson, L.R. (ed.) *Physiology of the Gastrointestinal Tract*, 2nd edn. Raven Press, New York, pp. 1469–1487.

Ballard, S.T., Hunter, J.H. and Taylor, A.E. (1995) Regulation of tight-junction permeability during nutrient absorption across the intestinal epithelium. *Annual Review of Nutrition* 15, 35–55.

Baly, D.L. and Horuk, R. (1988) The biology and biochemistry of the glucose transporter. *Biochimica et Biophysica Acta* 947, 571–590.

Bergman, E.N. (1990) Energy contributions of volatile fatty acids from the gastrointestinal tract in various species. *Physiological Reviews* 70, 567–590.

Bird, A.R., Croom, W.J., Jr, Fan, Y.K., Black, B.L., McBride, B.W. and Taylor, I.L. (1996) Peptide regulation of intestinal glucose absorption. *Journal of Animal Science* 74, 2523–2540.

Birnbaum, M.J. (1992) The insulin-sensitive glucose transporter. *International Review of Cytology* 137A, 239–297.

Cheeke, P.R. (1987) *Rabbit Feeding and Nutrition*. Academic Press, New York.

Cheng, K.-J., Forsberg, C.W., Minato, H. and Costerton, J.W. (1991) Microbial ecology and physiology of feed degradation within the rumen. In: Tsuda, T., Sasaki, Y. and Kawashima, R. (eds) *Physiological Aspects of Digestion and Metabolism in Ruminants*. Academic Press, New York, pp. 595–624.

Church, D.C. (1988) *The Ruminant Animal: Digestive Physiology and Nutrition*. Prentice Hall, Englewood Cliffs, New Jersey.

Clark, J.H., Klusmeyer, T.H. and Cameron, M.R. (1992) Microbial protein synthesis and flows of nitrogenous fractions to the duodenum of dairy cows. *Journal of Dairy Science* 75, 2304–2323.

Coulson, R.A. and Hernandez, T. (1983) *Alligator Metabolism: Studies on Chemical Reactions* in vivo. Pergamon Press, New York.

Crutzen, P.J. (1995) The role of methane in atmospheric chemistry and climate. In: von Engelhardt, W., Leonhard-Marek, S., Breves, G. and Giesecke, D. (eds) *Ruminant Physiology: Digestion, Metabolism, Growth and Reproduction*. Ferdinand Enke Verlag, Stuttgart, Germany, pp. 291–315.

Cummings, J.H., Rombeau, J.L. and Sakata, T. (1995) *Physiological and Clinical Aspects of Short-chain Fatty Acids*. Cambridge University Press, Cambridge, UK.

Czerkawski, J.W. (1986) *An Introduction to Rumen Studies*. Pergamon Press, New York.

Drake, H.L. (1994) *Acetogenesis*. Chapman and Hall, New York.

Duke, G.E. (1986a) Alimentary canal: anatomy, regulation of feeding, and motility. In: Sturkie, P.D. (ed.) *Avian Physiology*, 4th edn. Springer-Verlag, New York, pp. 269–288.

Duke, G.E. (1986b) Alimentary canal: secretion and digestion, special digestive functions, and absorption. In: Sturkie, P.D. (ed.) *Avian Physiology*, 4th edn. Springer-Verlag, New York, pp. 289–302.

Elsas, L.J. and Longo, N. (1992) Glucose transporters. *Annual Review of Medicine* 43, 377–393.

Ensminger, M.E. (1991) *Animal Science*, 9th edn. Interstate Publishers, Inc., Danville, Illinois.

Erfle, J.D., Sauer, F.D. and Mahaddevan, S. (1986) Energy metabolism in rumen microbes. In: Milligan, L.P., Grovum, W.L. and Dobson, A. (eds) *Control of Digestion and Metabolism in Ruminants*. Prentice-Hall, Englewood Cliffs, New Jersey, pp. 81–99.

Erni, B. (1992) Group translocation of glucose and other sugars by the bacterial phosphotransferase system. *International Review of Cytology* 137A, 127–148.

Ferraris, R.P., Yasharpour, S., Kent-Lloyd, K.C., Mirzayan, R. and Diamond, J.M. (1990) Luminal glucose concentrations in the gut under normal conditions. *American Journal of Physiology* 259, G822–G837.

Fine, K.D., Santa-Ana, C.A., Porter, J.L. and Fordtran, J.S. (1993) Effect of D-glucose on intestinal permeability and its passive absorption in human small intestine *in vivo*. *Gastroenterology* 105, 1117–1125.

Gabel, G. (1995) Transport of short-chain fatty acids in the ruminant forestomach. In: Cummings, J.H., Rombeau, J.L. and Sakata, T. (eds) *Physiological and Clinical Aspects of Short-chain Fatty Acids*. Cambridge University Press, Cambridge, UK, pp. 133–147.

Gray, G.M., Lally, B.C. and Conklin, K.A. (1979) Action of intestinal sucrase–isomaltase and its free monomers in an α-limit dextrin. *Journal of Biological Chemistry* 254, 6038–6043.

Guyton, A.C. (1971) *Textbook of Medical Physiology*, 4th edn. W.B. Saunder Company, Philidelphia, Pennsylvania.

Harmon, D.L. (1992) Dietary influences on carbohydrases and intestinal capacity for starch hydrolysis in ruminants. *Journal of Nutrition* 122, 203–210.

Hill, T.M., Schmidt, S.P., Russell, R.W., Thomas, E.E. and Wolfe, D.F. (1991) Comparison of urea treatment with established methods of sorghum grain preservation and processing on site and extent of starch digestion by cattle. *Journal of Animal Science* 69, 4570–4576.

Hobson, P.H. and Stewart, C.S. (1997) *The Rumen Microbial Ecosystem*, 2nd edn. Blackie Academic & Professional Press, New York.

Hopfer, U. (1987) Membrane transport mechanisms for hexoses and amino acids in the small intestine. In: Johnson, L.R. (ed.) *Physiology of the Gastrointestinal Tract*, 2nd edn. Raven Press, New York, pp. 1499–1526.

Hungate, R.E. (1966) *The Rumen and Its Microbes.* Academic Press, New York.

Huntington, G.B. (1997) Starch utilization by ruminants: from basics to the bunk. *Journal of Animal Science* 75, 852–867.

Karasov, W.H. and Hume, I.D. (1997) Vertebrate gastrointestinal system. In: Dantzler, W.H. (ed.) *Handbook of Physiology, Section 13, Comparative Physiology, Volume 1.* American Physiological Society, Oxford University Press, New York, pp. 409–480.

Kidder, D.E. and Manners, M.J. (1980) The level and distrubition of carbohydrases in the small intestine of pigs from 3 weeks to maturity. *British Journal of Nutrition* 43, 141–152.

Konings, W.N., Otto, R. and Ten Brink, B. (1986) Energy transduction and solute transport in streptococci. In: Milligan, L.P., Grovum, W.L. and Dobson, A. (eds) *Control of Digestion and Metabolism in Ruminants.* Prentice-Hall, Englewood Cliffs, New Jersey, pp. 100–121.

Madara, J.L. (1988) Tight junction dynamics: Is paracellular transport regulated? *Cell* 53, 497–498.

Mathison, G.W., Okine, E.K., Vaage, A.S., Kaske, M. and Milligan, L.P. (1995) Current understanding of the contribution of the propulsive activities in the forestomach to the flow of digesta, In: von Engelhardt, W., Leonhard-Marek, S., Breves, G. and Giesecke, D. (eds) *Ruminant Physiology: Digestion, Metabolism, Growth and Reproduction.* Ferdinand Enke Verlag, Stuttgart, Germany, pp. 23–41.

McNitt, J.I., Patton, N.M., Lukefahr, S.D. and Cheeke, P.R. (1996) *Rabbit Production*, 7th edn. Interstate Publishers, Inc., Danville, Illinois.

Miller, T.L. (1995) Ecology of methane production and hydrogen sinks in the rumen. In: von Engelhardt, W., Leonhard-Marek, S., Breves, G. and Giesecke, D. (eds) *Ruminant Physiology: Digestion, Metabolism, Growth and Reproduction.* Ferdinand Enke Verlag, Stuttgart, Germany, pp. 317–331.

Muller, V., Blaut, M. and Gottschalk, G. (1993) Bioenergetics of methanogenesis. In: Ferry, J.G. (ed.) *Methanogenesis: Ecology, Physiology, Biochemistry and Genetics.* Chapman & Hall, New York, pp. 360–406.

Newsholme, E.A. and Leech, A.R. (1989) *Biochemistry for the Medical Sciences.* John Wiley & Sons, New York.

Olson, A.L. and Pessin, J.E. (1996) Structure, function, and regulation of the mammalian facilitative glucose transporter gene family. *Annual Review of Nutrition* 16, 235–256.

Owens, F.N., Zinn, R.A. and Kim, Y.K. (1986) Limits to starch digestion in the ruminant small intestine. *Journal of Animal Science* 63, 1634–1648.

Pappenheimer, J.R. (1993) On the coupling of membrane digestion with intestinal absorption of sugars and amino acids. *American Journal of Physiology* 265, G409–G417.

Pappenheimer, J.R. (1998) Scaling of dimensions of small intestines in nonruminant eutherian mammals and its signficance for absorptive mechanisms. *Comparative Biochemistry and Physiology* 121, 45–58.

Pessin, J.E. and Bell, G.I. (1992) Mammalian facilitative glucose transporter family: structure and molecular regulation. *Annual Review of Physiology* 54, 911–930.

Planas, J.M., Villa, M.C., Ferrer, R. and Moreto, M. (1986) Hexose transport by chicken cecum during development. *Pflugers Archiv* 407, 216–220.

Rechkemmer, G., Gabel, G., Diernaes, L., Sehested, J., Moller, P.D. and von Engelhardt, W. (1995) Transport of short chain fatty acids in the forestomach and hindgut. In: von Engelhardt, W., Leonhard-Marek, S., Breves, G. and Giesecke, D. (eds) *Ruminant Physiology: Digestion, Metabolism, Growth and Reproduction.* Ferdinand Enke Verlag, Stuttgart, Germany, pp. 95–116.

Rodriguez, I.R., Taravel, F.R. and Whelan, W.J. (1984) Characterization and functions of pig intestinal sucrase-isomaltase and its separate subunits. *European Journal of Biochemistry* 143, 575–582.

Russell, R.W. and Schmidt, S.P. (1984) Measurement of fractional absorption of glucose from the gut. *Journal of Dairy Science* 67 (Suppl. 1), 162.

Semenza, G., Kessler, M., Hosang, M., Weber, J. and Schmidt, U. (1984) Biochemistry of the Na$^+$, D-glucose cotransporter of the small-intestinal brush-border membrane. *Biochimica et Biophysica Acta* 779, 343–379.

Shirazi-Beechey, S.P., Wood, I.S., Dyer, J., Scott, D. and King, T.P. (1995) Intestinal sugar transport in ruminants. In: von Engelhardt, W., Leonhard-Marek, S., Breves, G. and Giesecke, D. (eds) *Ruminant Physiology: Digestion, Metabolism, Growth and Reproduction.* Ferdinand Enke Verlag, Stuttgart, Germany, pp. 117–133.

Simpson, P.G. and Whitman, W.B. (1993) Anabolic pathways in methanogens. In: Ferry, J.G. (ed.) *Methanogenesis: Ecology, Physiology, Biochemistry and Genetics.* Chapman & Hall, New York, pp. 445–472.

Steven, D.H. and Marshall, A.B. (1970) Organization of the rumen epithelium. In: Phillipson, A.T. (ed.) *Physiology of Digestion and Metabolism in the Ruminant.* Oriel Press, Newcastle upon Tyne, UK.

Stevens, C.E. and Hume, I.D. (1995) *Comparative Physiology of the Vertebrate Digestive System,* 2nd edn. Cambridge University Press, New York.

Taraval, F.R., Datsura, R., Woloszuk, W., Marshall, J.J. and Whelan, W.J. (1983) Purification and characterization of a pig intestinal α-limit dextrinase. *European Journal of Biochemistry* 130, 147–158.

Thauer, R.K., Hedderich, R. and Fischer, R. (1993) Reactions and enzymes involved in methanogenesis from CO_2 and H_2. In: Ferry, J.G. (ed.) *Methanogenesis: Ecology, Physiology, Biochemistry and Genetics.* Chapman & Hall, New York, pp. 209–252.

Thorens, B. (1992) Molecular and cellular physiology of GLUT-2, a high-K_m facilitated diffusion glucose transporter. *International Review of Cytology* 137A, 209–238.

Thorens, B. (1993) Facilitated glucose transporters in epithelial cells. *Annual Review of Physiology* 55, 591–608.

Ugolev, A.M. (1968) *Physiology and Pathology of Membrane Digestion.* Plenum Press, New York.

Ulyatt, M.J., Dellow, D.W., John, A., Reid, C.S.W. and Waghorn, G.C. (1986) Contribution of chewing during eating and rumination to the clearance of digesta from the ruminoreticulum. In: Milligan, L.P., Grovum, W.L. and Dobson, A. (eds) *Control of Digestion and Metabolism in Ruminants.* Prentice-Hall, Englewood Cliffs, New Jersey, pp. 498–515.

Van Soest, P.J. (1994) *Nutritional Ecology of the Ruminant,* 2nd edn. Cornell University Press, Ithaca, New York.

Vinardell, M.P., Lopera, M.T. and Moreto, M. (1986) Absorption of 3-oxy-methyl-D-glucose by chicken cecum and jejunum *in vivo. Comparative Biochemistry and Physiology* A85, 171–173.

von Engelhardt, W. (1995) Absorption of short-chain fatty acids from the intestine. In: Cummings, J.H., Rombeau, J.L. and Sakata, T. (eds) *Physiological and Clinical Aspects of Short-chain Fatty Acids.* Cambridge University Press, Cambridge, UK, pp. 149–170.

Vonk, H.J. and Western, J.R.H. (1984) *Comparative Biochemistry and Physiology of Enzymatic Digestion.* Academic Press, New York.

Webster, T.K.M. and Hoover, W.H. (1998) Nutrient analyses of feedstuffs including carbohydrates. *Animal Science Report No. 1.* West Virginia University.

Widdas, W.F. (1988) Old and new concepts of the membrane transport for glucose in cells. *Biochimica et Biophysica Acta* 947, 385–404.

Wolin, M.J. (1960) A theoretical rumen fermentation balance. *Journal of Dairy Science* 43, 1452–1459.

Wright, E.M. (1993) The intestinal Na$^+$/glucose cotransporter. *Annual Review of Physiology* 55, 575–589.

Yokoyama, M.T. and Johnson, K.A. (1988) Microbiology of the rumen and intestine. In: Church, D.C. (ed.) *The Ruminant Animal: Digestive Physiology and Nutrition.* Prentice Hall, Englewood Cliffs, New Jersey, pp. 125–144.

Chapter 7
Aspects of Cellular Energetics

N.S. Jessop
*Institute of Ecology and Resource Management,
The University of Edinburgh, Edinburgh, UK*

Introduction

All animals start life as a single cell from which complex organisms develop by processes of cell multiplication, cellular differentiation and cellular growth. For mammals, there is an enormous diversity in final body size and shape, yet all share similar body constructive architecture. At a cellular level, these widely differing animal species are remarkably similar. For example, cell size in comparable organs or tissues does not vary appreciably between animals of widely differing size when compared at similar stages of maturity. What does differ is the number of cells each organism possesses.

In order to develop from a single fertilized egg into a complex organism, the supply of considerable quantities of nutrients is required. One need for nutrients is to provide a supply of energy for survival. When considering the energy requirements of farm animals, it is conventional to divide the total energy requirement into those for different processes or factors such as maintenance, growth, pregnancy and lactation. At this holistic level, empirical equations have been

developed that enable the quantification of these requirements. Further subdivision of these factors is necessary in order to gain more understanding of requirements and how these might change over the course of an animal's life. For example, maintenance costs are quantitatively the most important – in an animal living out its full life-span they will make up around 98% of total lifetime energy requirements. Even in animals slaughtered before they reach maturity, maintenance costs can be around 50% of total nutrient requirements. Maintenance includes many functions. Firstly, it includes the basal metabolic rate (BMR) which is the energy required in order to maintain cells within an animal's body in a functional state, together with minimal activity such as respiration and circulation enabling the animal to survive. It is measured as the heat production in a rested animal in the post-absorptive state, i.e. when there is minimal processing of food within the digestive tract. Next, maintenance includes energy costs of muscular activity above those included in BMR (such as beating of the heart, expansion of the chest wall). These might include locomotory costs or muscular activity associated with eating and processing of food within the digestive tract. Other maintenance functions include operation of the immune system and fighting infection, as well as costs of thermoregulation should environmental factors result in the rate of heat loss from an animal's body exceeding the rate of heat production. In such cases, heat production is increased by shivering or non-shivering thermogenesis to maintain body temperature, resulting in increased energy usage.

Components of Cellular Energy Requirements

In order to understand the requirements for energy and how they change across an animal's life, or between animals of different sexes or different species, we need to consider energy requirements at the level of the cell. The overall requirement of an animal is the sum of the requirements of all individual cells. By considering such processes at a cellular level, we can begin to understand what factors influence these requirements.

Maintenance costs have been estimated by many authorities (e.g. AFRC, 1993; NRC, 1996) to be a function of the weight of an animal. Since body composition can vary widely and since adipose tissue is metabolically relatively inactive when compared with other tissues, fat-free mass or protein weight is a better determinant (Emmans, 1994). Table 7.1 shows early proposals of how maintenance costs can be subdivided further, although this relates principally to subdivision of BMR. The broad division is in terms of energetic costs of organ systems, termed service functions, and those of individual cells. However, the former constitute the additional cellular costs of a particular organ or tissue. For example, circulation or heart work is the additional energy requirement of the muscle cells of the heart above those termed cell maintenance. At a cellular level, many experiments have supported these proposals.

Table 7.1. Apportionment of BMR (from Baldwin *et al.,* 1980).

Function	% BMR
Service functions	
Kidney work	6–7
Heart work	9–11
Respiration	6–7
Nervous functions	10–15
Liver functions	5–10
Total	36–50
Cell maintenance	
Ion transport	30–40
Protein synthesis	9–12
Lipid synthesis	2–4
Total	41–56

Ion Transport

These estimates come from experiments performed *in vitro* in which the proportion of a cell's rate of oxygen use required for sodium pump (Na$^+$,K$^+$-ATPase, EC 3.6.1.3) activity is measured. This enzyme is present in the plasma membrane of all animal cells and serves to maintain the observed ionic gradient of Na$^+$ between intra- and extracellular space at the expense of ATP (see also Chapters 1 and 6). Such measurements make use of the specific inhibitor of the sodium pump, ouabain. Isolated cells are suspended in appropriate incubation medium in a closed and temperature-regulated chamber of a Clark-type oxygen electrode. The oxygen content of the medium is recorded continuously and falls as the cells consume oxygen. The rate of oxygen use is linear and depends on the type and quantity of tissue being studied. During the course of the incubation (after a sufficient period of time that allows the rate of oxygen use to be measured), ouabain is added to the medium. Sodium pump activity is inhibited and thus ATP, and hence oxygen, usage declines. The proportional decrease in the rate of oxygen consumption is assumed to represent the ATP, and hence oxygen, use of the sodium pump.

The activity of the sodium pump is responsive to the intracellular concentration of sodium ions, and hence serves to maintain intracellular sodium ion concentration within certain limits (Smith and Rozengurt, 1978). It has been reported that the activity of the sodium pump varies between different tissues and between different physiological states.

The research group of Milligan and McBride have made extensive measurements of ion transport costs, mainly that of the sodium pump. It has been shown that the activity of this pump utilizes a substantial proportion of the cell's ATP production and that this cost varies with physiological state, hormonal status, environmental temperature and diet. Gregg and Milligan (1982b) measured O_2 consumption and the percentage of this inhibited by ouabain in muscle from calves of different ages and breeds. In the youngest animals (2–3 weeks old), total O_2 consumption was higher than in older animals (7 months old) and breed was found to have little effect. Sodium pump activity accounted for 40% of total O_2 consumption and did not vary with age or breed. McBride and Milligan (1984, 1985a) made similar measurements in duodenal mucosa taken from cows at different stages of lactation or from sheep on different planes of nutrition. In both cases, total O_2 consumption varied relatively little between treatments, but Na^+,K^+-ATPase activity increased from 35% in non-lactating or end of lactation cows to 55% during the peak of mid-lactation. With sheep, sodium pump activity accounted for 28, 50 and 61% of total O_2 consumption at feeding levels of zero, maintenance and twice maintenance, respectively. In studies with liver, McBride and Milligan (1985b) again found no difference in total O_2 consumption between samples taken from sheep that were starved or fed and non-lactating, at peak lactation or at a late stage of lactation. However, Na^+,K^+-ATPase activity was lowest (at 18% of total) for starved animals and highest (at 45% of total) for animals at peak lactation.

Other reported measurements of sodium pump activity vary widely, accounting for between 60 and 10% of total cellular energy production. One cause of this variation is the nature of the incubation medium used (Milligan and Summers, 1986; Jessop, 1988), with higher activities observed when HCO_3^-/CO_2-buffered, simple salt solutions were used and lower activities when more complex, HEPES-buffered cell culture media were used. There has been one reported study in which Na^+,K^+-ATPase activity has been measured *in vivo* (Swaminathan *et al.*, 1989). In this study, guinea-pigs were injected intraperitoneally with ouabain which caused a 40% reduction in whole-body metabolic rate.

The studies reviewed above have all been observational in nature, often termed empirical. They illustrate that variation in such processes occurs, but they do not provide any understanding of the causes of such variation. For example, changes in Na^+,K^+-ATPase activity imply that the rate of sodium ion entry into cells differs accordingly. Why might this be so? One major problem might be that of *in vitro* measurement, in that tissues or cells have been removed from the environment *in vivo*. Hormonal levels will be different, as might the concentration of substrates and other ions. Care has to be taken in order to ensure that the plasma membranes of the cell suspensions have not been damaged by the isolation procedure, as any changes in membrane permeability will give rise to large changes in sodium pump activity. In many cases, cell viability is assessed by means of dye exclusion. What causes sodium to enter cells? Figure 7.1 shows the major causes of Na^+ entry into a cell across its plasma membrane. As each Na^+ ion enters, so it must be removed by the sodium pump in order to maintain the intracellular Na^+ concentration. Since one mole of ATP is hydrolysed for every 3 moles of Na^+ pumped, every Na^+ entering the cell costs one-third of an ATP.

Consider a cell in its environment. It contains within its plasma membrane, nucleic acids (DNA and RNA) and many proteins. Proteins and nucleic acids are negatively charged when hydrated and these molecules, because of their size, cannot pass across the cell membrane. Hence they are often referred to as the cell's fixed negative charge. The negative

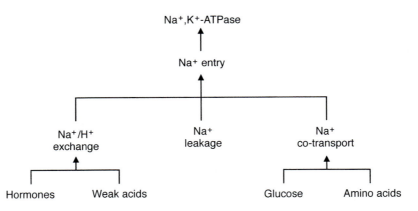

Fig. 7.1. Schematic diagram illustrating how various factors represented along the bottom row can influence the rate at which Na$^+$ enters a cell across the plasma membrane. To maintain steady-state concentrations of Na$^+$ within the cell, the rate at which Na$^+$ is pumped from the cell by Na$^+$,K$^+$-ATPase must equal the rate of entry of Na$^+$. The energetic cost of such pumping is one-third of a molecule of ATP per Na$^+$ expelled.

charge has to be balanced with positive charges in order to maintain electroneutrality, and potassium ions are used for this. The plasma membrane is relatively permeable to potassium ions but sodium ions are actively extruded by the sodium pump. Thus a gradient is maintained, with extracellular and intracellular concentrations of Na$^+$ being 120 and 10 mM, respectively, and of K$^+$ being 2.5 and 140 mM, respectively. This gradient or disequilibrium of sodium ions provides the driving force that cells are able to use to control and alter their intracellular environment. Maintenance of this Na$^+$ gradient in the face of both active and passive influx of Na$^+$ into the cell is energetically expensive. Additionally, the concentration gradient of K$^+$, together with the relative permeability of the plasma membrane to K$^+$, generates the resting electrochemical gradient across the plasma membrane of cells as K$^+$ diffuses out more quickly than other positively charged ions can diffuse in (Eckert and Randall, 1983).

Sodium/Proton Exchange

All cell membranes contain embedded proteins that exchange sodium ions for protons across the plasma membrane in a fixed ratio of one Na$^+$ for one H$^+$. It is accepted that the main mechanism for proton extrusion is the Na$^+$/H$^+$ antiporter which uses energy stored in the Na$^+$ gradient to pump protons out from the intracellular space (Graf et al., 1988). The activity of this antiporter is determined by the intracellular pH (pH$_i$) and it serves to protect cells against acidification of the cytosol (Pouyssegur et al., 1988). At pH$_i$ >7.4, this antiporter is virtually inactive but, as the pH$_i$ decreases from 7.4, the activity of the antiporter increases, reaching a maximum at a pH$_i$ of 6.0.

Hormones

Many of the hormones which stimulate anabolic processes in cells (mitogens or growth factors) have been shown to cause an increase in pH$_i$. This change is typically 0.15–0.3 pH units, representing a considerable decrease in the intracellular proton concentration. Such a change will, by itself, influence the activity of many metabolic pathways due to the pH sensitivity of many key enzymes. Pouyssegur et al. (1988) proposed a mechanism whereby binding of these hormones to receptors on the cell surface caused activation of protein kinase C (in the case of thrombin, bombesin, vasopressin and bradykinin) or activation of tyrosine kinase (in the case of epidermal growth factor and fibroblast growth factor), both resulting in modification to the Na^+/H^+ antiporter, changing its pH sensitivity. Insulin and insulin-like growth factor also cause similar changes in pH_i (Moore, 1983), probably through similar mechanisms (Bryer-Ash, 1988). The increase in sodium ions entering the cell is met by an increase in the rate of Na^+ extrusion by the sodium pump. There is an inhibitor of Na^+/H^+ exchange, amiloride, which has enabled studies of the activity of this process, although it has been reported that its inhibitory action is not specific for this antiporter but that it may inhibit Na^+,K^+-ATPase activity as well (Park *et al.*, 1992). Such studies have been undertaken in a similar manner to those described above for the sodium pump. Instead of ouabain being added to the cell suspension, amiloride is added and the reduction in oxygen consumption observed is assumed to be due to a decrease in sodium pump activity brought about by a decrease in Na^+/H^+ exchange.

Thyroid hormone levels have been shown to alter the rate of ion transport across the cell membrane. Gregg and Milligan (1987) measured Na^+,K^+-ATPase activity in sheep that had their thyroid gland removed surgically. Supplementation of the thyroid hormone T_3 to these animals, increased the activity of this enzyme by one-third. Gregg and Milligan (1982a) showed increases in Na^+,K^+-ATPase activity in muscle of cold-exposed sheep when compared with animals kept in warmer conditions. Cold stress causes increased thyroid hormone levels (Park *et al.*, 1992), and increasing the energy use for sodium pumping would be one mechanism whereby heat production could be increased. It is not clear how these hormones exert their effect, but they must increase Na^+ entry into cells substantially.

Weak acids

Intracellular pH can be affected directly by weak acids. Weak acids, such as acetic and carbonic acids, exist in equilibrium in aqueous solution:

Acetic acid:
$$CH_3COOH \rightleftharpoons H^+ + CH_3COO^-$$
Carbonic acid:
$$CO_2 + H_2O \rightleftharpoons H_2CO_3 \rightleftharpoons H^+ + HCO_3^-$$

The undissociated (and uncharged) forms of these acids can cross biological membranes readily by diffusion. Ketelaars and Tolkamp (1992) proposed that weak acids such as acetic and carbonic acids can act as proton ionophores, and thus their presence in extracellular media would incur an energy cost to the cell in counteracting acidification of the cytosol in the manner depicted for acetic acid in Fig. 7.2. Increased activity of Na^+/H^+ exchange will lead to an increase in the intracellular concentration of Na^+, stimulating Na^+,K^+-ATPase activity (Smith and Rozengurt, 1978). What is new about the explanation put forward by Ketelaars and Tolkamp is that it requires the plasma membrane to be permeable to small anions, e.g. acetate$^-$, to a significant degree. It has been argued that the plasma membrane is permeable to HCO_3^- and NH_4^+ (Boron and De Weer, 1976) with permeabilities of 5×10^{-7} and 10^{-6} cm s^{-1}, respectively (compared with the much greater permeabilities of 6×10^{-3} cm s^{-1} for both CO_2 and NH_3 – molecules which carry no charge and therefore cross biological membranes relatively easily), and that leakage of HCO_3^- occurs independently of carrier-mediated transport (Boron, 1983).

Jessop and Leng (1993) examined the effect of nutrient balance on Na^+,K^+-ATPase activity. Sheep were fed on poor-quality diets limiting in rumen-degradable nitrogen (the effective rumen-degradable protein to fermentable metabolizable energy ratio, eRDP:FME, was 6.0), which were either supplemented with additional rumen-undegradable protein (UDP) or not. Thus the protein to energy ratio of absorbed nutrients was expected to vary between the two dietary treatments. Hepatocytes were prepared and incubated over a range of acetate concentrations from 0 to 2.5 mM. Total respiration was unchanged, but the proportion of total

Extracellular space

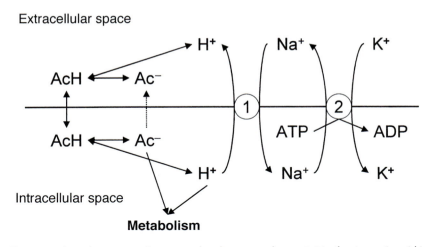

Fig. 7.2. Representation of acetate cycling across the plasma membrane. AcH refers to acetic acid in its undissociated form, Ac⁻ the acetate anion, membrane protein 1 is the Na⁺/H⁺ antiporter and membrane protein 2 is Na⁺,K⁺-ATPase.

respiration inhibited by ouabain (and hence assumed to represent Na⁺,K⁺-ATPase activity) varied with both dietary treatment and acetate concentration. Supplying additional UDP (at constant eRDP:FME) lowered ($P < 0.01$) the proportion of total respiration attributable to sodium pump activity by a constant amount at each acetate level whilst increasing acetate increased it linearly such that the percentage inhibition could be described by the following equation: %inhibition = 16.6 + 4.05 × acetate concentration (mM) (R^2 = 0.65, $P < 0.001$). This represents a change in the pattern of use of energy by liver tissue since, as total respiration rate did not alter as acetate level increased, so a greater proportion of energy production had to be diverted towards sodium pump activity.

From these results, it can be calculated that for acetate to cause an increase in sodium pump activity via the mechanism shown in Fig. 7.2, the rate of efflux of acetate⁻ would have to be 4.3 nmol min⁻¹ mg⁻¹ protein, equivalent to a permeability of 1×10^{-7} cm s⁻¹. This value is very close to those calculated for HCO_3^- and NH_4^+ and is in good agreement with one report of a measured permeability of the plasma membrane to acetate⁻ of 3.4×10^{-7} cm s⁻¹ (Sharp and Thomas, 1981; Hume and

Thomas, 1989). For efflux of acetate⁻ to take place, there must be a suitable 'driving force'; this would be provided by the substantial electrochemical gradient (positively charged on the extracellular surface and negatively charged on the intracellular one, thus repelling negatively charged ions from the cell) that exists across the plasma membrane (equivalent to a concentration gradient of ~100 mM for acetate⁻).

Carbon dioxide is produced continually within mitochondria from oxidative metabolism. It diffuses down its concentration gradient to the extracellular fluid. The potential exists for hydration of CO_2 to carbonic acid and then dissociation to H⁺ and HCO_3^-. Many tissues possess the enzyme catalase which greatly speeds up attainment of this equilibrium. The production of protons and bicarbonate from CO_2 results in what is termed facilitated diffusion of CO_2 from tissues (Gros et al., 1988). The HCO_3^- anion exchanges for Cl⁻ across the plasma membrane and the H⁺ is pumped out of the cell by the Na⁺/H⁺ antiporter. In studies with muscle tissue, where the rate of CO_2 production can increase substantially during exercise, this process of facilitated diffusion has been estimated to account for 70% of CO_2 removal from the tissue (Gros et al., 1988).

As noted earlier, measured activities of Na^+,K^+-ATPase were higher when the main pH buffer of the incubation medium was HCO_3^-/CO_2. In such studies, the CO_2 concentration in the extracellular fluid would be relatively high, reducing the concentration gradient of CO_2 between the incubation medium and intracellular fluid. Since CO_2 diffuses out of cells down this concentration gradient, this results in lower rates of CO_2 loss from cells and would increase the potential for facilitated diffusion of CO_2, increasing Na^+,K^+-ATPase activity. Extracellular CO_2 levels will be lower when alternative pH buffers, such as HEPES, are used.

Sies *et al.* (1973), from measurements of the change in pH of media draining perfused rat liver, have shown that addition of acetate (0–5 mM) to the perfusate (pH 7.4) caused a rapid change in proton uptake into hepatocytes, and using data supplied in this and an earlier publication (Sies and Noack, 1972) it can be calculated that the rates of proton uptake observed would cause changes in Na^+,K^+-ATPase activity similar to those reported above, assuming the previously discussed linkage between proton uptake and sodium pumping. The data from Sies' group do not differentiate between rapid initial extrusion of protons caused by equilibration of acetate across the plasma membrane and the proposed steady-state efflux of protons caused by acetate cycling. A similar response was seen when the perfused liver was exposed to differing levels of CO_2/HCO_3^-.

The ability of acetate to act as a proton ionophore will depend on the concentration of acetate in the extracellular fluid relative to the cell's ability to metabolize it. Thus the balance of nutrients available will determine metabolic efficiency, and it is to be expected that the optimal balance of nutrients will vary from tissue to tissue. Scollan and Jessop (1995) showed that in sheep given diets which would result in an imbalance of ingested nutrients (and would be expected to be used with a lower efficiency), blood acetate was markedly higher than in those fed on a more balanced diet. Cronjé *et al.* (1991) have shown that nutrient balance has a marked effect on acetate clearance, and Leng (1990) has discussed the influence of nutrient balance on the efficiency of use of metabolizable energy, pointing out the importance of the protein:energy ratio on the overall efficiency of energy use, as well as on the level of feed consumption.

Leakage

Biological membranes are composed of lipid bilayers in which many different proteins are embedded. Due to their arrangement, they have a hydrophobic inner layer which is presumed to be impermeable to charged or ionic species (or more specifically to molecules with high charge densities). As discussed above, this is not strictly true and many detailed electrophysiological studies have shown that the permeabilities of cell membranes to various ions, whilst low, are not zero (e.g. Hume and Thomas, 1989). It is not clear to what extent such permeabilities are due to the presence of specific ion channels or to non-specific leakage of ions across the lipid bilayer – maybe at regions where the lipid bilayer interacts with embedded proteins – or indeed to the processes outlined above. Studies from Hulbert's group in Australia have made detailed, comparative studies of the leakiness of biological membranes. They have studied the leakiness of both the plasma membrane to Na^+ and the mitochondrial membrane to H^+ and have shown that it varies markedly between cold-blooded reptiles and mammals (e.g. Else and Hulbert, 1987; Brand *et al.*, 1991). This may be due to much higher levels of unsaturated fatty acids in the mammal's membranes and differences in levels of thyroid hormones (Hulbert, 1987). This group have proposed that it is the higher rate of both Na^+ flux across the plasma membrane and H^+ leak across the mitochondrial membrane in warm-blooded animals that is important for maintaining higher rates of heat production, and hence the ability to keep body temperature at constant levels.

Thus there will be the potential for ionic flux across cell membranes which will be proportional to the surface area of the membrane, the difference in concentration of that ion across the membrane and the permeability of the membrane to the particular ion.

Coupled Transport

For many nutrients, e.g. glucose and some amino acids, transport into a cell is coupled to sodium entry. The transport mechanism only allows transport of the particular nutrient together with a sodium ion and thus utilizes the large concentration gradient of sodium ions to drive uptake of these nutrients from the extracellular water to the intracellular compartment. The sodium ions that are drawn into the cell in this manner are then pumped out on the sodium pump.

Adeola *et al.* (1989) measured Na^+,K^+-ATPase activity in muscle of pigs given diets that varied in protein content such that the rates of protein synthesis were altered. They reported an increase in Na^+,K^+-ATPase activity in direct proportion to increases in protein synthesis. Part of this increase may have been due to increased uptake of amino acids and glucose into muscle cells but part may also have been due to hormonal influences on pH_i, as discussed earlier.

Cell Volume Regulation

Plasma membranes do not provide any rigidity, and changes in the ionic environment can cause movement of water across the cell membrane. Within narrow limits, cells are able to compensate for this by altering the intracellular Na^+ concentration, thereby changing their osmolarity with respect to the extracellular environment.

Thus, rates of ion transport are essentially dependent on the hormonal and ionic environment together with the cell surface area. *In vivo*, the ionic environment is tightly controlled, although *in vitro* there

is the potential for it to vary more widely and it may change appreciably over time in a closed system (e.g. as end-products of metabolism accumulate). As cells grow, it is predicted that the cost of ion pumping will increase. This is due to both the hormonal environment necessary to mediate growth (increased pH_i) and the fact that cell surface area and hence Na^+ leakage per cell will also be increasing. The extent to which this might influence the rate at which cells grow is considered below and will depend on the rate at which energy in the form of ATP can be produced, i.e. the metabolic rate of the cell.

Energy Production

Across species of widely differing body size (e.g. mouse to elephant), cell size does not vary appreciably whereas cell number does. Therefore, species of larger mature size are characterized by having a greater number of cells than animals of smaller mature size. It has long been recognized that BMR varies with animal size. As animal size increases so does BMR, although not in direct proportion to the increase in size. From experimental observations, it has been shown that BMR increases in proportion to body weight raised to the power 0.73. Therefore as animal size increases across species, cell number increases in direct proportion to weight but metabolic rate increases in proportion to weight to the power 0.73. Thus metabolic rate per cell decreases as animal size increases (cellular metabolic rate will change in proportion to weight raised to the power of minus 0.27). Does this mean that cells from a large animal are incapable of metabolizing at rates equivalent to those from a small animal? Studies by Wheatley and Clegg (1994) suggest that this is not the case. They compiled data from a number of sources which compared metabolic rates of isolated cells or tissue slices taken from animals varying in size from 0.012 (mouse) to 780 (horse) kg. Whilst there was some reduction in metabolic rate measured *in vitro* as animal size increased, the magnitude of the differences *in vitro* were relatively small when compared with the differences in metabolic rates *in vivo*. Indeed, in the studies of O_2 consumption and sodium pump activity referred to earlier (Gregg and Milligan, 1982; McBride and Milligan, 1984, 1985a, b), there were few if any treatment effects on total O_2 consumption of different tissues incubated *in vitro*. Coulson (1993) argues that the differences in metabolic rates *in vivo* on a per cell basis are due to differences in the rate of supply of oxygen to these cells. For many metabolic pathways, the supply of oxygen is the rate-limiting step and delivery of it depends primarily on blood flow (oxygen extraction rates as tissues are perfused are remarkably similar across species). His argument, which he refers to as the 'Flow Theory', is based on certain physical constraints imposed on animal design (Coulson, 1993). Firstly, that blood pressure has to be maintained within certain limits (high enough to ensure that red blood cells can pass through capillary beds and plasma can perfuse cells, but not so high as to cause damage to blood vessels). Secondly, since blood volume is approximately 6.5% of body weight in animals (Schmidt-Nielsen, 1984), as animals increase in size, for blood volume to remain a fixed proportion of size, the diameter of the major blood vessels must decrease. As the diameter of blood vessels decreases, then the rate of flow of blood through them must also decrease in order to prevent blood pressure increasing dramatically.

Coulson uses the Flow Theory to argue that the rate of oxygen supply to tissues thus decreases as animal size increases, resulting in lower metabolic rates, expressed on a per cell basis, in larger animals. He uses this argument to explain differences between species of differing mature size and also to explain changes in the rate of growth as an animal matures. In this case, the cells within an animal's body will have a certain requirement for energy in order to meet their basal costs. Whilst oxygen supply is sufficient to ensure rates of energy production in excess of this fixed cost, the potential exists for the cells or tissues to grow. Therefore, as the animal grows, the diameter of major blood vessels must decrease in order to maintain blood volume at a fixed proportion of body weight. As this happens, so blood flow rates decrease, and hence the rate of oxygen supply to the tissues within the animal's body also falls. The resting metabolic rate of cells and thus their potential to produce ATP will decline, reducing the rate of growth. Additionally, as cells grow, their surface area increases, causing higher rates of Na^+ leakage. Therefore, as fixed costs increase and the potential metabolic rate of the cells decreases, the excess energy production over the fixed costs decreases, and hence the potential for growth reduces. Mature size is reached for a particular animal when fixed costs and potential energy supply coincide.

The potential for growth will depend on the difference between fixed costs of cells and their metabolic rate. Since fixed costs are determined in part by cell size (and this does not vary appreciably across species) and metabolic rate declines as mature size increases (as discussed above), the fractional or proportional rate of growth also declines across species as mature size increases. The fractional rate of growth is effectively the rate of growth on a per cell basis. Although this is lower in an animal of larger mature size than it is in a smaller one, the absolute rate of growth of the whole animal will be greater as larger animals contain many more cells than smaller ones do.

Conclusions

Care needs to be taken in the interpretation of measurements of Na^+,K^+-ATPase activity made *in vitro*. The incubation medium used, whether it employs CO_2/HCO_3^- as the main buffer or not (increasing the potential for cycling of carbonic acid across the plasma membrane), whether it contains a single energy substrate or a more balanced set of nutrients, and how tightly controlled pH and osmolarity can all influence the rate of Na^+ entry into the cell, and hence Na^+,K^+-ATPase activity. Nearly all measurements of ion transport have been made on isolated cells or pieces of tissue removed from the animal and incubated *in vitro*. The incubation medium used is usually devoid of hormones and contains standardized (and often high) levels of substrate. The differences observed indicate that some intrinsic property of cells has been altered and that this persists for the period of time between tissue removal and the measurements being made.

Consideration of physiological processes at the level of individual cells enables the understanding of energy use. It can be appreciated that many energetic costs are consequences of particular metabolic or physical processes, and thus the opportunity to manipulate them is limited. High rates of metabolic activity equate with increased basal metabolic requirements of individual cells. For example, high rates of CO_2 production will increase the rate of H^+ efflux from cells as part of facilitated diffusion of CO_2, in turn increasing energy use by Na^+,K^+-ATPase. The ability of cells to divide or to grow is dependent on hormonal stimuli that increase pH_i as part of the sequence of events they trigger. This increases basal energy use by increasing the rate of H^+ efflux, again increasing Na^+,K^+-ATPase activity.

Ensuring that the balance of nutrients is optimal will ensure that the potential for wasteful cycling of acetate across the cell membrane is minimized. Acetate cycling will be greater when the concentration of acetate in blood is high relative to the cell's ability to metabolize it. The availability of other nutrients can influence this (Illius and Jessop, 1996).

Therefore, the ability of weak acids such as acetic and carbonic acids to act as proton ionophores is worthy of further investigation as a new concept which might offer the possibility of a unifying theory to account for previously contradictory observations. It may explain the changes in efficiency of use of metabolizable energy with differing diets, the causes of which have not yet been elucidated satisfactorily. Understanding the causes of reduced metabolic efficiency and the associated heat increment would be of tremendous advantage, for example in developing improved feeding strategies when combating heat stress. The possibility of metabolic energy dissipation as a result of a physical transmembrane influence of metabolites could yield a very profound new insight into the energy metabolism of many species beyond ruminants. Such information will be required in order to assess the causes of differences in energy use between animals of differing genotype. Taylor *et al.* (1987) reported that maintenance needs of cattle varied with breed. Such differences cannot be accounted for by changes in the proportions of metabolically active tissues (Taylor *et al.*, 1991; Webster, 1993), thus indicating that differences in metabolic efficiency exist. Identification of nutrients and hormones that have a direct influence on metabolic efficiency will be necessary to understand the causes of such variation.

References

Adeola, O., Young, L.G., McBride, B.W. and Ball, R.O. (1989) *In vitro* Na^+,K^+-ATPase dependent respiration and protein synthesis in skeletal muscle of pigs fed at three dietary protein levels. *British Journal of Nutrition* 61, 453–465.

AFRC (1993) *Energy and Protein Requirements of Ruminants.* An advisory manual prepared by the AFRC Technical Committee on Responses to Nutrients. CAB International, Wallingford, UK.

Baldwin, R.L., Smith, N.E., Taylor, J. and Sharp, M. (1980) Manipulating metabolic parameters to improve growth rate and milk secretion. *Journal of Animal Science* 51, 1416–1428.

Boron, W.F. (1983) Transport of H^+ and of ionic weak acids and bases. *Journal of Membrane Biology* 72, 1–16.

Boron, W.F. and De Weer, P. (1976) Intracellular pH transients in squid giant axons caused by CO_2, NH_3 and metabolic inhibitors. *Journal of General Physiology* 67, 91–112.

Brand, M.D., Couture, P., Else, P.L., Withers, K.W. and Hulbert, A.J. (1991) Evolution of energy metabolism: proton permeability of the inner membrane of liver mitochondria is greater in a mammal than in a reptile. *Biochemical Journal* 275, 81–86.

Bryer-Ash, M. (1988) Rat insulin-receptor kinase activity correlates with *in vivo* insulin action. *Diabetes* 38, 108–116.

Coulson, R.A. (1993) The flow control theory of enzyme-kinetics – role of solid geometry in the control of reaction velocity in live animals. *International Journal of Biochemistry* 25, 1445–1474.

Cronjé, P.B., Nolan, J.V. and Leng, R.A. (1991) Acetate clearance rate as a potential index of the availability of glucogenic precursors in ruminants fed on roughage-based diets. *British Journal of Nutrition* 66, 301–312.

Eckert, R. and Randall, D.J. (1983) *Animal Physiology; Mechanisms and Adaptations.* W.H. Freeman and Co., New York, pp. 148–149.

Else, P.L. and Hulbert, A.J. (1987) Evolution of mammalian endothermic metabolism: 'leaky' membranes as a source of heat. *American Journal of Physiology* 253, R1–R7.

Emmans, G.C. (1994) Effective energy: a concept of energy utilization applied across species. *British Journal of Nutrition* 71, 801–821.

Graf, J., Henderson, R.M., Meier, P.J. and Boyer, J.L. (1988) Regulation of intracellular pH in hepatocytes. In: Häussinger, D. (ed.) *pH Homeostasis, Mechanisms and Control.* Academic Press, London, pp. 43–60.

Gregg, V.A. and Milligan, L.P. (1982a) Role of Na^+,K^+-ATPase in muscular energy expenditure of warm and cold exposed sheep. *Canadian Journal of Animal Science* 62, 123–132.

Gregg, V.A. and Milligan, L.P. (1982b) *In vitro* energy costs of Na^+,K^+-ATPase activity and protein synthesis in muscle from calves differing in age and breed. *British Journal of Nutrition* 48, 65–71.

Gregg, V.A. and Milligan, L.P. (1987) Thyroid induction of thermogenesis in cultured hepatocytes and sheep liver. In: Moe, P.W., Tyrrell, H.F. and Reynolds, P.J. (eds) *Energy Metabolism in Farm Animals.* European Association of Animal Production, Publication No 32. Rowman and Littlefield, Totowa, New Jersey, pp. 10–13.

Gros, G., Forster, R.E. and Dodgson, S.J. (1988) CO_2/HCO_3^- equilibria in the body. In: Häussinger, D. (ed.) *pH Homeostasis, Mechanisms and Control.* Academic Press, London, pp. 203–231.

Hulbert, A.J. (1987) Thyroid hormones, membranes and the evolution of endothermy. In: McLennan, H., Ledsome, J.R., McIntosh, C.H.S. and Jones, D.R. (eds) *Advances in Physiological Research.* Plenum Publishing Corporation, New York, pp. 305–319.

Hulbert, A.J., Mantaj, W. and Janssens, P.A. (1991) Development of mammalian endothermic metabolism: quantitative changes in tissue mitochondria. *American Journal of Physiology* 261, R561–R568.

Hume, R.I. and Thomas, S.A. (1989) A calcium- and voltage-dependent chloride current in developing chick skeletal muscle. *Journal of Physiology* 417, 241–261.

Illius, A.W. and Jessop, N.S. (1996) Metabolic constraints on voluntary intake in ruminants. *Journal of Animal Science* 74, 3052–3062.

Jessop, N.S. (1988) Estimation of energy expenditure associated with Na^+, K^+ ATPase activity in ovine liver. *Proceedings of the Nutrition Society* 47, 118A.

Jessop, N.S. and Leng, R.A. (1993) The influence of acetate and nutrient balance on ouabain-sensitive respiration in ovine liver. *Proceedings of the Nutrition Society* 52, 56A.

Ketelaars, J.J.M.H. and Tolkamp, B.J. (1992) Toward a new theory of feed intake regulation in ruminants 3. Optimum feed intake: in search of a physiological background. *Livestock Production Science* 31, 235–258.

Leng, R.A. (1990) Factors affecting the utilization of 'poor-quality' forages by ruminants particularly under tropical conditions. *Nutrition Research Reviews* 3, 277–303.

McBride, B.W. and Milligan, L.P. (1984) The effect of lactation on the ouabain-sensitive respiration of the duodenal mucosa of cows. *Canadian Journal of Animal Science* 64, 817–824.

McBride, B.W. and Milligan, L.P. (1985a) Influence of feed intake and starvation on the magnitude of Na^+,K^+-ATPase (EC 3.6.1.3)-dependent respiration in duodenal mucosa of sheep. *British Journal of Nutrition* 53, 605–614.

McBride, B.W. and Milligan, L.P. (1985b) Magnitude of ouabain-sensitive respiration in the liver of growing, lactating and starved sheep. *British Journal of Nutrition* 54, 293–303.

Milligan, L.P. and Summers, M. (1986) The biological basis of maintenance and its relevance to assessing responses to nutrients. *Proceedings of the Nutrition Society* 45, 185–193.

Moore, R.D. (1983) Effects of insulin upon ion transport. *Biochimica et Biophysica Acta* 737, 1–49.

NRC (1996) *Nutrient Requirements of Beef Cattle*, 7th edn. National Academy Press, Washington, DC.

Park, H.S., Kelly, J.M. and Milligan, L.P. (1992) Energetics and cell membranes. In: Kinney, J.M. and Tucker, H.N. (eds) *Energy Metabolism: Tissue Determinants and Cellular Corollaries*. Raven Press Ltd, New York, pp. 411–435.

Pouyssegur, J., Franchi, A., Paris, S. and Sardet, C. (1988) Mechanisms of activation and molecular genetics of the mammalian Na^+/H^+ antiporter. In: Häussinger, D. (ed.) *pH Homeostasis, Mechanisms and Control*. Academic Press, London, pp. 61–78.

Scollan, N.D. and Jessop, N.S. (1995) Diet-induced variation in acetate metabolism of ovine perirenal adipose tissue *in vitro. Journal of Agricultural Science, Cambridge* 125, 429–436.

Schmidt-Nielsen, K. (1984) *Scaling: Why is Animal Size so Important?* Cambridge University Press, Cambridge.

Sharp, A.P. and Thomas, R.C. (1981) The effects of chloride substitution on intracellular pH in crab muscle. *Journal of Physiology* 312, 71–80.

Sies, H. and Noack, G. (1972) Proton movement accompanying monocarboxylate permeation in hemoglobin-free perfused rat liver. *FEBS Letters* 22, 193–196.

Sies, H., Noack, G. and Halder, K.H. (1973) Carbon dioxide concentration and the distribution of monocarboxylate and H^+ ions between the intracellular and extracellular spaces of hemoglobin free perfused rat liver. *European Journal of Biochemistry* 38, 247–258.

Smith, J.B. and Rozengurt, E. (1978) Serum stimulates the Na^+,K^+ pump in quiescent fibroblasts by increasing Na^+ entry. *Proceedings of the National Academy of Science of the United States of America* 75, 5560–5564.

Swaminathan, R., Chan, E.L.P., Sin, L.Y., Ng, S.K.F. and Chan, A.Y.S. (1989) The effect of ouabain on metabolic rate in guinea-pigs: estimation of energy cost of sodium pump activity. *British Journal of Nutrition* 61, 467–473.

Taylor, St.C.S. and Murray, J.I. (1991) Effect of feeding level, breed and milking potential on body tissues and organs of mature, non-lactating cows. *Animal Production* 53, 27–38.

Taylor, St.C.S., Thiessen, R.B. and Murray, J.I. (1986) Inter-breed relationship of maintenance efficiency to milk yield in cattle. *Animal Production* 43, 37–61.

Webster, A.J.F. (1993) Energy partitioning, tissue growth and appetite control. *Proceedings of the Nutrition Society* 52, 69–76.

Wheatley, D.N. and Clegg, J.S. (1994) What determines the basal metabolic rate of vertebrate cells *in vivo? Biosystems* 32, 83–92.

Chapter 8
Trace Element Dynamics

W.T. Buckley

Agriculture and Agri-Food Canada, Brandon Research Centre, Brandon, Canada

Introduction

Trace element dynamics in animals refers to the quantitative metabolism and kinetics of trace element absorption, distribution, storage and excretion. Control of these processes normally yields a reasonably constant and optimum internal environment with respect to trace element functions in metabolism. Within a range of conditions, trace element homeostasis may be achieved and maintained. Trace element dynamics may be viewed as the shifting or maintenance of trace element status, which depends on numerous factors including the element and species in question, and the influence of homeostatic mechanisms. It is the objective of this chapter to summarize current knowledge of trace element dynamics with respect to the responses of whole-body trace element metabolism to changes in dietary intake. The reader is also referred to other reviews on the topic (Miller, 1973; Kirchgessner, 1993).

Trace elements can be divided into two groups with respect to their route of endogenous excretion: those for which homeostasis is partially dependent on endogenous faecal excretion, controlled by the intestinal tract, liver and pancreas, and those for which homeostasis is dependent upon renal excretion, controlled by resorption in the proximal renal tubule. Cationic elements including Cu, Mn and Zn fall into the first category while elements present in the body as anions including Cr, F, Mo and Se fall into the second category. In the cation group, control of homeostasis through variation in absorption usually is the most significant factor, although variation in excretion is also important. Iron, though, is unique because its homeostasis is dependent essentially, if not entirely, on control of absorption. In the anionic group, control of excretion predominates and absorption plays a minor role. In this chapter, we will discuss Zn, Cu, Mn, Fe and Se.

The trace element content of tissues may respond in basically two ways to changes in a dietary trace element intake: (A) no change over a range of intakes, beyond which a decrease or increase of tissue content occurs; or (B) a continuous change in tissue content over a range of intakes. In case A, a homeostatic plateau occurs, which is not apparent in case B. There are various combinations of tissue responses within individuals because some tissues maintain homeostasis more readily than others. Furthermore, there is a large variation among species. Responses to changes in dietary intake usually vary with level of intake, and several elements have specific storage tissues while others do not. One objective of this chapter is to identify the variations in homeostatic responses of trace elements among tissues and species.

Many studies of trace element dynamics, especially in larger animals and humans, have given little consideration to the dietary intake prior to the experimental period and to the effect of previous diet on body stores at the time of initiating the study. The effect of previous history on Zn metabolism was investigated by Johnson *et al.* (1988). By studying rats for two sequential dietary periods, it was shown that Zn absorption was affected only by the current dietary Zn intake, but that endogenous excretion was influenced by both current and past intake. Rats previously fed a deficient Zn diet, 1.5 µg Zn g^{-1}, had lower rates of endogenous excretion over a range of Zn intakes than rats previously fed 12.5 or 50.3 µg Zn g^{-1} diet (Johnson *et al.*, 1988). The differences in endogenous excretion allowed the previously deficient rats to recover body Zn more rapidly during the second dietary period.

Larger animals and humans may take months or even years to establish a new steady-state for some trace elements following a change in intake (Buckley, 1996). Although adaptive changes in rates of absorption may occur relatively rapidly, endogenous excretion will be in a state of flux until a new steady-state has been established. Furthermore, steady-state cannot be achieved in growing animals with respect to major trace element pools, which are constantly increasing in size. Although measurements of endogenous excretion can be made under non-steady-state conditions, investigators should be aware that the results apply only at the time of making the measurements. A goal of this chapter is to develop an appreciation of the rate of change of trace element status and its impact on interpretation of tracer and balance studies.

An isotope dilution technique (Weigand and Kirchgessner, 1976) has been used frequently for measuring true absorption and endogenous faecal excretion in studies of trace element dynamics. The technique depends on sampling a reference tissue or fluid which contains the labelled element assumed to be at the same specific activity as endogenous secretions. Endogenous faecal excretion is calculated from the quantity of tracer in faeces and the specific activity in the reference tissue or fluid. The validity of selecting certain tissues or fluids for the isotope dilution technique has been tested for several elements and species. Although support for acceptable reference tissues and fluids has been obtained, not all sources of error have been investigated, and some caution is required. For example, liver Mn specific activity has been used to represent specific activity of endogenous secretions; however, liver specific activity was shown recently to be indistinguishable from biliary specific activity in Mn-replete rats, but it was only about one-third of biliary-specific activity in Mn-deficient rats (Malecki *et al.*, 1996). Since bile is a significant source of endogenous Mn secretions, estimates of endogenous faecal excretion based on liver specific activity may be in error in Mn-deficient rats. On the other hand, endogenous secretions of Mn are very low in deficient rats, and correction for the potential error would only make the estimates lower and may have little effect on interpretation of the results. The effect of the choice of reference tissue and time of sampling on the accuracy of determinations of endogenous excretion has been discussed by Weigand *et al.* (1988a). Some aspects of trace element dynamics related to measurement technique are mentioned in this chapter.

The homeostatic control of Zn in rats has been studied much more intensively than other element and species combinations; consequently, Zn dynamics is emphasized in this chapter. Knowledge of Zn metabolism in the rat is sufficient to construct a kinetic simulation of whole-body and tissue responses to changes in dietary intake. Such a simulation of Zn metabolism was constructed for this chapter from the results of numerous Zn metabolism studies. The objective of the simulation is to compile results of studies which have addressed different aspects of Zn metabolism or different ranges of conditions. It is hoped that the whole-body simulation of Zn metabolism will help to identify productive areas of investigation for other elements as well as Zn. Simulation of whole body metabolism provides a method of reviewing Zn dynamics as well as providing unique insight into trace element dynamics in general.

Zinc

Metabolism

Zinc metabolism in animals and man has been the subject of extensive reviews (e.g. Chesters, 1997). Zinc is absorbed mainly by the small intestine, although the major section(s) from which absorption takes place have not been identified. During absorption, the rate of intramucosal Zn transport may be controlled by an interaction between cysteine-rich intestinal protein (CRIP), serving as an intracellular carrier, and metallothionein, which appears to inhibit intracellular transport (Chesters, 1997). As a result of desquamation of mucosal cells, more Zn enters the mucosa than is transported to plasma. This mechanism appears to be important in the regulation of Zn absorption. Zinc absorption determined by the isotope dilution technique (Weigand and Kirchgessner, 1976) does not include the fraction of Zn which enters, but does not cross, the mucosal lining to the bloodstream. Once in the plasma, Zn is transported predominantly in association with albumin and to a lesser extent with a high-molecular weight protein fraction. Transfer of Zn to liver from plasma is 5–6 times faster than transfer to other major tissues (House and Wastney, 1997). Although the liver is very active in Zn metabolism, it represents <5% of whole-body Zn, while bone and muscle

are normally the largest Zn pools. In small animals, however, the integument becomes quantitatively significant. In the rat, the Zn pool in the pelt (skin plus hair) may exceed that in the bone or muscle. Sources of endogenous Zn entering the gastrointestinal tract include saliva, gastric secretions, pancreatic secretions, bile and intestinal secretions. Of these, pancreatic secretions may be the most quantitatively significant. In normal pigs, more Zn was secreted in pancreatic fluid than in bile, but this order was reversed in Zn-deficient pigs since pancreatic secretion was reduced to a greater extent than biliary secretion, indicating that regulation of both pancreatic and biliary secretion of Zn is important in Zn homeostasis (Sullivan *et al.*, 1981). The quantity of Zn secreted into the intestine from all sources may be as much as dietary Zn intake. Although biliary Cu is known to be absorbed with much lower efficiency than dietary Cu, there has been insufficient work to determine if Zn responds in a similar manner. A lower rate of resorption of biliary and/or pancreatic Zn compared with dietary Zn could be a factor in maintaining homeostasis.

Growth depression is characteristic of Zn deficiency in the young of all species studied. Zinc deficiency normally results in the loss of Zn from bone and liver, but not from skeletal muscle. Integument losses also are a significant fraction of whole-body loss during Zn deficiency in rats and presumably other small animals. Loss of bone Zn has been found as a result of Zn deficiency in rats, calves, chickens and quail, but not in monkeys or cows. Loss of liver Zn has been reported for rats, calves, chickens, quail and monkeys, but not cows. Except for the stability of Zn in skeletal muscle, variable responses to Zn deficiency have been found in other tissues.

Above the nutritional requirement, whole-body Zn and Zn content of tissues appear to be regulated over a range of Zn intakes, although homeostatic control varies with species and physiological state. A small increase in digestive tract tissue Zn was observed in rats fed 104 compared with 24 µg Zn g^{-1} diet, while there was no effect on Zn content of liver, kidneys, spleen, brain, lungs, reproductive tissues, muscle, skeleton or pelt (Windisch and Kirchgessner, 1993). These and other studies have indicated that rats are able to maintain relatively constant tissue Zn concentration up to 600 µg Zn g^{-1} diet; however, higher intakes lead to substantial increases in Zn content of most internal organs and bone. Based on limited reports, the ability to maintain tissue Zn homeostasis with increasing dietary Zn concentration varies considerably among species, with quail and chickens having little ability to maintain homeostasis, calves and rats having moderate ability and mice having the greatest dietary range of species reported. Although the congruence is less than desirable among studies, species and physiological states with respect to tissues affected by excess Zn and the dietary range over which homeostasis can be maintained, it is possible to conclude that a homeostatic plateau exists for some range of Zn intakes above the nutritional requirement for most species.

Tissue Zn turnover varies among tissues and is a factor in mobilization of Zn and in its excretion from the body. Rapidly turning over tissues can respond more rapidly to a reduction in Zn intake. Disappearance curve analysis of individual tissues from sequentially sacrificed rams following intravenous ^{65}Zn administration showed that liver, heart, pancreas, salivary glands, kidney cortex and spleen had rapid Zn turnover ≥18% day^{-1}, while skeletal muscle and bone had slow turnover, <2% day^{-1} and other tissues had intermediate values (McKenney et al., 1962). Comparison of Zn kinetics in mice, rats, dogs and humans shows that the biological half-life of Zn increases as the size of the species increases.

Simulation of zinc dynamics – model development

Model simulation provides a means of compiling existing knowledge of metabolism from numerous studies to yield a more comprehensive view than can be provided by individual investigations. Based on the results of published studies, a model of Zn metabolism (Fig. 8.1) was constructed in order to simulate Zn dynamics. The simulation was prepared with the aid of a compartmental modelling program, SAAM II (SAAM Institute, 1994). The simulation has been constructed for male, growing rats consuming diets varying in Zn concentration from deficient to adequate. Although constructed for rats, similarities with other species are apparent in the results of the simulation.

Williams and Mills (1970) thoroughly documented feed intake, body weight changes and whole-body Zn concentrations over time with growing rats fed varying Zn concentrations from deficient (3 µg g^{-1}) to adequate (12 µg g^{-1}). Much of these data have been incorporated into the model, providing basic Zn data for growing rats. Dietary Zn intake varies with time (body size) and dietary Zn concentration (Fig. 8.2). Several other studies have shown that feed intake and growth rate no longer vary with dietary Zn concentration for a considerable range above the nutritional requirement. Thus, feed intakes for 15 and 18 µg Zn g^{-1} diet were included in the model equal to the intake at 12 µg Zn g^{-1} diet (Fig. 8.2). Whole-body Zn of young rats increased with age and dietary Zn concentration up to the nutritional requirement (Williams and Mills, 1970) (Fig. 8.3). Since Williams and Mills (1970) and others have shown repeatedly that whole-body Zn or tissue Zn does not increase with increases in dietary Zn above the minimum requirement up to relatively high intakes, dietary concentrations of 15 and 18 µg Zn g^{-1} diet were included in the simulation with no increase in whole-body Zn compared with rats fed 12 µg Zn g^{-1} diet (Fig. 8.3).

Johnson et al. (1988) investigated the effect of dietary Zn concentration on the coefficient of absorption of Zn using growing male rats similar in age to those studied by Williams and Mills (1970). Their measurements of Zn absorption included the dietary Zn range of 3.6–50 µg g^{-1}. A substantial reduction in coefficient of

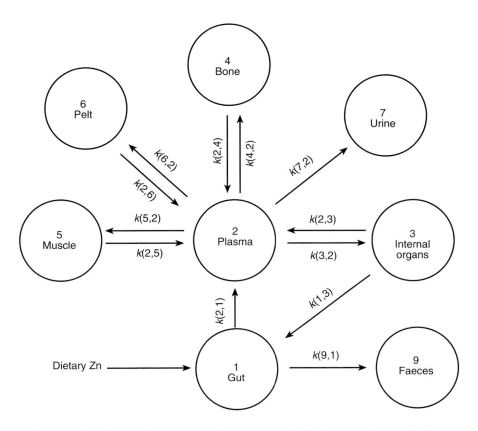

Fig. 8.1. Kinetic model of Zn metabolism in rats. Circles represent body Zn compartments, which are numbered arbitrarily. Arrows are fractional transfer coefficients (day^{-1}), $k(i,j)$, indicating transfer to compartment i from compartment j; for example, $k(2,1)$ is the fraction of compartment 1 (gut Zn) which is transferred to compartment 2 (plasma Zn) per day.

absorption occurred with increasing dietary Zn concentration. Their data (Johnson *et al.*, 1988) were subjected to non-linear regression, to yield the following relationship which was incorporated into the model:

$$\text{Abs} = 0.986 - 0.0233 \times \text{Zn p.p.m.} + 0.0002 \times \text{Zn p.p.m.}^2 \quad (8.1)$$

where Abs = coefficient of absorption and Zn p.p.m. = dietary Zn concentration, μg g^{-1} (Fig. 8.4).

Plasma Zn was held in steady-state in the simulation because it is only about 0.5% of whole-body Zn in the rat, and variations in the plasma Zn pool size, which are observed during deficiency, are negligible with respect to changes in the major tissue Zn pools. It was assumed that

the relative distribution of plasma Zn to tissues in the body of the growing rat would be similar to that found for mature rats in a recent compartmental modelling study (House and Wastney, 1997). Thus, values for the fractional transfer coefficients to tissues from plasma (determined by House and Wastney, 1997) are incorporated into the current simulation. The values utilized were 7.1 day^{-1} for transfer of plasma Zn to muscle ($k(5,2)$ in Fig. 8.1), 5.62 day^{-1} for transfer to skin and hair ($k(6,2)$), 35.7 day^{-1} for transfer to internal organs ($k(3,2)$) and 7.22 day^{-1} for transfer to bone ($k(4,2)$). Thus, Zn transfer from plasma to internal organs, mainly liver, in the simulation is relatively rapid, which is consistent with other observations on the

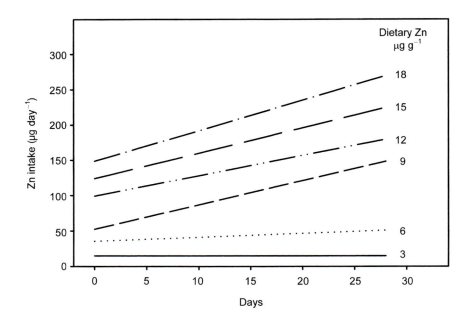

Fig. 8.2. Dietary Zn intake in young growing male rats fed a semi-synthetic diet with varying Zn concentrations. Adapted from Williams and Mills (1970).

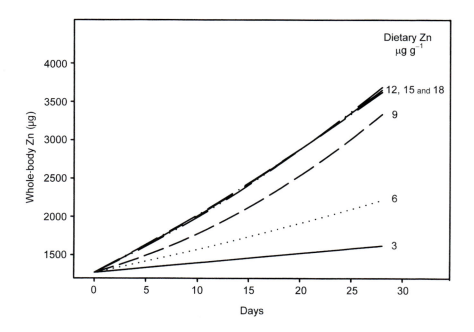

Fig. 8.3. Whole-body Zn accumulation in young growing male rats fed a semi-synthetic diet with varying Zn concentrations. Adapted from Williams and Mills (1970).

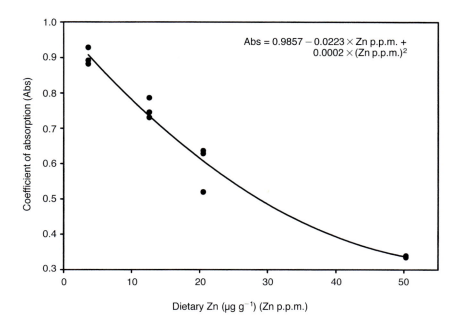

$$Abs = 0.9857 - 0.0223 \times Zn\ p.p.m. + 0.0002 \times (Zn\ p.p.m.)^2$$

Fig. 8.4. Absorption of Zn by young growing male rats fed a semi-synthetic diet with varying Zn concentrations. Adapted from Johnson *et al.* (1988).

rate of transfer of plasma ^{65}Zn to liver in humans, rats and cattle.

Tracer studies with rats, cows and calves show enhanced retention and/or increased specific activity of tracer in tissues of Zn-deficient animals compared with Zn-adequate animals, which indicates that Zn transfer from tissue to plasma is decreased in Zn deficiency (e.g. Windisch and Kirchgessner, 1994). On the other hand, excessive Zn intake leads to a reduction in tissue tracer specific activity or retention. These results indicate that tissue Zn turnover is decreased in Zn deficiency and increased when Zn supply is excessive. Thus, variations in tissue Zn mass in the simulation were accomplished through changes to tissue Zn egress transfer coefficients. The value of each coefficient was controlled by a function designed to adjust the compartment size, expressed as a percentage of whole-body Zn, to match tissue Zn contents obtained from several studies (Giugliano and Millward, 1984; Windisch and Kirchgessner, 1994; House and Wastney, 1997). The tissue egress

coefficients decreased with decreasing Zn intake in the simulation, as would be expected from published observations of changes in tissue Zn turnover. Percentages of whole-body Zn in muscle and bone of Zn-adequate growing rats used in the simulation were 26.7 and 27.9%, while percentages for Zn-deficient growing rats were 40.0 and 13.4%, respectively (from Giugliano and Millward, 1984, after correcting for pelt Zn). The percentage of whole-body Zn in the internal organs was fixed at 15.1 (from Giugliano and Millward, 1984, after correcting for pelt Zn). The percentage of Zn in the pelt was fixed at 30.5 (House and Wastney, 1997). Percentages of whole-body Zn in internal organs and in the pelt were fixed in the simulation because they were unaffected by variations in dietary Zn (Giugliano and Millward, 1984; Windisch and Kirchgessner, 1994).

Measurements of urinary Zn excretion for growing rats at various dietary Zn intakes from the study of Johnson *et al.* (1988) were subjected to non-linear regression to yield the following relationship:

Urinary Zn = 7.4
$$\times\ (1\ -\ e^{-0.0074\ \times\ \text{Zn intake}}) \qquad (8.2)$$

where units of urinary Zn and Zn intake are µg day^{-1} (Fig. 8.5). This expression was utilized in the simulation to describe the loss of Zn via urine.

All aspects of the model were derived from published results except for the rate of endogenous faecal excretion, which was determined for various nutritional states by solving the model. The model was solved for endogenous faecal excretion rather than using available data from the literature because endogenous faecal excretion cannot be varied independently from changes in whole-body Zn mass, and changes in whole-body mass were entered into the model from the data of Williams and Mills (1970) as discussed above.

Simulation of zinc dynamics – model output

The model was solved for dietary Zn intake by young growing male rats consuming diets varying from 3 µg g^{-1} (deficient) to 18 µg g^{-1} under conditions in which 12 µg g^{-1} provided adequate Zn. Urinary and faecal Zn excretion are shown in Figs 8.6 and 8.7. As has been well documented in animals, the simulation shows that faeces are the main route of excretion of dietary Zn. However, at lower dietary Zn intakes, urinary Zn excretion became a significant percentage of total Zn excreted (Fig. 8.8). Similar results have been found in humans and calves.

As might be expected, Zn balance varied considerably in response to dietary intake according to the simulation (Fig. 8.9). Except for the lowest level of dietary Zn (3 µg g^{-1}), Zn balance, expressed as µg day^{-1}, varied with time in the growing rats, and was highest for 9–18 µg Zn g^{-1} diet at 28 days. The simulation shows that measurement of balance alone may not be sufficient to distinguish an adequate from a deficient diet. At 28 days, balance for rats fed 9 µg Zn g^{-1} diet was as great as for 12–18 µg Zn g^{-1} diet, even though 9 µg Zn

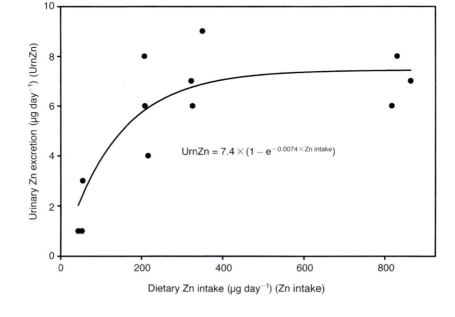

Fig. 8.5. Urinary excretion of Zn by young growing male rats fed a semi-synthetic diet with varying Zn concentrations. Adapted from Johnson *et al.* (1988).

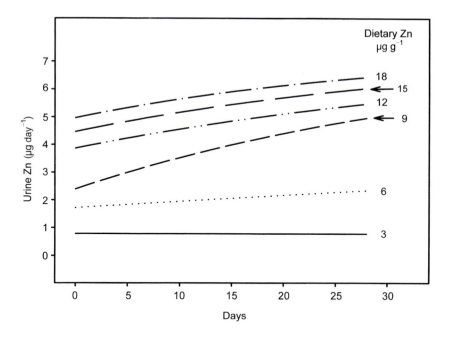

Fig. 8.6. Urinary Zn excretion by young growing male rats. The figure is a simulation based on a kinetic model of Zn metabolism (Fig. 8.1) and published data for rats fed a semi-synthetic diet with varying Zn concentrations as described in the text.

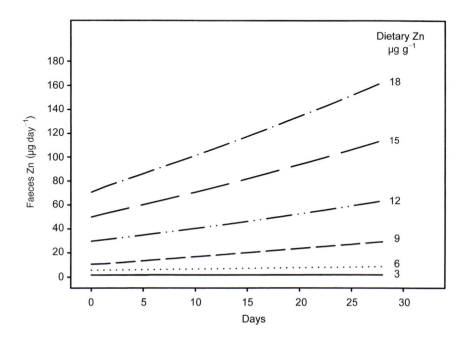

Fig. 8.7. Faecal Zn excretion by young growing male rats. The figure is a simulation as described in Fig. 8.6.

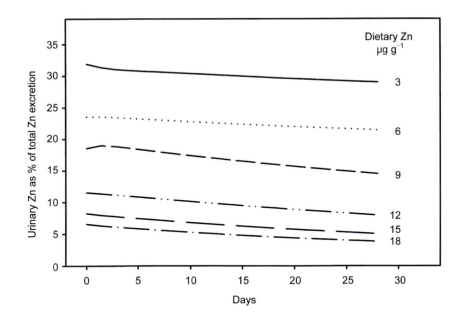

Fig. 8.8. Percentage of total Zn excretion (faeces + urine) excreted in the urine of young growing male rats. The figure is a simulation as described in Fig. 8.6.

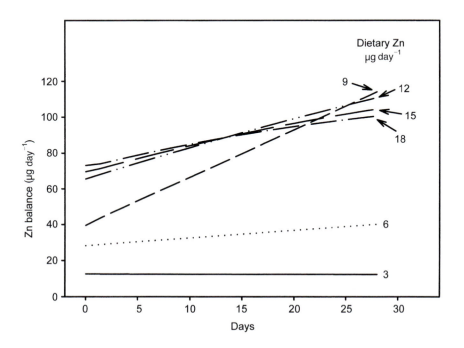

Fig. 8.9. Zinc balance of young growing male rats. The figure is a simulation as described in Fig. 8.6.

g^{-1} diet was unable to support as rapid growth as 12–18 µg Zn g^{-1} diet during the full 28-day period. During the last days of the simulation, whole-body accumulation of Zn at 9 µg Zn g^{-1} diet was nearly parallel to that at 12 µg Zn g^{-1} diet (Fig. 8.3), leading to nearly equivalent balance values. Thus, due to observed differences in feed intake, percentage absorption and percentage excretion, the simulation reveals that 9 µg Zn g^{-1} diet should be able to meet the nutritional requirement for Zn at the end of the 28-day period but not at the beginning.

Control of endogenous faecal Zn excretion is recognized as an important mechanism of Zn homeostasis. In the current simulation, endogenous faecal excretion was almost negligible at 3, 6 and 9 µg Zn g^{-1} diet in the growing rat (Fig. 8.10). The whole-body retention of Zn found by Williams and Mills (1970) was achieved by the nearly complete inhibition of endogenous faecal excretion. It shows that the rat has considerable capacity for

regulating loss of Zn from the body, since there was very little loss at intakes less than the nutritional requirement. The ability of organisms to minimize endogenous faecal excretion of Zn in response to dietary deficiency has been reported in studies with rats, calves, goats and human infants.

Although the coefficient of absorption decreases as dietary Zn concentration increases (Fig. 8.4), quantitative true absorption (µg day^{-1}) increases because the elevated Zn intake is not fully matched by the reduction in the coefficient of absorption. This relationship was observed by Weigand and Kirchgessner (1978) and is shown by solving the simulation for dietary concentrations up to 48 µg g^{-1} (Fig. 8.11). Since there was no further increase in whole-body Zn concentration above the nutritional requirement, the additional absorbed Zn was excreted in the faeces. Apparent absorption remained relatively constant above the nutritional requirement (Fig. 8.11), while both true absorption (µg

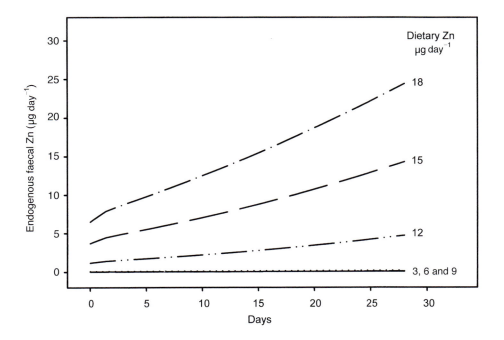

Fig. 8.10. Endogenous faecal excretion of Zn by young growing male rats. The figure is a simulation as described in Fig. 8.6.

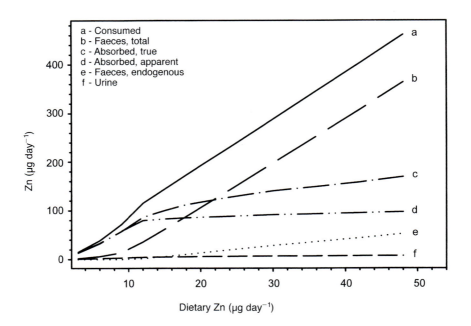

a - Consumed
b - Faeces, total
c - Absorbed, true
d - Absorbed, apparent
e - Faeces, endogenous
f - Urine

Fig. 8.11. Consumption, absorption and excretion of Zn in young growing male rats. The figure is a simulation as described in Fig. 8.6.

day^{-1}) and endogenous faecal excretion continued to rise, which is the pattern observed by Weigand and Kirchgessner (1978). As dietary Zn intake was increased to 141 µg Zn g^{-1} diet in the study of Weigand and Kirchgessner (1978), the quantity of endogenous faecal Zn excretion also increased until it was 90% of the value of apparent Zn absorption. Thus, regulation of endogenous excretion plays a critical role in conservation of body Zn during Zn deficiency and, also, in the elimination of Zn when excess Zn is absorbed.

Although regulation of absorption alone was not sufficient to maintain homeostasis in response to elevated dietary intake (Fig. 8.11), the threefold reduction in coefficient of absorption over the range of dietary intakes investigated is substantial (Fig. 8.4). A reduction in the coefficient of absorption with increasing dietary consumption of Zn has been observed repeatedly in rats, and also in calves, sheep, human infants and human adults. Changes in absorption may be of greater

significance at higher dietary Zn concentrations in ruminants than in monogastrics. Studies with ewes and calves indicate that homeostasis was maintained predominantly by changes in absorption, with very little if any change in endogenous faecal excretion when dietary Zn ranged from adequate to excessive.

Redistribution of Zn within the major Zn pools of the body has been observed several times in response to Zn deficiency in growing rats (e.g. Giugliano and Millward, 1984) as well as in mature rats and chicks. Redistribution involves the relatively greater loss of Zn from bone compared with other tissues during deficiency. Loss of bone Zn has also been demonstrated in Zn-deficient young pigs, although changes in other tissues have not been measured. Redistribution appears to be a mechanism of maintaining Zn concentration in preferred tissues at the expense of others and, as such, may be an important metabolic strategy influencing the health of deficient animals. Changes in skin and hair Zn as well as bone, muscle and internal organ Zn were simulated for growing rats receiving adequate (Fig. 8.12) or deficient (Fig. 8.13) dietary Zn. Rats fed a deficient Zn diet accumulated less Zn overall in tissues, but muscle accumulated relatively more zinc than the other tissues, mainly at the expense of bone. The tissue distribution of Zn shown at day 28 in Figs 8.12 and 8.13 is from Giugliano and Millward (1984). The redistribution of Zn was simulated using modelling techniques for regulating Zn tissue mass as described above. The rate of redistribution was assumed to take about one-half of the 28-day period simulated, which is consistent with the time course of ^{65}Zn redistribution observed in another study with marginally deficient rats.

Copper

Copper metabolism has been the subject of extensive reviews (e.g. Linder, 1991).

Copper absorption is quite variable depending on species and dietary factors. Absorption by humans varies from about 12 to 55%, whereas absorption by ruminants varies from about 1 to 13%. At low absorption percentages, changes of a few percent can double or triple absolute Cu absorption, which can have profound affects on Cu nutrition. Absorbed Cu is bound mainly to plasma albumin, and possibly transcuprein and amino acids. It is transported to the liver where it is removed efficiently from circulation. Within the liver, Cu is incorporated into the protein ceruloplasmin and released into the general circulation. Ceruloplasmin Cu is tightly bound, does not exchange readily with ionic Cu in plasma and comprises 80–97% of plasma Cu in species surveyed. Tissue Cu turnover leads to release of Cu to the bloodstream, where it is assumed to travel in association with plasma albumin, transcuprein and amino acids. Excretion of Cu is mainly via the bile

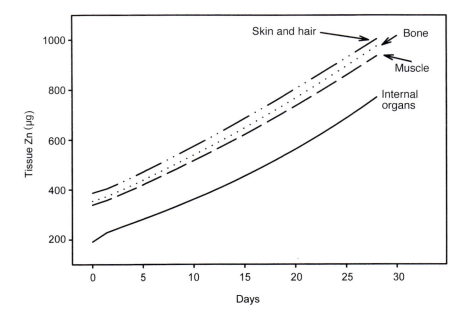

Fig. 8.12. Tissue Zn accumulation of young growing male rats fed adequate dietary Zn (12 µg g^{-1}) in a semi-synthetic diet. The figure is a simulation based on a kinetic model of Zn metabolism (Fig. 8.1) and published data as described in the text.

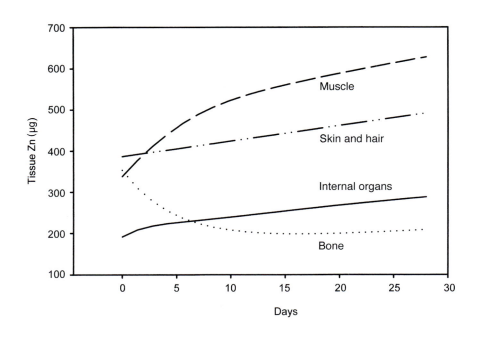

Fig. 8.13. Tissue Zn accumulation of young growing male rats fed deficient dietary Zn (3 µg g^{-1}) in a semi-synthetic diet. The figure is a simulation as described in Fig. 8.12.

and other gastrointestinal secretions, with only a small percentage of endogenous loss in the urine. Surface losses from sweat, skin and hair or feathers are small, but exceed urinary losses, at least in humans. Biliary Cu is reabsorbed poorly in mammals and chickens, which increases the efficiency of endogenous excretion.

The liver plays an important role in the quantitative whole-body metabolism of Cu, especially in ruminants. Up to 80% of whole-body Cu is found in the liver of healthy sheep and cattle, as opposed to 8 or 9% in the liver of monogastrics. Bone also is a major Cu pool in all species, varying in Cu content from about 18% of whole-body Cu in cattle to 40% in humans. Muscle comprises about 13% of whole-body Cu in cattle, 23% in humans and 31% in rats. In small animals, the skin also becomes a major component of whole-body Cu, about 23% in rats.

There is considerable variability among species in their ability to maintain liver Cu homeostasis (Fig. 8.14). Sheep appear to have little or no ability to regulate liver Cu concentration. Even small increments in dietary Cu to unsupplemented diets yield substantial increases in liver Cu. Sheep are very susceptible to chronic Cu poisoning, which is probably a result of their inability to regulate liver Cu accumulation. Pre-ruminant calves, which also are susceptible to chronic Cu poisoning, have a limited ability to control liver Cu accumulation, although that ability improves after weaning. Although the liver Cu of adult cattle increases with increasing Cu supplementation above the nutritional requirement, the concentration tends to level off at subtoxic accumulations, indicating some homeostatic regulation. Rats, on the other hand, demonstrate the same characteristic plateau in response to increasing dietary intake as has been observed with Zn. Liver Cu increases up to the nutritional requirement of about 5–10 µg Cu g^{-1} diet and thereafter remains constant up to about 100 µg Cu g^{-1} diet, beyond which a substantial increase in

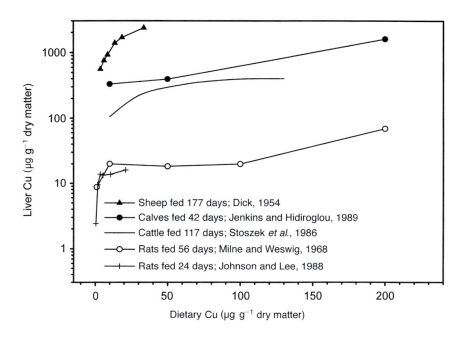

Fig. 8.14. Affect of dietary Cu concentration on liver Cu accumulation by animals. Data were taken from the published reports indicated. Mean data are plotted as symbols. Data extracted from graphs are plotted without symbols. Dietary Cu for cattle (Stoszek *et al.*, 1986) is supplemental Cu without the basal diet contribution.

liver Cu occurs. Laying hens maintain a constant liver Cu concentration up to a relatively high dietary concentration of 600 μg Cu g^{-1} diet, above which homeostatic control breaks down. Ponies also have an ability to maintain Cu homeostasis over a range of dietary intake.

Absorption of Cu decreases with increasing dietary Cu concentration. The results of a number of studies of dietary Cu absorption by humans were compiled by Turnlund (1989) and show an exponential reduction in absorption from about 55% in humans consuming 0.8 mg Cu day^{-1} to about 15% in humans consuming about 7.5 mg day^{-1}. Apparent and true absorption of Cu by rats also decreases with increasing dietary intake (e.g. Johnson and Lee, 1988). While the coefficient of true absorption decreased about twofold in rats fed 21 compared with 0.4 μg Cu g^{-1} diet, endogenous Cu excretion increased from 1 to 46 μg g^{-1} (Johnson and Lee, 1988). These results and others show that rats are

efficient at conserving Cu when fed a deficient diet. The response is similar to that found with Zn and Mn. The biological half-life of ^{67}Cu decreased from 2.36 to 1.96 days with increasing dietary Cu concentration in the study of Johnson and Lee (1988), indicating that turnover of tissue Cu accelerated with increasing absorbed Cu. It appears that only intestinal endogenous losses are important in homeostatic regulation of Cu, since urinary and salivary Cu were unaffected by changes in dietary Cu in humans. Biliary Cu secretion increases with increasing dietary Cu in rats, cattle and chickens, but not in sheep. At adequate Cu intakes, changes in absorption may play less of a role than endogenous faecal excretion in maintaining Cu homeostasis. Endogenous excretion of Cu by humans was reduced from 1.0 to 0.5 mg day^{-1} when dietary intake was reduced from 1.4 to 0.9 mg day^{-1}, while there was no measurable change in percentage absorption of Cu (Milne *et al.*, 1990).

Simulations of Cu metabolism in humans also predict quantitatively greater changes in endogenous excretion than absorption in response to changes in dietary intake (Buckley, 1996).

Manganese

Bone and muscle are the major body pools of Mn. Manganese concentration in humans, cattle and rats varies from 1.5 to 2.6 µg g^{-1} fresh weight in bone and from 0.06 to 0.80 µg g^{-1} fresh weight in muscle (Hurley and Keen, 1987). Manganese concentration in various body tissues is 0.1–0.005 times that of Zn. The lower tissue concentrations of Mn compared with Zn appear to be associated with more rapid tissue turnover, greater endogenous faecal excretion and lower percentage absorption. Divalent Mn entering the portal circulation system is removed rapidly and efficiently by the liver. The liver plays a major role in Mn homeostasis, with biliary excretion being the main route of endogenous loss. Non-biliary secretion, including pancreatic secretion, into the duodenum, jejunum and, to a lesser extent, the ileum also occurs. Urinary excretion of Mn is very small and plays a negligible role in maintaining homeostasis.

In studies with growing rats, the deposition of Mn in body tissues, including liver and skeletal muscle, increased moderately up to 35 µg Mn g^{-1} diet and thereafter remained relatively constant up to the highest dietary concentration tested, 100 µg Mn g^{-1} (Weigand et al., 1986). Exceptions were bone Mn (femur), which appeared to reach a plateau sooner at 4.5 or 11.2 µg Mn g^{-1} diet, and serum Mn, which reached a plateau at 4.5 µg Mn g^{-1} and also increased again at 100 µg Mn g^{-1} (Weigand et al., 1986). Other studies at higher Mn intakes show that rats are able to maintain a homeostatic plateau with respect to liver and bone Mn from the minimum dietary requirement up to at least 600 µg Mn g^{-1} diet.

Early work in Mn dynamics was interpreted mistakenly to indicate that percentage absorption of dietary Mn remained relatively constant and homeostatic control was established predominantly by variation in endogenous faecal excretion. Later work, though, showed that variation in percentage absorption with changes in dietary Mn intake was quantitatively significant, especially at lower dietary concentrations (Weigand et al., 1986). True Mn absorption in the growing rat decreased exponentially with increasing dietary Mn concentration from 29% at 1.5 µg Mn g^{-1} diet to 2.0% at 100 µg Mn g^{-1} (Weigand et al., 1986). At adequate dietary intake, true absorption is greater than apparent absorption, indicating that endogenous excretion is also significant. Turnover of Mn, estimated by loss of ^{54}Mn from various tissues or the whole body, increases with increasing dietary intake. Serum and liver show the greatest change in turnover with increasing intake, and skeletal muscle and bone the least. The increase in tissue Mn turnover is consistent with a nearly threefold increase in excretion of ^{54}Mn by rats consuming 100 µg Mn g^{-1} diet compared with 1.5 µg Mn g^{-1} (Weigand et al., 1986). Studies of direct collection of biliary Mn as well as tracer investigations show that variations in absorption as well as endogenous excretion are important in Mn homeostasis in the rat. Regulation of Mn homeostasis in calves appears to be similar to that in rats. Calves with higher Mn intake have greater tissue and whole-body Mn turnover, reduced percentage absorption and increased biliary excretion.

Studies with the chick show a linear relationship between dietary and tibia Mn concentration with dietary levels up to 3000 µg Mn g^{-1} diet (Henry et al., 1989). This relationship has been used in an assay to determine availability of dietary Mn supplements. Manganese can be stored in avian bone and other tissues to be available during a subsequent period of deficiency. Linear accumulation of Mn in liver, kidney, pancreas and muscle with increasing dietary Mn in the chick has also been observed. While these results might be interpreted to indicate that there is no homeostatic plateau in chicks with respect to Mn metabolism, the Mn levels investigated were high and the steps between successive dietary concentrations were large. On the other hand, chick liver Mn concentrations remained relatively constant at dietary Mn levels of 9.1, 25.8 and 59.7 µg g^{-1}, compared with reduced concentrations at 2.8 µg Mn g^{-1} diet (Weigand *et al.*, 1988b), indicating a homeostatic plateau in liver over a small range of dietary concentrations.

Manganese in other tissues, including bone and skin, feathers, head and feet, increased significantly. Endogenous Mn excretion in chicks increases with increasing dietary intake, indicating that regulation of endogenous excretion plays a role in Mn metabolism.

Iron

Although Fe metabolism has been studied extensively, including various indirect methods of measuring absorption and status, there has been relatively little work done on the quantitative dynamics of Fe (for reviews of Fe metabolism, see Bothwell, 1995; Beard and Dawson, 1997). Iron deficiency is of limited practical importance in farm animals except for suckling pigs, whereas it is one of the most common deficiencies in humans. Iron absorption takes place mainly in the duodenum and upper jejunum. Haem Fe is absorbed more readily than non-haem Fe, the absorption of which is affected by many factors. Mucosal ferritin appears to act as an iron sink in enterocytes and plays a major role in the regulation of Fe absorption. Absorbed Fe is distributed to tissues bound predominantly to the plasma transport protein, transferrin. Most body iron is cycled continuously from plasma to erythroid marrow to red cells, and from senescent red cells back to plasma. Most of the body pool of iron is in the form of haemoglobin in red cells and represents 85–90% of non-storage Fe. The main storage form of Fe is ferritin, of which about 60% is found in the liver and about 40% in muscles and the reticuloendothelial system. The amount of storage Fe can vary

considerably. Typically, the adult human male has a body Fe content of 4 g of which about 25% is in storage (Bothwell, 1995).

The rate of absorption of dietary Fe is an inverse function of the size of body Fe stores. However, when Fe stores are depleted and anaemia is present, a further increase in efficiency of absorption occurs, which suggests that iron absorption is regulated by demands for erythropoiesis in addition to the level of stores (Bothwell, 1995). It has been well established, although mostly by indirect procedures, that Fe homeostasis is determined by changes in rate of absorption. Fe absorption can vary considerably. Absorption of Fe by 126 subjects consuming wheat rolls with varying levels of Ca varied from 2.4 to 30% as determined by whole-body counting of ^{59}Fe (Hallberg *et al.*, 1991). The same subjects given ^{59}Fe with ascorbic acid while fasting absorbed 23–45% of the dose. The body has limited ability to excrete iron, and endogenous Fe loss is derived mainly from normal gastrointestinal blood loss, desquamated cells and bile. Such losses are small and represent only about 0.025% of body Fe per day in healthy human males. From this figure, a biological half-life of Fe in humans of about 7.6 years can be calculated. Other losses from menses, pregnancy, wounds and parasite infestation are significant and reduce the half-life. Although some correlation of Fe losses with Fe status has been observed, the changes in loss are small, and it has been proposed that the variations in loss simply reflect variations in the Fe content of desquamated cells rather than a regulatory process (Bothwell, 1995). Early tracer studies indicated no relationship between endogenous Fe loss and dietary intake in rats, indicating the absence of a role for endogenous excretion in the homeostasis of iron. More recently, increases in endogenous faecal Fe excreted per day (determined by the isotope dilution method) were negligible compared with the reduction in the percentage true absorption of Fe by young, growing male rats fed a high-Fe diet (400 µg g^{-1}) compared with an adequate-Fe diet (40 µg g^{-1}) (Kreuzer and

Kirchgessner, 1991). Thus, it appears that Fe is unique among the essential trace elements in that endogenous excretion by either faeces or urine does not play a significant role in homeostasis.

Selenium

The metabolism of Se varies with its chemical form (Sunde, 1997). Se in animal tissue is predominantly in the form of protein-bound selenocysteine, whereas plant Se is predominantly selenomethionine. Selenium in inorganic supplements is normally selenite or selenate. Circulating selenite is taken up by erythrocytes and rapidly reduced to selenide, which is a common intermediate in the metabolism of both inorganic and amino acid forms of Se. Selenocysteine and selenomethionine may be incorporated directly into proteins or also converted to selenide prior to incorporation of Se as selenocysteine into Se-specific selenoproteins such as glutathione peroxidase. Since animals are able to synthesize selenocysteine but not selenomethionine and since dietary selenomethionine may be incorporated into protein (mainly muscle protein), there are two kinetically distinct components of Se metabolism in animals: selenite-exchangeable Se and selenomethionine Se (Sunde, 1997). Since the selenomethionine pool cannot be labelled with selenite, the kinetics of labelled selenomethionine differ from those of labelled selenite. A selenite-exchangeable metabolic pool has been found to be highly correlated with whole-body Se in rats and to respond to dietary Se restriction by decreasing in size in humans. Most whole-body Se is found in muscle. Analysis of 12 major tissues of lactating dairy cows showed that 61% of Se in tissues analysed was in skeletal muscle, 7% in the hide, 6% in the liver, 5% in the udder, 4% in bone, 4% in smooth muscle of the reticulorumen and 3% or less in each remaining tissue.

Stable isotope tracer studies with selenite and selenomethionine in humans have helped to elucidate certain aspects of Se metabolism (Patterson *et al.*, 1989; Swanson *et al.*, 1991). According to kinetic models developed from the tracer experiments, 84% of orally administered selenite Se was absorbed and 90% of absorbed selenite Se was taken up by the liver. More than half, 58%, of the Se taken up by the liver was secreted into the gastrointestinal tract via the bile, from where most of it was reabsorbed. Selenium tracer released from the liver into plasma was taken up by a peripheral tissue compartment which eventually released the tracer for excretion into the urine without further recycling to liver or other tissues. Within 12 days, 18% of ingested dose was recovered in the faeces, including unabsorbed tracer, and 17% was recovered in the urine. Metabolism of selenomethionine Se differed from selenite Se in the kinetic model. Ninety-eight per cent of orally administered selenomethionine was absorbed and it was removed more rapidly from the blood by the liver than selenite Se. Slightly less tracer was returned to the gastrointestinal tract via the bile. Forty-three per cent of the selenomethionine Se released from the liver to plasma was taken up by a slowly turning over peripheral tissue compartment not accessed by the selenite tracer. Virtually all of the selenomethionine Se released from tissue compartments was recycled back to the liver. Over 12 days, 4% of ingested selenomethionine tracer was recovered in faeces and 11% was recovered in urine. In both the selenite and selenomethionine models, endogenous Se was excreted predominantly in the urine, which agrees with other studies. The combined effect of the differences in metabolism of the two Se forms was that the whole-body half-life of selenomethionine Se was 252 days while that of selenite selenium was 102 days. The percentage absorption and differences in endogenous faecal excretion of selenite and selenomethionine in rats are similar to the results obtained with humans.

Absorption of Se can be high, but it varies considerably among species. Se absorption by rats is >90% (Kirchgessner *et al.*, 1997), whereas measurements of absorption in humans vary between 53 and 98%, and absorption by ruminants is somewhat lower, between 11 and 46%.

Homeostatic regulation of Se retention has been investigated in rats (Kirchgessner *et al.*, 1997). Growing rats fed 40–3000 ng Se g^{-1} diet absorbed 93–97% of Se, which showed that there was no homeostatic regulation of Se metabolism at the site of gastrointestinal absorption. Endogenous faecal excretion played a relatively minor role and was responsible for elimination of only 6.4–9.0% of Se consumed. Homeostatic control of Se retention was achieved mainly by regulation of urinary excretion. Urinary excretion was small (75–140 ng day^{-1}) up to 100 ng Se g^{-1} diet and then jumped to 671 ng day^{-1} for rats fed 150 ng Se g^{-1} diet, which was interpreted as a transition from deficient to sufficient Se intake. Thereafter, urinary Se excretion increased from 32 to 63% of dietary intake, or 671–26,700 ng day^{-1}. However, urinary elimination was not 100% efficient and dietary retention varied from 55% of intake at 150 ng Se g^{-1} diet to 26% at 3000 ng Se g^{-1} diet, leading to excessive whole-body retention especially at the highest dietary concentrations. Nevertheless, whole-body Se increased only 20% over the range of 150–600 ng Se g^{-1} diet, indicating reasonably effective homeostatic control. The selenium concentration of most tissues, especially the liver, increased with increasing dietary intake. As has been observed with other elements (Zn, Mn), whole-body turnover of the element increased, which indicated that excessive Se intake exchanged with tissue Se prior to elimination from the body.

Selenium dynamics in ruminants is poorly understood and research reports to date have been somewhat conflicting. Ruminants excrete a higher proportion of dietary Se in the faeces than the urine, possibly due to the formation of unavailable forms of Se in the gastrointestinal tract, which may explain the lower absorption of Se by ruminants compared with monogastrics. Sheep responded to changes in dietary Se concentration with changes in urinary excretion, while faecal excretion remained relatively constant (Langands *et al.*, 1986), which is consistent with monogastric metabolism. Examination of gastrointestinal contents of sheep showed that two to three times the quantity of Se ingested entered the anterior portion of the small intestine each day, indicating that endogenous secretions of Se were substantial, although the secretions were reabsorbed in lower sections of the small intestine (Langands *et al.*, 1986). On the other hand, biliary secretion of ^{75}Se measured directly in cattle following intravenous injection of labelled selenite was <10% of that recovered in urine, suggesting that endogenous secretions are small (Symonds *et al.*, 1981). Recent studies revealed a significantly higher percentage absorption of dietary Se by ewes fed Se-deficient hay (46%) compared with ewes fed Se-adequate hay (18%) (Krishnamurti *et al.*, 1997), which does not agree with the constant percentage absorption observed in rats. Further work will be required to clarify the roles of absorption and excretion in the homeostasis of Se.

Concluding Remarks

The study of trace element dynamics provides insight into the significance of various body pools of elements as well as the regulation of their routes of absorption and excretion. It is apparent that the large pools of an element, often in muscle, bone or liver, play an important role in homeostasis and whole-body metabolism. However, except for Zn and Fe, the metabolism of the major body pools of trace elements has received little attention. Large pools may serve as a source or sink during periods of dietary insufficiency or excess. On the other hand, as in the case of muscle Zn in rats, the body attempts to maintain a constant concentration of the element at the expense of other pools during periods of deficiency. Compartmental modelling is an effective tool for compiling information on trace element dynamics. It also serves as a planning assistant in the design of studies and greatly facilitates understanding the complexities of whole-body metabolism. A fairly complete picture of the dynamics of Zn metabolism in young rats receiving deficient to adequate diets is now available, although the upper ranges of the homeostatic plateau for individual tissues and the whole animal have not been well established. Much work yet needs to be done on Cu, Mn and Se, particularly with respect to the regulation of body compartments and, especially for Se, the roles of absorption and endogenous excretion in homeostasis. The effects of various physiological states, other than growth, on trace element dynamics were not addressed in this chapter; however, research on the affects of ageing, gestation and lactation shows that these are productive areas of research in trace element dynamics. For all the elements discussed in this chapter, the quantity of research conducted in dynamics with rats and humans exceeds that performed with farm animals, but an effort was made to include farm animal results as much as possible. Until a greater body of knowledge is accumulated, extrapolation of the principles to farm animals will be necessary, although caution is required because of substantial differences in the metabolism of some elements among species.

References

Beard, J.L. and Dawson, H.D. (1997) Iron. In: O'Dell, B.L. and Sunde, R.A. (eds) *Handbook of Nutritionally Essential Mineral Elements*. Marcel Dekker, New York, pp. 275–334.

Bothwell, T.H. (1995) Overview and mechanisms of iron regulation. *Nutrition Reviews* 53, 237–245.

Buckley, W.T. (1996) Application of compartmental modeling to determination of trace element requirements in humans. *Journal of Nutrition* 126, 2312S–2319S.

Chesters, J.K. (1997) Zinc. In: O'Dell, B.L. and Sunde, R.A. (eds) *Handbook of Nutritionally Essential Mineral Elements*. Marcel Dekker, New York, pp. 185–230.

Dick, A.T. (1954) Studies on the assimilation and storage of copper in crossbred sheep. *Australian Journal of Agricultural Research* 5, 511–544.

Giugliano, R. and Millward, D.J. (1984) Growth and zinc homeostasis in the severely zinc-deficient rat. *British Journal of Nutrition* 52, 545–560.

Hallberg, L., Brune, M., Erlandsson, M., Sandberg, A.-S. and Rossander-Hultén, L. (1991) Calcium: effect of different amounts of nonheme- and heme-iron absorption in humans. *American Journal of Clinical Nutrition* 53, 112–119.

Henry, P.R., Ammerman, C.B. and Miles, R.D. (1989) Relative bioavailability of manganese in a manganese–methionine complex for broiler chicks. *Poultry Science* 68, 107–112.

House, W.A. and Wastney, M.E. (1997) Compartmental analysis of zinc kinetics in mature male rats. *American Journal of Physiology* 273, R1117–R1125.

Hurley, L.S. and Keen, C.L. (1987) Manganese. In: Mertz, W. (ed.) *Trace Elements in Human and Animal Nutrition*, 5th edn, vol. 1. Academic Press, Orlando, Florida, pp. 185–223.

Jenkins, K.J. and Hidiroglou, M. (1989) Tolerance of the calf for excess copper in milk replacer. *Journal of Dairy Science* 72, 150–156.

Johnson, P.E. and Lee, D.-Y. (1988) Copper absorption and excretion measured by two methods in rats fed varying concentrations of dietary copper. *Journal of Trace Elements in Experimental Medicine* 1, 129–141.

Johnson, P.E., Hunt, J.R. and Ralston, N.V.C. (1988) The effect of past and current dietary Zn intake on Zn absorption and endogenous excretion in the rat. *Journal of Nutrition* 118, 1205–1209.

Kirchgessner, M. (1993) Homeostasis and homeorhesis in trace element metabolism. In: Anke, M., Meissner, D. and Mills, C.F. (eds) *Trace Elements in Man and Animals – TEMA 8*. Verlag Media Touristik, Gersdorf, Germany, pp. 4–21.

Kirchgessner, M., Gabler, S. and Windisch, W. (1997) Homeostatic adjustments of selenium metabolism and tissue selenium to widely varying selenium supply in ^{75}Se labeled rats. *Journal of Animal Physiology and Animal Nutrition* 78, 20–30.

Krishnamurti, C.R., Ramberg, C.F., Jr, Shariff, M.A. and Boston, R.C. (1997) A compartmental model depicting short-term kinetic changes in selenium metabolism in ewes fed hay containing normal or inadequate levels of selenium. *Journal of Nutrition* 127, 95–102.

Kreuzer, M. and Kirchgessner, M. (1991) Endogenous iron excretion: a quantitative means to control iron metabolism? *Biological Trace Element Research* 29, 77–92.

Langands, J.P., Bowles, J.E., Donald, G.E. and Smith, A.J. (1986) Selenium excretion in sheep. *Australian Journal of Agricultural Research* 37, 201–209.

Linder, M.C. (1991) *Biochemistry of Copper*. Plenum Press, New York.

Malecki, E.A., Radzanowski, G.M., Radzanowski, T.J., Gallaher, D.D. and Greger, J.L. (1996) Biliary manganese excretion in conscious rats is affected by acute and chronic manganese intake but not by dietary fat. *Journal of Nutrition* 126, 489–498.

McKenney, J.R., McClellan, R.O. and Bustad, L.K. (1962) Early uptake and dosimetry of Zn[65] in sheep. *Health Physics* 8, 411–421.

Miller, W.J. (1973) Dynamics of absorption rates, endogenous excretion, tissue turnover, and homeostatic control mechanisms of zinc, cadmium, manganese, and nickel in ruminants. *Federation Proceedings* 32, 1915–1920.

Milne, D.B. and Weswig, P.H. (1968) Effect of supplementary copper on blood and liver copper-containing fractions in rats. *Journal of Nutrition* 95, 429–433.

Milne, D.B., Johnson, P.E., Klevay, L.M. and Sandstead, H.H. (1990) Effect of copper intake on balance, absorption, and status indices of copper in men. *Nutrition Research* 10, 975–986.

Patterson, B.H., Levander, O.A., Helzlsouer, K., McAdam, P.A., Lewis, S.A., Taylor, P.R., Veillon, C. and Zech, L.A. (1989) Human selenite metabolism: a kinetic model. *American Journal of Physiology* 257, R556–R567.

SAAM Institute (1994) *SAAM II User Guide*. SAAM Institute, Seattle, Washington.

Stoszek, M.J., Mika, P.G., Oldfield, J.E. and Weswig, P.H. (1986) Influence of copper supplementation on blood and liver copper in cattle fed tall fescue or quackgrass. *Journal of Animal Science* 62, 263–271.

Sunde, R.A. (1997) Selenium. In: O'Dell, B.L. and Sunde, R.A. (eds) *Handbook of Nutritionally Essential Mineral Elements*. Marcel Dekker, New York, pp. 493–556.

Sullivan, J.F., Williams, R.V., Wisecarver, J., Etzel, K., Jetton, M.M. and Magee, D.F. (1981) The zinc content of bile and pancreatic juice in zinc-deficient swine. *Proceeedings of the Society for Experimental Biology and Medicine* 166, 39–43.

Swanson, C.A., Patterson, B.H., Levander, O.A., Veillon, C., Taylor, P.R., Helzlsouer, K., McAdam, P.A. and Zech, L.A. (1991) Human [74Se]selenomethionine metabolism: a kinetic model. *American Journal of Clinical Nutrition* 54, 917–926.

Symonds, H.W., Mather, D.L. and Vagg, M.J. (1981) The excretion of selenium in bile and urine of steers: the influence of form and amount of Se salt. *British Journal of Nutrition* 46, 487–493.

Turnlund, J.R. (1989) Stable isotope studies of the effect of dietary copper on copper absorption and excretion. In: Kies, C. (ed.) *Copper Bioavailability and Metabolism*. Plenum Press, New York, pp. 21–28.

Weigand, E. and Kirchgessner, M. (1976) [65]Zn-labeled tissue zinc for determination of endogenous faecal zinc excretion in growing rats. *Nutrition and Metabolism* 20, 314–320.

Weigand, E. and Kirchgessner, M. (1978) Homeostasic adaptation of Zn absorption and endogenous Zn excretion over a wide range of dietary Zn supply. In: Kirchgessner, M. (ed.) *Trace Element Metabolism in Man and Animals – 3*. Arbeitskreis für Tierernährungsforschung, Weihenstephan, pp. 106–109.

Weigand, E., Kirchgessner, M. and Helbig, U. (1986) True absorption and endogenous faecal excretion of manganese in relation to its dietary supply in growing rats. *Biological Trace Element Research* 10, 265–279.

Weigand, E., Kirchgessner, M. and Kiliç, A. (1988a) Determination of endogenous manganese excretion in broiler chicks by an isotope-dilution method. *Archives of Animal Nutrition* 38, 879–892.

Weigand, E., Kiliç, A. and Kirchgessner, M. (1988b) Influence of different manganese supply on manganese retention in broiler chicks. *European Poultry Science* 52, 30–36.

Williams, R.B. and Mills, C.F. (1970) The experimental production of zinc deficiency in the rat. *British Journal of Nutrition* 24, 989–1003.

Windisch, V.W. and Kirchgessner, M. (1993) Zinc exchange in adult rats at different zinc supply. In: Anke, M., Meissner, D. and Mills, C.F. (eds) *Trace Elements in Man and Animals – TEMA 8*. Verlag Media Touristik, Gersdorf, Germany, pp. 351–355.

Windisch, V.W. and Kirchgessner, M. (1994) Distribution and exchange of zinc in different tissue
fractions at deficient and excessive zinc supply. 3. Effect of different zinc supply on quantitative
zinc exchange in the metabolism of adult rats. *Journal of Animal Physiology and Animal
Nutrition* 71, 131–139.

Part II

Feed Evaluation Methodologies

Chapter 9

Use of Near Infrared Reflectance Spectroscopy

Nutrient Conservation and Metabolism Laboratory,
Livestock and Poultry Sciences Institute,
Agricultural Research Service, USDA, Beltsville, Maryland, USA

Introduction

Most of us are familiar with the use of spectrometers for quantitative determinations. In these applications, one generally runs a set of standards containing various concentrations of the analyte, for example protein, and then compares the results of unknowns with the standard results using a standard curve. In such cases, the assumption is made that only the concentration of the analyte of interest (protein, P, etc.) is changing, and that the absorbance changes linearly with the changing concentration of the analyte according to Beer's Law, which states that:

$$A = abc \qquad (9.1)$$

where A = absorbance or ($\log_{10}(1/\text{transmittance})$), b = the cell pathlength, c = concentration and a = the molar extinction coefficient for the analyte at the wavelength used (constant telling how strongly the analyte absorbs at the wavelength chosen). In such determinations, the wavelengths used are generally in the ultraviolet (UV) or visible portion of the electromagnetic spectrum (EMS), and the wavelength needed for each determination is known.

The near infrared (NIR, 1100–2500 nm) portion of the EMS occurs at wavelengths longer than the visible (VIS, 400–760 nm) and shorter than the mid-infrared (MIDIR, 2500–25,000 nm) regions. Although the MIDIR is again very familiar, being used to identify unknown materials by comparing their MIDIR spectra with published works on group absorptions, i.e. ketone carbonyl at 5800–6100 nm, etc. (Colthup *et al.*, 1990), the NIR region has only gained prominence in the last 20 years or so. There is also a region (760–1100 nm) between the visible and NIR which has sometimes been included in the NIR and is used similarly. This region will be considered as the short-wave-NIR (SWNIR) for the discussion at hand. It should be noted that this region is often at least partially available on many UV–VIS or VIS spectrometers designed to use test tubes and cuvettes; however, these are not NIR spectrometers as used to perform feed analysis.

Near infrared spectroscopy (NIRS) is based on the absorptions of C-H, N-H and O-H groups found in organic constituents. These absorptions are the overtones and combination bands of the much stronger absorptions found in the MIDIR spectral region (Murray and Williams, 1987). Since NIR absorptions are weaker, longer path-lengths can be used for liquids (particularly where water is involved) and for solids; unlike the MIDIR, dilution with KBr or preparation of KBr pellets is unnecessary.

The NIR spectral region, in various spectroscopic forms (diffuse reflectance, transmission, etc.) over the last decade has been used increasingly to determine the composition and quality of many products and to monitor the progress of various biological or chemical processes (Marten *et al.*, 1989; Kemeny, 1992). With solids, NIRS in the reflectance mode has been used extensively to determine the composition/quality of materials such as hays (Marten *et al.*, 1989), silages (Reeves *et al.*, 1989; Reeves and Blosser, 1991), grains (Osborne *et al.*, 1987; Tkachuk, 1987) and food products (Osborne and Fearn, 1986). In the pharmaceutical industry, NIRS has also being used to monitor the identity of the raw materials arriving at loading docks (Ciurczak, 1992b). Transmission NIRS has been used extensively to monitor biological processes, such as fermentations and chemical reactions (Kemeny, 1992).

The successful application of NIRS to problems in such diverse areas is due to the nature of the absorptions in the spectral region, and the variety of instrumentation available. Near infrared spectrometers based on the use of filters, gratings, acoustics, interferometers and crystals are in use (McClure, 1987; Williams, 1987; Workman and Burns, 1992). Sampling devices include rotating and stationary sample cups and fibre optic probes (Kemeny, 1992).

Despite the widespread acceptance and use of NIRS, there is still a great deal of mis-understanding about its use and a need for more research on the basis of NIR spectra. On the spectroscopic side, decades of work have been carried out to identify spectral bands in the MIDIR (Colthup *et al.*, 1990) and programs are even available which automate the process (Sadtler IR Mentor, Bio-Rad Sadtler Division, Philadelphia, Pennsylvania). Conversely, NIR spectral interpretation can be described as prelimin-ary at best (Murray and Williams, 1987;

Ciurczak, 1992a). This can be largely traced to the fact that most of the work in NIR has been done by non-spectroscopists who were and are more interested in the final results than in theory.

In Fig. 9.1, a diagram of a diffuse reflectance accessory for a NIR spectrometer is shown. For animal feed samples, this is one of the primary methods used to obtain spectral information. Although work is per-formed using transmission spectroscopy, the majority of feed analysis is performed using this diffuse reflectance method. As shown in Fig. 9.1, several types of events occur when light is shone on a sample contained in a sealed sample cell. Only the NIR radiation which penetrates fragments of the sample, is scattered randomly from particle to particle (diffuse reflectance) and eventually leaves the sample cell in various directions is of interest. Depending on the composition of the sample, energy at various wavelengths will be absorbed to various degrees, and it is this absorption which provides information on the composition of the sample. Unlike the determinations previously discussed, to determine the composition of feedstuffs by NIR, a half dozen to hundreds of wave-lengths are used, depending on the samples, instrument used and constituent in question. Thus, instead of a data set of absorbances at a specific wavelength, one obtains an array of absorbances for each sample, where each element of the array consists of an absorbance at a given wavelength. When data are collected over a range of wave-lengths at specific intervals and the absorbances are plotted against the range of wavelengths, the result is a spectrum, as in Fig. 9.2 for lucerne hay and wheat straw. While not all NIR determinations require a complete spectrum as shown in Fig. 9.2, this is the place where calibration development begins.

Calibration Development

General aspects

Just as a calibration curve is necessary for determining the protein or P content of a

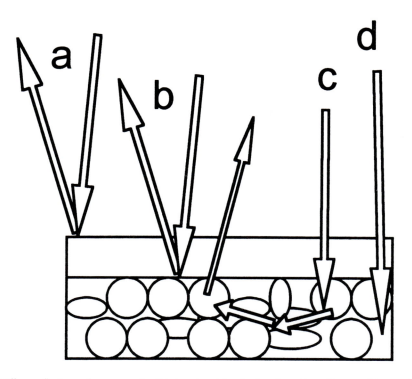

Fig. 9.1. Diffuse reflectance for a ground solid showing: (a) reflection from the cell cover; (b) specular reflection from the sample; (c) absorption and diffuse reflection from the sample; and (d) total absorption by the sample.

sample, it is necessary to develop a calibration for the determination of solid feed composition by NIRS. However, the two procedures are as different as the samples in question. In the case of protein or P in solution, for all intents and purposes one has a single analyte (protein or P content) changing in an otherwise constant media (water, buffers, etc.). Also, the analyte at best represents a very small percentage of the total system. When using NIRS to determine feed composition (i.e. neutral and acid detergent fibre (NDF and ADF), crude protein (CP), lignin, etc. (Van Soest, 1994)), one has a solid medium (feed itself) in which the analyte (NDF, etc.) is not only the object of the determination, but also constitutes a significant fraction of the medium itself. Also, unlike the earlier calibrations for protein or P in which the media (water, buffers, etc.) are generally non-absorbing at the wavelength chosen,

with feeds the media consists of other components of the feedstuff which also have absorption bands in the NIR, and generally at the same wavelengths as the component of interest. This can be seen in Fig. 9.3, where the NIR spectra of casein and cellulose are shown. For a hay or silage, the NIR spectrum thus consists of overlapping spectra of the many different constituents present, each one different, but, like cellulose and casein, often having absorptions in the same or similar regions. Except for pure and simple materials such as acetone, spectra do not consist of sharp, individual peaks. Thus, developing a calibration becomes a very complicated process. As a result, calibration development has resulted in NIRS becoming almost synonymous with the terms multivariate statistics and chemometrics.

Multivariate simply means that there are multiple variables (wavelengths in the

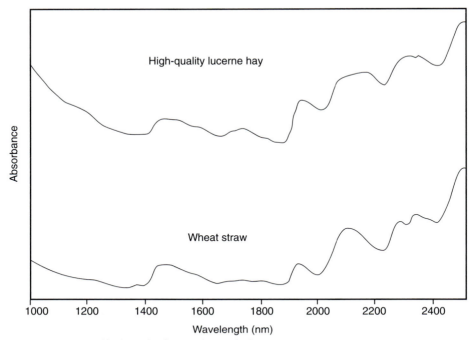

Fig. 9.2. NIR spectra of high-quality lucerne hay and wheat straw.

case of NIRS) involved in finding a calibration equation for the constituent of interest. The field of using multivariate statistical procedures for the quantitative and qualitative analysis has come to be known as chemometrics, and is an integral part of utilizing NIRS.

Since the constituent of interest is both the analyte being determined and part of the media or matrix, and since all the other constituents in the sample are most probably also changing in relative amounts from sample to sample, it is extremely important that the proper samples be used when developing a calibration. Because all the organic constituents in a feed sample are likely to absorb NIR radiation at all wavelengths to at least some degree, and because all or most of the constituents will vary simultaneously in relative amounts present, one determines the values for a given constituent not only in terms of itself, but also in terms of everything else present. As a result, the structure of a data set is probably the most important part of developing and utilizing NIRS, and the

misunderstanding of this point probably leads to more problems and disillusionment with NIRS than anything else.

Sample sets and calibration development

In using a single wavelength, it is easy to see that anything (other than changes in the analyte) that might alter the absorbance will result in some error in the determination of the analyte. For example, in Fig. 9.4, if spectrum A were to be shifted to the right to give the results in B (temperature changes can easily cause such peak shifts), then the absorbance value read at the wavelength where the peak should be would result in an incorrect value for the analyte. In Fig. 9.4C and D, we see the effects of two kinds of baseline shift. In Fig. 9.4C, the entire spectrum has shifted upwards (this is very common in NIR spectra due to particle size differences between samples), resulting in higher absorbance values, although a simple baseline correction can be made. In Fig. 9.4D, the baseline

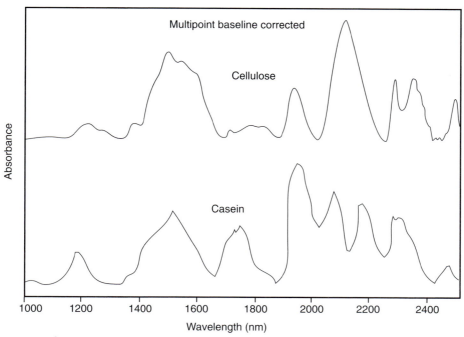

Fig. 9.3. Baseline-corrected NIR spectra of cellulose and casein.

is tilting from left to right, also resulting in incorrect absorbance values, but, in this case, the error varies in intensity from 0 on the left to a maximum on the right side of the peak. This type of error is called multiplicative scatter (Isaksson and Kowalski, 1993) and is also common among ground feed samples due to particle size and absorbance differences, but requires more than a simple baseline shift for correction. In reality, as opposed to this simplification, multiplicative scatter is a function of the absorbance values (i.e. the greater the absorbance the larger the shift). Finally, in Fig. 9.4E, we see the result when a second component is present (F), and the resulting spectrum E is a combination of the two component spectra (A and F). In this case, using the absorption at the peak also gives incorrect results. This could occur if, for example, a sample was tested using a calibration built from samples which had no component F. Since no F was ever present in the calibration set, there would be no compensation built into the calibration for it. This, combined with the fact that virtu-

ally anything different about samples (physical or compositional) or the conditions under which spectra were obtained (instrumental, environmental, etc.) can alter NIR spectra and thereby influence the accuracy of a calibration, probably explains more about the nature and problems of NIR calibration development, maintenance and use than anything else. Since NIR calibrations often use many wavelengths, one can imagine the total effect of many such spectral alterations on a calibration.

Although developing a calibration or equation to determine the composition of feed samples from their NIR spectra, one is trying to find relationships between the spectra obtained and the component of interest (NDF, ADF, etc.) in order to determine the composition of new samples using only their spectra. Therefore, anything which is different between the spectra used to develop the calibration initially, and the spectra of future samples, which is not due only to compositional variations which have been included in the calibration, can result in errors. A list of

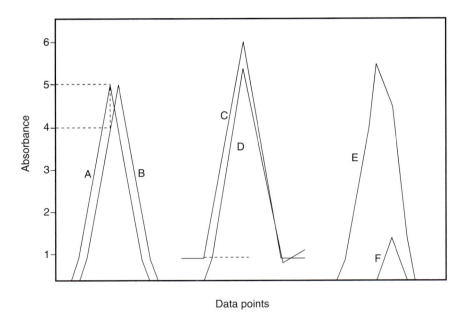

Fig. 9.4. Hypothetical effects of peak shift (B), baseline shifts (C and D) and a second component (E and F) on an NIR spectrum (A).

those things which commonly cause problems is shown in Table 9.1.

While any of these factors can vary from one sample to the next, the problem arises when they vary between the samples used to develop a calibration, and new samples on which the calibration is used. Ultimately, the objective in developing a calibration is to find a set of samples whose spectra/composition are representative of a larger set of samples, i.e. one does not want any systematic differences. Thus, one does not want to develop a calibration using samples ground to one mesh size or scanned at one temperature, and then use that calibration to determine the values for samples ground to a different mesh (or even ground on a different type of grinder) or scanned at a different temperature. While it may not be possible to take into account the repair of an instrument, one can avoid the problems caused by the other factors by scanning the calibration samples over a range of temperatures or scanning each sample at several different temperatures, and so forth. Thus, to a large degree, variations likely to influence spectra can be

built into the calibration set. The calibration process will then avoid those wavelengths where, for example, variations due to temperature have too great an influence. Also, spectral pre-treatments, such as multiplicative scatter correction (Isaksson and Kolwalski, 1993), can be used to eliminate some effects, such as those due to particle size differences. The real problems occur with differences in spectrometers and samples. Spectrometer to spectrometer variation is difficult and expensive to build into a calibration because it requires running the same samples on many different instruments and using all the spectra obtained to develop the calibration. Even then, another spectrometer may vary too greatly from those used for the calibration for it to work properly. Therefore, generally, the problem is handled outside the calibration development process in what is called 'Calibration Transfer'. Sample differences lie at the heart of calibration development, and revolve around 'Sample Populations'. In developing calibrations, many effects (temperature variations, etc.) can be eliminated or

Table 9.1. Some factors (as differences between samples) which can alter spectra and influence calibration accuracy.

Factor	Spectral effect	Solution
Particle size	Baseline shifts, multiplicative scatter	Mathematical pre-treatments of spectra
Temperature	Spectral peak shifts	Include temperature differences in calibration
Sample packing	Spectra do not represent sample	Pack uniformly, scan a larger sample
Sample homogeneity	Non-representative sample	Grind more finely or scan a larger sample
Constituent out of range	Inappropriate for calibration	Add a sample with wider range of values
Different feed or samples	Inappropriate for calibration	Add samples to old or develop new calibration
Spectrometer repaired or changes somehow	Peak shifts, absorbance changes, multiplicative effects, etc.	Redevelop calibration or use calibration transfer
Different spectrometer used	Peak shifts, absorbance changes, multiplicative effects, etc.	Redevelop calibration or use calibration transfer
Stray light in instrument	Inaccurate determination	Fix instrument or use constant lighting at all times

reduced by deliberately including the variation in the calibration; the difficult problem lies in the nature of the samples themselves and the variations that occur over a growing season, between seasons, between growing locations, between varieties, etc.

Closed and open populations

Closed populations and calibration development

A closed population is one in which one has all the samples of interest, e.g. 2000 lucerne samples from a pasture feeding experiment. After grinding the samples, the samples should be scanned in a random order to avoid any pattern between the samples and the order of scanning, i.e. avoid scanning all the highest quality samples on one day, at one temperature, and the lowest quality samples on another day, at a different temperature. The more any differences due to personnel, room conditions, instrument conditions, etc. are randomly distributed across all the samples, the better. The next step is to select the samples for which the analyte of interest

will be measured by the standard technique, i.e. NDF, ADF by extraction procedures (Van Soest, 1994). It is these values which will be used to determine the wavelengths needed for the NIR-based determination of the remaining samples. A smaller set of test samples is also needed in order to test the calibration after development. These are only to determine if the calibration/equation developed works properly on samples not in the original calibration set.

The question then is how to find samples in the set which represent all 2000 samples. Several methods have been used over the years. First, N samples can be randomly selected. Second, every nth sample can be used. If this is done, it is important to avoid a structured data set: i.e. a set of 2000 samples consisting of 100 sets of 20 samples, each set in order of increasing NDF content, and every 20th sample taken for the calibration set. This would result in only the samples with the lowest NDF content being included in the calibration. Under such circumstances, it is unlikely that the calibration developed would work on the test set or very many of the remaining samples. The third method and probably the best requires scanning all the samples first, and then choosing samples on the basis of their spectral differences.

Since the spectra are supposed to be determined by the composition, choosing the 100 most spectrally different samples can be a good place to start. This of course supposes that 100 samples can represent the remaining 1900 samples. Depending on the diversity of the samples, this may or may not be true. For example, if one had a sample set of 2000 lucerne hays from one growing season and one farm, it would be much more likely that 100 samples could represent the entire group than if one had 2000 samples consisting of 100 different feedstuffs each collected over 5 years from four different locations. The diversity in such a sample set might require many more (or even all) samples to be tested. The latter was found to be true for a set of 325 chemically/physically treated samples, in which no two samples were the same feedstuff treated in the same way. The samples produced were so diverse that even using all 325 samples did not produce a satisfactory NIR calibration (Reeves, 1994b). Unfortunately, only by testing the calibration can one determine if enough samples were used. If the results are unsatisfactory, more samples can be added to the calibration and the process repeated. Unfortunately, it is also true that only experience and knowledge of one's samples can be used for guidance.

Open populations

While in a closed population, one has all the samples there will ever be at the start of the process, in an open population, this is never true. For example, one of the successes of NIR has been its use to determine the nutritive value of forages. By using a van carrying a NIR spectrometer, and the means to collect and grind hay samples on the spot, NIRS has even been used at hay auctions. In such cases, it is obvious that one can never have all the possible samples. This is the case for many of the most useful applications of NIR.

The problems arising from open populations give rise to the biggest misunderstanding of NIR and subsequent disillusionment and that is the belief that if one buys an NIR spectrometer or finds someone with one, then one never needs to perform a wet chemical analysis again. On the contrary, as new samples arise, one must periodically run a few samples by both the standard and the NIR methods and compare the results to determine if the calibration is performing properly. If not, then one can add some of the new samples to the calibration, and perhaps remove some of the old ones (i.e. a variety or feed no longer grown), and redevelop the calibration. This is what the private feed testing companies utilizing NIR do. However, even if one out of every ten samples were to be checked, this would still reduce the need for the standard analysis by 90%.

One point about results performed by commercial feed testing laboratories using NIRS should be understood: such results are likely to be accurate only if the firm has developed equations which cover your geographic area, your type of samples and the season of interest.

Research samples

The questions revolving around open and closed populations probably have a great impact on the usefulness of NIRS for research samples. For example, for a farmer, the ability to get a rapid analysis of his feedstuff, a matter of minutes at a hay auction, may outweigh the need for extreme accuracy, and thus the use of a general hay calibration may be more than acceptable. In the research environment, the problem is that accuracy is generally paramount, and the samples may represent rather unique population sets containing rather small numbers of sample. For such sample sets, it is unlikely that NIRS will be of great benefit.

On the other hand, if either a large sample set is available or will be accumulated over time as a result of repetitive efforts, developing an NIR calibration may well be worth the time. As an example, we recently had 1800 samples which contained several forages, treated with different levels of manure and collected at four or five cuttings over a 2-year period. Using only 120 calibrations (based on spectral diversity) and 24 test samples, excellent calibrations for NDF and CP were obtained, resulting in a reduction of almost 95% in the number of chemical determinations.

Two other considerations should be taken into account when considering NIR for assaying research samples. The first relates to the calibration nature of an NIR spectrometer. An NIR calibration is based on the reference method used to provide the assay values needed for building the calibration. As such, NIR determinations are often stated to be, at best, no better than the calibration standards (assays) used to develop the calibration. While there is debate about this, many feel this to be generally true. Thus, if one has the choice between NIR determinations and accurate chemically determined values, the latter may be preferable. On the other hand, it is highly likely that if several operators are involved the NIR results may well be more consistent than will be the reference method. This is because there are fewer steps involved in using an existing calibration than in performing many chemical procedures, and different individuals always do things slightly differently, introducing errors and biases. The second consideration deals with error distributions in NIR calibrations. It has been reported (Buxton and Mertens, 1991) that the errors in NIR calibrations are not always randomly distributed across samples. Such an effect is demonstrated in Fig. 9.5 (hypothetical). If the samples in sets 1 and 2 were matched sets whose true values were the same, the conclusion that there is a difference between the sets (i.e. varieties or treatments) would be incorrect. Examination of the statistics alone (R^2 of 0.971, mean value of 5.5 for all samples) would give no indication of a problem. Even by examination of the plotted data (Fig. 9.5) a problem might not be indicated, unless the samples were labelled in the plot as to source (A or B). Then, as shown,

one would notice all the As were predicted high and all the Bs low. In the real world, one needs to check some test samples to see that this is not occurring.

The point of this is not to show that NIR is useless and should not be used, only that like all procedures, one should not simply assume that NIR solves all one's problems at the press of a button. Finally, it should be noted that work to improve NIR calibrations has done a lot to show how poor the wet chemical procedures, against which NIR is rated, can be. Many NIR calibrations have been improved simply by cleaning up or changing the procedures used to obtain the calibration values.

Chemometrics and NIR

As previously discussed, the area of statistics used to develop NIR calibrations has come to be known as chemometrics and is a vital part of using NIR spectroscopy. While a subject unto itself, at least a brief discussion is needed to understand what NIR is all about and what is involved in its use. For a more in-depth discussion, the reader is advised to check one or more of the following references or software packages: Sharaf *et al.* (1986); Massart *et al.* (1988); PLSplus (1992); Shenk and Westerhaus (1993); or Unscrambler (1994). There is also a web site at *http://newton.foodsci.kvl. dk/chdb_asc.html* which contains a searchable database containing >1200 references on chemometrics.

The basic objective of calibration development is to find a relationship between spectral information and the analyte of interest. In the beginning, much of the NIR data were obtained from filter instruments, and thus consisted of a dozen or few dozen wavelengths at most. In addition, the computers available were limited in speed and memory which limited the algorithms which could be used practically. As a result, most of the early work used stepwise multiple linear regression (MLR) techniques. Today, a wide range of tools and statistical procedures, which serve three basic functions (data exploration,

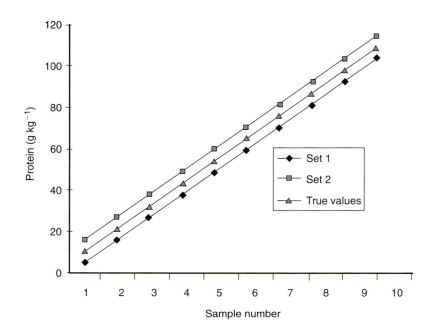

Fig. 9.5. Demonstration of effect of non-random partitioning of NIR errors between two truly identical sample sets.

regression analysis and calibration validation and testing) are available for analysing NIR data.

Data exploration

Once a set of NIR spectra is obtained, one needs to examine the spectra and see if there are any apparent problems, as demonstrated in Fig. 9.6. As can be seen, one of the five spectra differs in several ways from the others: first, the peaks are different, especially in the 400–600 nm region, and second the baseline is shifted upwards. Such baseline shifts are often due to particle size differences between the samples but, in this case the samples were scanned on different spectrometers. Since NIR spectra of a given material tend to be very similar, such spectral differences indicate potential problems. The last thing about all the spectra is the discontinuity

visible at 1100 nm, due to the use of two detectors: one for 400–1098 nm, and the second for 1100–2498 nm. By examining spectra before performing a calibration, bad spectra can be found and corrective actions taken, i.e. rerun the sample, do not use the region around 1100 nm, etc. Although it is highly likely that such problems will be discovered during the calibration process (i.e. a single bad sample will be tagged as either a spectral or compositional outlier), they would influence the results and require redevelopment of the calibration after removal or replacement of the bad spectra.

Data exploration can also include examination of plots showing the correlations at each wavelength between the spectra and the analyte of interest. Such 'Correlation Plots' can be used to select regions of the spectra to use or avoid when

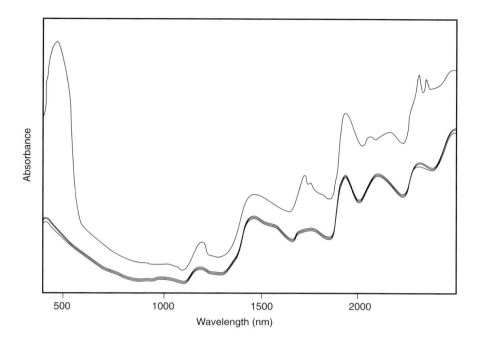

Fig. 9.6. Demonstration of the value of examining spectra before calibration development.

developing a calibration, which can sometimes result in improved calibrations. Also, some chemometric procedures, such as Neural Networks, still require considerable computer time even on the fastest personal computer, and, by reducing the wavelengths to be examined, the process can be sped up considerably (McClure *et al.*, 1992).

Data exploration also includes determining which samples are to provide the analyte calibration and test values. As previously discussed, although random selection can be used, it is also possible and best to select samples on the basis of spectral similarities and differences. Using a spectrally diverse set of samples offers the best chance of developing a calibration which will be applicable to other samples. The techniques used can be visual (cluster analysis based on spectral similarity) or numerical (regressing one spectrum against the other). The objective is the same: to find groups of samples that are similar and pick one to represent each group. Unfortunately, there is no magical way to know how many

samples will be needed. Most of the techniques used normalize the data before starting in such a way that only relative differences are determined. Thus, the result might be the 50 most diverse out of 100 or 1000 or 10,000 samples. Whether 50 will be enough or too many for any of these three sets depends on how similar the samples are, something which is very difficult to determine absolutely *a priori*.

Regression analysis

Once the samples needed for calibration development and testing have been determined, and the analyte values determined by the reference method, the process moves to finding the relationship between the spectral data and analyte. Many procedures have been tried and are being used to various degrees. While an in-depth discussion would require a book unto itself (see earlier references), a short discussion is necessary.

One of the problems with MLR is the possibility of over-fitting the data. In such a case, relationships are found between the calibration spectra and data, which are based partially on random correlations and not true chemical/spectral relationships, or are very specific to the calibration sample. This can occur because there are so many wavelengths available. In theory, if one has 700 wavelengths and only 100 samples, by using enough wavelengths (100 unknowns require 100 knowns) one gets a perfect fit. One solution has been to limit the number of wavelengths selected (i.e. one for every ten samples in the calibration to a maximum of ten or so). The problem then is that there is a lot of potentially useful spectral information available which is not being used. The solution used to address both problems simultaneously has been to use what are generally known as 'whole spectrum'-based procedures.

As a result, most of the chemometric efforts over the last 10 years or so have revolved around procedures such as factor analysis, principal components (PCR) and partial least squares (PLS) regression (Sharaf *et al.*, 1986). PCR and PLS, in particular, have enjoyed great success. In these two procedures, the entire spectrum is used. The spectra are decomposed into a series of factors which represent the variance in the spectra. In such a manner, the information in the spectra is compressed into a reduced series of factors which can then be used in a regression process to determine the analyte of interest. Other procedures used include Neural Networks (McClure *et al.*, 1992), genetic algorithms (Goldberg, 1989, used to reduce the number of wavelengths to be considered) and just about any method ever devised to extract predictive information from data. At present, efforts based on PLS, PCR and Neural Networks seem to be the most popular, with genetic algorithms used to select wavelengths. Considerable theoretical work has been carried out using factor analysis, but it has not found much use because one needs to know what the spectra of the factors (components in the samples) are before starting and, in complex samples, such as feedstuffs, that is virtually impossible.

Calibration validation and testing

Regardless of what method is used to develop the calibration, there are many steps which need to be performed in determining the final calibration. For example, how many wavelengths in an MLR are needed. If five are enough, then using more just results in over-fitting. The same applies to PLS; the number of factors possible is one less than the number of samples, but rarely are more than a dozen or so needed, even for large data sets. How does one decide how many to use? For each procedure, PLS or MLR, and even in many cases for each software package, a number of statistical tests are available, which in essence determine when the increase in accuracy obtained by adding an additional factor reaches the point of diminishing returns.

One simple method used with MLR is to divide the calibration set into two sets of data, a calibration and validation set. The equations are then developed using the calibration samples and the validation samples are predicted. In developing calibrations, it is not uncommon to try various data pre-treatments (i.e. derivatives, scatter corrections, etc., which are used to help extract the information from the spectra); the result is that one often has many different calibrations to examine and choose from. Since the validation set is involved in the development process, it becomes likely that one will find a set of terms which also randomly does well on the validation set, but not on future samples. By placing restrictions on the criteria for selecting how many terms one can use, experience has shown that one improves the likelihood that the final equation selected will be valid for future samples. The final test comes when one applies the selected equation to a new set of samples (test set).

Very similar procedures are used for Neural Net calibrations. For PLS and PCR a slight variation, called one-out cross-validation, is used. In this procedure, each sample is removed from the data set and a calibration developed using the remaining samples. This is repeated N times (each sample left out once) with the sample left out used as the validation set. The results are used to estimate the prediction error and to provide guidance in selecting the final number of factors to use. This procedure is felt to provide the best way to find the optimal equation and avoid over-fitting to the calibration data, although again an independent test set should also be used.

An obvious question which arises is, what happens if everything looks great, until the equation is used on the test set? Unfortunately, there is no easy answer to this question. One of the problems, which has become more apparent as NIR use has expanded beyond the laboratory, is that developing and maintaining NIR calibrations, while economically beneficial, is not a simple thing to learn. It takes a lot of experience and knowledge to know both what to do and what to look for. At a recent meeting, it was stated that it was felt that a year working in a chemometrics laboratory was needed to really know how to develop calibrations.

Part of the problem arises from the black box nature of NIR; take the spectra, apply the statistical procedure and see what happens. Unlike the case where we know that proteins absorb in the UV at 280 nm, data on NIR absorption bands are scattered throughout the literature and are very fragmented. While there are sections in various books (e.g. Murray and Williams, 1987), there are no books dedicated to the subject, as is true in the MIDIR (Colthup *et al.*, 1990 and many others). Only recently have efforts turned to the better understanding of NIR spectra in an effort to better understand calibrations.

Black box versus understandable NIR
While black box calibrations may be adequate when dealing with closed populations, it can be quite a different matter with open populations. For example, take the case of acetone–water mixtures; as the amount of acetone decreases, there are peak shifts particularly at 2390 and 2412 nm. A simple linear regression (percentage acetone = a + b × wavelength position) yielded an R^2 of 0.994 using the position of the peak at 2390 nm and 0.984 using that at 2414 nm, based on eyeball peak positions. Therefore, an accurate calibration could be developed based on peak position alone. This might be fine, unless the peak positions shifted for reasons other than water content, e.g. temperature changes. A similar effect has been used to determine salt concentrations in water. Salt does not have any absorption bands in the NIR, but does cause changes in the spectra of water, which can be used to determine the amount of salt present (Hirschfeld, 1985). However, it is important to understand that other salts (KCl, KNO_3, etc.) can easily cause the same effects, and that one is not determining salt concentration directly. Therefore, the calibration would not detect a substitution based on the spectral information alone. While this may be a simple case, similar things have occurred with calibrations, and the more one understands about the process and spectra, the less likely they are to occur.

For this reason, more and more effort is going into understanding the spectra and the basis for calibrations. Such knowledge can also explain why something does not work in order to eliminate the waste of trying something in the first place.

Calibration transfer

The final issue to be discussed dealing with calibrations is calibration transfer. As discussed above, almost anything which differs between the samples used to develop a calibration and the samples upon which it is to be used can cause errors, and this includes differences in the instrument at the times the samples were scanned, and applying a calibration to samples scanned on different machines. This represents a big problem when, for example, one wishes to develop a network of instruments to determine forage quality. One certainly does not want to scan all the samples on each instrument, and go through the calibration procedure for each, and then to have to repeat the process periodically due to repairs or even wear and tear over time. In reality, the problem is even worse because, for feedstuffs, it is difficult to maintain a set of samples over long periods of time without changes occurring in the samples.

The area of chemometrics dealing with this subject has come to be known as 'Calibration transfer', or how to transfer (or use) a calibration developed on one instrument to another, or to the same instrument after changes have occurred. Many procedures have been tried and considerable research is still being carried out to solve this problem (Wang and Kolwalski, 1992). The two central approaches used are: (i) to make all the instruments as identical as possible; and (ii) to alter the spectra so they look as though they came off the same instrument.

Approach number one is being used on many Fourier transform NIR spectrometers (FTNIR). One of the big problems with transferring calibrations is differences in wavelength accuracy. For example, a scanning monochromator may be designed to collect data starting at wavelength 1100 nm. However, due to instrumental variations, the actual wavelengths being collected are off a little, so data point one may be 1100.5 or 1099.5 nm. Only by scanning a standard and comparing the results with known values can the actual wavelengths scanned be known. The problem is that the wavelengths can be off by varying degrees from wavelength to wavelength. Thus, one might be able to make 1100 exactly 1100, but then 1800 might be 1799.5 nm and 2498, 2498.5 nm, etc. Instruments based on filters can have similar problems due to the difficulty of mass-producing identical filters. Fourier transform spectrometers (Griffiths and de Haseth, 1986) have the ability to lock in all wavelengths accurately using a laser as the standard. Since wavelength shift is one of the biggest problems, some feel that FTNIRs have an advantage with respect to calibration transfer. At present, however, their use has been virtually limited to discriminate analysis of raw materials and not for quantitative determinations of feedstuffs.

The general approach to making spectra look alike has been to use regression analysis to determine how the spectra vary and to correct the variation. One weakness with this technique is that a set of samples similar in nature to those being tested is needed for matching the spectra between instruments. Even when using sealed sample cups, it is difficult to produce samples which do not change over time. However, this appears to be one of the better approaches at the present time. The procedure is to run the set of standards periodically and then the software regresses the spectra against a master set of spectra, finds where differences exist and designs a regression equation to convert the new spectra to the masters on a point by point basis. Using this method, not only peak position, but also changes in band shape and photometric response (absorbances), etc. can be handled. Once the equation is determined, the spectra of all newly scanned samples can be converted automatically. This procedure can be used on one instrument, so that spectra taken next year should look like spectra taken today. It can also make several instruments produce the same spectra for a given set of samples. It is the latter which has been used in networks of instruments. The procedure has even been used to convert spectra across vastly different types of instruments. Recently, efforts have concentrated on using a single sample to perform the same transfer.

The biggest weakness with the procedure mentioned above is its dependence on a set of standard samples or sample. The standards need to be similar to the types of samples being tested since they correct for band shape, etc. Efforts have been made to seal forages in plastics, but these efforts have not been successful. While it is a very important subject, and research is continuing, it is difficult to determine how much success has been achieved to date.

Instrumentation

Instrumentation for NIR comes in a wide variety of sizes, shapes and forms. There are also several ways to classify such instruments, which unfortunately often overlap. For example, instrumentation can be classified by sampling mechanisms (fibre optics, rotating cups for ground samples, bulk samplers for unground samples, liquid samplers), by function (general purpose or dedicated to a single analyte or several similar analytes), by portability (bench top, luggable, meter), by optical design (grating, filter, light-emitting diodes, FTNIR, single detector, integrating spheres, diode array, charged coupled devices, etc.), or by wavelength range (NIR, SWNIR, SWNIR/NIR, MIDIR, etc.). While there can be considerable overlap, all possible combinations are not available, at least not for analysing feedstuffs.

The user of NIR for analysing feedstuffs has many options at the present time. In addition, there are many other instruments still in use which were made by companies that no longer exist or have been purchased by other companies. For example, the model 6500 scanning monochromator presently manufactured by FOSS-NIRSystems is the successor to instruments in the 6000 series made by previous owners of NIRSystems (Perstorp, Pacific Scientific, Neotec). While some of these older instruments may be in working condition and perfectly suitable for a given project, one should consider that these instruments may not be repairable without heroic efforts and, unless precautions are taken to allow calibration transfer, one may end up with a useless collection of spectra. The problem is not with the instrument manufacturers, so much as with the advances in electronics which have made many spare parts impossible to get. Also, many systems once relied on proprietary computer systems for which keyboards, monitors, power supplies, etc. are no longer available (personal experience).

Finally, in purchasing an instrument for NIR work, the potential buyer should carefully consider future plans in addition to the immediate needs. Portable instruments using fibre optic cables might seem a great overall choice since they can be used in the laboratory or in the field, but they generally have very small fibre optic bundles which means a small area of illumination. This can be fine for solutions or even finely ground homogeneous powders or solids, but would not be optimal for work with bulk quantities of heterogeneous materials. Also, they are often limited to the SWNIR or lower part of the NIR, although this is changing. If one wants or needs the region from 1800 to 2500 nm, then many of these are not adequate. The same applies to the LED-based instruments.

The same type of thinking applies to dedicated versus general purpose instruments. If all one needs is an instrument to measure moisture in feedstuffs, why purchase a general purpose instrument costing ten times more, which would also be more difficult to use and maintain? Alternatively, many general purpose scanning monochromators can be purchased with accessories to use a wide variety of cells (liquid, powders, bulk), attachments (diffuse reflectance, transmission, fibre optic probes), spectral ranges (visible through the NIR), software packages and so on. The only drawbacks are cost and lack of easy portability.

Finally, while FTNIRs appear to be making big inroads in the NIR field, they have not as yet been directed at feedstuff analysis. The companies producing them are aiming almost completely at the industrial need for quality checking of incoming raw material using discriminate analysis and, since virtually no work has been done using FTNIRs on feedstuffs, it is difficult to judge their suitability.

For further information on instrument designs, advantages, disadvantages, etc. the reader is referred to some of the following references: Griffiths and de Haseth (1986); McClure (1987); Marten *et al.* (1989); Workman and Burns (1992) or the Internet, where many companies provide a wealth of information.

Applications to Feed Chemistry

In Table 9.2 are listed some of the feedstuff determinations for which NIR has been

Table 9.2. Applications of NIR to animal feedstuffs.

Type of feed	Determination(s)
Forages and by-products including those treated chemically or physically	Dry matter
	Total crude protein (CP), acid detergent fibre-CP, heat-damaged protein
	Fibre (neutral and acid detergent, cellulose, hemicelluose, crude fibre, organic cellular content, total non-structural carbohydrates, etc.)
	Digestibility (*in situ* and *in vitro*, cell wall and dry matter, low and high digestible fibre fraction)
	Lignin (72% H_2SO_4 $KMnO_4$, $NaClO_2$, acetyl bromide, etc.)
	Lignin composition (nitrobenzene oxidation products)
	Energy (net and other measures)
	Intake
	Alkaloids
	Fungal contaminants (chitin and glucosamine)
	Dysprosium marker
	Minerals (Ca, Cu, Fe, K, Mg, Na, P, S), Si and ash
	Botanical composition determinations
Mixed rations and feed ingredients, including poultry and swine feeds	See forage above as appropriate
	Energy (*in vitro* digestible, metabolizable, net)
	Digestible crude protein
	Lysine in swine feeds
	Oil
	Starch
	Sugars
	Sulphur
Silages	See forage above as appropriate
	Cellulase digestibility
	NH_3, acid detergent- and hot-water insoluble N, insoluble N
	pH
	True dry matter
	Volatile fatty acids
	Effect of soil contamination on NIR analysis
	Fermentation characteristics
Other materials Oesophageal fistula and faeces samples	Any of the above as appropriate

used. As can be seen, an entire book could be written summarizing the results obtained for feedstuffs alone. The examples which follow were chosen because, while demonstrating how NIR can be applied to the area of feedstuffs, they also demonstrate many of the important concepts previously discussed. For the reader who wishes to know more on a specific determination, e.g. how well can I expect to determine NDF in forage samples, there are several means to get started. The book by Williams and Norris, *Near-Infrared Technology in the Agricultural and Food Industries* (Williams, 1987), although 10 years old, is excellent, as is the monograph *Analysis of Agricultural and Food Products by Near Infrared Reflectance Spectroscopy* (Shenk and Westerhaus, 1993). Also, on the Internet, many companies have web sites with tutorials and even data sets available, journals are listing the titles of published articles and, while there may not be a free database of NIR articles similar to the chemometrics database previously listed, there are many sites with references listed. As demonstrated in Table 9.2, NIRS has been used for a wide range of feedstuff analysis. Basically, it can be said that if there is a determination presently being used in the analysis of animal feedstuffs, then someone has probably investigated the use of NIR to carry out the determination.

Sample populations and effect on calibrations

The tall fescue results in Table 9.3 (Blosser *et al.*, 1988) demonstrate the result of some of these effects. Samples were collected over three consecutive growing years from the same fields, ground with the same grinder, scanned in the same cells, on the same instrument under similar conditions, with chemistries performed by the same technician using the same equipment and chemicals. Thus, many of the variations which affect a calibration developed or used over a period of years did not exist. Yet as can easily be seen, the equations developed using samples collected in one year, often would not work on samples collected in a different year. One possible explanation is that if samples from one year all contain the same percentage of some constituent, such as hemicellulose, then the calibration equation does not need to include wavelengths to account for variations in hemicellulose concentration. The result is that if that equation is applied to samples from a year where the hemi-cellulose content varies, the values for fibre will probably be incorrect. It is similar events which make samples from one year different from those of another, thus causing many of the calibration problems.

Calibration improvement and redevelopment

When an existing calibration fails to perform satisfactorily on new samples, one can often correct the problem by including some of the new samples in the calibration set, followed by redevelopment of the calibration. Typically, only a few of the new samples are needed. An example using two closed population sets may be seen in Table 9.4 (Reeves *et al.*, 1991). These samples were residues of hays from two nylon bag *in situ* digestion studies. While the original hays were the same for both studies, the animals used and their diets were different. As can be seen, the determination of constituents in samples in study 2 from equations developed using samples from study 1 often resulted in reasonable correlations, but extremely large biases. To correct this, six samples for each feed (9%) from study 2 were added to the study 1 samples and new equations developed, with the results shown.

It is also important to avoid continually adding new and unique samples to a calibration set. This produces not only a very large and therefore difficult set to work with, but also a set which may determine all samples equally, but few samples particularly well. Therefore, the development and main-tenance of calibrations is a continuous job, the reward of which is the reduced time, waste and costs of performing wet chemical analyses.

Table 9.3. Analysis of ADF in tall fescue by NIRS using equations prepared from samples of various growing years (Blosser *et al.*, 1988).

VAL year	Mean	SD	CAL year	N VAL	PMean	PSD	SEA	Bias	r^2
1976	34.6	2.07	1976	21	34.2	2.07	0.72	0.40	0.88
1976	34.6	2.35	1977	64	35.5	2.66	1.66	−0.89	0.61
1976	34.6	2.35	1978	64	33.4	1.94	1.90	1.25	0.34
1978	37.0	3.30	1978	20	37.1	3.63	0.63	0.14	0.96
1978	36.9	3.63	1976	61	33.9	2.81	1.63	3.00	0.82
1978	36.9	3.63	1977	61	36.1	3.91	1.08	0.81	0.92

VAL = validation set, CAL = calibration set, *N* = no. of samples, P = predicted, SD = standard deviation, SEA = standard error of analysis, Bias = mean − Pmean.

Table 9.4. Results of NIRS determination of study 2 *in situ* samples using calibration set from study 1[a] (Reeves *et al.*, 1991).

Forage	CS[b] source	VS[c] source	Assay[d]	Calibration R^2	Calibration SEC[e]	Validation R^2	Validation SEP[f]	Bias
Lucerne	Second	None	DIG	0.99	1.77			
($n = 64$)			CP	0.99	0.42			
	First	Second	DIG			0.69	8.95	28.32
			CP			0.97	1.07	−13.74
	First+	Second	DIG	0.94	3.59	0.95	3.41	−0.01
			CP	0.99	0.61	0.98	0.60	−0.12
Orchard-grass	Second	None	DIG	0.99	1.69			
			CP	0.98	0.46			
($n = 64$)	First	Second	DIG			0.94	4.52	−72.35
			CP			0.97	0.98	−1.28
	First+	Second	DIG	0.98	2.45	0.98	2.91	−0.70
			CP	1.00	0.26	0.98	0.61	−0.13

[a]Study 2 samples digested and analysed at the University of Maryland, study 1 at Beltsville.
[b]CS = calibration set: second = all study 2 samples, first = all study 1 samples, First+ = all of the study 1 samples plus six of lucerne and/or orchardgrass samples from study 2 as appropriate.
[c]Validation set: second = all samples from study 2.
[d]DIG = percentage digested, CP = crude protein.
[e]SEC = standard error of calibration.
[f]SEP = standard error of performance.

Chemical dependence

At present, NIRS is inherently limited by its dependence on the calibration process, and thus the chemically or physically determined calibration values. This leads to two basic limits to the use of NIRS. First and foremost, NIRS-determined values are on average no more accurate than the chemically determined values upon which they are based. The second and more subtle limit relates to the basis of the chemical values. Most of the chemistries used for animal feeds are largely, if not completely, empirical in nature. Therefore, measures such as NDF and ADF determine whatever is insoluble in that particular solution. This leads to the possibility that only partial extraction of components occurs. The question of how this fractional extraction varies among samples, and whether the fraction extracted is spectrally the same or different from the fraction not extracted, is one which has yet to be answered. At present, the effect of the empirical nature of many of the presently used measures of composition and quality on the accuracy and long-term stability of calibrations is largely unknown. However, it is generally felt that better chemical analyses (more accurate and precise and less empirical in nature) will lead to better NIRS calibrations. Support for this exists in the fact that NIRS calibrations are generally best for dry matter and protein and decrease in quality, in order, for measures of fibre, digestibility and lignin. While lignin is in fact a definable material composed of polymerized propenyl-benzene units, lignin as measured can be a mixture of true lignin, protein, waxes and carbohydrates, the exact combination of which depends on the sample in question and the procedure being used (Reeves, 1993).

High moisture samples

While the previously noted effects also apply to high moisture samples, these materials have particular problems.

Populations of silage samples often contain samples of high moisture content and possess a wide range of moisture contents. Even though NIR radiation is better able than MIDIR to handle samples containing a large amount of water, water still causes considerable problems. In a sample containing a large amount of water, the water bands present are quite large and tend to overlap and obscure other spectral features. This can also cause non-linear responses due to instrumental limitations. Thus doubling the concentration of a component does not necessarily cause an absorption doubling. The end result, as shown in Table 9.5 (Reeves and Blosser, 1991), is that the results found for high moisture samples, such as silages, are not as good as those for the same or similar samples when dried. The former USDA NIRS Network and former Pacific Scientific Co. (now FOSS NIRSystems, Inc.) sponsored studies of this problem which showed that, no matter how wet silages were ground or scanned (data not shown), the results were never as good as for the same samples when dried. However, as shown in Table 9.6, NIRS is capable of measuring many, but not all components of interest in wet samples (Reeves *et al.*, 1989). The choice seems either to use NIRS on dried and, therefore, modified samples (loss of volatiles such as short-chain fatty acids and ammonia on drying) or to use wet unmodified samples and accept the loss in accuracy. Another alternative is to use NIR to determine some variables using dry samples, and other methods, such as titration, on volatiles.

Many researchers are exploring the SWNIR region for samples containing a large amount of water. Just as radiation in the NIR can penetrate deeper than can radiation in the MIDIR range, so radiation in the SWNIR penetrates still deeper. However, as will be shown, penetration depth is not the only problem when dealing with silages.

Mixed rations

Compared with forages and silages, mixed rations have an added problem. For these samples, in addition to all the other considerations already discussed, it is necessary to account for variations present in all the ration ingredients, in developing the calibration equations.

Theoretical Considerations

As previously discussed, because of the way NIRS has developed, most of the research efforts have been in the area of practical applications and ways to avoid or eliminate problems encountered. Considerably less effort has been applied to theoretical aspects of NIRS. Thus, while it

Table 9.5. NIRS results[a] for acid detergent fibre and total Kjeldahl nitrogen for dried and untreated silages with 10 nm between wavelengths using a circular cell (Reeves and Blosser, 1991).

Grind[b]	Calibration (*n* = 98)		Validation (*n* = 47)		
	R^2	SEC	r^2	SEP	Bias
Acid detergent fibre					
VIT	0.94	2.03	0.94	2.03	−0.04
DRY	0.96	1.49	0.96	1.48	−0.01
Crude protein					
VIT	0.98	0.96	0.97	1.05	−0.07
DRY	0.99	0.58	0.99	0.61	0.01

[a]NIRS results: R^2 = calibration *r*-square; SEC = standard error of calibration; r^2 = validation *r*-square; SEP = standard error of prediction; Bias = difference in predicted and actual mean for validation set samples.
[b]Grinds: VIT = Vita-Mix using dry ice; DRY = ground dried material using a Wiley grinder.

Table 9.6. Accuracy of NIRS in analysing undried silages[a] (Reeves *et al.*, 1989).

Component	Calibration set (*n* = 98)		Validation set (*n* = 48)		
	R^2	SEC[b]	r^2	SEP[c]	Bias[d]
Dry matter (DM)	0.97	2.07	0.95	3.15	−0.05
Crude protein	0.97	1.02	0.96	1.25	−0.11
Acid detergent fibre	0.91	2.59	0.90	2.78	0.70
Neutral detergent fibre	0.87	3.18	0.87	3.75	0.83
In vitro digestible DM	0.87	2.39	0.73	3.78	0.28
Ammonia N	0.87	0.35	0.82	0.39	−0.05
Hot water-insoluble N	0.95	0.68	0.82	1.28	−0.42
ADF-insoluble N	0.71	0.65	0.59	1.40	0.31
pH	0.85	0.28	0.55	0.45	0.09
Acetic acid	0.74	0.56	0.57	0.79	−0.05
Butyric acid	0.68	0.18	0.57	0.29	−0.01
Lactic acid	0.71	1.41	0.74	1.30	0.01

[a]Chemical composition expressed on a dry matter basis.
[b]Standard error of calibration.
[c]Standard error of performance.
[d]Deviation of NIRS mean from chemistry laboratory mean.

is known that the spectra found in the NIR are due to overtone and combination bands of absorptions found in the MIDIR (Murray and Williams, 1987), the consequences of the overlapping of the many bands present in a multicomponent system are much less understood. This overlapping may, for example, account for the fact that NIRS does not in general perform well for minor constituents.

Minerals

One application area for which theoretical concerns are known to place limits is determination of minerals by NIRS. While NIRS can be used to determine analytes such as K, Na and P in forages, the bases for these determinations are correlations between the minerals and organic constituents (Clark, 1989). This is because these minerals do not have absorptions in the NIR spectral region. Therefore, the accuracy of mineral determination by NIRS depends entirely on the degree of correlation between organic constituents, which do absorb in the NIR, and the mineral in question. For example, it has been shown that one can predict Ca, K, Mg and P from

the ADF and CP content of forages with an accuracy equal to that achieved using NIRS (Shenk *et al.*, 1992).

High moisture samples

As shown earlier, NIRS does not perform as well on high moisture samples as it does for dried materials, even for the same assay on the same samples. The question can then be asked: are there fundamental reasons why this is so and can they be addressed? Research using simple systems of water and single compounds, such as sugars, amino acids, polysaccharides, ketones, alcohols, amines, etc., has shown (Reeves, 1993) that while as dry crystalline solids, they give spectra which have sharp peaks and which are unique to each sugar, in solution, the spectra lack sharp peaks and look much more alike, resembling polysaccharides such as cellulose and starch to a great degree. It was also found that for ketones and alcohols in particular that the addition of water caused peak shifts, the degree of which was dependent on the water concentration.

A second study (Reeves, 1994a) showed that variations in pH, ionic strength and physical state can also have spectral effects similar to those caused by water. Thus amorphous and molten sugars look very much like sugars in solution, indicating a loss in crystallinity as the cause. The question then remains as to whether these effects are the reason that NIRS does not operate as well on high moisture materials.

Efforts to quantify the loss of spectral information caused by water were carried out by comparing water-subtracted spectra with other water-subtracted spectra and with spectra of amorphous and dry crystalline materials (Reeves, 1995). Results showed that spectra for dry crystalline materials are in general much less similar than spectra of dissolved or amorphous materials. However, the loss of information typically is so large that the question then becomes how NIRS operates at all on high moisture samples. Examining the effects of water on the various compounds by class showed that polymeric materials, such as cellulose, starch, pectins, hemicelluloses and proteins, were the least effected by water, pH and physical state variations. The fact that such polymers make up a large percentage of the total dry matter in either dry forages or wet silages may account for why NIRS works reasonably well with high moisture materials. Thus, for wet samples, NIRS may only have trouble determining the composition of the relatively small fraction of the sample comprised of monomeric materials.

Solid state matrix effects

Another possible reason why NIRS performs better with high moisture samples than the work with model compounds would indicate, may lie in the nature of spectra found for dry materials. In reality, dry samples such as forages are complex mixtures of the various components, and may contain compartmentalized fractions and fractions which behave more like solid solutions than simple mixtures of pure components. For example, the soluble monomers in plant leaves are likely to be compartmentalized either in vacuoles or in the sap. In samples which have been crushed or fermented (silages), the sap or vacuoles may well be mixed with the more structural parts of the plant tissue. In either case, one is unlikely to find an isolated solution of glucose which can crystallize well.

The question is what happens to spectra under these circumstances. If a solution of glucose is dried in the presence of cellulose, does the spectrum of the resulting dry mixture look like the spectrum obtained if dry cellulose and dry crystalline glucose are simply mixed together? Results have shown that it is easy to see the spectrum of glucose in simple mixtures of cellulose and glucose using spectral subtraction. However, when a solution of glucose is added to cellulose and the mix dried under vacuum while being stirred continuously, it becomes difficult to find the glucose. Thus, even for dry materials, there are spectral interactions which resemble those found with high moisture mixtures and solutions. Only further efforts with both dried and high moisture samples are likely to answer the question of how the presence of water in high moisture samples degrades NIRS results.

Conclusions

While there is still the need for research on NIRS and the limits to its use, it is a useful technique. With proper planning and care, it can reduce the need and time required for chemical analysis. At present, NIRS works best on dried materials and requires constant checking to maintain the accuracy of calibration equations. How much the present limits to analysis by NIRS can be reduced by improvements in instrumentation, chemometric techniques and wet chemical analysis procedures remains to be seen. If the techniques used to determine fibre were as precise and as non-empirical as those used for protein, would the accuracy for fibre determination by NIRS be as high as that obtained for protein, and if not why? These and many other questions still remain to be answered. One point is certain: with all the pressure, both direct and financial, to reduce the genera- tion of chemical wastes, there will be a steady increase in the demand for instrumental methods of analysis, such as NIRS.

References

Blosser, T.H., Reeves, J.B., III and Bond, J. (1988) Factors affecting analysis of the chemical composition of tall fescue with near infrared reflectance spectroscopy. *Journal of Dairy Science* 71, 398–408.

Buxton, D.E. and Mertens, D.E. (1991) Errors in forage-quality data predicted by near infrared reflectance spectroscopy. *Crop Science* 31, 212–218.

Ciurczak, E.W. (1992a) Principles of near-infrared spectroscopy. In: Burns, D.A. and Ciurczak, E.W. (eds) *Handbook of Near-Infrared Analysis.* Marcel Dekker, Inc., New York, pp. 7–12.

Ciurczak, E.W. (1992b) NIR analysis of pharmaceuticals. In: Burns, D.A. and Ciurczak, E.W. (eds) *Handbook of Near-Infrared Analysis.* Marcel Dekker, Inc., New York, pp. 549–564.

Clark, D.H. (1989) Other forage and feed nutrients. In: Marten, G.C., Shenk, J.S. and Barton, F.E., II (eds) *Near Infrared Reflectance Spectroscopy (NIRS): Analysis of Forage Quality.* Agriculture Handbook No. 643. National Technical Information Series. Springfield, Virginia, p. 58.

Colthup, N.B., Daly, L.H. and Wiberley, S.E. (1990) *Introduction to Infrared and Raman Spectroscopy*, 3rd edn. Academic Press, Inc., New York.

Goldberg, D.E. (1989) *Genetic Algorithms in Search, Optimization and Machine Learning.* Addison-Wesley Publishing Company, Inc., New York.

Griffiths, P.R. and de Haseth, J.A. (1986) *Fourier Transform Infrared Spectrometry.* John Wiley & Sons, New York.

Hirschfeld, T. (1985) Salinity determination using NIRA. *Applied Spectroscopy* 39, 740–741.

Isaksson, T. and Kowalski, B. (1993) Piece-wise multiplicative scatter correction applied to near-infrared diffuse reflectance data from meat products. *Applied Spectroscopy* 47, 702–709.

Kemeny, G.J. (1992) Process analysis. In: Burns, D.A. and Ciurczak, E.W. (eds) *Handbook of Near-Infrared Analysis.* Marcel Dekker, Inc., New York, pp. 53–106.

Marten, G.C., Shenk, J.S. and Barton, F.E., II (eds) (1989) *Near Infrared Reflectance Spectroscopy (NIRS): Analysis of Forage Quality.* Agriculture Handbook No. 643. National Technical Information Series. Springfield, Virginia.

Massart, D.L., Vandeginste, B.G.M., Deming, S.N., Michotte, Y. and Kaufman, L. (1988) *Chemometrics: a Textbook.* Elsevier Science Publishers, New York.

McClure, W.F. (1987) Near-infrared instrumentation. In: Williams, P.C. and Norris, K. (eds) *Near-Infrared Technology in the Agricultural and Food Industries.* American Association of Cereal Chemists, Inc., St Paul, Minnesota, pp. 89–106.

McClure, W.F. (1992) Making light work: lighting new frontiers. In: Murray, I. and Cowe, A. (eds) *Making Light Work: Advances in Near-Infrared Spectroscopy.* VCH, New York, pp. 1–13.

Murray, I. and Williams, P.C. (1987) Chemical principles of near-infrared technology. In: Williams, P.C. and Norris, K. (eds) *Near-Infrared Technology in the Agricultural and Food Industries.* American Association of Cereal Chemists, Inc., St Paul, Minnesota, pp. 17–34.

Osborne, B.G. and Fearn, T. (1986) *Near Infrared Spectroscopy in Food Analysis.* John Wiley and Co., New York.

Osborne, B.G., Fearn, T. and Stevenson, S.G. (1987) Near-infrared research in Europe. In: Williams, P.C. and Norris, K. (eds) *Near-Infrared Technology in the Agricultural and Food Industries.* American Association of Cereal Chemists, Inc., St Paul, Minnesota, pp. 185–200.

PLSplus V2.1G (1992) Galactic Industries, Corporation, 395 Main Street, Salem, NH 03079.

Reeves, J.B., III (1993) Influence of water on the near infrared spectra of model compounds. *Journal of AOAC International* 76, 741–748.

Reeves, J.B., III (1994a) Influence of pH, ionic strength, and physical state on the near-infrared spectra of model compounds. *Journal of AOAC International* 77, 814–820.

Reeves, J.B., III (1994b) Use of near infrared reflectance spectroscopy as a tool for screening treated forages and by-products. *Journal of Dairy Science* 77, 1030–1037.

Reeves, J.B., III (1995) Efforts to quantify changes in near-infrared spectra caused by the influence of water, pH, ionic strength, and differences in physical state. *Journal of Applied Spectroscopy* 49(2), 181–187.

Reeves, J.B., III and Blosser, T.H. (1991) Near infrared spectroscopic analysis of undried silages as influenced by sample grind, presentation method, and spectral region. *Journal of Dairy Science* 742, 882–895.

Reeves, J.B., III, Blosser, T.H. and Colebrander, V.F. (1989) Near infrared reflectance spectroscopy for analyzing undried silages. *Journal of Dairy Science* 72, 79–88.

Reeves, J.B., III, Blosser, T.H., Balde, A.T., Glenn, B.P. and Vandersall, J. (1991) Near infrared spectroscopic analysis of forage samples digested *in situ* (nylon bag). *Journal of Dairy Science* 74, 2664–2673.

Sharaf, M.A., Illman, D.L. and Kowalski, B.R. (1986) *Chemometrics*. John Wiley & Sons, New York.

Shenk, J.S., Workman, J.J., Jr and Westerhaus, M.O. (1992) Application of NIR spectroscopy to agricultural products. In: Burns, D.A. and Ciurczak, E.W. (eds) *Handbook of Near-Infrared Analysis*. Marcel Dekker, Inc., New York, pp. 383–431.

Shenk, J.S. and Westerhaus, M.O. (1993) *Monograph: Analysis of Agricultural and Food Products by Near Infrared Reflectance Spectroscopy*. NIRSystems, Inc., 12101 Tech Road, Silver Spring, MD 20904.

Tkachuk, R. (1987) Analysis of whole grains by near-infrared reflectance. In: Williams, P.C. and Norris, K. (eds) *Near-Infrared Technology in the Agricultural and Food Industries*. American Association of Cereal Chemists, Inc., St Paul, Minnesota, pp. 233–240.

Unscrambler Ver. 5.5 User's Guide (1994) CAMO A/S, Olav Tryggvasonsgt, 24, 7011 Trondheim, Norway.

Van Soest, P.J. (1994) Forage evaluation techniques. In: *Nutritional Ecology of the Ruminant*, 2nd edn. Comstock Publishing Associates, Ithaca, New York, pp. 108–121.

Wang, Y. and Kowalski, B.R. (1992) Calibration transfer and measurement stability of near-infrared spectrometers. *Applied Spectroscopy* 46, 764–771.

Williams, P.C. (1987) Commercial near-infrared reflectance analyzers. In: Williams, P.C. and Norris, K. (eds) *Near-Infrared Technology in the Agricultural and Food Industries*. American Association of Cereal Chemists, Inc., St Paul, Minnesota, pp. 107–142.

Workman, J.J., Jr and Burns, D.A. (1992) Commercial NIR instrumentation. In: Burns, D.A. and Ciurczak, E.W. (eds) *Handbook of Near-Infrared Analysis*. Marcel Dekker, Inc., New York, pp. 37–52.

Chapter 10

Gas Production Methods

P. Schofield

Department of Animal Science, Cornell University,
Ithaca, New York, USA

Introduction

The energy metabolism of ruminant animals is based on their ability to digest plant structural carbohydrates such as cellulose. This digestion is carried out under anaerobic conditions in the rumen by a complex consortium of bacteria, fungi and protozoa. Cellulose is an exceptionally stable polymer of glucose units with a structure resembling reinforced concrete in some respects. It is therefore digested slowly. Limitations on the body size of ruminants mean that fibrous feeds can be retained in the rumen for only a limited period of time, 24–48 h for cattle, before passing to the lower tract where most fibre digestion ceases. There is thus a continuing competition between the processes of ruminal digestion and passage. For this reason, a study of ruminant nutrition must include the topics of fibre digestibility and digestion rates – how they are measured and interpreted. The goal of this chapter is to survey the application of *in vitro* gas production measurements to the study of these topics.

We first consider some quantitative aspects of gas production and their bearing on the historical development of the technique. We summarize general factors that affect gas measurements and discuss the merits and demerits of alternative techniques. Following a survey of equipment needs, we examine alternative models for fitting and interpreting gas curves and explore the relationship between the substrate pools hypothesized by these models and actual plant carbohydrate fractions.

Gas and microbial yields per unit of substrate digested are considered next. We survey applications of the gas method including the detection of plant secondary compounds that may interfere with digestion, the role of plant soluble carbohydrates in the fermentation process, and practical applications such as intake prediction. The appendix contains a brief review of non-linear curve fitting and a description of pressure sensor structures.

Quantitative Aspects

The process of fermentation involves a series of energy-yielding reactions catalysed by microbial cells in which organic compounds act as both oxidizable substrates and oxidizing agents. If we ignore microbial cell production, then fermentation of glucose in the rumen produces a stoichiometrically balanced mixture of acetate, propionate, butyrate, CO_2 and CH_4 (Wolin, 1960). It is helpful, at this stage, to look at an example of a theoretical balanced equation for this kind of glucose fermentation (Baldwin, 1970):

$$1 \text{ glucose} \rightarrow 1.2 \text{ acetate}$$
$$+ 0.4 \text{ propionate} + 0.2 \text{ butyrate}$$
$$+ 1 \text{ } CO_2 + 0.6 \text{ } CH_4 + 0.4 \text{ } H_2O \qquad (10.1)$$

In this example, fermentation of 1 mol of glucose produces 1.6 mol of gas (CO_2 + CH_4, direct gas) plus 1.8 mol of volatile fatty acid (VFA). If the fermentation takes place in a bicarbonate buffer at pH 6.5, then the VFA will react with the buffer to give an equimolar amount of CO_2 (indirect gas). The total gas yield will then be 3.4 mol mol^{-1} of glucose.

Let us also review the physical law that governs gas behaviour. The general gas law,

$$PV = nRT \qquad (10.2)$$

tells us that, for an ideal gas, pressure (P) and volume (V) are inversely related. If one of these is held constant, the other is directly proportional to both the molar amount (n) of a gas and the absolute temperature (T). The universal gas constant (R) has the units (pressure × volume × $moles^{-1}$ × $temperature^{-1}$) and the numerical value of R depends on the units selected for pressure, volume and temperature. Most students remember that 1 mol of a perfect gas occupies 22.4 litres at one atmosphere pressure and 0°C. We can use this information to calculate R from Equation 10.2:

$$R = (1 \text{ atm} \times 22.4 \text{ l})/(1 \text{ mol} \times 273°K) =$$
$$0.0821 \text{ atm l } mol^{-1}.°K^{-1}$$

Equation 10.2, or simplified forms of it, will be needed to convert measured gas volumes to a standard temperature and pressure, to derive volumes from pressure measurements, and to relate gas volumes to substrate disappearance. The gas law also reminds us that the volume of a fixed

molar amount of a gas is defined only when both temperature and pressure are defined.

If we now apply Equations 10.1 and 10.2 to the fermentation of 1 g of glucose equivalents (formula weight = 180 − 18 g mol^{-1}) at 39°C and one atmosphere pressure, the predicted gas volume is:

$$(1/162) \text{ mol} \times 22.4 \text{ l/mol}$$
$$\times 3.4 \text{ mol/mol} \times (312/273) °K/°K$$
$$= 537 \text{ ml}$$

In practice, the gas yield from fibre substrates such as cellulose and neutral detergent fibre is always less than this figure and is approximately 350–400 ml g^{-1} glucose equivalent (Pell and Schofield, 1993). The reasons for this discrepancy will be discussed later.

The above calculation provides a useful sense of the size of gas volumes produced in an *in vitro* system that measures the gas output from fibre fermentation. The design of the equipment is dictated to some degree by the volume considerations noted above. Several different approaches have been taken to measure the gas produced during *in vitro* fermentation. The paper by Blümmel *et al.* (1997b) contains references to the early history of the gas method. The following survey is restricted to techniques currently in use.

Techniques – an Overview

If an *in vitro* fermentation is carried out in a syringe, the volume of gas produced at the prevailing atmospheric pressure is automatically made evident by plunger displacement. The syringe technique has been used extensively by Menke and collaborators at the Institute for Animal Nutrition at the University of Hohenheim in Germany. The original method was described in 1974 and revised and reviewed in 1988 (Menke and Steingass, 1988). Some important features of the method are:

1. The standard incubation contains 10 ml of ruminal fluid, 20 ml of buffer and

200 mg of sample. Digestion takes place within a 100 ml graduated glass syringe installed on a rotor and maintained at 39°C. Gas volumes are read to ±0.5 ml. If a large volume of gas is to be measured, the syringe can be emptied after a measured volume is collected, and the fermentation can then be continued.

2. The system can be used both for digestibility measurements (24 h incubation) and for rate measurements (readings taken after 4, 8, 12, 24 and 32 h). Recent work has sometimes used more extensive sampling.

3. Blanks (four syringes with no substrate) and standards (three syringes with hay, hay + starch, concentrate) are run with each experiment. The standards each have a known gas production determined by averaging many replicates and using different ruminal fluid inocula. If the standard included within a run produces between 90 and 110% as much gas as the 'average' value for that standard, then the ruminal fluid is scored as normal and all the measured gas volumes are corrected by the factor 'average standard volume/run standard volume'. If, however, the run standard volume lies outside this 90–110% range, the run data are discarded on the grounds that the ruminal fluid was abnormal. The average blank volume is subtracted from all samples. This volume is normally 6–12 ml or 13–27% of the final reading, quite a high blank value.

4. The above treatment of blanks and standards is claimed to correct for atmospheric pressure differences between runs. As applied, the correction converts gas volumes to the average pressure at which the standards were determined. Unless this pressure is reported, it is difficult to compare gas volume data from different laboratories.

Manual methods of recording data, whether by reading a manometer or a syringe, necessarily restrict the amount of data collected. If one is interested in digestibility values, the problem is manageable because only a few readings need be taken from each sample. However, for a kinetic analysis of feedstuff digestion, many timed readings are necessary, and manual methods become burdensome. Research workers in this field therefore looked for an appropriate automatic data recording system. The first hint of a possible solution was published in 1974, well before Menke's syringe method appeared. This report described the use of an electronic pressure sensor and strip chart recorder to follow the growth of gas producing bacteria such as *Enterobacter aerogenes* and *Escherichia coli* in closed test tube cultures (Wilkins, 1974). Taya *et al.* (1980) reported an application of this technique. They studied the use of a pressure sensor to control the fermentation of cellulose by *Ruminococcus albus* on an industrial scale. These workers showed that the total gas yield was proportional to the amount of cellulose digested (480 ml g^{-1} at 39°C).

When microcomputers became readily available in the early 1980s, the stage was set for the electrical signal from a pressure sensor to be combined with a computer-based data collector. Beaubien *et al.* (1988) described a method to measure gas flow from a bioreactor. A schematic diagram of the method is shown in Fig. 10.1.

A three-way solenoid valve is controlled by a separate flow meter circuit that responds to a voltage signal from the pressure sensor. The valve is set so that ports 1 and 2 are normally open and communicate with the transducer and ballast. Port 3 is normally closed. When the pressure in the reactor and ballast rises to a pre-determined set point, the controller activates the valve for about 2 s, closing port 2 and opening port 3 to vent the ballast and restore atmospheric pressure. The valve is then deactivated and the cycle repeated. The computer records the time of each open–close cycle and counts the number of cycles. Each cycle will correspond to a fixed gas volume that depends on the ballast size and the pressure sensor trip point. This incremental volume can be varied over a wide range, depending upon the experimental need.

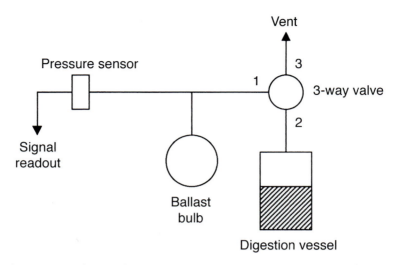

Fig. 10.1. Schematic view of a vented gas measurement system (redrawn from Beaubien *et al.*, 1988).

There are several important advances in this design:

1. Because the gas is measured in small increments, then released, we can use larger amounts of substrate in the reactor than would be possible in a closed system.
2. The system is very flexible. Its sensitivity can be adjusted by changing the response range and/or trip point of the pressure transducer, and by changing the ballast volume.
3. Data are logged on a computer. Once the experiment is started, no further human intervention is required until the experiment is finished.

A pressure sensor was used in a different way by Theodorou *et al.* (1994). The method used a three-way stopcock to connect a syringe (for gas volume measurement), a pressure sensor linked to a numerical display and a closed incubation bottle. The setup resembles that in Fig. 10.1 with the syringe connected to the ballast port. At pre-determined time intervals, the pressure was read and was reset to atmospheric by withdrawing gas into the syringe. This gas was then vented and the cycle repeated.

A new phase of equipment design began when less expensive pressure sensors and commercial computer software for data input became available in the 1990s. Pell and Schofield (1993) designed a closed system in which 16 sample bottles were each connected to a sensor and the data sent to a computer via a 16-channel analogue-to-digital (A/D) card. This system was novel because it measured the pressure increase in each bottle as a function of time and calculated the corresponding gas volumes from calibration curves. Bottle and sample sizes were chosen such that the maximum pressure increase was <0.6 atmospheres. Because the sample sizes were small (≤100 mg), these investigators introduced a micro-method for determining residual fibre. After digestion, neutral detergent solution (Goering and Van Soest, 1970) was added to each bottle, the bottles were sealed and autoclaved, and the residue was filtered, washed and dried on glass fibre filters (Pell and Schofield, 1993).

The most recent automated gas production apparatus was described by Cone *et al.* (1996). This apparatus is essentially a refinement of the design in Fig. 10.1. The article contains a detailed description of the apparatus, sources for parts and a useful discussion of experimental procedures. A similar system was developed independently in the UK (Theodorou *et al.*, 1998).

Summarizing the current state of affairs, there are three different approaches to measuring *in vitro* gas production for feedstuff evaluation. The early Menke syringe method is still used in many parts of the world, most notably at Hohenheim, Germany, its birthplace (Blümmel *et al.*, 1997a). Computer-linked electronic pressure sensors have been applied in two different ways. In the first of these, gas is allowed to accumulate in the digestion vessel and changes in gas pressure are recorded (Pell and Schofield, 1993). In the second, gas is vented at intervals determined by the pressure sensor and recorded by the computer. The volume/time profile is then calculated from the venting data.

Factors Affecting Gas Measurements

Before attempting to evaluate the respective merits and demerits of these different approaches, let us step back for a moment and consider some of the factors that must be taken into account in any protocol for gas measurement.

Sample size, physical state

As we have seen, the gas volume produced by complete digestion of 1 g of fibre is about 350 ml. Digestibility (rather than digestion rate) measurements will therefore require the use of either small samples or equipment able to handle large gas volumes. Many early studies using the syringe method were concerned with comparing *rates* of gas production from different substrates and, therefore, did not have to deal with large gas volumes. Gas volumes are proportional to sample size.

Because many animal feedstuffs are not homogeneous, they present sampling problems. These problems can be reduced by grinding the feedstuff. However, we must also remember that the digestion rates we measure *in vitro* may depend upon particle size. This dilemma is not peculiar to the gas technique but underlies any *in vitro* method involving an insoluble substrate. In practice, the usual approach

is to grind the feedstuff to pass a 1 mm sieve, to ferment multiple samples and to discount the particle size effect on the grounds that chewing and rumination in the animal will produce a result similar to grinding.

Ruminal fluid (RF)

There are two questions to be answered here, namely pre-treatment and amount. RF contains both the microorganisms (bacteria, fungi, protozoa) and soluble factors (VFAs, vitamins) needed for fibre digestion. The composition of this fluid will vary from day to day and from animal to animal, and these variations may affect *in vitro* digestion profiles. One way to reduce this variation is to filter the fluid through glass wool, pellet the microorganisms by centrifugation and resuspend them in a defined medium (Doane *et al.*, 1997b).

Ruminal fluid is usually diluted with a buffered salt solution before use. Previous *in vitro* studies (Hungate *et al.*, 1955; Tilley and Terry, 1963) showed that a buffered medium containing 20–25% RF gave the best results. A higher content of RF will produce higher blanks (samples incubated with RF but without substrate).

pH control

The standard buffer has been based on McDougal's analysis of sheep saliva (McDougal, 1949) and contains both bicarbonate and phosphate. Some variations on the exact buffer composition are seen among different laboratories. The primary buffering agent, bicarbonate, is consumed as VFAs are released during digestion and thus the pH declines. For quantitative gas measurements using this buffer, it is important that the pH be held within the range 6.8–6.2. At a lower pH, the cellulolytic bacteria become less active (Russell and Dombrowski, 1980) and the yield of CO_2 per mole of VFAs declines (Beuvink and Spoelstra, 1992).

Temperature control

Microbial activity, and gas volumes and pressures all change with temperature. Close temperature control, using either a water bath or an incubator maintained at 39°C, is therefore needed for *in vitro* digestion studies.

Atmospheric pressure changes

The amount of a gas in moles is defined by the volume, the temperature and the pressure (Equation 10.1), and all three of these quantities must be known or measured in a gas production experiment. We return later to the problem posed by changes in atmospheric pressure during the course of an experiment.

Stirring

Carbon dioxide has a strong tendency to form supersaturated solutions in aqueous media. If this occurs, then either pressure- or volume-based gas readings will be incorrect. Fortunately, this tendency is countered by the presence of particulate matter in an *in vitro* system and can be reduced further by occasional gentle stirring or shaking (Pell and Schofield, 1993).

Closed versus open systems

The amount of gas produced in a chemical reaction can be measured by holding the volume constant and observing the pressure change (closed system) or by maintaining a constant (usually atmospheric) pressure and measuring the volume change (open system). The vented system of Beaubien *et al.* (1988) can be considered a compromise between these two extremes. Factors affecting system choice are considered below.

Information desired

Possible applications of gas fermentation data include testing of plant varieties for plant breeding, feedstuff comparisons, digestion rates for modelling studies and feed component interactions including inhibitory effects of plant secondary compounds. The nature of the application will dictate the experimental design and may influence the choice of gas method.

Pros and Cons of Alternative Methods

For convenience, we divide the methods into three groups: the syringe method, and the open and closed automated methods.

Syringe method

- *Pro*. Simple and relatively inexpensive. No excess pressure accumulates and thus equal molar amounts of CO_2 and CH_4 give equal volume changes.
- *Con*. Insensitive (maximum precision ±0.5 ml) and subject to error from sticking plungers. Not convenient for detailed kinetic studies because of manual recording of data.

Closed automated method

- *Pro*. Simplest automated method to construct and maintain because it requires no valves. Good for measuring small gas volumes because the sensitivity of the system depends on the bottle size and the sensor range, both of which can be made small.
- *Con*. Not readily adapted to handle sample sizes >250 mg because of the need to keep the maximum pressure increase down to about 0.5 atmospheres. This arbitrary limit is imposed for two reasons. First, because gas leaks are less likely when the pressure is low. Second, because some data have suggested that more scatter in pressure readings occurs at higher pressures (Theodorou *et al.*, 1994). We have not observed a trend of this kind (Schofield and Pell, 1995a).

A correction may be required to deal with the different sensor response to a more water-soluble gas such as CO_2 and a less water-soluble gas such as CH_4 (Schofield and Pell, 1995b).

Open automated method

- *Pro.* Will accomodate larger samples. The sample size may be limited, however, by the buffering capacity of the medium. Measurements are made at an approximately constant pressure close to atmospheric and thus pressure effects on digestion are not an issue.
- *Con.* If the method is to be sensitive, the excess pressure needed to trigger valve opening must be small. The pressure sensors used by Cone *et al.* (1996) measure the pressure *difference* between the atmosphere and the digestion vessel and must record this difference over a 50 h period. Changes in atmospheric pressure may significantly change the volume of gas needed to trigger valve opening. Sudden changes will affect only a few readings, but a slow, steady change can affect many. One simple solution to this problem would be to use a 'differential' rather than a 'gauge' type of sensor and refer all pressure measurements to a closed standard (see Appendix for a description of these different types of sensors). This approach insulates the digestion bottle from any external pressure changes. It could also be used for the closed system.

Problems with mixtures of CO_2 and CH_4 are no different in the open system than in the closed automated method (see above). A small excess pressure must accumulate before venting. The volume of gas needed to generate this pressure increase will be greater for CO_2 than for CH_4 because of the difference in water solubility of these gases. The calibration factor (volume of gas needed to trigger valve opening) will thus change if the composition of the headspace gas changes. The error for a single reading is small but must be evaluated as a fraction of a total reading that also is small.

Appropriate Use of Blanks

The usual procedure in all gas systems is to subtract, at each time point, the gas produced in a 'blank' container from that produced in the sample bottle or syringe. The blank contains buffered RF in the same proportions as the sample. Some gas does appear in the blank because the RF inoculum (unless centrifuged, washed and re-suspended) inevitably contains feed particles. The size of this blank contribution to the total gas volume depends on the proportion of RF used. Some groups use a 1:2 ratio of RF to buffer (Menke and Steingass, 1988; Cone *et al.*, 1996), some a 1:4 ratio (Pell and Schofield, 1993) and others a 1:9 ratio (Theodorou *et al.*, 1994). For the 1:2 ratio, the blank contributed about 30% of the total reading after 10 h incubation of grass samples (Cone *et al.*, 1997). These authors have demonstrated that microbial turnover in the blank begins after about 1 h and that about 30% of the maximum blank reading can be attributed to this turnover. In the presence of substrate, turnover is delayed so that the blank does not reflect accurately what happens in the sample. For this reason, Cone *et al.* (1997) suggest omitting the blank correction altogether.

An alternative, less draconian, approach is to use a more diluted inoculum that will reduce the contribution of the blank. A second reason to retain the blank correction appears in the 'closed' system where pressure accumulates. The blank plays a dual role in this system. Besides correcting for fermentation products from the inoculum, the blank also corrects for atmospheric pressure changes occurring during the run (Pell and Schofield, 1993).

Equipment Needed for Computerized Gas Measurement

Digestion vessels

Figure 10.2 shows an example of serum bottles as digestion vessels and an incubator used for *in vitro* gas measurements. Any

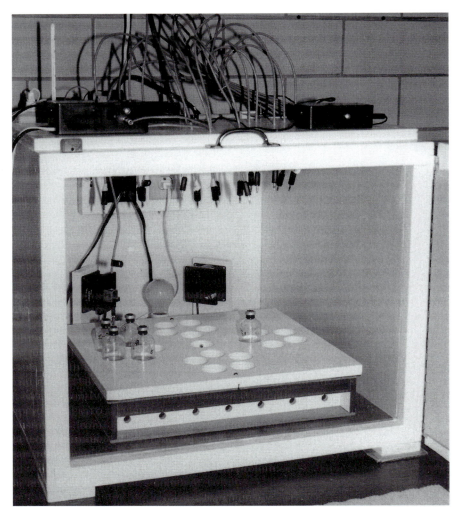

Fig. 10.2. Interior view of the Pell–Schofield box system containing a 20-place stirrer. The temperature is regulated to ±0.5°C by switching the light bulb on and off. Two fans disperse the heat from this source. The box is lined with 2.5 cm styrofoam. The temperature controller is on the top left and the sensor power source (+10 V DC) on the top right. Only one sensor is shown connected. Overall dimensions are 65 cm wide, 58 cm high, 72 cm deep. Directions for construction of the temperature controller and wood-walled incubator have been published (Schofield, 1996).

vessel with a gas-tight closure can be used for the digestion.

Computers, A/D cards, software

We must distinguish between the data acquisition and data analysis roles of the computer. For data acquisition, an unsophisticated computer will suffice as data logger. It should be able to support one or more A/D cards, run the data collection software and present a real-time graphic display of the voltage curves as they are recorded. An IBM-compatible machine, with a 386 or better CPU, running Windows 3.1 is adequate. There are many choices for the A/D card. The user should ensure that the data collection software is compatible with the card selected.

Data analysis requires, at minimum, a spreadsheet program with macro and good graphics capability. We currently are using Microsoft Excel 97© (Microsoft, Redmond, Washington). For numerical analysis of gas curves, a non-linear curve-fitting program such as SAS (SAS Inst., Inc., Cary, North Carolina) or TableCurve© from Jandel/SPSS (Chicago, Illinois) will be required (see Appendix). These programs will run much faster on a machine with a faster processor.

Hardware costs

Pressure sensors are relatively expensive (~US$40–100 each) and have a limited lifetime. They are usually designed for measurement of dry gases; the water-saturated atmosphere of an *in vitro* fermentation, coupled with traces of hydrogen sulphide, restricts their lifetime to between 6 months and 2 years. Multiple place systems such as those of Cone *et al.* (1996) (12 place) or Pell and Schofield (1993) (16 place) thus represent a significant investment in sensors. A/D cards are also relatively expensive (US$400–800 each, 16 channel) because the market for this hardware is more restricted than that for computers.

Availability

Both of the open systems discussed above are now available commercially. (Enquiries should be addressed to: Dr M.K. Theodorou, IGER, Plas Gogerddan, Aberystwyth, Ceredigion, SY23 3EB, UK or to Dr John W. Cone, ID-DLO, Department of Ruminant Nutrition, PO Box 65, NL-8200 AB Lelystad, The Netherlands.) Detailed directions for construction of the closed system have been published (Pell and Schofield, 1993; Schofield, 1996).

Models for Curve Fitting

In Fig. 10.3 are shown typical gas curves from the *in vitro* digestion of four different types of feed. These data illustrate the range of shapes commonly seen for such curves. At a qualitative level, one might conclude that:

(i) On a dry matter basis, soy hulls are the most, lucerne the least digestible of these feeds;

(ii) rates of digestion vary widely, both with feed and with time; and

(iii) maize silage and wheat straw produce more sigmoidal curves than soy hulls and lucerne.

For quantitative analysis, there would be a clear advantage if a mathematical model were available to analyse the detailed information hidden within these gas curves. There is no general agreement on a single model among workers in this field, and we briefly review proposed models and identify underlying assumptions.

Models, an initial distinction

Most animal feeds contain a complex mixture of carbohydrates that are digested at different rates. For kinetic analysis, we can treat the substrate either as a single pool, digesting at a fractional rate that varies with time, or as multiple pools, each of which has a characteristic fractional digestion rate. The latter multiple pool approach is appealing because chemical assays have been devised to measure separate carbohydrate pools (such as NDF, ADF, NSC) and these pools are digested at different rates *in vitro*. Multiple pools are also conceptually simpler to understand. We consider them first.

Simple exponential model

The *in vitro* fibre digestion method of Tilley and Terry (1963), as modified by Goering and Van Soest (1970), has been widely used to measure insoluble fibre digestion rates. The data from such experiments are usually fitted using a discontinuous exponential function (discontinuous because of the lag term) of the form:

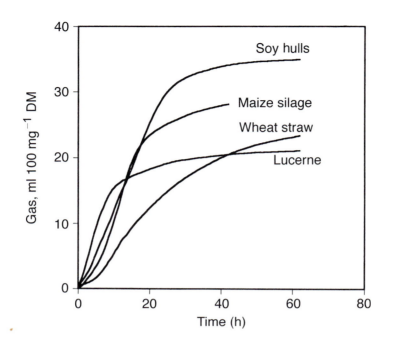

Fig. 10.3. Typical gas curves recorded using the closed system depicted in Fig. 10.2. Note the different curve shapes. Substrates (100 mg DM each) were lucerne, wheat straw, soy hulls and maize silage.

$$S_t = S_i + S_0 \quad (t < L)$$
$$S_t = S_i + S_0 \times \exp(-k \times (t - L))$$
$$(t > L) \qquad (10.3)$$

where S_t is the total residual fibre at time t, S_i is the indigestible fibre, S_0 is the initial digestible fibre, k is a rate constant (units time^{-1}) and L is a discrete lag term, a time during which no digestion occurs (Mertens and Loften, 1980).

If we use this kind of expression to model gas production, the equation must be modified because we are now measuring the appearance of a product rather than the disappearance of a substrate. The modified exponential equation becomes:

$$V_t = 0 \qquad (t < L)$$
$$V_t = V_f \times (1 - \exp(-k \times (t - L)))$$
$$(t > L) \qquad (10.4)$$

where V_t = volume of gas at time t, V_f = final asymptotic gas volume corresponding to complete substrate digestion, and k, t

and L have the same meanings as in Equation 10.3. Equation 10.4 produces curves of the shape shown in Fig. 10.4.

This simple exponential equation can be derived on the assumption that the rate of gas production, at times beyond the lag time, depends solely on the amount of digestible substrate available. The microbial population size is assumed not to limit the rate at any stage. The discrete lag term is something of an embarrassment but is necessary to get a good data fit in many cases. Some justification can be offered on the grounds that the cellulolytic bacteria must first attach to the fibre, and perhaps also express some cellulase genes, before digestion can begin. In principle, Equation 10.4 can be expanded to cover multiple pools:

$$V_t = \Sigma \, V_{Fn} \times (1 - \exp(-k_n \times (t - L_n)))$$

where the subscript n would be the pool number. However, summed exponential

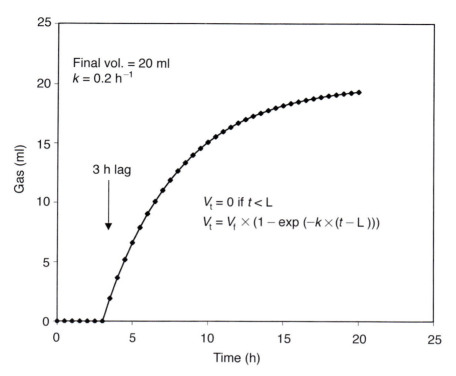

Fig. 10.4. Exponential curve with discrete lag.

curves of this kind do not differ enough in shape from a single curve to be able to reproduce the kinds of shapes shown in Fig. 10.4. They are not able to produce a sigmoidal shape.

Logistic curves

The exponential model assumes a single rate-limiting factor, the amount of digestible fibre. The logistic growth function, as applied in microbiology (Zwietering *et al.*, 1990), assumes that gas production is proportional to both the microbial population size and the digestible substrate (Schofield *et al.*, 1994). At the beginning of fermentation, the microbial population is the limiting factor, at the end the substrate plays this role. In consequence, the logistic curve is inherently sigmoidal and the maximum rate occurs when half the substrate has been digested. The single pool equation takes the form:

$$V_t = V_f \times (1 + \exp(2 - 4 \times S \times (t - L)))^{-1} \quad (10.5)$$

The symbols have the same meaning as in Equation 10.4 and S is a specific rate, similar to the fractional rate constant k. Equation 10.5 produces curves of the form shown in Fig. 10.5.

A multiple pool version of this equation would be:

$$V_t = \sum V_{fn} \times (1 + \exp(2 - 4 \times S_n \times (t - L_n)))^{-1} \quad (10.6)$$

This equation turns out to be very versatile for fitting gas curves and, in most cases, two pools suffice to describe a feed gas profile (Schofield *et al.*, 1994). One important difference between Equations 10.4 and 10.6 lies in the lag term L. Equation 10.4 is a discontinuous function and L determines the point of discontinuity. In contrast, Equation 10.6 is valid over all positive values of t.

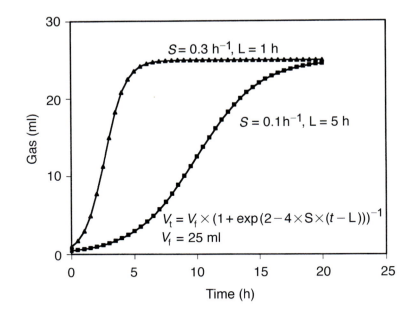

Fig. 10.5. Examples of single-pool logistic curves.

An empirical multi-pool model

To fit gas curves, Groot *et al.* (1996) proposed an equation of the form:

$$V = \sum V_{fi} \times (1 + (B_i/t)^{Ci})^{-1} \qquad (10.7)$$

in which V_f is the asymptotic gas volume and B and C are positive constants. The subscript i identifies the phase or pool. It can be shown that B (units, h) is the time at which one-half of the asymptotic gas volume has appeared. C is a dimensionless switching constant that, together with B, determines the shape of the gas profile. When $C \leq 1$, the curve has no point of inflection and resembles an exponential function; when $C \geq 1$, the curve is sigmoidal. Examples of these curve shapes are given in Fig. 10.6. Two or, at most, three pools will usually suffice to describe a gas curve.

Equation 10.7 is also very versatile and is best able to reproduce almost any gas curve encountered in practice. Unfortunately, the shape parameter C is difficult to interpret in biological terms.

An empirical single-pool model

The first equation published as an alternative to the simple exponential equation (Equation 10.4) treated the degradable substrate as a single pool undergoing degradation at a fractional rate that was time dependent (France *et al.*, 1993). The concept of a discrete lag (T, h) was retained and the fractional rate of degradation, μ (h^{-1}) was postulated to vary with time t as follows:

$$\mu = 0 \qquad\qquad\qquad t < T$$
$$\mu = b + c \times (2 \times \sqrt{t})^{-1} \qquad t \geq T$$

No reason was provided for this hypothetical relationship. If V_f is the asymptotic gas volume, the equation describing accumulated gas volume (V) with time (t) becomes:

$$V = V_f \times \{1 - \exp[-b \\ \times (t - T) - c \times (\sqrt{t} - \sqrt{T})]\} \qquad (10.8)$$

Equation 10.8 is quite limited in its application and gives fits that are less satisfactory than the multiple pool models described above. For example, if the data sets graphed

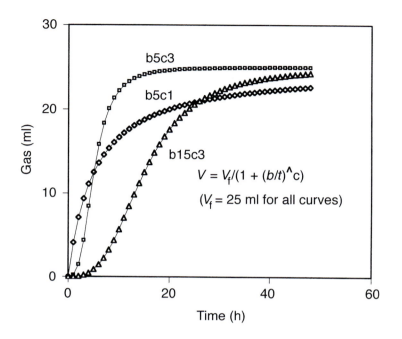

Fig. 10.6. Curves produced by the empirical equation of Groot *et al.* (1996). Different values of the parameters b and c produce quite different shapes (b5c3 means b = 5 h and c = 3).

in Fig. 10.3 are fitted using Equation 10.8, only one (wheat straw) gives a high *F* value combined with well-defined parameters (see Appendix: Non-linear curve fitting).

Do Multiple Pools Really Exist?

In forage analysis, we are used to the concept of multiple carbohydrate fractions. The classic detergent system of Goering and Van Soest (1970) divides carbohydrates into fractions soluble and insoluble in neutral and acid detergent (NDS, NDF and ADF, respectively). These fractions can be characterized further in terms of their content of soluble sugars, starch, pectin, hemicellulose and cellulose. *In vitro* studies on individual components have shown that the rates of fermentation of these fractions differ widely. Soluble sugars and pectin ferment more quickly than most forms of starch and much more quickly than cellulose and hemicellulose (Sniffen *et al.*, 1992).

The multi-pool kinetic analysis of gas curves also predicts up to three pools with varying sizes, digestion rates and (sometimes) lag terms. The relationship, if any, between these mathematically derived pools and the chemical fractions in a given forage is potentially of interest.

Models with different mathematical structures can yield quite disparate results from the same gas curve. This point is illustrated in Fig. 10.7 where the data for wheat straw and soy hulls (Fig. 10.3) have been fitted using either the multi-pool model of Groot *et al.* (1996) (Equation 10.7) or the logistic model of Schofield *et al.* (1994) (Equation 10.6). The Groot model requires two pools for soy hulls, one for wheat straw; the logistic model requires exactly the reverse. For purely descriptive applications, the choice of model will be dictated by the closeness of fit. In a more detailed analysis, the validity of pool assignments may become important.

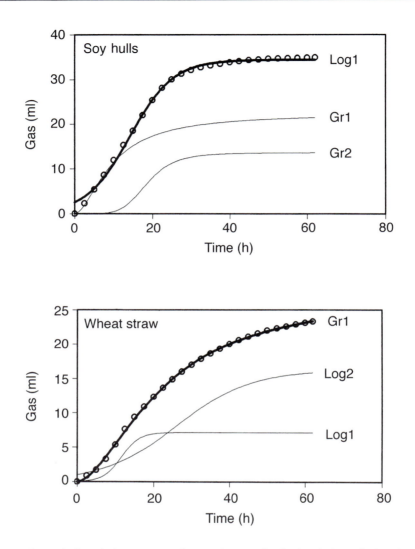

Fig. 10.7. Data for soy hulls and wheat straw (circles, see Fig. 10.4) fitted using single- or dual-pool equations. Log = logistic (Equation 10.5), Gr = Equation 10.7 (Groot *et al.*, 1996). When a two-pool model was required, the curves for the individual pools were plotted separately (the sum of these curves fits the data points almost exactly). Numbers 1 and 2 for the individual pools (lighter lines) identify the faster and slower digesting components respectively. The solid line tracking the data points represents the single-pool fit. For clarity, only 20% of the experimental data points are shown.

One way to test the validity of these assignments is to examine mixtures of simple homogeneous substrates as reported by Schofield *et al.* (1994). These investigators used mixtures of processed cellulose and bacterial cellulose. The gas curves from *in vitro* digestion of each individual cellulose could be fitted using a single pool logistic equation and the specific rate for the bacterial cellulose was higher than that for the processed cellulose. Gas curves from mixtures of known composition were analysed using a dual-pool logistic equation, and the pool sizes (faster, slower) correlated well with sample composition.

A second, less abstract, demonstration of the internal consistency of the logistic model was reported by Stefanon *et al.*

(1996). They isolated the water-soluble and water-insoluble fractions of lucerne (*Medicago sativa*) and bromegrass (*Bromus inermis*) and recorded gas curves during *in vitro* digestion of the whole forage and of the two fractions. All curves were fitted using a two-pool logistic model (Equation 10.6) and gas volumes corresponding to the faster- and slower-digesting components were derived from these data. The authors demonstrated a close correspondence between the total faster pool volume (from the whole forage) and the sum of the faster pool sizes in the water-soluble and water-insoluble fractions. They also compared the total gas curve from the whole forage with that created by adding the individual curves from the two component fractions. Discrepancies of up to ±10% were found, but the overall agreement was quite good. These results suggest that pool allocations under the logistic model are not unreasonable.

Cone *et al.* (1997) did a similar experiment but analysed the results differently. They used a three-pool model to fit digestion curves from grasses, clover, maize silage, corn cob mix and chopped ear corn silage. They hypothesized that pools 1 and 2 corresponded to the water-soluble and water-insoluble fractions of these feeds (pool 3 was equated to microbial turnover – see Appropriate Use of Blanks, p. 215). They compared the separately measured digestion curves of these isolated fractions with the curves corresponding to pools 1 and 2 in the intact feed and found some similarities among these sets of curves but noted that the match was not exact. More work is needed to explore the consistency of pool allocations using this model. We conclude that caution is appropriate in using multi-pool analysis of gas data. While it is clear that plants contain carbohydrate fractions that are digested at different rates, the 'pools' depicted in Fig. 10.7 should be viewed as purely mathematical constructs that may or may not correspond to chemical entities. The actual existence of such fractions should be documented by independent evidence.

Plant Carbohydrate Fractions and Nutritional Models

In vitro digestion rates from gas curves can be used in nutritional models. The Cornell Net Carbohydrate and Protein System (CNCPS) predicts nutrient supply based on the competition between ruminal digestion and passage. The carbohydrate composition of each feed ingredient is described by the following four fractions: (A) sugars and organic acids; (B1) starch and pectic substances; (B2) digestible fibre; and (C) indigestible residue (Sniffen *et al.*, 1992) (Fig. 10.8). Organic acids are treated, for convenience, as carbohydrates in this system.

The CNCPS model thus requires rate and pool size information on these four fractions. The B2 (digestible fibre) fraction is relatively easy to deal with because this fraction can be isolated chemically and its digestion behaviour measured *in vitro* (Schofield and Pell, 1995). If the digestion curve from NDF (or B2) is subtracted from the digestion curve for an equivalent amount of the intact forage, one obtains a curve corresponding to the digestion of the neutral detergent-soluble (NDS) fraction of the forage (Schofield and Pell, 1995a). This fraction contains both the A and B1 CNCPS fractions (Fig. 10.8).

The A fraction (sugars, organic acids) can be removed from a forage by treatment with 80% aqueous ethanol (Smith, 1981). The ethanol-insoluble residue (EIR) can also be fermented *in vitro*. Thus, if we ferment separately the whole forage (WF) and the EIR and NDF fractions (Fig. 10.8), curve subtraction will allow us to derive separate digestion curves for:

- A fraction = WF − EIR
- B1 fraction = EIR − NDF
- B2 fraction = NDF.

There are three main assumptions underlying this approach:

1. That the chemical treatments used to prepare the EIR and NDF fractions do not change the digestion behaviour of these fractions.

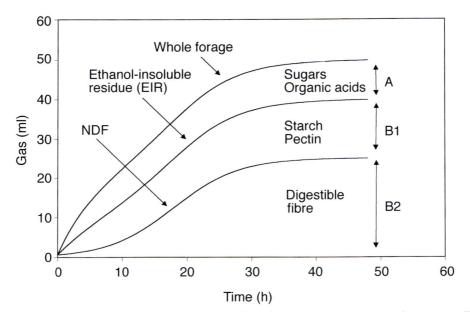

Fig. 10.8. A diagrammatic view of curve subtraction. Three digestion curves are measured experimentally for a given forage (whole forage, EIR and NDF). Hypothetical curves for the A and B1 fractions are then obtained by subtraction.

2. That associative effects (e.g. the effects of soluble sugars on fibre digestion) can be ignored.

3. That extraction with either aqueous ethanol or NDF does not remove substances inhibitory to *in vitro* digestion.

Extraction with aqueous ethanol at room temperature is, both chemically and physically, a mild process and would not seem likely to affect the digestibility of the EIR fraction provided that the whole forage does not contain ethanol-soluble inhibitory compounds (see below). The NDF fraction is prepared by extraction of the whole forage with neutral detergent in an autoclave at 105°C. Small increases of the order of 5% in fibre digestibility may result from this treatment with temperate forages (Schofield and Pell, 1995a; Doane *et al.*, 1997b). Comparative studies on NDF digestion in the whole forage versus in the isolated NDF suggest that both rates and extents of digestion are similar (Doane *et al.*, 1997b). Associative effects in this *in vitro* system appear to be small. Good agreement was seen between the digestion

curves for whole lucerne and bromegrass and for the sum of the separately digested water-soluble and water-insoluble fractions (Stefanon *et al.*, 1996; Cone *et al.*, 1997). Errors in curve subtraction resulting from associative effects will cause an *under-estimation* of the A fraction and an *over-estimation* of the B2 fraction. Assumption 3 above is certainly invalid for many tropical legumes that may contain tannins and saponins (see Plant Secondary Compounds, p. 227).

The pools studied in the curve subtraction approach described above differ from those derived by multi-pool analysis of a whole forage gas profile. Within the limitations of curve subtraction, these pools represent actual chemical entities and each pool may be a complex mixture and require a multi-pool kinetic analysis. The object of curve subtraction is to obtain a digestion curve for a given, chemically defined, forage fraction that cannot itself be isolated and fermented readily. This digestion curve may then be analysed using any of the mathematical models already discussed. In contrast, the mathematical pools obtained from the whole-forage profile may or may not correspond to a given chemical fraction.

Gas Yield and Microbial Yield

Feeds in the rumen are converted to short-chain fatty acids (SCFAs), to CO_2, to CH_4 and to microbial mass plus water. In our earlier discussion of gas yields, we chose to ignore the microbial mass. We now return to consider two different quantitative measures in forage digestion. The gas yield is the volume of gas produced by digestion of 1 g of substrate. The microbial yield is the microbial mass produced from this same digestion.

The gas system measures waste products (mostly CO_2 and CH_4). We make no distinction here between CO_2 and CH_4 since the latter arises directly from the former. Carbon dioxide comes from two sources, direct and indirect. The direct source is the fermentation of glucose by various pathways yielding VFAs, ATP and CO_2. The indirect source is the reaction of VFAs with bicarbonate. Both sources provide a benefit to the animal. The ATP is used for microbial growth in the rumen, the VFA as a substrate for metabolism in other organs. The gas measured in an *in vitro* experiment is thus an indirect measure of nutritionally important events.

The scheme in Fig. 10.9 shows the relationship between carbohydrate digested (CHO_dig) and its products. We now consider separately the production of gas and of microbial mass.

Gas yield

We have already noted that the yield of gas per g of substrate digested is generally less than that expected for complete conversion to direct and indirect gas. A wide range of yields may be encountered in practice, ranging from 200 to 480 ml g^{-1} (Table 10.1).

Part of the reason for this variation is that some of the substrate is used to produce microbial mass. Another reason is that the actual yield of gas per g of substrate digested may vary with the chemical nature of the substrate and with the microbial population. Different populations of rumen microorganisms may use several different metabolic pathways for digestion (Van Soest, 1994). Variations in these pathways will result in variations in the composition of the VFA mixture produced and will cause a corresponding variation in gas from both direct and indirect sources (Beuvink and Spoelstra, 1992). Readily digested soluble carbohydrates will tend to produce more propionate and less direct gas (Sarwar *et al.*, 1992).

A third reason why indirect gas yields are less than unity is because the *in vitro* buffer contains phosphate as well as bicarbonate (Beuvink and Spoelstra, 1992).

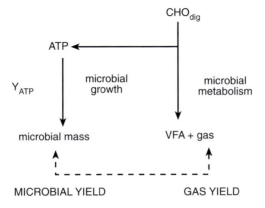

Fig. 10.9. Relationship between carbohydrate digested (CHO_dig) and its products.

Table 10.1. Gas yield from different carbohydrates.

Substrate	Gas yield (ml g^{-1})	Reference
Non-starch polysaccharide	200	Longland *et al.* (1995)
Various mixed	215–365, mean = 288	Blümmel *et al.* (1997)
Aqueous soluble fraction from grass, legume hay	240–280	Stefanon *et al.* (1996)
Cellulose, processed	320	Schofield *et al.* (1994)
Glucose	369	Cone *et al.* (1997)
NDF	360	Stefanon *et al.* (1996)
NDF	390	Pell and Schofield (1993)
Cellulose	384	Cone *et al.* (1997)
Pectin	437	Cone *et al.* (1997)
Cellulose, bacterial	440	Schofield *et al.* (1994)
Cellulose + *R. albus*	480	Taya *et al.* (1980)

The phosphate anion reacts with some of the protons that otherwise would generate CO_2. Feeds with a high protein content may also produce some ammonia on fermentation that reacts with VFAs and reduces the indirect gas yield. If samples with widely different protein content are to be compared, it may be necessary to measure and correct for ammonia production (Cone, 1998) and for direct gas from protein.

Microbial yield

The pathways used by the microorganisms for CHO degradation will determine the amount of ATP available for microbial cell production. The microbial yield, Y_{ATP}, is the mass of microorganisms produced from 1 mol of ATP, and can vary from about 10 to 20 g under rumen conditions. This yield varies with the microbial species and tends to be higher when bacteria are growing quickly, slower when growing slowly (Hespell and Bryant, 1979).

It is clear that the relationship between microbial mass and gas volume is complex. It may vary with the type of substrate, with the nature of the inoculum, with the growth conditions and with the time of observation (Blümmel *et al.*, 1997a). This relationship was first explored in the gas system by Krishnamoorthy *et al.* (1991). Using a syringe technique and defined substrates (starch, cellulose and a glucose–starch–cellulose mixture), these authors

recorded gas volumes before and 2 h after pulse-labelling the culture with ^{32}P. The total microbial protein synthesis during this 2 h period was calculated from the specific activity of the extracellular phosphate pool and from the N:P ratio in the bacterial pellet. They found a curvilinear relationship between the rate of microbial protein synthesis and the rate of gas production. High rates of gas production corresponded to high rates of protein synthesis, but the curvature of this relationship varied with the type of substrate; cellulose produced a steep upward curve, starch a less steep curve. With the mixed carbohydrate substrate, they also found a linear relationship between microbial protein synthesis and cumulative gas production over an 8 h time span. The important conclusion from this work was that one should not rely solely on cumulative gas production as an index of the microbial growth potential of feeds.

Blümmel *et al.* (1997a) used different methods to measure microbial yield in the digestion of roughage. Incubations were carried out in syringes for 24 h. The insoluble residue was then collected by centrifugation, washed, lyophilized and weighed. A known mass of this material was then refluxed with neutral detergent solution and the residue again washed and weighed. The microbial mass was calculated as the loss of mass caused by the detergent treatment (Blümmel *et al.*, 1997a). These data were then used to relate microbial mass to gas volumes and gave values from 1.07 to 2.65 mg ml^{-1}. The same authors also used ^{15}N incorporation as a measure of biomass yield and found that substrates with proportionally higher gas production showed lower ^{15}N incorporation. Experimental data thus support the idea that the biomass yield may depend on the type of substrate used *in vitro*.

We must now confront the question of how to deal with this yield variation in interpreting gas data. The logistic model (Schofield *et al.*, 1994) incorporates the relationship α between substrate digested and gas volume into the specific rate constant *S*. *S* and α are inversely proportional to one another. The model assumes that different forage fractions can be treated as separate pools, each having a different, but constant, specific rate of digestion. A large value of *S* may thus mean either a fast digestion rate or a low value for α, or some combination of the two. Independent measurements of α are required to distinguish among these possibilities (Blümmel *et al.*, 1997a). Other models assume a constant gas yield (France *et al.*, 1993) or incorporate the gas yield into a biologically undefined parameter (Groot *et al.*, 1996).

To make good nutrition decisions based on gas data, we thus need to be aware that gas yield and microbial yield are substrate-dependent variables. If the *gas volume* from digestion of a given feed is low, we should measure the *gas yield* (based on organic matter disappearance) and the *microbial yield* (based on microbial mass produced) before concluding that the feed value necessarily is low.

Plant Secondary Compounds

Tropical forage plants may contain secondary compounds such as the polyphenolic tannins, the terpene- or steroid-based saponins and the nitrogenous alkaloids. Tannins are the major components of this group of compounds (Morris and Robbins, 1997). Chemical assays for polyphenols (Hagerman and Butler, 1989) have not shown a close correlation with biological activity as

measured by inhibition of microbial growth or by effects on *in vitro* digestion (Nelson *et al.*, 1997). *In vitro* digestion assays offer an important additional tool to assess the feed value of tropical forages.

The usual way to investigate tannin effects has been to digest tannin-containing forages *in vitro* in the presence and absence of binding agents such as polyvinylpolypyrrolidone (PVP) or polyethylene glycol (PEG). These agents are believed to bind the tannins preferentially and make them unavailable to react with competing targets such as microbial cells and extracellular enzymes. The inhibitory effect of the tannins is thus measured as the difference in gas produced with and without the agent. PEG has replaced PVP as the more effective tannin-binding agent (Khazaal *et al.*, 1996). Makkar *et al.* (1995) used a syringe method and added an approximately equal weight of PEG (average mol wt 6000 kDa) to the tannin-rich feed. They found an increase in gas production after 24 h incubation that correlated well ($r = 0.95$) with the protein-precipitating capacity of the plant tannin. Temperate browse species such as heather (*Calluna vulgaris*) may show a substantial (51%) increase in gas production in response to PEG treatment (Tolera *et al.*, 1997).

Other Applications

Plant soluble components

The main advantage of the gas system, other than the ready automation of readings, is that it can be applied to study the digestion of soluble materials. These studies can be conducted using curve subtraction (e.g. for the NDS fraction, see Plant Carbohydrate Fractions and Nutritional Models, p. 223) or by isolating and digesting the fraction of interest (e.g. for the water- or ethanol-soluble fraction). The results have tended to challenge the current assumption that all soluble material, if digestible, is digested rapidly (Stefanon *et al.*, 1996).

Forage ensiling converts plant soluble sugars into acids and would thus be expected to change the digestion profile and the feed value of silage compared with forage. Doane *et al.* (1997a) used a curve subtraction approach to compare the gas yield from the NDS (neutral detergent-soluble) fraction of freeze-dried, oven-dried and ensiled forages and reported decreases in gas yield of 7–36% in this fraction on ensiling.

Correlation with in sacco *method*

In sacco methods are discussed in Chapter 11. Degradation rates of a grass (*Lolium perenne*), measured using nylon bags *in situ* and also measured using an open gas system, were reasonably well correlated ($r^2 = 0.74$) (Cone *et al.*, 1998). For this comparison, the gas curve corresponding to the fibre fraction (extracted using a three-pool Groot equation (Cone *et al.*, 1997)) was fitted to an exponential model so that these data could be compared with the *in sacco* results. Some of the lack of perfect agreement may lie in the assumption that the digestion curve extracted from the three-pool equation is equivalent to that measured directly *in sacco*.

Intake predictions

Dry matter intake depends upon so many different factors (see Part III of this volume, Intake and Utilization), many of them strongly dependent on the individual animal, that it is difficult to correlate intake and any single measured feed property (Van Soest, 1994). Blümmel and Bullerdieck (1997) have attempted to make this correlation using intake data from legume and grass hays (all high NDF) and *in vitro* gas production data on the same forages. They found no significant correlation between intake and the gas parameters *a*, *b* and *c* from the exponential equation $y (\text{gas}) = a + b \times (1 - e^{-ct})$ (compare Equation 10.4). However, if a partitioning factor (the reciprocal of the gas yield discussed above, measured at 24 h) was included, the r^2 increased to 0.74. The

inclusion of low NDF feeds would provide a more critical test of this correlation.

Summary

The gas system is an alternative analytical technique to study feed digestion *in vitro*. Instead of measuring the dissolution of insoluble plant components, as in the Tilley–Terry and *in sacco* methods, we measure the appearance of gaseous products. This change of focus yields two principal advantages. The first is that, with electronic pressure sensors, measurements can be recorded by computer. The second advantage is that digestion of soluble feed components can be studied in a way that permits a direct comparison with insoluble components.

There is general agreement that the limited data from *in sacco* methods are best interpreted using a simple exponential equation. No such agreement presently exists for the richly detailed data from the gas system.

Questions have been raised about the relevance of gas data to microbial cell production. The answer seems to be that gas data need to be supplemented with measurements of substrate disappearance, VFA profiles and microbial yield before they can supply the maximum nutritional information.

In this brief review, we have discussed only a few of the possible applications of gas data. These have included the study of the feed soluble components, the measurement of digestion rates for model testing and the investigation of 'anti-nutritional' plant secondary compounds such as tannins. One important nutritional topic that has received little attention by investigators using the gas technique is that of 'associative effects', the interaction between feed fractions during digestion. The gas technique is well suited to this type of investigation.

Acknowledgements

The author wishes to thank Dr Michael Blümmel, University of Hohenheim, Stuttgart, Germany, Dr John Cone, ID-DLO,

Lelystad, The Netherlands, and Dr Michael Theodorou, IGER, Aberystwyth, UK for providing material prior to publication. Much of the work discussed originated in the laboratories of Dr Alice N. Pell at Cornell University.

References

Baldwin, R.L. (1970) Energy metabolism in anaerobes. *American Journal of Clinical Nutrition* 23, 1508–1513.

Beaubien, A., Jolicoeur, C. and Alary, J.F. (1988) Automated high sensitivity gas metering system for biological processes. *Biotechnology and Bioengineering* 32, 105–109.

Beuvink, J.M.W. and Spoelstra, S.F. (1992) Interactions between substrate, fermentation end-products, buffering systems and gas production upon fermentation of different carbohydrates by mixed rumen microorganisms *in vitro. Applied Microbiology and Biotechnology* 37, 505–509.

Blümmel, M. and Bullerdieck, P. (1997) The need to complement *in vitro* gas production measurements with residue determinations from *in sacco* degradabilities to improve the prediction of voluntary intake of hays. *Animal Science (Pencaitland)* 64, 71–75.

Blümmel, M., Makkar, H.P.S. and Becker, K. (1997a) *In vitro* gas production: a technique revisited. *Journal of Animal Physiology and Animal Nutrition* 77, 24–34.

Blümmel, M., Steingass, H. and Becker, K. (1997b) The relationship between *in vitro* gas production, *in vitro* microbial biomass yield and ^{15}N incorporation and its implications for the prediction of voluntary feed intake of roughages. *British Journal of Nutrition* 77, 911–921.

Cone, J.W. (1998) The development, use and application of the gas production technique at ID-DLO. In: In vitro *Techniques for Measuring Nutrient Supply to Ruminants.* Occasional Paper. British Society of Animal Science, Penicuik, UK.

Cone, J.W., van Gelder, A.H., Visscher, G.J.W. and Oudshoorn, L. (1996) Influence of rumen fluid and substrate concentration on fermentation kinetics measured with a fully automated time related gas production apparatus. *Animal Feed Science and Technology* 61, 113–128.

Cone, J.W., van Gelder, A.H. and Driehuis, F. (1997) Description of gas production profiles with a three-phasic model. *Animal Feed Science and Technology* 66, 31–45.

Cone, J.W., van Gelder, A.H. and Valk, H. (1998) Prediction of nylon bag degradation characteristics of grass samples with the gas production technique. *Journal of the Science of Food and Agriculture* 77, 421–426.

Doane, P.H., Pell, A.N. and Schofield, P. (1997a) The effect of preservation method on the neutral detergent soluble fraction of forages. *Journal of Animal Science* 75, 1140–1148.

Doane, P.H., Schofield, P. and Pell, A.N. (1997b) NDF disappearance, gas and VFA production during the *in vitro* fermentation of six forages. *Journal of Animal Science* 74, 3342–3352.

France, J., Dhanoa, M.S., Theodorou, M.K., Lister, S.J., Davies, D.R. and Isac, D. (1993) A model to interpret gas accumulation profiles associated with *in vitro* degradation of ruminant feeds. *Journal of Theoretical Biology* 163, 99–111.

Goering, H.K. and Van Soest, P.J. (1970) Forage fibre analysis (apparatus, reagents, procedures, and some applications). *Agricultural Handbook No. 379.* ARS-USDA, Washington, DC.

Groot, J.C.J., Cone, J.W., Williams, B.A., Debersaques, F.M.A. and Lantinga, E.A. (1996) Multiphasic analysis of gas production kinetics for *in vitro* fermentation of ruminant feeds. *Animal Feed Science and Technology* 64, 77–89.

Hagerman, A.E. and Butler, L.G. (1989) Choosing appropriate methods and standards for assaying tannin. *Journal of Chemical Ecology* 15, 1795–1810.

Hespell, R.B. and Bryant, M.P. (1979) Efficiency of rumen microbial growth: influence of some theoretical and experimental factors on Y_{ATP}. *Journal of Animal Science* 49, 1640–1659.

Hungate, R.E., Fletcher, D.W., Dougherty, R.W. and Barrentine, B.F. (1955) Microbial activity in the bovine rumen: its measurement and relation to bloat. *Applied Microbiology* 3, 161–173.

Khazaal, K., Parissi, Z., Tsiouvaras, C., Nastis, A. and Ørskov, E.R. (1996) Assessment of phenolics-related antinutritive levels using the *in vitro* gas production technique: a comparison between different types of polyvinylpolypyrrolidone or polyethylene glycol. *Journal of the Science of Food and Agriculture* 71, 405–414.

Krishnamoorthy, U., Steingass, H. and Menke, K.H. (1991) Preliminary observations on the relationship between gas production and microbial synthesis *in vitro. Archives of Animal Nutrition, Berlin* 41, 521–526.

Longland, A.C., Theodorou, M.K., Sanderson, R., Lister, S.J., Powell, C.J. and Morris, P. (1995) Non-starch polysaccharide composition and *in vitro* fermentability of tropical forage legumes varying in phenolic content. *Animal Feed Science and Technology* 55, 161–177.

Makkar, H.P.S., Blümmel, M. and Becker, K. (1995) Formation of complexes between polyvinyl pyrrolidones or polyethylene glycols and tannins, and their implication in gas production and true digestibility in *in vitro* techniques. *British Journal of Nutrition* 73, 897–913.

McDougal, E.I. (1949) Studies on ruminant saliva. 1. The composition and output of sheep's saliva. *Biochemical Journal* 43, 99.

Menke, K.H. and Steingass, H. (1988) Estimation of the energetic feed value obtained from chemical analysis and *in vitro* gas production using rumen fluid. *Animal Research and Development* 28, 7–55.

Mertens, D.R. and Loften, J.R. (1980) The effect of starch on forage fiber digestion kinetics *in vitro. Journal of Dairy Science* 63, 1437–1446.

Morris, P. and Robbins, M.P. (1997) Manipulating condensed tannins in forage legumes. In: McKersie, B.D. and Brown, O.C.W. (eds) *Biotechnology and the Improvement of Forage Legumes.* CAB International, Wallingford, UK, pp. 147–173.

Motulsky, H.J. and Ransnas, L.A. (1987) Fitting curves to data using nonlinear regression: a practical and nonmathematical review. *FASEB Journal* 1, 365–374.

Nelson, K.E., Pell, A.N., Doane, P.H., Giner-Chavez, B. and Schofield, P. (1997) Chemical and biological assays to evaluate bacterial inhibition by tannins. *Journal of Chemical Ecology* 23, 1175–1194.

Pell, A.N. and Schofield, P. (1993) Computerized monitoring of gas production to measure forage digestion *in vitro. Journal of Dairy Science* 76, 1063–1073.

Ross, G.J.S. (1987) *MLP, Maximum Likelihood Program, Version 3.08.* Numerical Algorithms Group, Oxford.

Russell, J.B. and Dombrowski, D.B. (1980) Effect of pH on the efficiency of growth by pure cultures of rumen bacteria in continuous culture. *Applied and Environmental Microbiology* 39, 604–610.

Sarwar, M., Firkins, J.L. and Eastridge, M.L. (1992) Effects of varying forage and concentrate carbohydrates on nutrient digestibilities and milk production by dairy cows. *Journal of Dairy Science* 75, 1533–1542.

Schofield, P. (1996) An inexpensive incubator for the biology laboratory. *American Biology Teacher* 58, 494–498.

Schofield, P. and Pell, A.N. (1995a) Measurement and kinetic analysis of the neutral detergent-soluble carbohydrate fraction of legumes and grasses. *Journal of Animal Science* 73, 3455–3463.

Schofield, P. and Pell, A.N. (1995b) Validity of using accumulated gas pressure readings to measure forage digestion *in vitro*: a comparison involving three forages. *Journal of Dairy Science* 78, 2230–2238.

Schofield, P., Pitt, R.E. and Pell, A.N. (1994) Kinetics of fiber digestion from *in vitro* gas production. *Journal of Animal Science* 72, 2980–2991.

Smith, D. (1981) Removing and analyzing total nonstructural carbohydrates from plant tissue. PhD thesis, University of Wisconsin College of Agriculture and Life Sciences, Madison, Wisconsin.

Sniffen, C.J., O'Connor, J.D., Van Soest, P.J., Fox, D.G. and Russell, J.B. (1992) A net carbohydrate and protein system for evaluating cattle diets: II. Carbohydrate and protein availability. *Journal of Animal Science* 70, 3562–3577.

Stefanon, B., Pell, A.N. and Schofield, P. (1996) Effect of maturity on digestion kinetics of water-soluble and water-insoluble fractions of alfalfa and brome hay. *Journal of Animal Science* 74, 1104–1115.

Taya, M., Ohmiya, K., Kobayashi, T. and Shimizu, S. (1980) Monitoring and control of a cellulolytic anaerobe culture by using gas evolved as an indicator. *Journal of Fermentation Technolology* 5, 463–469.

Theodorou, M.K., Lowman, R.S., Davies, Z.S., Cuddeford, D. and Owen, E. (1998) In: *In vitro Techniques for Measuring Nutrient Supply to Ruminants.* Occasional Paper. British Society of Animal Science, Penicuik, UK.

Theodorou, M.K., Williams, B.A., Dhanoa, M.S., McAllan, A.B. and France, J. (1994) A simple gas production method using a pressure transducer to determine the fermentation kinetics of ruminant feeds. *Animal Feed Science and Technology* 48, 185–197.

Tilley, J.M.A. and Terry, R.A. (1963) A two stage technique for the *in vitro* digestion of forage of forage crops. *Journal of the British Grassland Society* 18, 104–111.

Tolera, A., Khazaal, K. and Ørskov, E.R. (1997) Nutrititive evaluation of some browse species. *Animal Feed Science and Technology* 67, 181–195.

Van Soest, P.J. (1994) *Nutritional Ecology of the Ruminant*, 2nd edn. Cornell University Press, Ithaca, New York.

Wilkins, J.R. (1974) Pressure transducer method for measuring gas production by microorganisms. *Applied Microbiology* 27, 135–140.

Wolin, M.J. (1960) A theoretical rumen fermentation balance. *Journal of Dairy Science* 43, 1452–1459.

Zwietering, M.H., Jongenburger, I., Rombouts, F.M. and van't Tiet, K. (1990) Modeling of the bacterial growth curve. *Applied and Environmental Microbiology* 56, 1875–1881.

Appendix

Non-linear curve fitting

Useful numerical information is extracted from gas data by means of non-linear curve fitting. To understand the significance of such information, it is helpful to have an overview of the curve-fitting process and some appreciation of the statistical tests used to evaluate the quality of a fit (Motulsky and Ransnas, 1987).

At least three different pieces of software have been applied for this fitting. France *et al.* (1993) used the Maximum Likelihood Program (Ross, 1987). Cone *et al.* (1996) used a program called NLREG (non-linear regression analysis). Schofield *et al.* (1994) used a commercial program called TableCurve (published by Jandel Scientific, now incorporated into SPSS Science, Chicago, Illinois) that is powerful, graphically oriented and easy to use. The following description applies to TableCurve.

After importing the data set (as an *xy* curve) into the program, one first constructs or imports an equation, called a user-defined function, to use for fitting. Taking the single pool logistic equation (Equation 10.5) as an example, the equation would be entered as:

$$Y = \#A \times (1 + \exp(2 - 4 \times \#B \times (x - \#C)))^{-1} \quad (10.9)$$

Here, Y is the gas volume at time *x*, #A is the asymptotic gas volume (units, ml), #B is the specific rate (units, h^{-1}) and #C is the lag (units, h). #A, #B and #C are parameters to be calculated by the program such that the function represented by Equation 10.9 passes through, or close to, as many of the data points as possible. The next step is to assign starting values to #A, #B and #C and to set limits on possible values. For the logistic equation, we can specify that all parameters must be >0. The asymptotic volume #A is easily estimated from the data curve. The specific rate #B usually lies within the range 0.02–0.2 h^{-1}, and the lag #C is also readily estimated from the data curve. The program allows one to see the visual effects on the curve shape of changes in these starting values. In addition, the program can perform a 'limited' fit to help obtain these values. With starting values assigned to produce a curve of approximately the right shape, we are now ready to do a full-scale fit. During this process, the parameters are adjusted iteratively to minimize the sum of the squared errors (the difference between the calculated and actual data points, SSE). The fitting process is extremely fast and takes <1 s for most of the functions and data sets we use.

Fitting stops and convergence is assumed when the coefficient of determination (r^2) did not change in the sixth significant figure for five consecutive iterations. Among the statistics reported by TableCurve, *F* statistic and r^2 were used to evaluate a fit. The *F* statistic (mean square regression/mean square error: larger values mean a better fit) and r^2 (maximum = 1.0, values within the range 0.97–1.0 are acceptable) give a measure of the overall fit. In addition, one should examine the standard error (SE), 95% confidence limits and t values of the parameters (parameter value/standard error). Multiple-pool models usually give a higher F statistic and r^2 than a single-pool model because there is more 'wiggle room'. However, this extra flexibility is sometimes purchased at the expense of less well-defined parameter values (lower t).

The t value reflects the importance of a given parameter in determining the overall function value. If t is low, then the function is insensitive to changes in that parameter value. In Equation 10.5, for example, the lag term L is less important than the specific rate or asymptotic volume in determining V_t. The t value for L will always be less than that for S. If we wish to use curve fit parameters for comparative purposes, rather than simply to summarize a data set, then the preference is to produce a good fit with the smallest possible number of well-defined parameters.

Simple inspection of the appearance of the calculated curve compared with the data points provides a useful, though not a sufficient, criterion for a good fit. It is important to supplement numerical analysis with common sense!

Some thought should be given to the choice of data points used for curve fitting. If the data approach an asymptote, then points much beyond the asymptotic value should be excluded from the fit. There is otherwise a danger that 'the tail may wag the dog' and that these constant or very slowly changing data may unduly influence the program's choice of best parameters to fit regions of the curve where the data are changing rapidly.

Pressure sensors, types and construction

We live in a pressurized world and pressure measurements must therefore always involve pressure *differences*. Pressure sensors vary in the standard against which an unknown pressure is measured. 'Absolute' sensors use a sealed vacuum reference; 'differential' sensors use a second pressure source; 'gauge' sensors use atmospheric pressure as the reference. The most common sensors are of the differential type. These become gauge sensors if the reference port is left open to the atmosphere.

The sensing element of a solid-state pressure sensor consists of four nearly identical piezo-resistors (resistors whose value changes with strain) buried within the surface of a thin silicon diaphragm. A pressure applied to this diaphragm causes it to flex and to change its resistance. If a voltage is applied across the resistor network, resistance changes are transformed into voltage changes. These changes can then be amplified and used to measure pressure.

Sensors are calibrated by attaching them to a sealed bottle of known volume containing medium and measuring the changes in voltage output as known volumes of CO_2 are injected into the bottle. This calibration result will depend both on the bottle size and on the atmospheric pressure at the time of calibration. In this way, the sensor output (Volts) can be translated simply and directly into a gas volume (Schofield and Pell, 1995b).

Chapter 11
In Sacco Methods

P. Nozière and B. Michalet-Doreau[1]
Département Elevage et Nutrition des Animaux,
Unité de Recherches sur les Herbivores, INRA Theix, France

Introduction

As predictive models for estimating the nutritive value of feeds for ruminant livestock have become increasingly complex in their approach, they have highlighted the need for an accurate characterization of the degradation kinetics of different feed fractions. A direct method of measuring the rumen degradation of feeds consists of placing a small amount of foodstuff in an undegradable porous bag, suspending the bag in the rumen and measuring the disappearance of feed components after incubation. This technique is very old, and was used for the first time by Quin *et al.* (1939). They used silk bags which were introduced in the rumen via a cannula. This technique was used again later to investigate the ruminal degradation of cellulose and the dry matter (DM) digestibility of a range of feeds. However, in all the studies, no attempt to describe the degradation curves by regression was made. It was not until the 1980s that this technique was used to obtain an evaluation of the rate and extent of degradation in the rumen. New ruminant rationing models (protein system) require determination of

the dynamic aspects of feed nitrogen (N) degradation in the rumen and have adopted the *in sacco* technique to characterize it.

One of the limitations of the *in sacco* technique is its low repeatability and its lack of reproducibility, as is confirmed by the results of the ring-tests carried by Oldham in the UK, Vérité in France and by Madsen and Hvelplund in the EC, as reported by Michalet-Doreau and Ould-Bah (1992). To be able to take data from different laboratories in feed tables and use them to interpret the results from production experiments in different countries, a standardized *in sacco* method was proposed following on the EEC-EAAP meeting in 1986 where the present situation regarding protein evaluation systems for ruminants was presented. The first part of this chapter will examine methodological aspects.

Many *in sacco* data are provided by the numerous kinetic studies of N disappearance which were used to elaborate the modern systems for evaluation of feed and protein requirements for ruminants. Increasingly this technique is also used to describe the kinetics of degradation of other feed components such as starch and

[1]Corresponding author.

structural carbohydrates. In the second part of this chapter, we will survey the different uses of this technique and their limits.

Sources of Variation in the *in Sacco* Technique

The key to the usefulness of this technique focuses on the ability to standardize it. We will investigate the factors associated with the use of this technique, especially the factors likely to introduce a bias in the range of feeds according to their rumen degradability. In order to make discussion of pertinent sources of variation clearer, this chapter has been divided into three parts, bag and sample characteristics, ruminal environment and exchanges between bag and rumen, and modelling degradation kinetics.

Bag and sample characteristics

Milling
The types of cloth generally used are polyester, nylon or dacron, with the latter two being used most often (see review by Huntington and Givens, 1995). However, the weave structure of the cloth, multi-filamentous or monofilamentous, is of greater importance. With monofilamentous woven cloth, the aperture size is defined with precision, which means that the pores are uniform and do not change with mechanical stress. Conversely, the aperture size of dacron threads is more variable and seems to be affected by physical pressure during incubation (Marinucci *et al.*, 1992). Another important characteristic of bags is their pore size. It must permit the influx of digesting agents and buffers, but prevent the efflux of undegraded sample whilst allowing the removal of degradation end-products. Generally speaking, the degradation of dietary components increases with pore size (Weakley *et al.*, 1983). These results were obtained with large variations in pore size (5–50 μm). Now researchers use bags whose pore size is between 35 and 55 μm (Huntington and Givens, 1995), and

the pore size proposed in the recommended experimental procedure is between 30 and 50 μm.

Choice of bag porosity is also conditioned by the processing of the sample, and more particularly by the fineness of grinding. Grinding is carried out in order to obtain a homogeneous sample and also to mimic the effect of mastication. Mastication decreases particle size and thereby exposes more surface area. Additionally, the crimping and crushing action of the mastication process exposes more area of digestible tissue within a given particle size, and facilitates rupture of the anatomical barriers of plant structures to allow subsequently increasing microbial enzyme accessibility. In a comparison between three forages, masticated or not, Olubobokun *et al.* (1990) showed that the mastication allowed a greater release of soluble nutrients. For cereals, ingestive mastication increased DM digestion from 16, 26 and 30% to 53, 69 and 66% for barley, maize and wheat, respectively, in comparison with whole grain (Beauchemin *et al.*, 1994). Incubation of masticated feeds would be the best method for *in sacco* studies, but it is also a very laborious method. A less perfect but easier simulation of mastication can be obtained by grinding of feedstuff prior to ruminal incubation.

Feed degradation rate tends to increase with fineness of grinding, and variations depend on rumen incubation time and feed. The influence of grinding increases when the incubation time is short (see review by Michalet-Doreau and Ould-Bah, 1992), and differences between feeds are also important. When the fineness of grinding increased from 1 to 3 mm, the DM and/or N degradability of barley was not modified, whereas that of maize, oat, pea, fababean or soybean meal decreased (Nordin and Campling, 1976; Michalet-Doreau and Cerneau, 1991). For forages, when the grinding screen was increased from 0.8 to 6 mm, N degradability was not modified (Michalet-Doreau and Cerneau, 1991), but the kinetic parameters varied: compared with the chopped material, grinding of hay markedly increased the rate of DM and NDF disappearance or decreased the lag time, i.e. the time between the introduction of the bag into the rumen and the beginning of degradation. The influence of grinding on the rate and extent of sample degradation in the rumen is contradictory, probably because grinding does not affect the particle size of feeds to the same extent. Thus a given increase in particle size causes the same increase in *in sacco* N degradability (Michalet-Doreau and Cerneau, 1991).

After milling at the same screen mesh size, particle size distribution is different between forages (Emanuele and Staples, 1988) and between concentrates (Michalet-Doreau and Cerneau, 1991). For the 0.8 mm screen, the mean particle size of pea was 5, barley 52, maize 186, soybean meal 292, lucerne hay 321 and cocksfoot hay 348 µm (Michalet-Doreau and Cerneau, 1991). The chemical composition of different sized particles varies. In this last experiment, the smallest particles of lucerne hay contained a higher proportion of N than the coarser particles, probably because the leaves highest in N are the most fragile parts of this plant and so are ground most finely. Similarly Gerson *et al.* (1988) observed that when meadow grass hay was chopped and subsequently wet sieved, the proportion of lipid (cuticle) increased as the size of sieve decreased and, conversely, as sieve size increased the proportion of lignified (stem) material increased. These variations of particle size distribution with grinding of a specific feedstuff have implications for the *in situ* technique. There is a linear relationship between the proportion of N in the smallest particles, measured by wet sieving and weighing, and N particulate losses through the pore bags (Michalet-Doreau and Ould-Bah, 1992). On 20 feeds with 0.8 mm grinding fineness, N losses were a mean of 10%, ranging from 4% for soybean to 32% for oat. For starch, the proportion of particles lost through the bag pores without being degraded is also important and very variable. With immature maize, oven dried and ground at 3 mm screen, the starch

losses represented 11% of starch initially introduced in the bags, and ranged from 5 to 25% according to stage of maturity and genotype. However, this proportion was much greater when samples were freeze-dried (Philippeau and Michalet-Doreau, 1997). In agreement with these results, Lopez *et al.* (1995) determined that for 1 mm ground forages, greater DM losses occurred after freeze-drying than after oven-drying below 60°C.

Particle size also has an influence on the accessibility of dietary components to the microorganism enzymes. Emanuele and Staples (1988) studied the *in situ* degradation kinetics of different sized particles of the same feed. The solubilized fraction or the lag time significantly increased with an increase in particle size. Similarly, Nocek and Kohn (1988) noted that chopping and then sieving lucerne or timothy hay through a 3.2 mm screen resulted in a shift in the proportion of insoluble and non-degradable DM towards a larger particle size. In a trial using meadow grass hay (Gerson *et al.*, 1988), *in vitro* gas production was 30% lower for the large particles, but the surface area was 10% that of the small particles. External surface area per unit of mass and an intact cuticle could be determinants of ruminal degradation kinetics.

Another aspect of the effect of mastication on feeds is the increase in feed wetting, and thus solubilization rate and accessibility of feed components to microorganisms. In order to facilitate the attack of feeds by rumen microorganisms, some researchers pre-soak samples in water or in buffer. The time of pre-soaking varied between 1 and 15 min. Little information is available to study the advantages of pre-soaking bags before their incubation. This treatment should nevertheless enable the degradation rates of insoluble nutrient components to be determined more easily.

In conclusion, the aim of sample preparation is to simulate the resultant particle distribution that would be achieved by mastication. However, there may be considerable differences in particle sizes between feeds ground using the same sized screen. The chemical composition of different sized particles is different, and fractions of different particle size potentially have different rates and extents of degradation. Therefore, it is necessary to control the extent of particle losses that are sometimes important, and which could result in: (i) an overestimated extent of degradation; (ii) an underestimated rate of degradation if the lost particles have a faster rate of degradation than those remaining in the bag; and (iii) an over-estimation of the immediately soluble fraction. A more rational approach to the use of milling would be to characterize the processing of feeds not by the grinding screen aperture, but rather by foodstuff particle size (Michalet-Doreau and Cerneau, 1991), and to establish some degree of uniformity in particle size within foodstuff categories.

Drying

For fresh forages, the lacerated form prior to rumen incubation is probably the sample preparation which best reproduces chewing. However, the use of fresh sample is difficult; it is necessary to have the animal and the forage samples at the same moment. Therefore, samples commonly are conserved by freezing or drying. Several drying methods have been proposed, and they affect ruminal degradation in different ways. The nature and content of various constituents may be influenced by the drying process, and long drying times are required when a low temperature is used in order to avoid thermochemical degradation of the sample. In comparison with freeze-drying or fresh forage, oven-drying between 45 and 60°C decreased the soluble N content and *in situ* N degradability (Lopez *et al.*, 1995; Dulphy *et al.*, 1999), and this decrease was due essentially to a smaller rapidly degradable fraction. The freezing of chopped forage does not affect the N degradability (Dulphy *et al.*, 1999). However, when samples are ground after freeze-drying, N degradability increases (Michalet-Doreau and Ould-Bah, 1992), the freezing probably inducing a disruption of plant structures.

Exchanges between bag and rumen

Bags must be placed in the rumen so as to permit free movement within the rumen liquor and so that the bags are squeezed during muscular contractions, facilitating fluid exchange between the internal environment of the bag and the rumen. The bacteria present in the more aqueous regions of the rumen, the ventral sac, could colonize and attack freshly exposed feed surface more easily than the microflora in the dorsal sac. In most studies cited by Huntington and Givens (1995), the authors incubated the bags in the ventral sac. However, the distribution of microorganisms in the ruminal content depends on the physical and chemical conditions inside each rumen compartment, and these conditions themselves vary during the nycthemeral period. Therefore, the site of bag incubation and the incubation sequence in relation to animal feeding can influence digestion rates inside bags.

As it is necessary for microorganisms to enter the bag in order for feed degradation to take place, it is also essential that they be eliminated from the bag after incubation to avoid underestimation of DM and N degradation.

To begin with, we will show diurnal fluctuations of digestive ruminal capacity in relation to time after feeding and site of sampling in the rumen, and the implications of these spatial variations within the rumen on degradation rates in the bags. Then we will study microbial colonization of feed samples and exchanges between bags and the surrounding digesta.

Effect of bag procedure

Ruminal contents are very heterogeneous. The DM content drops considerably from the dorsal rumen to the ventral rumen, whereas the bottom of the ventral sac and the reticulum show comparable values. These differences in DM between compartments can be explained by the considerable differences in size and density of food particles in them. A matted mass of large particles occupies the dorsal sac, whereas small, high-density particles accumulate after fermentation in the ventral sac. This vertical stratification continues throughout the nycthemeral period, reaching a maximum after the meal. Moreover, it has been shown that particle microbial colonization increased when particle size decreased (Gerson *et al.*, 1988). Therefore, the higher bacterial colonization of the small particles in the lower parts of the rumen involves higher microbial enzyme activity in this part of the rumen (Martin *et al.*, 1999 ; Fig. 11.1A).

The digestive ruminal capacity shows spatial variations within the rumen. The relative locations of nylon bags suspended within the rumen can also affect digestion rates. Several methods of suspending the bags in the rumen are used; currently, the

bags are fastened along a string weighted with a sinker to ensure that they do not float on top of the rumen contents. The anchor weight, from 0.5 to 2 kg for cows and 75 to 300 g for sheep, does not affect DM degradability of feeds (Huntington and Givens, 1997). Some researchers use a template to allow maximal exchanges between the feed sample and the incubation environment, but the results obtained with this apparatus have not been compared with those obtained by a more classical process. The length of the string along which bags are fastened is also an important factor because it determines the location of the bags in the rumen. A 25 cm string would be a sufficient length to allow free movement of bags in the rumen of

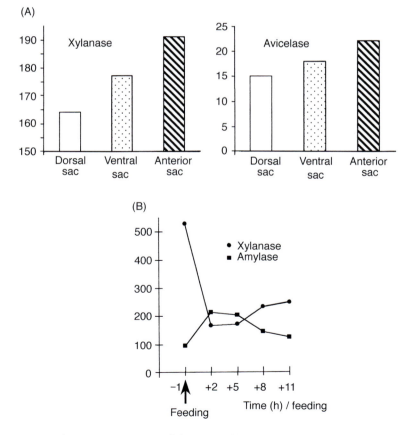

Fig. 11.1. Variations of enzyme activities in solid-associated bacteria. (A) Effect of rumen sampling site (Martin *et al.*, 1999) (μmol reducing sugars g^{-1} DM h^{-1}). (B) Effect of sampling time (Martin *et al.*, 1993) (nmol reducing sugars mg^{-1} protein h^{-1}).

sheep (Mehrez and Ørskov, 1977), but the DM disappearance after ruminal incubation varies according to the location of the bags in the rumen (Stritzler et al., 1990). Stritzler et al. (1990) reported an increase of disappearance in response to increased string length, in relation to increased microbial activity measured by the ATP concentration within the bags. These variations are related to the stratification of digesta and the variations in the concentration of microorganisms with sampling site, dorsal and ventral sac.

The bag incubation sequence can also influence digestion rates. Nocek (1985) compared two bag incubation sequences: all bags were placed in the rumen at once and removed at designated time intervals, or bags were introduced in reverse sequence and removed all at once. The former procedure resulted in lower variation and slower digestion rates, perhaps because the digestion process is interrupted when bags are removed then replaced in the rumen. However, if the bags are not introduced at the same time in the rumen, they will not be submitted to the same degradation conditions. In most studies, animals are fed in two meals per day, and the rumen environment cannot be considered as stable. After feeding, the rapidly changing rumen conditions such as osmotic pressure, entrance of oxygen or dilution and passage rate involve diurnal changes in the microbial ecosystem (see review by Dehority and Orpin, 1988) and in its enzyme activity (Martin et al., 1993; Fig. 11.1B). To compare degradation rates, it is probably better to introduce all the bags at the same time in the rumen, but Huntington and Givens (1997) did not report an effect of incubation sequence on DM degradability of feeds.

Microbial colonization of bag samples: input of microorganisms

The pore size and open area of the cloth used for in situ bags needs to be such that the cloth permits the influx of digesting agents and buffers. From the synthesis of Huntington and Givens (1995), researchers have favoured the use of two distinct aperture ranges, <15 and >35 µm, and this suggests two approaches to the problem: those authors who are looking for minimization of loss of undegraded particles, and those who favour equating the internal microbial microenvironment of the bag with that of the rumen.

A more diverse microbial colonization of feed samples is indicated in 40 µm as compared with 20 µm bags, and may relate to increased numbers of protozoa (Lindberg et al., 1984) entering the bag. Meyer and Mackie (1986) showed that maximum influx of protozoa occurred after 12 h (50% after 4 h) of rumen incubation. The number of protozoa increases as the pore size of the bags increases (Huntington and Givens, 1995). Even when pore size is sufficient for protozoal influx, the bacterial population inside the bag differs from that of the surrounding rumen digesta, and more particularly the cellulolytic population (Meyer and Mackie, 1986). Therefore, the fibrolytic activity of solid-adherent microorganisms is lower in bag residues than in rumen digesta (Nozière and Michalet-Doreau, 1996). These differences can be explained by the shorter time spent in the rumen by the bag particles, the lack of mastication of incubated forages and the confining conditions of feed inside the bag. In bags, the possibilities of exchange between the feed particles and the rumen medium are limited by the surface area of the pores in the bag material (Lindberg et al., 1984), which accounts for the acidification of the medium inside the bags. The pH in the bags is lower than the pH of the rumen contents, at least for the longest incubation time (Nozière and Michalet-Doreau, 1996), and this difference may be due to an accumulation of volatile fatty acids inside the bags (Marinucci et al., 1992). The amylolytic enzyme activity of solid-adherent microorganisms is higher in bags containing barley than in bags containing maize, at least for the first hours of incubation (Nozière and Michalet-Doreau, 1997). The amylase activity of microorganisms colonizing cereals in the bags would depend on the nature of the substrate in the bag, and more specifically on the amount of available starch. The differences in proteolytic activity of solid-adherent microorganisms between bags and the surrounding digesta are slight (Michalet-Doreau and Nozière, 1998). In the bags, the proteolytic activity varies with the incubated feeds, but differences between feeds are observed only for longer incubation times, and would not limit the use of the *in situ* method to characterize feed N degradability.

Microbial colonization of bag samples: output of microorganisms

The washing of bags after rumen incubation has two main objectives: to stop microbial activity and to free feed residues from rumen microorganisms, without increasing the loss of feed particles through bag pores. Several mechanical methods have been proposed for rinsing post-incubation bags: hand rinsing of bags until the water is clear, about 90 s per bag, or mechanical rinsing of bags in a washing machine for a variable duration from 2 to 15 min (Michalet-Doreau and Ould-Bah, 1992). Cherney *et al.* (1990) compared the two rinsing methods. Machine rinsing twice for 2 min or hand rinsing of bags gave similar results, but higher DM disappearance and higher standard error for DM disappearance were observed when bags were machine rinsed twice for 5 min than when bags were either machine rinsed twice for 2 min or hand rinsed.

Despite washing, the bag residue can still contain significant quantities of microbial matter after incubation. Different markers of microbial population (diaminopimelic acid (DAPA), ^{15}N or ^{35}S) or feed (^{15}N) can be employed for measuring the microbial contamination of incubated feeds (see Chapter 12). The marker technique nevertheless is difficult and the results are probably affected by the type of marker used. Moreover, the use of a marker for the microbial population requires a reference bacterial sample in order to calculate the percentage of bacterial DM or N from the concentration of marker in the residue. This reference bacterial sample is isolated either from the liquid or the solid

phase of rumen content, or directly from nylon bag residues. The chemical composition and the marker concentration of bacteria vary according to the microbial population. Marker concentration for the fluid-phase microbial population is higher than that for solid-phase microbial population (Merry and McAllan, 1983; Craig *et al.*, 1987). However, Olubobokun and Craig (1990) and Beckers *et al.* (1995) found little or no difference in N degradability between values corrected for fluid or adherent microbes.

The bacterial DM in the bag, as a percentage of residual DM, increases rapidly in the first hours of incubation, and either remains steady (Beckers *et al.*, 1995) or declines with ruminal incubation time (Wanderley *et al.*, 1993). The time necessary for the appearance of the peak of contamination and the maximum value of this peak, expressed as a percentage of microbial DM in bag residual DM, varies considerably between feeds. Several hypotheses have been proposed to explain the microbial contamination variations between feeds. For example, the cell wall content of bag residues: however, it was not possible to find a relationship between the fibre fraction of bag residues and their colonization rate by the microorganisms. It is also possible that the differences in particle size between feeds could explain the differences in microbial contamination. The microbial colonization of feed particles in the rumen is related negatively to their size (Gerson *et al.*, 1988). However W.Z. Yang and C. Poncet (France, 1991, personal communication) reported no relationship between microbial colonization of particles and their size inside the bags. Furthermore mastication, which increases the bacterial colonization of particles in the rumen, did not affect microbial colonization of particles inside the bags (Olubobokun *et al.*, 1990).

The bacterial contamination of bags leads to considerable and variable underestimation of the N degradability of feeds, and this underestimation is greater when the feed N content is low (Fig. 11.2). In a study conducted on 51 forages, the

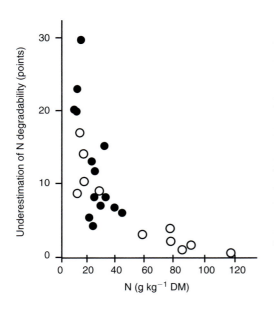

Fig. 11.2. Relationship between underestimation of N degradability due to bacterial contamination and N content of forage (●) and concentrate (○) (Michalet-Doreau and Ould-Bah, 1992; Wanderley *et al.*, 1993; Beckers *et al.*, 1995).

In summary, microbial contamination of forage residues can result in a substantial underestimation of degradability value, and this effect is particularly important for feeds in which the N content of the feed constitutes only a small proportion of the DM. To take the bacterial contamination into account, a marker technique of the microbial population can be used, but it is laborious and expensive. In routine experiments, treatments for decontamination can be useful to dislodge bacterial DM fixed to the bag residues, but they generally tend to underestimate N degradability. Another promising method consists of predicting microbial contamination of the bag residue by near infrared spectrometry (Lecomte *et al.*, 1994).

underestimation of N degradability varied from 8 to 15 points when the crude protein content of forages decreased from 18 to 8% DM (Michalet-Doreau and Ould-Bah, 1992).

Different techniques are used to dislodge the bacteria attached to the bag residues: physical treatments such as the freezing–rethawing technique associated with stomaching (Michalet-Doreau and Ould-Bah, 1992) or not associated with stomaching (Kamel *et al.*, 1995); or chemical treatments using the properties of surfactants, salts or detergents associated with stomaching (Beckers *et al.*, 1995) or not associated with stomaching (Hof *et al.*, 1990). The efficiency of these techniques in detaching associated bacteria from bag residues is variable, but no procedure completely removes microbial contamination. Moreover, these treatments not only remove bacteria fixed to the residues, but also partially remove N feed residues from the bags (Beckers *et al.*, 1995).

Modelling of kinetics of degradation

The ruminal degradation kinetics of dietary DM or any component may be described by a curvilinear regression according to incubation time. The exponential model, described by Ørskov and McDonald (1979) for N degradation, is the most commonly used. This model, the biological significance of its parameters and their determination will be presented and discussed in this chapter. We will then briefly present the main methods used to determine the ruminal degradability of feeds from the *in sacco* degradation profiles and the turnover rate of particles in the rumen.

The exponential model

First-order degradation kinetics, reported by Ørskov and McDonald (1979), have been commonly used to describe ruminal N degradation kinetics, and more recently for cell walls and starch degradation kinetics. This model supports the existence of three dietary fractions (Fig. 11.3).

1. The undegradable fraction represents the amount of residue remaining in the bag after a long incubation time. For starch, it is generally believed that there is no undegradable fraction, as observed by several authors (review of Sauvant *et al.*, 1994).

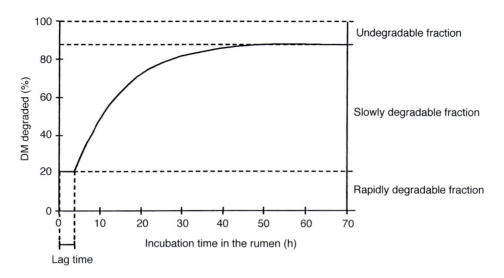

Fig. 11.3. *In sacco* degradation of forage DM: adjustment to first-order kinetics.

2. The insoluble but potentially degradable fraction is considered to be degraded by microorganisms according to first-order kinetics, implying that substrate digested at any time is proportional to the amount of potentially digestible matter remaining at that time. An important assumption in using first-order kinetics is that this pool of slowly degradable material is homogeneous.
3. The rapidly degradable fraction corresponds to the fraction which disappears prior to the earliest removal of bags from the rumen. This fraction includes not only soluble material but also undegraded small particles that are washed out of the bags.

The degradation kinetics of DM or any component of the incubated feedstuff may be described by curvilinear regression of the amount which has disappeared from the bag with time:

$$D(t) = a + b \times (1 - \exp(-c \times t)) \quad (11.1)$$

where $D(t)$ is the amount of feedstuff which has disappeared from bag at incubation time t, a is the rapidly degradable fraction, b is the slowly degradable fraction and c is the fractional digestion rate constant (h^{-1}) of the fraction b.

When substrate is incubated in the rumen, degradation is usually not con-sidered to begin instantaneously. The period during which either no digestion occurs or digestion occurs at a greatly reduced rate is generally referred to as the lag phase. A modification of the model of Ørskov and McDonald (1979), incorporating a lag phase time, has been given by Dhanoa (1988):

$$D(t) = a \text{ for } t \leq \theta \quad (11.2)$$

$$D(t) = a + b \times (1 - \exp(-c \times (t - \theta)))$$
$$\text{for } t > \theta \quad (11.3)$$

where $D(t)$, a, b, c and t are as defined in Equation 11.1, and θ is the discrete lag time (h). This model is used mainly to describe the kinetics of forage DM and cell wall degradation.

Subsequently, these simple models were improved and completed in order to take better account of the dynamic processes of digestion. A possible method for correcting degradation data for the small particles lost at time zero is dividing the a-term into two subfractions: (i) the water-soluble fraction; and (ii) the particles sufficiently small to pass through the bag pores, this subfraction being considered as degraded at the same rate as the particles within the bag (Huntington and Givens, 1995). The amount of residue in the bag at each incubation time is thus corrected by adding the amount of small particles that would still be in the bag at the same time if no particle loss had occurred. However, these corrections are based on the asumption that the particle losses through the bag pores are representative of the incubated sample, which is not proven.

In this first-order process of degradation, the slowly degradable fraction is assimilated to a homogeneous fraction. Another way to tackle substrate heterogeneity is to consider that the degradation rate is a continuous variable, assuming the existence of a gamma distribution of the degradation rate (see review by Sauvant, 1997). This simple empirical approach improves the statistical fit of experimental data; however, it has the drawback of ignoring the partitioning of substrate into well-defined subfractions.

In the exponential model including a lag phase, digestion of the slowly degradable fraction is considered to start only and instantaneously when factors limiting digestibility, i.e. hydration, attachment and colonization, are overcome, i.e. at lag time, assuming implicitly that the lag phase has a zero slope. However, because these limitations can be overcome within certain microenvironments (e.g. surface of particles, points of physical damage), it could be considered that there is partial substrate availability when describing digestion. Substrate may thus be digested as soon as it is placed in the rumen, but at a very reduced rate. As more substrate is hydrated and more microorganisms attach, the rate of disappearance will increase. Hydration of forage has been shown to reduce the lag time before *in vitro* degradation, and frequent measurements of *in sacco* degradation have shown that there is actually not a discrete but a progressive lag phase which can be modelled empirically or mechanistically (Sauvant, 1997). A simple approach consists of assuming that the degradation rate is the outcome of two basic components, one of accelerating degradation (i.e. no resistance) and one of resistance. However, studies are needed to assess precisely the value of such an approach for describing *in situ* kinetics.

Some authors developed more mechanistic models of the initial lag phase (Sauvant, 1997). These were based on a compartmental description, assuming that the substrate is firstly in a pool of matter with a lag phase prior to degradation. This compartment is transformed progressively, according to first-order kinetics, into another compartment containing the degradable form of the substrate which is subjected to digestion with first-order kinetics. This statement is realistic because processes of particle hydration and microbial colonization are progressive. Compared with the model with the discrete lag phase, the compartmental model reduces the residual mean squares for predicting the rate of disappearance.

Calculation of parameters

Two main methods are often used for fitting data to the first-order kinetic model: logarithmic transformation followed by linear regression (lnLIN) and non-linear least square regression (NLIN). The GLM and NLIN procedures of SAS (Statistical Analysis Systems, 1985) are often used. Errors and differences in parameters can arise according to the method of fitting data to the kinetic model. This is due to differences in the statistical error structure assumed in each model and differences between sequential and simultaneous estimation of parameters (reviewed by Mertens, 1993).

With the lnLIN method, the undegradable fraction is determined using data from the last incubation time and subtracted from the residue at each incubation time. A regression analysis is then conducted on log-transformed residues according to incubation time, assuming that error is proportional to the size of the residue for each observation (Mertens, 1993). The slope of the relationship corresponds to the constant degradation rate. A curve-peeling method could be conducted if the presence of prominent inflexions is detected. The major disadvantage of the lnLIN approach is that indigestible residue must be estimated experimentally using data from the last incubation time observed. Any error in estimating this fraction introduces a bias into the estimates of fractional rate and lag time. Choice of an incubation time which is too short may produce an over-estimation of the indigestible residue, an underestimation of the potentially digestible fraction and an overestimation of its degradation rate. Sometimes an incubation which is too long results in a concave semi-logarithmic curve indicating than more than one digestible pool exists. Observations during lag time must be removed from the data set before semi-logarithmic regression, to prevent an underestimation of the degradation rate. If the discrete lag time cannot be determined visually, an iterative approach may have to be used to determine which data to use for determining the rate after an initial lag time (Mertens, 1993).

In most cases, NLIN regression methods are preferred because they result in the smallest residual sum of squared deviations from the model. Model parameters are adjusted to the exponential model with (Dhanoa, 1988) or without (Ørskov and McDonald, 1979) lag time, through an iterative procedure until the change in the residual sums of square meets a convergence criterion, assuming equal error at each observation (Mertens, 1993). Advantages of this technique are that all parameters are estimated simultaneously. The Marquardt method in the NLIN procedure of SAS (1985) is used most often.

The different methods of calculation of degradation rates of DM, N and cell wall components have been compared by some authors. The same data and model may give different parameter estimates when fit by lnLIN compared with NLIN regression, but both will provide acceptable estimates of kinetic parameters when data are collected during well-designed experiments, i.e. a large number of incubation times adequately spaced out. Optimal and minimal incubation schedules have been proposed by Mertens (1993) (Table 11.1).

Determination of effective degradability
The nylon bag technique offers the possibility of measuring the extent and rate of degradation of feed during specific intervals. However, digestion rate relative to rate of passage is a critical dynamic property affecting digestibility: most non-cell wall components in feeds are digested rapidly with rates that are 3–10 times faster than rates of passage; conversely, the rate of cell wall digestion typically is of the same magnitude as the rate of passage

Table 11.1. Recommended incubation intervals (h) to obtain a precise estimate of sample degradation kinetics for degradation models containing three parameters (Mertens, 1993).

Rapidly degradable feeds		Slowly degradable feeds	
Optimum	Minimum	Optimum	Minimum
0[a]		0[a]	
0	0	0	0
2	2	3	3
4	4	6	6
8	8	9	9
12	12	12	12
16		18	
20	20	24	24
24		30	
32	32	36	36
40		48	
48	48	72	72
64	64	96	96

[a] Determination of the water-soluble fraction.

(Mertens, 1993). Thus, as feed particles have the opportunity to pass out of the rumen undegraded, the extent of degradation in the bag will not give a correct estimate for the effective degradation under normal rumen conditions. In this respect, it is necessary to consider both the rate of degradation and the turnover of particles in the rumen. To take account of the turnover rate in the estimation of feed ruminal digestion, mathematical methods based on interpretation of the *in sacco* degradation profile including a fixed turnover rate were proposed, by summing up step by step the amount of feed degraded before leaving the rumen during each incubation period (Kristensen *et al.*, 1982), or by integration of the *in sacco* degradation profile in relation to the ruminal particulate outflow rate (Ørskov and McDonald, 1979).

With the step by step method, the rate of degradation in the rumen as well as the outflow rate of the feed are combined to express the effective degradability (ED) by the following equation (Kristensen *et al.*, 1982):

$$\text{ED} = \Sigma(\text{D}(t_{i+1}) - \text{D}(t_i)) \times f(t_i, t_{i+1}) \quad (11.4)$$

where $(\text{D}(t_{i+1}) - \text{D}(t_i))$ is the amount of feed degraded during the time interval from t_i to t_{i+1}, and $f(t_i, t_{i+1})$ is the average proportion of feed remaining in the rumen from t_i to t_{i+1}. The amount of feed remaining in the rumen $(f(t_i))$ is estimated from the outflow rate (k, h^{-1}) by the following equation:

$$f(t_i) = \exp(-k \times t_i) \quad (11.5)$$

The effective degradability can also be calculated from the parameters of kinetics obtained from exponential adjustment without (Ørskov and McDonald, 1979) or with (Dhanoa, 1988) lag time, both by the following equation:

$$\text{ED} = a + (b \times c \times \exp(-k \times \theta)/(c + k)) \quad (11.6)$$

where a, b, c and θ are as defined in Equations 11.1 and 11.3, and k is the rumen small particle outflow rate (h^{-1}).

The adequacy of the calculation of effective degradability between these two methods obviously depends on how good the fit is to the regression, and this is essentially linked to the pertinence of the incubation schedule.

As discussed previously, numerous factors affect degradability data obtained with the *in sacco* technique. In order to allow comparisons between laboratories, a standard procedure of measurement has been proposed to measure N degradation rate of feeds (Madsen and Hvelplund, 1994), but some points such as processing of wet samples, taking account of microbial contamination in bags, etc., have not yet been the subject of specific recommendations. In spite of efforts to standardize the methodology for measurements, intra- and inter-laboratory variability remains high (Michalet-Doreau and Ould-Bah, 1992; Madsen and Hvelplund, 1994). Use of reference samples as internal standards has been proposed to reduce variability by incubating a standard sample of known degradation alongside test substrates (Michalet-Doreau and Ould-Bah, 1992). Increasing use of a single standard sample in the various laboratories carrying out *in sacco* degradation measurements should help to reduce variability between laboratories, but also to understand the origin of these variations when the degradation results for this standard sample are compared.

Utilization of the *In Sacco* Technique

To predict rumen escape and small intestine digestion

N escape

The most recent methods to evaluate the N values of feeds are based on estimation of the quantity of amino acids that can be absorbed by the small intestine. These amino acids have two possible origins: dietary or microbial. The feed N which escapes rumen degradation is one of the major elements in the determination of feed N value. For these systems to be effective, reliable procedures must be developed to provide rapid and realistic estimates of ruminal protein degradation for a wide variety of dietary feed ingredients. *In vivo* measurements of ruminal degradation of dietary protein require that animals be surgically prepared with cannulas in the rumen and duodenum. This method also requires suitable markers for calculating the flow rate of digesta and a reliable microbial marker for differentiation between microbial and dietary protein flowing to the small intestine. *In vivo* estimates of protein degradation are expensive, labour intensive, time consuming and subject to error associated with the use of markers of digesta flow rate, microbial markers and animal variation. Therefore, alternative procedures for measuring ruminal digestion of dietary protein are needed. Among the many proposed methods, the bag technique has been used widely.

The closest relationships between *in vivo* (measured by difference between N intake and non-microbial non-NH$_3$ duodenal N divided by N intake) and *in sacco* degradation were reported by Madsen and Hvelplund (1985) with 11 feeds ($R^2 = 0.79$) and by Vérité *et al.* (1987) with eight feeds ($R^2 = 0.90$). More recently, Poncet *et al.* (1995) compared *in vivo* measurements with *in situ* estimates from five experiments pooling 21 comparisons. The intercept of the linear relationship differs between experiments but, in all trials, the slope is the same and does not differ from 1.

In the *in sacco* technique, N which disappears from the bag is considered to have been degraded in the rumen, and the term 'disappearance' is synonymous with 'degradation'. As discussed previously, an overestimation can be due to undegraded particle losses through the bag pores, introducing a bias in the range of feeds according to their N degradability. Numerous methodological reviews recently have dealt with these factors, and it is now possible to appreciate this bias in relation to feed in the bag. *In situ* degradability measurement can also underestimate dietary N supply with leguminous seeds. A significant amount of soluble dietary proteins and small peptides from dietary protein degradation are found and can accumulate

in the rumen during the first hours after feeding (Williams and Cockburn, 1991). With these feeds, Poncet *et al.* (1998) also reported a discrepancy between *in sacco* and *in vivo* data because the peptides and soluble proteins are included in the *in vivo* N by-pass and considered as degraded proteins in the *in sacco* technique.

Another more recent application of the *in sacco* technique is the mobile bag technique. This is developed for estimation of intestinal availability of rumen-undegraded dietary protein (Hvelplund, 1985; De Boer *et al.*, 1987). After incubation in the rumen for a variable period, the food is placed in a bag and introduced via a duodenal cannula into the intestine where it transits freely, then is recovered at the end of the small intestine or in the faeces, when the quantity of residual N is determined. A relationship between digestibility of N in the bags and digestibility in the small intestine was reported by Hvelplund (1985). However, the intestinal N digestibility of rumen-degradable N depends on many factors: the duration of the preceding rumen incubation time; the retention time in the intestine; the location of bag recovery (ileum or faeces); etc. Therefore, this technique can give only an indication of the intestinal availability of rumen-undegradable protein.

Starch escape

Research in starch utilization by ruminants was reviewed recently. Although starch in cereal grains is almost completely digested in the whole digestive tract, the rate and extent of ruminal fermentation vary widely with grain source and cereal processing (reviewed by Huntington, 1997). The site of starch digestion has implications for the nature and amount of nutrients delivered to the animal. The absorbed nutrients, volatile fatty acids or glucose, are used with different efficiencies for energy production (ATP synthesis) during catabolic reactions and for anabolic processes such as fat and protein synthesis. The rapid fermentation of starch in the rumen increases the acidity in this compartment and increases the incidence of acidosis and feed intake problems related to digestive upsets, hence the need to evaluate starch escaping rumen digestion.

Sauvant *et al.* (1994) list rumen-degradable starch for various feedstuffs, and propose the use of the *in sacco* technique to characterize starch degradability. However, *in sacco* degradability tends to underestimate the degradability of slowly degraded starches (Fig. 11.4). This discrepancy could be the result of the failure of this technique to account for a reduction in the particle size of grains through mastication. The differences between cereals or between cultivars in ruminal starch degradation rate depend on the starch accessibility to microorganisms, i.e. starch which is protected by the protein matrix surrounding the starch granules. As an increase in cereal particle size involves a decrease in starch ruminal digestion, its effect is more important for slowly degradable cereal than for rapidly degradable cereal (Huntington, 1997). Therefore, when cereals are coarsely cracked, *in sacco* measurements give the same values as *in vivo* results (Philippeau *et al.*, unpublished data). In the bag technique, the cereals are ground, and it is not possible to take account of this effect of particle size.

To predict cell wall digestion

Organic matter digestibility of forages depends mainly on their cell wall digestibility, and thus on the amount of cell walls undigested within the digestive tract. Because ruminal cell wall digestion represents on average 80% of their digestibility in the total gastrointestinal tract, the amount of cell walls escaping ruminal digestion is a good estimate of the digestibility of forages. In the same way, the ingestibility of forages depends on the amount undegraded in the rumen which induces the ruminal fill. As the *in sacco* method makes it possible to assess the quantity of cell walls undegraded in the rumen, it appears an interesting method for the prediction of forage digestibility and ingestibility.

Digestibility and cell wall ruminal digestion
The *in sacco* technique has been used to estimate digestibility of forages (reviewed by Michalet-Doreau, 1990). The percentage

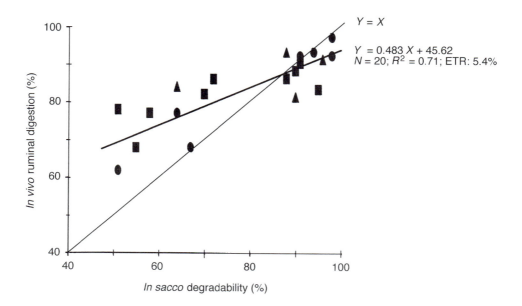

Fig. 11.4. Relationship between *in sacco* and *in vivo* methods for determining rumen-degradable starch for various feedstuffs (Sauvant *et al.*, 1994).

of DM digested after a long period of incubation in the rumen (48 or 72 h) was taken as an index of organic matter digestibility of forages. More recently, the *in sacco* technique has also been used to forecast ruminal digestion of the cell walls of forages. In an attempt to validate the use of the *in sacco* technique for estimation of ruminal digestion of cell walls, a few studies have been carried out where both *in sacco* and *in vivo* degradation were measured. Validations were based on the comparison of the duodenal flows of structural carbohydrates measured *in vivo* and the effective degradability calculated from *in sacco* degradation and outflow rate. Using *in sacco* digestion kinetic data leads to an underestimation of ruminal cell wall digestion (Archimède, 1992), but the slope of the relationship between effective degradability and the pre-duodenal digestibility does not differ significantly from 1 (Fig. 11.5). The underestimation of ruminal digestion by *in sacco* measurements can be due to an underestimation of the rate of digestion by *in situ* incubation, as suggested by several authors (Archimède, 1992; Stensig *et al.*, 1994). The lower number of cellulolytic bacteria (Meyer and Mackie, 1986) and the lower fibrolytic enzyme activities (Nozière and Michalet-Doreau, 1996) within the bags than in the surrounding digesta would appear to be responsible for the underestimation of degradation rate by the *in sacco* method. However, a threshold activity value above which variations in xylanase and cellulase microbial activity no longer induce variations in the hemicelluloses and cellulose degradation rates has been demonstrated (Nozière *et al.*, 1996). With forage-based diets, the fibrolytic activity of solid-associated microorganisms in the bags was above this threshold activity, so the underestimation of degradation rate by the *in sacco* method may be not related to the lower potential microbial activity within the bags. Another hypothesis to explain the underestimation of the ruminal digestion of cell walls by the *in sacco* technique can be suggested. As shown previously, the forage is ground

prior to incubation in order to reproduce the effect of mastication, to reduce the size of forage particles and to increase the accessibility of cell walls to microbial enzymes. In the bags, the accessibility of digestible cell wall components to microbial enzymes is lower than that of forage particles in the rumen content (Olubobokun *et al.*, 1990). This lower accessibility could be the main factor responsible for the underestimation of the degradation rate by the *in sacco* method.

Forage ingestibility and fill value
Ingestibility of forages is dependent on their cell wall content and on the lignification of these cell walls, i.e. the same parameters as those conditioning their digestibility. Thus ingestibility and digestibility of forages are closely linked, and methods used for prediction of digestibility can also be used for prediction of ingestibility. The nylon bag technique has thus been used as a method for prediction of the ingestibility of forages, with DM or cell wall residues used in the estimations (Michalet-Doreau, 1990). More recently, the dynamic aspects of DM and cell wall ruminal digestion, and its impact on rumen fill, have been taken into account by the *in sacco* degradation rate (Stensig *et al.*, 1994). The fill index, defined as the ratio between the amount of rumen content (g DM) and the amount of DM voluntary intake (g day^{-1}), can be estimated by the ruminal retention time (RRT, day) of DM or NDF calculated by the following equation:

$$RRT = (((1 - a - b)/k) + (b/(c + k)))/24 \quad (11.7)$$

where a, b, c and k are as defined in Equations 11.1 and 11.3. Such a definition of RRT is based on the following hypothesis: the rapidly degradable fraction (a) does not fill the rumen; the potentially degradable fraction (b) fills the rumen in proportion to its degradation rate (c) and the turnover rate (k); and the undegradable fraction ($1 - a - b$) fills the rumen in proportion to the turnover rate. RRT appears to be a good estimate of both fill index and ingestibility (see review by Faverdin *et al.*,

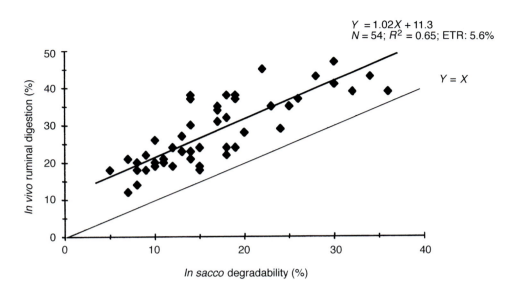

Fig. 11.5. Relationship between *in sacco* and *in vivo* methods for determining forage cell wall digestion in the rumen (Archimède, 1992).

1995). This approach seems to be promising for predicting the fill effect of a feedstuff. However, this equation does not take into account the particle size distribution of the feeds, which is well known to affect the rate of passage, rumen fill and, in turn, ingestibility. The fill effect of large particles can be assumed to be constant, as they cannot flow out of the rumen and their microbial degradation modifies their volume only slightly. The increase in the retention time due to comminution time (CT) of large particles could be estimated by the index of fibrousness, and/or by particle size measurement. The RRT could thus be calculated by the following equation (Faverdin *et al.*, 1995):

$$\text{RRT} = (((1 - a - b)/k_{sp}) + (b/(c + k_{sp})) + \text{CT})/24 \qquad (11.8)$$

where *a*, *b* and *c* are as defined in Equations 11.1 and 11.3 and k_{sp} is the rate of passage of small particles (h^{-1}).

Fibrolytic activity of ruminal microorganisms
The *in sacco* method has been used in research in order to follow the variations in digestive activity of ruminal microorganisms, by measuring variations in

ruminal degradability and/or the degradation rate of a given feedstuff in different conditions varying according to characterics of the animals (species, physiological stage, feeding level, etc.), or to characteristics of the diet (additives, N content, level and nature of concentrate, etc.). In this chapter, only results related to feeding level and energetic supplementation with carbohydrates or lipids are reported as an illustration of the limits of the *in sacco* method for quantifying variations in fibrolytic activity of rumen microorganisms.

The depressive effect of an increasing level of intake on forage fibre ruminal degradation is attributed classically to the decrease in ruminal retention time of particles, without significant variation in microbial fibrolytic activity, as estimated by *in sacco* degradation. However, with an increasing feeding level for sheep, the xylanase and cellulase enzyme activities of solid-associated microorganisms have been shown to decrease in the rumen, without significant variations in the forage fibre degradation rate *in sacco* (Kabré *et al.*, 1994). This result illustrates the lack of sensitivity of the *in sacco* method for the assessment of variations in microbial fibrolytic activity induced by changes in feeding level.

The *in sacco* method has been used extensively for quantification of the associative effects between forage and readily fermentable carbohydrates. However, results have to be interpreted with caution. The amplitude of depression of the fibre degradation rate depends on the variations in microbial fibrolytic activity but also on the nature of the forage in the bag (reviewed by Huhtanen, 1991), and more precisely on the amount and the nature of the cell wall components, carbohydrates and lignin. The effect of a decrease in microbial activity on the cell wall degradation rate depends largely on the accessibility of cell wall components to the enzymes. A relationship has been observed between fibrolytic enzyme activity of solid-associated microorganisms and cell wall polysaccharide degradation rate, but the impact of variations in microbial activity on cell wall degradation appeared to increase with greater accessibility of cell wall components to microbial enzymes (Nozière *et al.*, 1996). In experiments where forage incubated in bags was the same as in the diet, some authors focused on comparisons between *in vivo* and *in sacco* methods, and reported that the *in sacco* method overestimates the decrease in cell wall ruminal digestion for diets supplemented with rapidly or slowly degradable starch or with digestible fibres (Archimède, 1992; Stensig *et al.*, 1994). Nozière and Michalet-Doreau (unpublished data) observed a decrease in fibrolytic enzyme activities of the solid-associated microorganisms in relation to supplementation of the diet with up to 60% barley, and this decrease was more marked in incubated nylon bags containing the dietary hay than in rumen content. Part of these differences can be explained by a more significant decrease in pH inside the bags than in the digesta (Table 11.2). This could be due to an accumulation of end-fermentation products within the bags. Quantification by the *in sacco* method of ruminal digestive interactions induced by fat supplementation has been the subject of

less study. Variations in forage ruminal degradation induced by fat supplements have been shown to be underestimated by the *in sacco* method (Doreau *et al.*, 1991). The depressive effect of lipids on forage degradation is not due to water-soluble factors such as those observed when diets are supplemented with cereals (increase in readily fermentable substrates, drop in pH), but rather to an adsorption of lipids on forage particles which may reduce their microbial colonization in the rumen. It can be expected that lipids do not enter the bag and that the colonization of feed particles within the bags occurs in a normal way.

In conclusion, variations in the fibrolytic activity of solid-associated micro-organisms can be more marked (highly digestible carbohydrates supplementation) or less marked (increase of level of intake, fat supplementation) in the bags than in the rumen. This could be attributed to problems of exchange between the rumen digesta and the bag, including both input of ruminal milieu and output of end-fermentation products.

Conclusions

With N rationing systems for ruminants, the use of the *in sacco* technique to predict dietary N by-pass has become common. A large number of methodological studies have been carried out to pinpoint the factors which vary and their respective importance, and also to establish the limits for use of this technique. At present, the technique is used increasingly to predict not only degradation of feed N in the rumen, but also degradation of other feed components and more especially that of starch and the cell walls of forage.

The principle of the technique means that *in sacco* degradation of feeds represents their degradation *in vivo* if the exchanges between the ruminal milieu and the bag, i.e. the influx of degradation agents and the outflux of microorganisms and of degradation products, are adequate and if the feed components potentially degradable by rumen microorganisms are accessible to the microbial enzymes.

Table 11.2. Differences in pH and fibrolytic enzyme activities in solid-associated microorganisms (μmol reducing sugars released g^{-1} DM h^{-1}) between rumen content and bags, with cows fed various levels of concentrate (Nozière and Michalet-Doreau, unpublished data).

	Barley content of diet (g kg^{-1})		
	0	300	600
pH			
Rumen	7.16	6.99	7.09
Bag	6.64	6.19	5.78
Difference	0.52	0.80	1.31
Avicelase			
Rumen	17.7	23.3	17.7
Bag	15.7	14.3	5.9
Difference	2.0	9.0	11.8
Xylanase			
Rumen	263	318	248
Bag	251	231	69
Difference	12	87	179

The main factors which govern exchanges between the rumen contents and the bag are the bag characteristics, pore size and open area. Recommended procedures are generally agreed between users and relatively well standardized. The problems of exchanges between the bags and the ruminal milieu have become better understood over the past few years due to studies of the microbial ecosystem involving techniques of numeration and enzymology. The main questions which remain today concerning the exchanges between the bag and the ruminal contents are the chemical composition and degradation characteristics of the fraction lost through the pores of the bag, which naturally vary according to the nature of the feed and how to account for microbial contamination relative to dietary N degradability measurements, because this contamination may introduce a non-negligible bias for feedstuffs with little N.

Different degrees of accessibility of components to microbial enzymes may also be at the origin of a bias in classification of feedstuffs according to their degradability in the rumen. Accessibility of components depends on how the sample is presented. Whereas dry feedstuffs are presented in more or less standard fashion

and therefore do not pose any major problems, the same cannot be said for moist feedstuffs and in particular for forage. Lack of knowledge of the dynamic processes involved in accessibility of digestible components to microbial enzymes during and after the lag time is a major hurdle yet to be overcome for more accurate modelling of the degradation processes.

Validation of the *in sacco* technique to predict degradability of dietary N in the rumen is now well established thanks to the concordant studies aimed at establishing the relationship between *in vivo* and *in sacco* measurements. The *in sacco* technique is now also used to predict ruminal degradability of starch and cell walls. However, comparisons between *in vivo* and *in sacco* degradation measurements are few as yet, and this aspect needs to be studied more closely. Finally, in the light of knowledge today, the *in sacco* technique would seem capable of revealing variations in the fibrolytic activity of ruminal microorganisms in relation to changes in the diet, the level of intake, etc., but not of quantifying them. Indeed, the variations in *in sacco* degradation amplify or minimize the variations in fibrolytic activity according to changes in dietary conditions.

References

Archimède, H. (1992) Etude des facteurs impliqués dans les interactions digestives entre les fourrages et les aliments concentrés chez les ruminants. Thèse, Institut National Agronomique Paris-Grignon, France.

Beauchemin, K.A., Mc Allister, T.A., Dong, Y., Farr, B.I. and Cheng, K.J. (1994) Effects of mastication on digestion of whole cereal grains by cattle. *Journal of Animal Science* 72, 236–246.

Beckers, Y., Thewis, A., Madoux, B. and François, E. (1995) Studies on the *in situ* nitrogen degradability corrected for bacterial contamination of concentrate feeds in steers. *Journal of Animal Science* 73, 220–227.

Cherney, D.J.R., Patterson, J.A. and Lemenager, R.P. (1990) Influence of *in situ* rinsing technique on determination of dry matter disappearance. *Journal of Dairy Science* 73, 391–397.

Craig, W.M., Brown, D.R., Broderick, G.A. and Ricker, D.B. (1987) Post-prandial compositional changes of fluid- and particle-associated ruminal microorganisms. *Journal of Animal Science* 65, 1042–1048.

De Boer, G., Murphy, J.J. and Kennelly, J.J. (1987) Mobile nylon bag for estimating intestinal availability of rumen indegradable protein. *Journal of Dairy Science* 70, 977–982.

Dehority, B.A. and Orpin, C.G. (1988) Development of, and natural fluctuations in, rumen microbial populations. In: Hobson, P.N. (ed.) *The Rumen Microbial Ecosystem*. Elsevier Applied Science, London and New York, pp. 151–183.

Dhanoa, M.S. (1988) On the analysis of dacron bag data for low degradability feeds. *Grass and Forage Science* 43, 441–444.

Doreau, M., Chilliard, Y., Bauchart, D. and Michalet-Doreau, B. (1991) Influence of different fat supplements on digestibility and ruminal digestion in cows. *Annales de Zootechnie* 40, 19–30.

Dulphy, J.P., Demarquilly, C., Baumont, R., Jailler, M., L'Hotelier, L. and Dragomir, C. (1999) Study of modes of preparation of fresh and conserved forage samples for measurement of their dry matter and nitrogen degradation in the rumen. *Annales de Zootechnie* 48, 275–288.

Emanuele, S.M. and Staples, C.R. (1988) Effect of forage particle size on *in situ* digestion kinetics. *Journal of Dairy Science* 71, 1947–1954.

Faverdin, P., Baumont, R. and Ingvartsen, K.L. (1995) Control and prediction of feed intake in ruminants. In: Journet, M., Grenet, E., Farce, M.H., Thériez, M. and Demarquilly, C. (eds) *Recent Developments in the Nutrition of Herbivores. Proceedings of the IVth International Symposium on the Nutrition of Herbivores*. INRA Editions, Paris, France, pp. 95–120.

Gerson, T., King, A.S.D., Kelly, K.E. and Kelly, W.J. (1988) Influence of particle size and surface area on *in vitro* rate of gas production, lipolysis of triacylglycerol and hydrogenation of linoleic acid by sheep rumen digesta or *Ruminococcus flavefaciens*. *Journal of Agricultural Science, Cambridge* 110, 31–37.

Hof, G., Kouwenberg, W.J.A. and Tamminga, S. (1990) The effect of washing procedure on the estimation of the *in situ* disappearance of amino acids from feed protein. *Netherlands Journal of Agricultural Science* 38, 719–724.

Huhtanen, P. (1991) Associative effects of feeds in ruminants. *Norwegian Journal of Agricultural Science* 5 (Suppl.), 37–57.

Huntington, G.B. (1997) Starch utilization by ruminants: from basics to the bunk. *Journal of Animal Science* 75, 852–867.

Huntington, J.A. and Givens, D.I. (1995) The *in situ* technique for studying the rumen degradation of feeds: a review of the procedure. *Nutrition Abstracts and Reviews (Series B)* 65, 63–93.

Huntington, J.A. and Givens, D.I. (1997) Studies on *in situ* degradation of feeds in the rumen: 1 – effect of species, bag motility and incubation sequence on dry matter disappearance. *Animal Feed Science and Technology* 64, 227–241.

Hvelplund, T. (1985) Digestibility of rumen microbial protein and undegraded dietary protein estimated in the small intestine of sheep and by sacco technique. *Acta Agriculturae Scandinavica, Supplement* 25, 132–144.

Kabré, P., Martin, C. and Michalet-Doreau, B. (1994) Enzyme activities of rumen solid-adherent microorganisms in chronically underfed ewes. *Journal of the Science of Food and Agriculture* 65, 423–428.

Kamel, H.E.M., Sekine, J., Suga, T. and Morita, Z. (1995) The effect of frozen–rethawing technique on detaching firmly associated bacteria from *in situ* hay residues. *Canadian Journal of Animal Science* 75, 481–483.

Kristensen, E.S., Moller, P.D. and Hvelplund, T. (1982) Estimation of the effective protein degradability in the rumen of cows using the nylon bag technique combined with the outflow rate. *Acta Agriculturae Scandinavica* 32, 123–127.

Lecomte, P., Kamoun, M., Agneessens, R., Beckers, Y., Dardenne, P., Thewis, A. and François, E. (1994) Approach to the use of near infrared spectrometry for the estimation of microbial nitrogen contamination of forages during ruminal incubation of nylon bag. *Proceedings of the Society of Nutrition Physiology* 3, 44 (abstract).

Lindberg, J.E., Kaspersson, A. and Ciszuk, P. (1984) Studies of pH, number of protozoa and microbial ATP concentrations in rumen-incubated nylon bags with different pore sizes. *Journal of Agricultural Science, Cambridge* 102, 501–504.

Lopez, S., Hovell, F.D. DeB., Manyuchi, B. and Smart, R.I. (1995) Comparison of sample preparation methods for the determination of the rumen degradation characteristics of fresh and ensiled forages by the nylon bag technique. *Animal Science* 60, 439–450.

Madsen, J. and Hvelplund, T. (1985) Protein degradation in the rumen. *Acta Agriculturae Scandinavica, Supplement* 25, 103–124.

Madsen, J. and Hvelplund, T. (1994) Prediction of *in situ* protein degradability in the rumen. Results of a European ringtest. *Livestock Production Science* 39, 201–212.

Marinucci, M.T., Dehority, B.A. and Loerch, S.C. (1992) *In vitro* and *in vivo* studies of factors affecting digestion of feeds in synthetic fibre bags. *Journal of Animal Science* 70, 296–307.

Martin, C., Devillard, E. and Michalet-Doreau, B. (1999) Influence of sampling site on concentrations and carbohydrate-degrading enzyme activities of protozoa and bacteria in the rumen. *Journal of Animal Science* 77, 979–987.

Martin, C., Michalet-Doreau, B., Fonty, G. and Williams, A. (1993) Postprandial variations in the activity of polysaccharide-degrading enzymes of fluid- and particle-associated ruminal microbial populations. *Current Microbiology* 27, 223–228.

Mehrez, A.Z. and Ørskov, E.R. (1977) A study of the artificial fibre bag technique for determining the digestibility of feeds in the rumen. *Journal of Agricultural Science, Cambridge* 88, 645–650.

Merry, R.J. and McAllan, A.B. (1983) A comparison of the chemical composition of mixed bacteria harvested from the liquid and solid fractions of rumen digesta. *British Journal of Nutrition* 50, 701–709.

Mertens, D.R. (1993) Kinetics of cell wall digestion and passage in ruminants. In: Jung, H.G., Buxton, D.R., Hatfield, R.D. and Ralph, J. (eds) *Forage Cell Wall Structure and Digestibility*. American Society of Agronomy, Crop Science Society of America and the Soil Science Society of America, Madison, Wisconsin, pp. 535–570.

Meyer, J.H.F. and Mackie, R.I. (1986) Microbiological evaluation of the intraruminal *in sacculus* digestion technique. *Applied and Environmental Microbiology* 51, 622–629.

Michalet-Doreau, B. (1990) New methods for estimating forage feed values: in sacco. In: *XVIth International Grassland Congress*, Nice. AFPF, INRA, Route de St-Cyr, Versailles, France, pp. 1850–1852.

Michalet-Doreau, B. and Cerneau, P. (1991) Influence of foodstuff particle size on *in situ* degradation of nitrogen in the rumen. *Animal Feed Science and Technology* 35, 69–81.

Michalet-Doreau, B. and Nozière, P. (1998) Validation of *in situ* nitrogen degradation measurements: comparative proteolytic activity of solid-adherent microorganisms isolated from rumen content and nylon bags containing various feeds. *Animal Feed Science and Technology* 70, 41–47.

Michalet-Doreau, B. and Ould-Bah, M.Y. (1992) *In vitro* and *in sacco* methods for the estimation of dietary nitrogen degradability in the rumen: a review. *Animal Feed Science and Technology* 40, 57–86.

Nocek, J.E. (1985) Evaluation of specific variables affecting *in situ* estimates of ruminal dry matter and protein digestion. *Journal of Animal Science* 60, 1347–1358.

Nocek, J.E. and Kohn, R.A. (1988) *In situ* particle size reduction of alfalfa and timothy hay as influenced by form and particle size. *Journal of Dairy Science* 71, 932–945.

Nordin, N.Y. and Campling, R.C. (1976) Digestibility studies with cows given whole and rolled cereal grains. *Animal Production* 23, 305–315.

Nozière, P. and Michalet-Doreau, B. (1996) Validation of *in sacco* method: influence of sampling site, nylon bag or rumen contents, on fibrolytic activity of solid-associated microorganisms. *Animal Feed Science and Technology* 57, 203–210.

Nozière, P. and Michalet-Doreau, B. (1997) Effects of amount and availability of starch on amylolytic activity of ruminal solid-associated microorganisms. *Journal of the Science of Food and Agriculture* 73, 471–476.

Nozière, P., Besle, J.M., Martin, C. and Michalet-Doreau, B. (1996) Effect of barley supplement on microbial fibrolytic enzyme activities and cell wall degradation rate in the rumen. *Journal of the Science of Food and Agriculture* 72, 235–242.

Olubobokun, J.A. and Craig, W.M. (1990) Quantity and characteristics of microorganisms associated with ruminal fluid or particles. *Journal of Animal Science* 68, 3360–3370.

Olubobokun, J.A., Craig, W.M. and Pond, K.R. (1990) Effects of mastication and microbial contamination in ruminal *in situ* forage disappearance. *Journal of Animal Science* 68, 3371–3381.

Ørskov, E.R. and McDonald, I. (1979) The estimation of protein degradability in the rumen from incubation measurements weighted according to rate of passage. *Journal of Agricultural Science, Cambridge* 92, 499–503.

Philippeau, C. and Michalet-Doreau, B. (1997) Influence of genotype and stage of maturity of maize on rate of ruminal starch degradation. *Animal Feed Science and Technology* 68, 25–35.

Poncet, C., Michalet-Doreau, B., McAllister, T. and Rémond, D. (1995) Dietary compounds escaping rumen digestion. In: Journet, M., Grenet, E., Farce, M.H., Thériez, M. and Demarquilly, C. (eds) *Recent Developments in the Nutrition of Herbivores. Proceedings of the IVth International Symposium on the Nutrition of Herbivores.* INRA Editions, Paris, France, pp. 167–204.

Poncet, C., Rémond, D., Bernard, L. and Peyronnet, C. (1998) Nitrogen value of protein and leguminous seeds in ruminants: ruminal degradability of raw and extruded pea and lupin. *Third European Conference on Grain Legumes.* Valladolid, Spain.

Quin, J.I., van der Wath, J.G. and Myburgh, S. (1939) Studies on the alimentary tract of merino sheep in South Africa. IV. Description of experimental technique. *Onderstepoort Journal of Veterinary Science and Animal Industry* 11, 341–360.

SAS Institute (1985) *SAS User's Guide: Statistics.* SAS Institute, Inc., Cary, North Carolina.

Sauvant, D. (1997) Rumen mathematical modelling. In: Hobson, P.N. and Stewart, C.S. (eds) *The Rumen Microbial Ecosystem.* Blackie Academic & Professional, London, pp. 685–708.

Sauvant, D., Chapoutot, P. and Archimède, H. (1994) La digestion des amidons par les ruminants et ses conséquences. *Productions Animales* 7, 115–124.

Stensig, T., Weisbjerg, M.R., Madsen, J. and Hvelplund, T. (1994) Estimation of voluntary feed intake from *in sacco* degradation and rate of passage of DM or DNF. *Livestock Production Science* 39, 49–52.

Strizler, N.P., Hvelplund, T.A. and Woelstrup, J. (1990) The influence of the position in the rumen on dry matter disappearance from nylon bags. *Acta Agriculturae Scandinavica* 40, 363–366.

Vérité, R., Chapoutot, P., Michalet-Doreau, B., Peyraud, J.L. and Poncet, C. (1987) Révision du système des protéines digestibles dans l'intestin (PDI). *Bulletin Technique CRZV Theix, INRA* 70, 19–34.

Wanderley, R.C., Huber, J.T., Wu, Z., Pessarakli, M. and Fontes, C., Jr (1993) Influence of microbial colonization of feed particles on determination of nitrogen degradability by *in situ* incubation. *Journal of Animal Science* 71, 3073–3077.

Weakley, D.C., Stern, M.D. and Satter, L.D. (1983) Factors affecting disappearance of feedstuffs from bags suspended in the rumen. *Journal of Animal Science* 56, 493–507.

Williams, A.P. and Cockburn, J.E. (1991) Effect of slowly and rapidly degraded protein sources on the concentrations of amino acids and peptides in the rumen of steers. *Journal of the Science of Food and Agriculture* 56, 303–314.

Chapter 12
Use of Markers

J.P. Marais

*Biochemistry Section, KwaZulu-Natal Department of Agriculture,
Pietermaritzburg, Republic of South Africa*

Introduction

The productivity of animals and ultimately the profitability of farm animal enterprises are closely linked to the nutrition of the animal which, in turn, is determined by the amount of feed consumed and the nutritive value of the diet. The accurate measurement of dry matter intake and the degree of selection of specific plant species in mixed pastures by the grazing animal are vital for evaluating the energy balance of the animal. The nutritive value of the feed is determined by its chemical composition and the degree to which these chemical substances are transformed in the gut into nutrients required by the animal. Fibre digestibility is determined by the potential extent and rate of digestion, and rate of passage. Microbial protein synthesis is the main source of α-amino nitrogen supply to the ruminant and is of particular importance for diet formulation of ruminants. The measurement of digesta volume and flow through the gut or through segments of the digestive tract provides information regarding the quantity of feed components in the gut and the efficiency of their utilization by the animal. These measurements, used for optimizing animal production, can all be made routinely by means of techniques using indigestible marker substances which are quantified in the faeces or in segments of the digestive tract, depending on the purpose of the study. This chapter is a critical evaluation of the more commonly used markers in animal nutrition.

Properties of Markers

Ideal markers are indigestible substances not absorbed or affected by the digestive tract. They should also not affect or be affected by the microbial population in the tract. Markers must be closely associated with or physically similar to the undigested nutrient in question, or must flow through the digestive tract at an identical rate and not separate from the respective labelled fractions. Attachment of a particle-bound marker is critical in digestive segments such as the rumen where particle flow varies, but adherence becomes less critical post-ruminally, where variation in particle flow is small. Furthermore, highly sensitive and specific analytical methods for quantifying markers must be available. The sensitivity of analysis determines the amount of marked material administered in order to obtain acceptable results, without exceeding the marker-binding capacity of the feed particles. Minor changes in marker concentration may have marked effects on kinetic estimates obtained from complex mathematical models.

No existing marker totally satisfies all requirements. Some particulate markers tend to migrate to particles not initially labelled. In this respect, liquid markers are generally more satisfactory than particulate markers. Marker migration is of concern because the label being followed would be unrelated to the component originally marked. Unless the integrity of the marked feed particle has been established, pool sizes and rate of passage should be discussed in terms of the marker employed, and not the fraction initially marked. Some markers such as lignin may be partly metabolizable and may therefore not be suitable for estimating residence time, since disappearance is not proportional to residence time. Some markers are slightly absorbable in the gastrointestinal tract, and are therefore not totally recoverable in the faeces. Finely milled particles used for labelling may pass from the rumen more quickly than feed particles as they are not delayed for reduction in size. Mordanted particles may also pass very rapidly from the rumen, due to their high density. Because binding affinities vary among feed components, feeds may be labelled unevenly. The importance of marker criteria such as indigestibility, however, depends entirely on the use to which the marker is put. Markers should therefore be selected with discretion in order to avoid serious errors in interpreting results. Markers are classified as internal or external markers.

Internal Markers

An internal marker is a chosen substance which forms an integral part of the forage or feed consumed by the animal. Internal markers have the advantage of being cheap and convenient, and may be particularly useful in experimentation with wild or free-ranging animals, which are difficult to dose with external markers. Although many internal markers appear promising, few have gained acceptance, mainly because the marker in the diet may be different from the marker analysed in the faeces due to changes occurring during digestion. Furthermore, erratic results frequently have been reported in evaluation studies of internal markers by different laboratories, or when a marker is applied across a wide range of forages. Of the internal markers, the alkanes have the most widespread application for estimating organic matter digestibility and forage species selection under grazing conditions, while purines appear to be the most promising for predicting microbial protein synthesis in the rumen.

Indigestible acid detergent fibre (IADF)

The usefulness of indigestible fibre as an internal marker has been limited by a lack of standardized analytical procedures. The treatment of plant material with neutral and acid detergents produces a fraction known as lignocellulose or acid detergent fibre (ADF) (Van Soest, 1963). IADF is determined gravimetrically after incubating ADF with cellulases for 10–14 days (Penning and Johnson, 1983), after rumen fluid fermentation in vitro for 4 days or after incubation in nylon bags in the rumen for 6–8 days. These fractions should, theoretically, be totally indigestible, rendering them suitable as markers, but in practice variable results are often obtained. Furthermore, faecal recoveries of in vitro IADF of 0.46 and 0.99, and recoveries of cellulase IADF of 0.47 and 0.97, were obtained with immature tall fescue and lucerne cubes, respectively, indicating that IADF fractions should be used with caution as markers in immature forage (Cochran et al., 1986).

Indigestible lignin

Because mammals do not appear to contain enzyme systems capable of degrading polymerized phenolic compounds, lignin should theoretically be indigestible and suitable as an internal marker. However, lignin has a complex structure, the chemical properties of which may vary from plant to plant and even from one plant part to another. A shortcoming of lignin as a marker is its low and inconsistent recovery in the faeces. Furthermore, lignin can give positive faecal recoveries by binding to components of indeterminate nature (Thewis *et al.*, 1989). Acid detergent lignin recoveries of between 0.52 and 1.16 were found by Cochran *et al.* (1986).

Acid detergent lignin is determined gravimetrically after cellulose has been removed from ADF by treatment with 26 M sulphuric acid and the ash content has been deducted (Van Soest, 1963). Alkaline peroxide lignin, a less digestible lignin fraction, prepared by treating the sample with alkaline hydrogen peroxide before the acid detergent step in the acid detergent lignin procedure, was proposed as internal marker for digestibility predictions. However, Momont *et al.* (1994) showed that although alkaline peroxide lignin was nearly totally recoverable from the faeces, the results on mature prairie grass hay were variable and adversely affected dry matter intake predictions. It was concluded that alkaline peroxide lignin does not appear to improve the accuracy of predicting the dry matter digestibility of grasses over acid detergent lignin (Sunvold and Cochran, 1991).

Insoluble ash

Acid-insoluble ash is often used as an indigestible marker for estimating apparent metabolizable energy in chickens and digestibility in ruminants. It is prepared by drying and ashing the sample, and boiling the ashed sample in 2 M hydrochloric acid for 5 min. The ash content is determined gravimetrically after the hot hydrolysate has been filtered, washed free of acid and re-ashed (Van Keulen and Young, 1977). Contamination of feed and faeces samples with dust or soil could lead to erroneous results.

Odd-chain n-alkanes

Plant *n*-alkanes are simple straight-chain hydrocarbons with carbon chain lengths ranging from pentacosane (C_{25}) to pentatriacontane (C_{35}). They are components of the cuticular wax layer covering all higher plants and occur in plant material mainly as odd-chain molecules. Individual alkanes in plants differ in concentration, resulting in each plant having a unique alkane profile, with hentriacontane (C_{31}) and tritriacontane (C_{33}) usually as the major components (Table 12.1). Alkanes are associated predominantly with the particulate matter in digesta, and some are virtually quantitatively excreted in the faeces. Their stability in the digestive tract of the ruminant appears to increase with the size of the molecule. The recovery in the faeces of C_{33} is about 0.87, while that of C_{35} has been estimated at 0.95. Alkanes appear to be completely stable in the digestive tract of mountain hares. Natural alkanes are used to estimate digestibility and species selection by the grazing animal.

Separation of alkanes from plant or faeces samples involves saponification in alcoholic potassium hydroxide and extraction with non-polar solvents such as heptane (Dillon and Stakelum, 1990). The extracted alkanes are purified by means of a silica gel column, and the alkanes are separated and quantified by means of capillary gas chromatography (Dove and Mayes, 1991).

2,6-Diaminopimelic acid (DAPA)

DAPA is an amino acid occurring in varying concentrations in bacterial cells. Since the DAPA to protein ratios of mixed ruminal bacteria are relatively constant, it has become the most commonly used internal marker for estimating microbial protein synthesis (Czerkawski, 1974). Broderick and Merchen (1992) pointed out that this marker has many serious shortcomings. Because DAPA only occurs in microbial cell walls, the DAPA to protein ratio could change depending on microbial cell size and shape. Of greater importance is the occurrence of substantial amounts of DAPA in certain feed

Table 12.1. Alkane profiles of a selection of forage species.

Species	Alkane content (mg kg^{-1} dry matter)								
	C_{27}	C_{29}	C_{30}	C_{31}	C_{32}	C_{33}	C_{34}	C_{35}	Total
Digitaria eriantha	28	32	0	37	4	24	1	4	130
Festuca arundinacea	48	278	0	594	12	114	0	0	1046
Lolium multiflorum	34	248	0	350	12	100	0	0	744
Lolium perenne	15	63	0	114	10	101	4	16	323
Paspalum dilatatum	3	7	0	36	3	16	1	2	68
Pennisetum clandestinum	17	29	7	124	9	300	13	241	740
Plantago lanceolata	47	34	0	24	0	9	0	0	114
Setaria sphacelata	40	116	6	68	1	7	0	0	238
Trifolium repens	34	168	40	443	46	134	6	15	886

sources. The DAPA to N ratio in common feedstuffs such as soybean meal could be as high as 37% of that in isolated rumen bacteria (Rahnema and Theurer, 1986). Abomasal DAPA flows should therefore be corrected for dietary DAPA intake. Due to catabolic activity, a varying and often large proportion (>50%) of DAPA leaving the rumen may not be associated with the bacterial fraction and may be free or in a non-cell-bound peptidal form (Masson et al., 1991). Disproportionately high DAPA outflow from the rumen may lead to overestimates of bacterial protein yields. High values obtained may also be due to the analytical procedure used.

It is difficult to resolve DAPA from other amino acids by means of the conventional amino acid analyser technique using a ninhydrin reagent at pH 5.5. However, by manipulating the pH of the eluting buffer, it can be separated from most interfering amino acids (Rahnema and Theurer, 1986; Sadik et al., 1990). DAPA can also be quantified by means of an amino acid analyser after converting interfering methionine to methionine sulphone with performic acid (Ibrahim et al., 1970).

D-Alanine

D-Alanine is more widely distributed among bacterial species than DAPA and forms part of the oligopeptides cross-linking bacterial cell wall peptidoglycans. It is often not present in feed samples and has been used successfully to estimate bacterial protein synthesis and flow (Garrett et al., 1987). However, reports of bacterial protein flow values exceeding total protein flow when estimates were based on D-alanine question its usefulness as a bacterial protein marker (Quigley and Schwab, 1988). It can be assayed by colorimetric procedures (Quigley and Schwab, 1988), or by means of an amino acid analyser.

Nucleic acids

High concentrations of nucleic acids, particularly RNAs in microorganisms, led to their recognition as potential rumen bacterial protein markers. Nucleic acids in digesta samples are often analysed as the purine bases, adenine and guanine, or their derivatives (mainly allantoin) by means of high-performance liquid chromatography (Balcells et al., 1992), or after perchloric acid hydrolysis of the sample (Martin Orue et al., 1995). Invasive techniques requiring experimental animals fitted with cannulas in the rumen and proximal duodenum are normally used for measuring protein flow. Recently, non-invasive methods based on the urinary excretion of purine derivatives such as allantoin have been developed (Perez et al., 1996).

External Markers

External markers are indigestible substances which are added or bonded to the feed or digesta. These markers commonly are administered by mouth, through fistulas or by means of controlled-release devices. Controlled-release devices offer the advantage of eliminating the need for repeated daily dosing or the continuous use of faecal bags during total faecal collection, which could interfere with normal animal behaviour. However, problems associated with these devices sometimes result in a lack of consistency in faecal output predictions (Buntinx *et al.*, 1992). Controlled-release devices often appear to overestimate faecal output when the manufacturer's prescribed release rates are used for calculations. External markers are administered either as a single pulse dose or continuously or frequently over a period of time in an attempt to reach steady-state conditions under which the digesta is labelled uniformly and the ratio of digesta to marker is constant. The time required for the excretion of a marker to reach a steady-state depends on the diet and the type of animal. An adaptation period usually of between 6 and 8 days for sheep and cattle is required before the experimental period.

Transition metals

Oxides and salts of trivalent and tetravalent metals such as titanium, chromium, cobalt, ruthenium and hafnium have characteristics of inert markers and have been used as such with varying degrees of success. Of these, chromium has been most widely employed.

Chromium
CHROMIUM SESQUIOXIDE (CR_2O_3). Chromium oxide is practically insoluble in water, but slightly soluble in alkalis and acids, and is one of the most commonly used markers for estimating faecal output. It is administered orally to ruminants, by means of gelatin capsules, or mixed with the ration. A controlled-release device for the continuous delivery of Cr_2O_3 to the ruminant is also available. The chromium release rate in the rumen has been shown to increase with decreasing dry matter digestibility of the feed and also varies from one animal to another, but not between devices within the same animal

(Pond *et al.*, 1990). These workers concluded that controlled-release devices are unsuitable for the accurate estimation of the intake of individual animals, but are suitable for mean animal intakes in group situations.

CHROMIUM MORDANTS. Trivalent and tetravalent metals, such as chromium, which form strong ligands with plant cell wall components, are commonly bonded onto fibre to form mordants used as particulate markers. Since the stable coordinate bonds of trivalent chromium result in slow rates of ligand exchange, chromium mordants are prepared preferably by reducing hexavalent dichromate compounds with ascorbic acid, rather than from the trivalent salts. However, the hydroxides of most of these elements, which are insoluble at rumen pH, make it difficult to establish whether the element is moving as a complex with the food ingredients or separately as the insoluble hydroxide. In order to give reliable results, metal mordants must be recovered on the plant matrix to which they are bonded.

Prior to mordanting, soluble interfering substances, which could reduce the binding of chromium to the fibre, should be removed by treating small batches of plant material with neutral detergents such as lauryl sulphate (Van Soest, 1963; Udén *et al.*, 1980). Larger batches could either be sealed in a cloth bag and put through the laundering cycle of a washing machine, or could be boiled in a laundry detergent in a large pressure cooker. The fibre preparations or neutral detergent residues (NDRs) should be rinsed thoroughly in water and acetone, and dried at 65°C.

Although chromium binds firmly to particulate matter, it may adversely affect particulate passage due to the increased density of the feed (Ehle *et al.*, 1984) and by rendering the cell wall virtually indigestible (Faichney and Griffiths, 1978; Udén *et al.*, 1980). Due to limited fermentation, the passage rate of chromium-mordanted neutral detergent fibre (Cr-NDF) particles has been shown to be significantly slower than more digestible tritium-labelled particles (Van Bruchem *et al.*, 1990). Udén *et al.* (1980) mordanted plant fibre in a solution with chromium at a concentration of 120–140 g kg^{-1} of fibre. In many subsequent studies, the chromium concentration in mordanting solutions was reduced to decrease the chromium content of mordants and minimize changes in feed density. Chromium concentrations of 10 g kg^{-1} on hay and 23 g kg^{-1} on feed pellets were considered sufficiently low not to affect adversely the density and kinetics of the feed in the digestive tract (Moore *et al.*, 1992). However, the disappearance from nylon bags in the rumen of silage and hay containing chromium at a concentration of 31 and 23 g kg^{-1} dry matter, respectively, was reduced by 36.7 and 56.4%, respectively (Beauchemin and Buchanan-Smith, 1989).

The digestibility of mordanted plant material has a marked effect on the recovery of marker in the faeces. The lowest recovery is associated with samples with the highest digestibility. Furthermore, the particle size of Cr-NDF has a marked effect on determined passage rates. A particle size of 0.6–1.0 mm gave a fractional passage rate of 2.0% h^{-1}, compared with a passage rate of 4.1% h^{-1} for particles <0.3 mm (Bruining and Bosch, 1992).

CHROMIUM-ETHYLENEDIAMINE TETRAACETIC ACID (CR-EDTA). Cr-EDTA, which is readily soluble in water, is used as a liquid phase marker. Udén *et al.* (1980) prepared Cr-EDTA as its lithium salt (the only salt that could be crystallized) by dissolving chromium(III)acetate monohydrate, EDTA and lithium hydroxide monohydrate in water on a steam bath. Cr-EDTA was crystallized by cooling and the addition of ethanol. The compound gave a yield of about 90% and was stable to drying at 100°C. Cr-EDTA is usually infused continuously into the rumen (Remillard *et al.*, 1990). If radiolabelled ^{51}Cr-EDTA is used, it is first diluted with carrier Cr-EDTA.

Like polyethylene glycol (PEG), Cr-EDTA is slightly absorbable through the rumen wall, but occupies a larger fluid space in the rumen than PEG. It is affected by fluctuations in osmotic pressure which could lead to an overestimation of the inflow or outflow of ruminal water. Low concentrations of Cr-EDTA may also bind to particulate matter in the rumen.

Chromium can be analysed by means of a titrimetric procedure (Christian and Coup, 1954), by spectrophotometry (Fenton and Fenton, 1979) or by atomic absorption spectrophotometry (Arthur, 1970). Unlabelled chromium can also be assayed as ^{51}Cr after neutron activation (Udén *et al.*, 1980) or plasma emission spectroscopy (Combs and Satter, 1992). Since ^{31}Si, the main contaminant, has a half-life of only 2.6 h, it does not interfere with the analysis. Advantages of this method are that radioactive contamination of animals is avoided and the dry faecal samples can be counted without prior preparation.

Cobalt

Cobalt-ethylenediamine tetraacetic acid (Co-EDTA) is prepared either as the sodium or lithium salt of the monovalent Co-EDTA anion (Udén *et al.*, 1980). The yield of LiCo-EDTA was about 90%, which was higher than the yield of the sodium salt. Both salts are stable to drying at 100°C. Cobalt is quantified by atomic absorption spectrophotometry, by neutron activation analysis or by plasma emission spectroscopy (Combs and Satter, 1992).

Ruthenium

Ruthenium is used as a particulate marker, usually in the form of ruthenium phenanthroline (Ru-phe), which has no adverse effects on the metabolic activity of the rumen microbiota at the concentrations used (Tan *et al.*, 1971). It is prepared by converting ruthenium chloride to potassium pentachlorohydroxyruthenate and refluxing the hydroxyruthenate with 1,10-phenanthroline and hypophosphite to form Ru-phenanthroline chloride (Tan *et al.*, 1971).

Ru-phe is infused continuously into the rumen, often as the isotope, ^{103}Ru-phe, or administered as a single dose. The dose can be prepared by dissolving the marker in water, mixing it with milled grass in a plastic syringe with a wide nozzle, and leaving it soaking overnight before administering it directly into the rumen. Administered Ru-phe is strongly adsorbed by the particulate fraction of the digesta. It is not absorbed to any significant extent in the digestive tract, and 93–102% is recovered in the faeces, while <0.4% is excreted in the urine of sheep (Tan *et al.*, 1971).

Ruthenium is assayed by atomic absorption spectroscopy or the isotope is measured by autogamma spectrometry. As ^{103}Ru-phe and ^{51}Cr-EDTA can be assayed simultaneously, these markers conveniently may be used together as particulate and fluid marker, respectively.

Titanium

Titanium oxide is insoluble in water and dilute acid and is not taken up into plants to any extent. It has no detrimental effect on sheep if ingested at a concentration of 2–3 g day^{-1}, and is completely excreted in the faeces (98% recovery). Titanium is assayed spectrophotometrically after oxidation with hydrogen peroxide (Brandt *et al.*, 1983).

Hafnium

Hafnium binds strongly to forages and concentrates, and is resistant to displacement in acidic media (pH 2) (Worley, 1987). It may therefore be a useful marker in acidic segments of the digestive tract. Because of its strong binding capacity (up to 5% of the dry matter), the concentration of hafnium used for mordanting feeds must be restricted in order to avoid an adverse increase in the density of the marked feed and an excessive reduction in digestibility. Its strong binding properties should render hafnium a suitable marker for concentrate feeds.

Rare earth elements

The rare earth elements appear to be indigestible and are not absorbed from the gastrointestinal tract of mammals. Several of these metals, such as lanthanum,

cerium, neodymium, samarium, europium, dysprosium, erbium and ytterbium, have been bound to plant material and used as indigestible markers. Since the rare earths give identical digesta kinetic estimates, they can be used for marking different particles (Quiroz *et al.*, 1988) or different ingredients (Moore *et al.*, 1990) in a single experiment. The strength of binding to fibre particles depends on the method of application. Spraying rare earths onto feed particles results in the saturation of strong as well as weak binding sites (Mader *et al.*, 1984) and can lead to substantial dissociation of the marker in the digestive tract unless the loosely bound marker is removed by thorough rinsing. The marker is prepared by soaking feed samples overnight in a solution of rare earth nitrate, acetate or chloride, rinsing in tap water and drying in a forced-air oven (Beauchemin and Buchanan-Smith, 1989; Remillard *et al.*, 1990; Moore *et al.*, 1992). A method has been developed in which rare earths are bound to feed particles in the presence of a soluble ligand such as citrate, ensuring that rare earths only attach to the strongest binding sites, thus preventing exchange during passage through the digestive tract (Faichney *et al.*, 1989).

There are relatively large differences among rare earth elements in their binding affinities. Ytterbium tends to form the strongest complexes with feed samples. Trivalent cerium does not form stable complexes with plant fibre. However, stable complexes are formed with tetravalent cerium. Dissociation losses appear to be minimal during a 24 h incubation period if concentrations of rare earths lower than the binding capacity of the fibre particles (<0.18%) are applied to feed samples (Hartnell and Satter, 1979; Teeter *et al.*, 1984).

The marker also tends to dissociate from the feed particle and migrate to unlabelled particles and soluble components in the digestive tract, especially in an acidic environment such as the abomasum (Crooker *et al.*, 1982). Displacement is of little consequence in digesta flow studies involving ruminants since no variation in flow between solute and particulate matter occurs in the acidic segment of the digestive tract. During *in vitro* incubation of ytterbium- or dysprosium-marked feeds, 6–23% of the marker dissociated from the particles, but only 0.3–1.4% of the marker re-associated with unmarked feeds, suggesting that dissociated marker largely passes with the liquid fraction of the digesta.

If rare earths (or any other marker) are used for estimating particle mean retention time, marker should only be applied to particles with a narrow size range. Faichney *et al.* (1989) described a wet-sieving procedure for sieving rumen digesta through a stack of vibrating sieves and using only one particle size fraction for labelling with marker. Marker can be administered by means of gelatin capsules or can be incorporated directly into the feed. Rare earths are analysed by atomic absorption spectrophotometry after wet ashing (Quiroz *et al.*, 1988; Luginbuhl *et al.*, 1994), by neutron activation analysis (Kennelly *et al.*, 1980) or by plasma emission spectroscopy (Combs and Satter, 1992). Cerium was also estimated by ashing the sample, oxidizing it to the Ce(IV) form and titrating it against ammonium iron(III) sulphate, using *O*-phenanthroline as indicator. Methods for extracting rare earths to avoid ashing have been developed (Hart and Polan, 1984).

Even-chain n-alkanes

Even-chain alkanes occur in plants in low concentrations only, but are available commercially and can be administered suspended on cellulose powder in gelatin capsules (Dove and Mayes, 1991; Vulich *et al.*, 1991), as alkane-impregnated shredded filter paper or paper stoppers (Giráldez *et al.*, 1997) or as an aqueous suspension of alkane-impregnated grass particles (Marais *et al.*, 1996). In some instances, even-chain alkane marker can be sprayed onto the forage (Mayes *et al.*, 1997). An intraruminal controlled-release device has also been developed and evaluated for sheep, and gave a constant release of even-chain alkane within 1.5–4.0% of the nominal release value and a coefficient of variation of release rate between animals of 4.07% (Dove *et al.*, 1991). Dotriacontane (C_{32}) is the most commonly used external alkane marker and has a recovery in the faeces of about 87%. Even- and odd-chain alkanes are quantified simultaneously by means of capillary gas chromatography.

Polyethylene glycol (PEG)

PEG is used as a liquid marker, but it has been shown to be excluded from a large proportion of water in beet tissue when used at a molecular weight of 4000 Da (Czerkawski and Breckenridge, 1969), and is precipitated by feeds rich in tannins (Kay, 1969). PEG is infused continuously into the rumen (De Smet *et al.*, 1992), and has a recovery in faeces and digesta of sheep and rabbits of about 95%, suggesting the partial absorption of PEG in the digestive tract. PEG in the liquid phases of undiluted digesta and faeces is assayed by turbidimetry according to Malawer and Powell (1967).

Bacterial spores

Bacillus stearothermophillus spores have been used to measure the rate of passage of both liquid and solid particles in a single procedure (Mir *et al.*, 1997). Bacterial spores were isolated from commercially available ampoules and cultured on agar plates. Cells and spores were washed from the plates and further propagated by repeated rounds of shock treatment in boiling water, and culturing on agar. Following administration to heifers or steers of the bacterial suspension containing 10^8 spores, rumen contents were sampled at regular intervals and strained through cheesecloth to give a solid and liquid fraction. Both fractions were plated on agar and incubated at 65°C. Microbial concentrations were expressed either as colony-forming units (c.f.u.) ml^{-1} of rumen fluid or c.f.u. g^{-1} dry matter.

Inorganic [15]nitrogen

Inorganic ^{15}N is often preferred to other isotopic markers for estimating microbial nitrogen synthesis since it is a stable isotope and does not present an environmental hazard. In order to obtain a uniform distribution of ^{15}N marker throughout the microbial nitrogen pools, 10–85% ^{15}N-enriched ammonium sulphate is infused continuously through the rumen fistula for a period of 48 h. After this period, there is little difference between the ^{15}N enrichment in ruminal and post-ruminal microbial pools sampled simultaneously, although it takes 7–8 days to obtain a plateau and constant specific enrichment of ruminal or post-ruminal nitrogen pools. If the ^{15}N is administered by including it in the feed, a feeding period of longer than 48 h is required (Broderick and Merchen, 1992).

Procedures for quantifying ^{15}N have been reviewed (International Atomic Energy Agency, 1985). Although the accuracy and precision of analysis by isotope ratio mass spectrometry is very good (enrichment of 0.01–0.05% is adequate for most studies), the procedure is tedious, as the nitrogen fraction under study must be isolated prior to analysis.

L-[4,5-^{3}H]Leucine

L-[4,5-^{3}H]Leucine, infused into the rumen for 36 h, is incorporated into the protein fraction of all microbial species, and presents an accurate means of estimating microbial nitrogen flow (Sinclair *et al.*, 1993). [^{3}H]Leucine is measured by liquid scintillation counting.

Inorganic [35]sulphur

Labelled sulphur can be infused continuously (14 days) into the rumen in the form of ^{35}S-labelled sodium sulphate (Kang-Meznarich and Broderick, 1981). After reduction to sulphide, the label is incorporated into bacterial protein by *de*

novo synthesis of the sulphur-containing amino acids, cysteine and methionine, or by incorporation into substances such as coenzyme A. Protozoa eventually become labelled by indirect means. Collected digesta samples are treated and analysed according to Elliott and Armstrong (1982). Although of relatively short half-life (87 days), ^{35}S is a potential health hazard and may accumulate in meat and milk, rendering it unsuitable for consumption.

Inorganic [32]phosphorus

Inorganic ^{32}P has also been used as a microbial marker by incorporating it into microbial phospholipids (Bucholtz and Bergen, 1973), but substantial precautions need to be taken for its use as a radioactive tracer.

Radionuclide-labelled microspheres

The microspheres are commercially available polymeric resin-covered, non-biodegradable, ion exchange beads labelled with [141]Ce, [57]Co, [95]Nb or [103]Ru (Young *et al.*, 1991). When administered directly into the rumen of sheep, the microspheres are injected as a dextran suspension. However, when fed to sheep, they are blended with finely ground fish meal and pelleted. The radionuclide content is determined in oven-dried samples of faeces compressed into cylinders and read directly in a neckless counting vial in a gamma counter.

Microspheres were shown not to pass through the wall of the gastrointestinal tract and gave a satisfactory recovery of 98.6% in the faeces (Young *et al.*, 1991). Microspheres do not represent the flow of any particular food particle in the digestive tract, but appear to be suitable for comparative studies. They have the advantages of uniformity of particle size and density which do not change during passage through the gut. They are available with different radionuclide labelling and are measured easily in faeces.

Intrinsically ^{14}C- and ^{3}H-labelled plant material

Plant cell walls can be labelled with ^{14}C by multiple-pulse [^{14}C]carbon dioxide dosing of plants grown in a plastic tent (Smith, 1989), or by immersing excised leaves in a 10 μM solution of ^{14}C-labelled acetate and exposing the leaves to a high-intensity tungsten light source for several 30 min periods alternated with 30 min dark periods (Kolattukudy, 1965). Tritium-labelled grass can be obtained by spraying young grass at regular intervals with tritiated water, as described by Van den Hoek *et al.* (1985). As the label is incorporated into potentially digestible and indigestible components, tritium and ^{14}C-labelled plant material do not meet the criterion of indigestibility, as required for markers used for rumen kinetic studies. Digestible components should be removed before employing relatively indigestible fractions such as NDF (after chromium or cobalt mordanting) and alkanes as isotopically labelled markers.

Tritiated gypsum

Gypsum labelled in its water of crystallization is prepared by mixing gypsum powder with an appropriate amount of water, the tritium content of which is adjusted to suit the level of supplementation required. After mixing to a smooth paste, the gypsum is spread out and allowed to dry. It is then milled to a powder, freeze-dried and added to the feed ingredients (Dove, 1984). Activity is measured by means of liquid scintillation counting.

Estimations Using Markers

Since marker techniques tend to give variable results depending on experimental conditions, the marker employed, the material analysed and the model used for processing the data should be verified, if possible, using alternative markers or procedures.

Digesta flow

Digesta consist of particles of various sizes suspended in a fluid, forming a number of interacting pools. Labelling and tracing each pool through the digestive tract is complex and a marker suitable for labelling one pool may not be suitable for another. By preparing animals with cannulas, digesta flow can be estimated at the points of cannulation. Since the estimation of flow requires measurement of the amount of marker consumed by the animal, both analytical and dosing errors will influence results. Furthermore, estimations depend on regular faecal sampling, but will only give accurate results if the flow of the marker is constant. However, marker concentration often shows considerable fluctuation depending on the feeding pattern of the animal.

To estimate digesta flow, a limited amount of marker such as chromium-mordanted or rare earth-labelled fibre is administered, usually as a single pulse dose followed by time-sequence sampling of digesta. However, the continuous dosing of marker as a component of the normal diet is preferred to pulse dosing because of poor mixing and differential flow of pulse-dosed marker from the rumen. After withdrawing the continuously injected marker, the declining marker concentration curves are fitted to appropriate models. Comprehensive comparisons of mathematical models used for estimating passage kinetics have been made (Lallés *et al.*, 1991; Ellis *et al.*, 1994; Huhtanen and Kukkonen, 1995). The most frequently used models are two-compartmental with two rates of decay, the slowest associated with rumen passage and the fastest with post-rumen flow (Grovum and Williams, 1973). The Grovum and Williams model assumes passage to have an exponential lifetime distribution and implies that there is an equal probability of particles leaving the rumen, regardless of their size or age. It is recommended for the estimation of the passage of liquids (Quiroz *et al.*, 1988). The gamma age-dependent models of Ellis *et al.* (1994) assume a gamma lifetime distribution and imply that the probability of a particle leaving the rumen increases with time. Gamma 2 two-compartment models are recommended for small and medium particles, and the gamma 3 two-compartment models for large particles (Quiroz *et al.*, 1988). Algebraic or multi-compartment models have also been used in an attempt to improve the description of marker excretion curves (Pond *et al.*, 1984; Dhanoa *et al.*, 1985; Quiroz *et al.*, 1988; Lallés *et al.*, 1991). The multicompartment models assume instantaneous mixing within and steady-state flow through successive compartments. Comparison of models showed that the two-compartment models require good initial parameter estimates but gave similar rumen turnover rates to that of the multicompartment models (Beauchemin and Buchanan-Smith, 1989). However, apparent turnover rates in the caecum and proximal colon were twice as long and transit times were 35% longer using the multicompartment model compared with the two-compartment model.

Reese *et al.* (1995) developed a multi-compartment digesta flow model with gamma-distributed retention times which allows the estimation of total digesta compartment retention time, rather than marker retention time. This model is used mainly to assess changes in digesta flow relative to changes in the environment, diet and physiological condition of the animal.

Susmel *et al.* (1996) fitted results obtained from a pulse dose of Cr-mordanted forage to both a gamma age-dependent model and a multicompartmental model to predict faecal output. Similar output predictions were obtained, but the multicompartmental model produced more accurate results.

Markers such as chromium oxide, which tend to behave independently of both particulate and fluid phases, will give erroneous estimates of flow rate when used on their own. These limitations are overcome by the commonly used double-marker technique of Faichney (1992, 1993). It involves the administration of a particulate phase marker, such as Ru-phe, and a liquid phase marker, such as Cr-EDTA, in the feed or through a fistula either as a pulse dose or

at a constant rate until a steady-state has been reached. Samples are taken at a point(s) where flow is to be measured. This procedure requires uniform distribution of marker within phases, but does not require the exclusive association of each marker with each phase.

The rare earth elements are used extensively for measuring the retention of solids in the gastrointestinal tract, while Cr-EDTA and Co-EDTA are used widely for measuring the retention time of the liquid phase. Rumen turnover rates based on ytterbium-labelled NDF are faster than those based on Cr-mordanted fibre as analysed by multi- and two-compartment models, and probably reflect a difference in particle size of the marked feed (Beauchemin and Buchanan-Smith, 1989). Rare earths tend to bind to particles in proportion to their surface area, giving mean retention times biased towards that of smaller feed particles in the rumen. Rare earth markers partly dissociated from the feed particles also tend to leave the rumen more rapidly than the feed particles. Direct comparison of rare earth- and chromium-mordanted-based passage rates is therefore not advisable. However, dissociation of rare earth markers in the abomasum may not invalidate kinetic estimates based on faecal marker concentrations. Rare earth elements may reduce the digestibility of feed particles. Labelling silage with ytterbium at a concentration of 35 g kg^{-1} DM reduced its rate of disappearance from the rumen by 26% (Beauchemin and Buchanan-Smith, 1989), but concentrations <6 g kg^{-1} DM had no effect on digestion (Siddons *et al.*, 1985).

The excretion curve of radionuclide-labelled microspheres in sheep fitted to a two-compartment model gave a mean retention time of 55 h compared with 51.2 h for the liquid phase marker, Co-EDTA, 61.8 h for Cr_2O_3, and 61.9 and 55.1 h for the particulate markers, ruthenium and ytterbium, respectively (Young *et al.*, 1991).

The mean retention time in the rumen, estimated using bacterial spores as markers, which may be more indicative of the transport of rumen digesta than inorganic markers, was found to be 5.5 h longer than with Co-EDTA, and could be due to the difference in specific gravity between bacterial spores and Co-EDTA (Mir *et al.*, 1997).

Faecal output can be estimated by the dilution of an orally dosed external marker using Equation 12.1.

$$\text{Faecal output} = M_d/M_c \qquad (12.1)$$

where M_d = daily dose rate of the marker and M_c = the marker concentration in the digesta or faeces.

The flow of a nutrient component in the digestive tract or part of it can be calculated using Equation 12.2.

$$\text{Component flow} = N_d(M_h/M_d) \qquad (12.2)$$

where N_d = the concentration of the nutrient component in the digestive tract, M_h = the concentration of the marker in herbage or diet and M_d = the concentration of the marker in the digestive tract.

Both internal and external alkane markers appear to be strongly associated with the particulate phase of abomasal digesta, but the carrier matrix used for external markers can affect the passage rate. Alkane-coated cellulose powder gives faster flow rates than alkane-impregnated shredded paper or paper bungs. Dosed alkanes appear to be as effective as ytterbium acetate as a digesta passage rate marker (Giráldez *et al.*, 1997). The natural alkanes, with their quantitative duodenal recovery and strong affinity for the solid phase of the digesta, appear to be suitable markers for studying digesta kinetics, particularly since they flow with undigested feed residues and the rate of breakdown of the marked particle in the gut will be similar to that of the digesta particles. In order to use natural alkanes as markers for this application, the plant can be labelled with ^{14}C and fed as a pulse dose. Digesta kinetics can be studied by following the ^{14}C label in the alkanes of digesta or faeces.

Microbial protein synthesis

Estimation of microbial nitrogen flow to the duodenum and the efficiency of microbial nitrogen synthesis depend largely on the marker used. By using ^{15}N as marker, the bacterial nitrogen fraction of the digesta nitrogen is calculated using Equation 12.3.

$$\text{Bacterial N fraction} = E_d/E_b \qquad (12.3)$$

where E_d = [15]N enrichment of the digesta and E_b = [15]N enrichment of the bacterial fraction.

For internal markers such as DAPA, the bacterial nitrogen fraction is calculated using Equation 12.4.

$$\text{Bacterial N fraction} = M_d/N_d \times N_b/M_b \qquad (12.4)$$

where M_d = the marker concentration in the digesta, N_d = total N in the digesta, N_b = total N in the bacterial fraction and M_b = the marker concentration in bacterial fraction.

Ideal protein markers should account for both bacterial and protozoal synthesis associated with the solid and liquid phases of the digest. At present, no simple ideal marker system exists. Bacterial plus protozoal crude protein flow from the rumen is computed from the marker to bacterial plus protozoal crude protein ratio of a sample of rumen microorganisms. Reviewing protein markers, Broderick and Merchen (1992) pointed out that because none proved completely satisfactory, yield estimates obtained are relative rather than absolute. The ^{15}N procedure gives more plausible and less variable results than the DAPA procedure (Sadik *et al.*, 1990). During short-term dosing studies with ^{15}N ammonium salts, only microbial nitrogen is labelled, since it is not found in the normal diet above natural enrichment. All nitrogen pools will be labelled, but with different enrichments since bacteria are labelled directly by the incorporation of [15]NH$_3$, while protozoal nitrogen is labelled indirectly through predation of labelled bacteria, thus rendering the basis for calculating microbial yield in ruminants uncertain.

Schönhusen *et al.* (1995) compared D-alanine, ^{15}N, DAPA, RNA and amino acid profiles as microbial markers and concluded that D-alanine and ^{15}N gave the best results for rumen and duodenal bacteria. Microbial nitrogen flows estimated from ^{15}N procedures have been shown to be lower than estimates based on purines (Perez *et al.*, 1996), but this finding has been ascribed to an inadequate isotope distribution or to difficulties in obtaining representative samples of microbial pools. The presence in the diet of fish meal, which contains relatively high concentrations of nucleic acids, could lead to erroneous predictions. With most other feeds, the intestinal passage of dietary nucleic acids appears to be insignificant. A further concern regarding the use of nucleic acids as markers is the finding that nucleic acid to protein ratios could differ in bacteria and protozoa and also among the fluid and particle-associated pools in the rumen. Since the rumen microbial biomass is largely associated with the particulate fraction in the rumen, it is recommended that the particulate fraction, or mixed rumen bacteria pooled over time after feeding, is used for measuring purine to nitrogen ratios of bacteria leaving the rumen. Although fluid-associated bacteria are much easier to isolate than bacteria associated with the particulate fraction, their use in determining purine to nitrogen ratios could lead to the underestimation of bacterial protein yields. The ruminal protozoal purine to nitrogen ratios are usually about half those of ruminal bacteria (Broderick and Merchen, 1992), and will lead to the underestimation of the protozoal protein contribution if total bacterial plus protozoal flow is estimated from bacterial purine to nitrogen ratios.

Non-invasive methods based on the urinary excretion of purine derivatives assume that duodenal nucleic acids are largely of microbial origin and are recovered proportionally in the urine mainly as allantoin and, to a lesser extent, as hypoxanthine, xanthine and uric acid after intestinal digestion. Reliable estimates of duodenal flow were obtained using this technique, provided the minor non-allantoin purine derivatives were also taken into account in the calculations. Dietary nucleic acids contribute little to purine derivative excretion as they are degraded extensively in the rumen. Estimation of microbial protein reaching the duodenum, based on urinary purine derivative assays, did not differ significantly from estimations based on purine nitrogen in duodenal digesta (Perez *et al.*, 1996).

Digestibility

Conventionally, the digestibility of a forage is the difference between the quantities consumed and excreted in the faeces, and involves the measurement of feed intake and total faecal excretion. Apparent digestibility of herbage or feeds can be estimated by using an internal marker, or incorporating an external marker into the diet at a known concentration and collecting faecal samples when a steady-state has been reached. The advantage of the use of markers in digestibility studies is that total quantitative faecal collection is replaced by random grab sampling, which saves costs and labour, especially in studies with large herbivores.

A combination of rumen evacuation-derived rate of digestion values and of two-compartmental passage models gave good estimates of rumen NDF digestibility (0.94–0.96 of the actual digestibility) (Huhtanen *et al.*, 1995). Partial digestibility coefficients have been estimated by the dual-marker reconstitution method of Faichney (1980) using Cr-EDTA and ytterbium as markers, or the single marker concentration method of Schneider and Flatt (1975), using ytterbium. The two methods gave similar results, but the reconstitution method required more sample preparation time and three times the number of atomic absorption spectrophotometer analyses than the single indicator method (Remillard *et al.*, 1990).

Digestibility can also be derived from Equation 12.5.

$$\text{Dry matter digestibility (g kg}^{-1}) = 1000(1 - M_h/M_f) \qquad (12.5)$$

where M_h = the marker concentration in herbage and M_f = the marker concentration in faeces.

This technique can also be used to estimate the apparent digestibility of nutrient components within the forage, using Equation 12.6.

Digestibility of nutrient component
$$(g\ kg^{-1}) = 1000 - 1000(M_h/M_f)(N_f/N_h)$$
(12.6)

where M_h = the marker concentration in the herbage, M_f = the marker concentration in the faeces, N_h = the concentration of the nutrient component in the herbage and N_f = the concentration of the nutrient component in the faeces.

These equations are based on the assumption that the marker is completely inert and not absorbed, and that marker concentration reached a steady-state in the digestive tract. Furthermore, if an external marker is used, feed intake should be known in order to calculate feed marker concentration.

Markers with incomplete faecal recoveries, such as the even-chain alkanes, can be used if the equation contains a correction factor to compensate for incomplete recovery. Since the loss of alkane through absorption from the small intestine tends to decrease with an increasing molecular weight of the alkane, the concentration of the natural alkane C_{35}, which has a constant recovery of 95% (Mayes et al., 1986), is used to estimate digestibility, provided it is present in the forage in sufficient quantities (Equation 12.7).

Dry matter digestibility $(g\ kg^{-1})$
$$= 1000(1 - (M_h/M_f) \times 0.95)$$
(12.7)

where M_f = the concentrations of C_{35} in the faeces and M_h = the concentration of C_{35} in the herbage.

The accuracy of the estimates depends on the degree of variation in recovery. Errors in digestibility estimates may be larger in cattle than in sheep due to an apparent lower and more erratic recovery of alkanes (Dove and Mayes, 1991). A disadvantage of C_{35} as marker is the relatively low C_{35} content of many plants and forages (Dove and Mayes, 1996). However, any of the natural alkanes present in sufficient concentrations may be used as a

marker provided its recovery is known. Comparing alkane C_{31} and chromium oxide as markers gave digestibility values of 605 and 633g kg^{-1}, respectively (Ohajuruka et al., 1991).

The recovery of a marker can be estimated by dosing grazing animals with known mixtures of even-chain alkanes and either comparing relative concentrations of alkanes in a faecal sample with the amounts dosed or by measuring even-chain alkane output by total faecal collection. Because of the low concentration of even-chain alkanes in forage, the recoveries of the dietary odd-chain alkanes can be calculated by interpolation. Recovery can also be estimated from a separate group of housed animals with known intakes and on which total faecal collections have been made (Mayes et al., 1994; Salt et al., 1994).

Penning and Johnson (1983) obtained variable results using acid-insoluble ash as marker for digestibility estimates. Accurate estimates of the digestibility of grasses have been obtained using acid-insoluble ash as marker (Van Keulen and Young, 1977; Sunvold and Cochran, 1991), but highly variable results have been obtained on hays. Hays were also ranked in a different order than that obtained with in vitro methods or in vivo procedures with beef cattle. The observed variation could have been partly due to contamination of samples with sand.

Acid detergent lignin and chromium oxide added to the feed as external digestibility marker in cows gave digestibility values 11.0 and 12.4% lower, respectively, than that calculated from total faecal collection (Morse et al., 1992). A comparison of the suitability of the internal markers, rumen-indigestible NDF, cellulase-indigestible ADF, Klasons lignin, potassium permanganate-soluble and insoluble Klasons lignin, and permanganate-insoluble ash, and the external markers, chromium-mordanted NDR and Co-EDTA, for estimating the digestibility of feed components showed that only chromium-mordanted NDR, Co-EDTA and cellulase-indigestible ADF can be regarded as suitable (Tamminga et al., 1989).

Chromium oxide has been used to determine the digestibility of amino acids in pigs by ileal and faecal methods of analysis (Li *et al.*, 1993; see also Chapter 13). Animals receiving a chromium oxide marker in their ration were fitted with a single T-cannula at the terminal ileum. Digesta were sampled through the cannula and digestibilities of amino acids calculated on the basis of the concentration of indigestible marker in the feed and digesta. The ileal method gave more reliable results than the faecal method. Comparison of the chromium oxide method with the direct method of measuring whole tract digestibility in pigs showed that the chromium oxide method gave lower results (digestibility three percentage units lower and ileal digestibility seven units lower), probably as a result of low recoveries (82–85%) of chromium in the faeces (Mroz *et al.*, 1996). Nevertheless, preference was given to the marker technique over direct measurement, since calculations based on markers were independent of losses of feed, digesta and faeces. Digestibility has also been estimated successfully in horses with chromium oxide as marker (Todd *et al.*, 1995b). Dysprosium is not satisfactory as a digestibility marker for horses but can be used to estimate relative rates of passage. The recovery of dysprosium in the faeces of horses was found to be 82.9%. Due to the incomplete recovery, the dry matter digestibility was six to seven digestibility units lower than that based on total collection or chromium oxide as marker (Todd *et al.*, 1995a).

Feed digestibilities based on the rare earth radionuclide ^{144}Ce as marker were similar to those based on total collection (Young *et al.*, 1991).

Herbage and supplement intake

The most commonly used method for estimating herbage intake by animals is based on the ratio between faecal output and herbage digestibility as represented in Equation 12.8.

$$\text{Herbage intake} = F/(1 - D) \qquad (12.8)$$

where: F = faecal output and D = herbage digestibility.

Faecal output can be measured directly by using faecal collection bags but, apart from affecting the grazing behaviour of the animal, losses from the bags may lead to the underestimation of intake. When animals cannot be restrained in pens or when it is undesirable to burden them with faecal collecting harnesses, faecal output can be estimated from the concentration in faeces of orally administered external markers (Equation 12.1), while digestibility is estimated either *in vitro* or by means of internal markers (Equation 12.6).

Before the advent of the alkane technique, dry matter intake was estimated mainly using Cr_2O_3 as marker to estimate faecal output and measuring digestibility by means of the *in vitro* technique. The main disadvantage of this approach is that the *in vitro* digestibility technique does not account for changes in digestibility of a forage due to the level of intake, supplementary feeding or parasite burden of the animal. Alkanes are ideally suited for estimating herbage intake in grazing animals from the daily dose rate, and the dietary and faecal concentrations of the dosed even-chain alkane and an odd-chain, natural alkane adjacent in chain length. Both internal and external markers are extracted and quantified simultaneously and the results are calculated using Equation 12.9.

$$\text{Dry matter intake} = (F_o/F_e)D_e/(H_o - (F_o/F_e)H_e) \qquad (12.9)$$

where: D_e = daily dose of even-chain alkane, F_o = faecal concentrations of odd-chain natural alkane, H_o = herbage concentration of odd-chain natural alkane, F_e = faecal concentration of even-chain dosed alkane and H_e = herbage concentrations of even-chain natural alkane.

Alkanes of adjacent chain lengths appear to have similar recoveries. The adjacent pair, C_{32} and C_{33}, which are most often used for intake predictions, have recoveries of 0.868 ± 0.0175 and 0.872 ± 0.0125, respectively (Dove and Mayes,

1991). It is noteworthy that provided a pair of alkanes of similar recoveries are used for intake predictions, their incomplete recoveries in the faeces would not matter, since these values would cancel out (see Equation 12.9).

It is important to ensure that the herbage sample analysed is representative of the herbage actually consumed by the experimental animal in terms of alkane composition. Hand-plucked samples may be adequate in the case of uniform, cultivated pastures, but may be inadequate for mixed pastures of complex composition. Representative extrusa samples may be obtained from oesophageal fistulated animals fitted with bags or remote-controlled oesophageal valves (Raats and Clarke, 1992; Raats *et al.*, 1993).

Faecal concentrations of dosed alkanes reach equilibrium after 5 or 6 days. However, diurnal variation in faecal marker concentration may occur, depending on the time and frequency of marker dosing and faecal collection. The diurnal variation in the faecal alkane concentration of sheep dosed once daily with alkane-impregnated paper or twice daily with alkane-coated cellulose powder is small, but may be higher with cattle (Dove and Mayes, 1996). With markers such as Cr_2O_3 and Ru-phe, the diurnal variation in absolute marker concentration is important, while in the case of alkanes an error will only be introduced if diurnal variation in the ratio of faecal concentrations of herbage and dosed alkanes exists.

Alkanes have many advantages over most other indigestible markers used for intake estimations in free-ranging animals. Intake estimates are not dependent on *in vitro* digestibility determinations. The actual feed digestibility of individual animals is calculated and the method is therefore well suited for studying genetic differences in animals regarding intake, digestibility and feed conversion. The feeding of supplements is accommodated by the method and has been validated by several studies (Mayes *et al.*, 1986; Dove *et al.*, 1995). Because alkanes are simple straight-chain hydrocarbons, their extraction, purification and quantitative separation by gas chromatography are relatively simple procedures and involve less work than the chromium oxide technique.

In ten validation studies reported by Dove and Mayes (1996), the largest discrepancy between known and estimated intake amounted to 2.6%. Piasentier *et al.* (1995) showed that the external alkane marker (C_{32}) in his study gave a higher faecal recovery than the natural odd-chain alkanes, C_{31} and C_{33}, which led to an underestimation of intake by 3% on average. In comparison, the chromium oxide method overestimated intake by 5% due to the incomplete faecal recovery of the marker.

Supplement intake in the field situation can be estimated by mixing a marker such as ytterbium with methyl cellulose and spraying it onto a grain supplement. After total faecal collection, supplement intake can be estimated from the recovery of marker in the faeces (Curtis *et al.*, 1994).

Intake of supplement by individual animals has been determined by labelling the supplement with Cr_2O_3 and measuring total faecal excretion (Dove and Coombe, 1992). A disadvantage of this method is the need to measure total faecal excretion. By using chromium oxide and tritiated gypsum as markers and measuring the accumulation of tritium in the body water pool of animals, the need to measure total faecal excretion is eliminated. Both methods gave similar results, although the chromium method had smaller standard errors, while the tritiated gypsum method gave more accurate results under field conditions at low levels of feed intake (Dove, 1984; Dove and Coombe, 1992).

Because of its near absence in feedstuffs and its high faecal recovery (0.95), hexatriacontane (C_{36}) could be used as a supplement marker by spraying it onto the supplement.

Herbage species selection

Before the advent of the alkane marker technique, it was extremely difficult, if not impossible, to assess accurately the botanical composition of herbage ingested by the grazing herbivore. The microscopic examination of indigestible plant cuticle fractions in the faeces of herbivores has been most widely used, but problems associated with this and other procedures have been discussed recently (Dove and Mayes, 1996).

It has long been known that differences in the alkane composition of different plant species could be used in chemotaxonomic studies. Diet composition in terms of plant species or plant parts can now be estimated from a knowledge of the alkane profile or 'fingerprint' of a representative sample of the mixed diet, in the form of oesophageal extrusa (Dove *et al.*, 1993) or faeces (Salt *et al.*, 1994), and the alkane profiles of the component plants or feeds making up the diet. When faecal samples are used, corrections for incomplete recovery may be necessary in order to prevent a bias towards dietary components with a predominance of longer chain alkanes (Mayes *et al.*, 1994; Salt *et al.*, 1994). Simultaneous equations (Dove, 1992) or least-squares optimization methods (Dove *et al.*, 1993; Salt *et al.*, 1994; Newman *et al.*, 1995) have been used for estimating diet composition. Least-squares optimization methods tend to minimize the squared deviations between the observed alkane pattern in the consumed herbage or faeces and that indicated by the predicted diet composition, but predicted results are otherwise similar to predictions obtained with simultaneous equations (Dove and Mayes, 1996). By using alkane concentrations in the least-squares minimization procedure, an estimate of whole diet digestibility can also be obtained.

Theoretically, the number of component species which could be determined in a mixture is limited to the number of alkane markers present, which may vary from eight to 15. However, in practice, the number may be smaller due to possible similarities in the alkane profile of different component species, or the possibility of certain component species having very low total alkane contents. Alkane

profiles of different plant parts such as leaf and stem may also differ and must be taken into account when representative samples of ingested forage are taken. These differences have been exploited to estimate the intake of plant parts by the animal (Dove *et al.*, 1992).

In order to validate diet composition estimates, known plant mixtures have been analysed for alkanes and their mixed ratios predicted by means of the alkane procedure (Fig. 12.1A). The species composition of three- and four-component mixtures has also been estimated (Dove, 1992). Several validation studies showed that alkane profiles can provide accurate estimates of the diet composition in grazing or browsing animals (Fig. 12.1B) (Dove and Mayes, 1996). The use of alkanes to estimate species selection is not restricted to ruminants, but has also been applied to non-ruminants such as pigs, horses and mountain hares (Dove and Mayes, 1996).

Conclusions

In recent years, major advances have been made in the use of indigestible markers for studying digesta kinetics, rumen protein synthesis, digestibility, herbage intake and species selection. Estimates of digesta flow rates are largely influenced by the marker and model used, and caution must be exercised in choosing experimental procedures. Due to a lack of agreement between procedures, estimates of digesta flow parameters must often be regarded as relative indices rather than absolute values. Quantifying microbial protein synthesis is hampered by unequal ^{15}N enrichment and internal marker to N ratios of protozoal and bacterial pools. A major advance has been the advent of *n*-alkanes as internal and external markers. Estimates of digestibility, intake and species selection by means of alkane markers appear to be more accurate than with other procedures. The use of markers has greatly enhanced our knowledge of farm animal nutrition and in particular the nutrition of free-ranging animals.

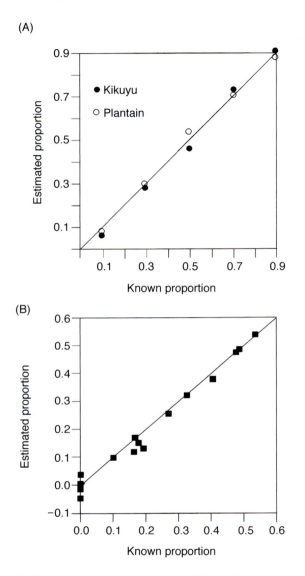

Fig. 12.1. (A) Relationship between the known proportions of kikuyu (*Pennisetum clandestinum*) and plantain (*Plantago lanceolata*) in herbage mixtures and the proportions predicted from the alkane concentrations of the component species and their mixtures. (B) Proportions of the rush *Juncus effusus* in the diet of goats fed mixtures of *Juncus* and *Lolium perenne* (data from Dove and Mayes, 1996), faecal recoveries estimated by dosing goats with C_{24}, C_{28}, C_{32} and C_{36} alkanes. Solid lines are the 1:1 lines.

References

Arthur, D. (1970) The determination of chromium in animal feed and excreta by atomic absorption spectrophotometry. *Canadian Journal of Spectroscopy* 15, 134–140.

Balcells, J., Guada, J.A., Peiró, J.M. and Parker, D.S. (1992) Simultaneous determination of allantoin and oxypurines in biological fluids by high-performance liquid chromatography. *Journal of Chromatography* 575, 153–157.

Beauchemin, K.A. and Buchanan-Smith, J.G. (1989) Evaluation of markers, sampling sites and models for estimating rates of passage of silage or hay in dairy cows. *Animal Feed Science and Technology* 27, 59–75.

Brandt, M., Poedjivo, G. and Allam, S.M. (1983) Zur Eignung von TiO_2-haltigem Polystyrol als Bezugssubstanz für Verdaulichkeitsbestimmungen. *Zeitschrift für Tierphysiologie, Tierernährung und Futtermittelkunde* 50, 10.

Broderick, G.A. and Merchen, N.R. (1992) Markers for quantifying microbial protein synthesis in the rumen. *Journal of Dairy Science* 75, 2618–2632.

Bruining, M. and Bosch, M.W. (1992) Ruminal passage rate as affected by CrNDF particle size. *Animal Feed Science and Technology* 37, 193–200.

Bucholtz, H.F. and Bergen, W.G. (1973) Microbial phospholipid synthesis as a marker for microbial protein synthesis in the rumen. *Applied Microbiology* 25, 504–513.

Buntinx, S.E., Pond, K.R., Fisher, D.S. and Burns, J.C. (1992) Evaluation of the Captec chrome controlled-release device for the estimation of fecal output by grazing sheep. *Journal of Animal Science, Cambridge* 70, 2243–2249.

Christian, K.R. and Coup, M.R. (1954) Measurement of feed intake by grazing cattle and sheep. VI. The determination of chromic oxide in faeces. *New Zealand Journal of Science and Technology* 36, 328–330.

Cochran, R.C., Adams, D.C., Wallace, J.D. and Galyean, M.L. (1986) Predicting digestibility of different diets with internal markers: evaluation of four potential markers. *Journal of Animal Science* 63, 1476–1483.

Combs, D.K. and Satter, L.D. (1992) Determination of markers in digesta and feces by direct current plasma emission spectroscopy. *Journal of Dairy Science* 75, 2176–2183.

Crooker, B.A., Clark, J.H. and Shanks, R.D. (1982) Rare earth elements as markers for rate of passage measurements of individual feedstuffs through the digestive tract of ruminants. *Journal of Nutrition* 112, 1353–1361.

Curtis, K.M.S., Holst, P.J. and Murray, P.J. (1994) Measuring supplement intake in the field using ytterbium as a marker. *Australian Journal of Experimental Agriculture* 34, 339–343.

Czerkawski, J.W. (1974) Methods for determining 2,6-diaminopimelic acid and 2-aminoethyl-phosphonic acid in gut contents. *Journal of the Science of Food and Agriculture* 25, 45–55.

Czerkawski, J.W. and Breckenridge, G. (1969) Distribution of polyethyleneglycol in suspensions of food particles, especially sugar-beet pulp and dried grass pellets. *British Journal of Nutrition* 23, 559–565.

De Smet, S., Demeyer, D.I. and Van Nevel, C.J. (1992) Effect of defaunation and hay:concentrate ratio on fermentation, fibre digestion and passage in the rumen of sheep. *Animal Feed Science and Technology* 37, 333–344.

Dhanoa, M.S., Siddons, R.C., France, J. and Gale, D.L. (1985) A multicompartmental model to describe marker excretion patterns in ruminant faeces. *British Journal of Nutrition* 53, 663–671.

Dillon, P. and Stakelum, G. (1990) The analysis of *n*-alkanes in faeces and herbage. *Proceedings of the VIIth European Grazing Workshop*. Wageningen, The Netherlands, October 1990.

Dove, H. (1984) Gypsum labelled with tritiated water as a marker for estimating supplement intake by individual sheep fed in groups. *Australian Journal of Experimental Agriculture and Animal Husbandry* 24, 484–493.

Dove, H. (1992) Using the *n*-alkanes of plant cuticular wax to estimate the species composition of herbage mixtures. *Australian Journal of Agricultural Research* 43, 1711–1724.

Dove, H. and Coombe, J.B. (1992) A comparison of methods for estimating supplement intake and diet digestibility in sheep. *Proceedings of the Australian Society for Animal Production* 19, 239–241.

Dove, H. and Mayes, R.W. (1991) The use of plant wax alkanes as marker substances in studies of the nutrition of herbivores: a review. *Australian Journal of Agricultural Research* 42, 913–952.

Dove, H. and Mayes, R.W. (1996) Plant wax components: a new approach to estimating intake and diet composition in herbivores. *Journal of Nutrition* 126, 13–26.

Dove, H., Mayes, R.W., Lamb, C.S. and Ellis, K.J. (1991) Evaluation of an intra-ruminal controlled-release device for estimating herbage intake using synthetic and plant cuticular wax alkanes. *Proceedings of the 3rd International Symposium on the Nutrition of Herbivores*. Penang, Malaysia, p. 82.

Dove, H., Siever-Kelly, C., Leury, B.J., Gatford, K.L. and Simpson, R.L. (1992) Using plant wax alkanes to quantify the intake of plant parts by grazing animals. *Proceedings of the Nutrition Society of Australia* 17, 149.

Dove, H., Freer, M. and Moore, A.D. (1993) Using plant wax alkanes to estimate diet selection by sheep. In: Farrell, D.J. (ed.) *Recent Advances in Animal Nutrition in Australia*. University of New England, Armidale, Australia, p. 5A.

Dove, H., Mayes, R.W. and Freer, M. (1995) Using cuticular wax alkanes to estimate herbage intake in animals fed supplements. *Annales de Zootechnie* 44, 237.

Ehle, F.R., Bas, F., Barno, B., Martin, R. and Leone, F. (1984) Particulate rumen turnover rate measurement as influenced by density of passage marker. *Journal of Dairy Science* 67, 2910–2913.

Elliott, R. and Armstrong, D.G. (1982) The effect of urea and urea plus sodium sulphate on microbial protein production in the rumens of sheep given diets high in alkali-treated barley straw. *Journal of Agricultural Science, Cambridge* 99, 51–60.

Ellis, W.C., Matis, J.H., Hill, T.M. and Murphy, M.R. (1994) Methodology for estimating digestion and passage kinetics of forages. In: Fahey, G.C. (ed.) *Forage Quality, Evaluation, and Utilization*. American Society of Agronomy, Crop Science Society of America and the Soil Science Society of America, Madison, Wisconsin, pp. 682–756.

Faichney, G.J. (1980) The use of markers to measure digesta flow from the stomach of sheep fed once daily. *Journal of Agricultural Science, Cambridge* 94, 313–318.

Faichney, G.J. (1992) Application of the double-marker method for measuring digesta kinetics to rumen sampling in sheep following a dose of the markers or the end of their continuous infusion. *Australian Journal of Agricultural Research* 43, 277–284.

Faichney, G.J. (1993) Digesta flow. In: Forbes, J.M. and France, J. (eds) *Quantitative Aspects of Ruminant Digestion and Metabolism*. CAB International, Wallingford, UK, pp. 53–85.

Faichney, G.J. and Griffiths, D.A. (1978) Behaviour of solute and particle markers in the stomach of sheep given a concentrate diet. *British Journal of Nutrition* 40, 71–82.

Faichney, G.J., Poncet, C. and Boston, R.C. (1989) Passage of internal and external markers of particulate matter through the rumen of sheep. *Reproduction, Nutrition, Développment* 29, 325–337.

Fenton, T.W. and Fenton, M. (1979) An improved procedure for the determination of chromic oxide in feed and feces. *Canadian Journal of Animal Science* 59, 631–634.

Garrett, J.E., Goodrich, R.D., Meiske, J.C. and Stern, M.D. (1987) Influence of supplemental nitrogen source on digestion of nitrogen, dry matter and organic matter and on *in vivo* rate of ruminal protein degradation. *Journal of Animal Science* 64, 1801–1812.

Giráldez, F.J., Mayes, R.W. and Lamb, C.S. (1997) Estudio de los alcanos sintéticos de cadena par como marcadores para estimar el ritmo de paso de los alimentos. *Asociación Interprofesional pas el Desarrollo Agrario. VII Jornadas Sobre Producción Animal*, 13–15.

Grovum, W.L. and Williams, V.J. (1973) Rate of passage of digesta in sheep. 4. Passage of marker through the alimentary tract and the biological relevance of rate-constants derived from the changes in concentration of marker in faeces. *British Journal of Nutrition* 30, 313–329.

Hart, S.P. and Polan, C.E. (1984) Simultaneous extraction and determination of ytterbium and cobalt ethylenediaminetetraacetate complex in feces. *Journal of Dairy Science* 67, 888–892.

Hartnell, G.F. and Satter, L.D. (1979) Extent of particulate marker (samarium, lanthanum and cerium) movement from one digesta particle to another. *Journal of Animal Science* 48, 375–380.

Huhtanen, P. and Kukkonen, U. (1995) Comparison of methods, markers, sampling sites and models for estimating digesta passage kinetics in cattle fed at two levels of intake. *Animal Feed Science and Technology* 52,141–158.

Huhtanen, P., Jaakkola, S. and Kukkonen, U. (1995) Ruminal plant cell wall digestibility estimated from digestion and passage kinetics utilizing mathematical models. *Animal Feed Science and Technology* 52, 159–173.

Ibrahim, E.A., Ingalls, J.R. and Bragg, D.B. (1970) Separation and identification of amino acids present in rumen microorganisms. *Canadian Journal of Animal Science* 50, 397–400.

International Atomic Energy Agency (1985) *Laboratory Training Manual on the Use of Nuclear Techniques in Animal Nutrition*. International Atomic Energy Agency, Vienna, Austria.

Kang-Meznarich, J.H. and Broderick, G.A. (1981) Efects of incremental urea supplementation on ruminal ammonia concentration and bacterial protein formation. *Journal of Animal Science* 51, 422–431.

Kay, R.N.B. (1969) Effect of dietary tannic acid on the solubility of polyethylene glycol. *Proceedings of the Nutrition Society* 28, 22A–23A.

Kennelly, J.J., Apps, M.J., Turner, B.V. and Aherne, F.X. (1980) Dysprosium, cerium and chromium marker determination by instrumental neutron activation analysis. *Canadian Journal of Animal Science* 60, 749–761.

Kolattukudy, P.E. (1965) Biosynthesis of wax in *Brassica oleracea*. *Biochemistry* 4, 1844–1855.

Lallés, J.P., Delval, E. and Poncet, C. (1991) Mean retention time of dietary residues within the gastrointestinal tract of the young ruminant: a comparison of non-compartmental (algebraic) and compartmental (modelling) estimation methods. *Animal Feed Science and Technology* 35, 139–159.

Li, S., Sauer, W.C. and Fan, M.Z. (1993) The effect of dietary crude protein level on ileal and fecal amino acid digestibility in early-weaned pigs. *Journal of Animal Physiology and Animal Nutrition* 70, 117–128.

Luginbuhl, J.M., Pond, K.R. and Burns, J.C. (1994) Whole-tract digesta kinetics and comparison of techniques for the estimation of fecal output in steers fed coastal bermudagrass hay at four levels of intake. *Journal of Animal Science* 72, 201–211.

Mader, T.L., Teeter, R.G. and Horn, G.W. (1984) Comparison of forage labeling techniques for conducting passage rate studies. *Journal of Animal Science* 58, 208–212.

Malawer, S.T. and Powell, W. (1967) An improved turbidimetric analysis of polyethylene glycol utilizing an emulsifier. *Gastroenterology* 53, 250–256.

Marais, J.P., Figenschou, D.L., Escott-Watson, P.L. and Webber, L.N. (1996) Administration in suspension-form of *n*-alkane external markers for dry matter intake and diet selection studies. *Journal of Agricultural Science, Cambridge* 126, 207–210.

Martin Orue, S.M., Balcells, J., Guada, J.A. and Castrillo, C. (1995) Endogenous purine and pyrimidine derivative excretion in pregnant sows. *British Journal of Nutrition* 73, 375–385.

Masson, H.A., Denholm, A.M. and Ling, J.R. (1991) *In vivo* metabolism of 2,2′-diaminopimelic acid from Gram-positive and Gram-negative bacterial cells by ruminal microorganisms and ruminants and its use as a marker of bacterial biomass. *Applied and Environmental Microbiology* 57, 1714–1720.

Mayes, R.W., Lamb, C.S. and Colgrove, P.M. (1986) The use of dosed and herbage *n*-alkanes as markers for the determination of herbage intake. *Journal of Agricultural Science, Cambridge* 107, 161–170.

Mayes, R.W., Beresford, N.A., Lamb, C.S., Barnett, C.L., Howard, B.J., Jones, B.-E.V., Eriksson, O., Hove, K., Pedersen, O. and Staines, B.W. (1994) Novel approaches to the estimation of intake and bioavailability of radiocaesium in ruminants grazing forested areas. *Science of the Total Environment* 157, 289–300.

Mayes, R.W., Giráldez, J. and Lamb, C.S. (1997) Estimation of gastrointestinal passage rates of different plant components in ruminants using isotopically-labelled plant wax hydrocarbons or sprayed even-chain alkanes. *Proceedings of the Nutrition Society* 56, 187A.

Mir, Z., Mir, P.S., Zaman, M.S., Selinger, L.B., McAllister, T.A., Yanke, L.J. and Cheng, K.-J. (1997) Use of *Bacillus stearothermophilus* spores as a marker for estimating digesta passage rate from the rumen in cattle. *Livestock Production Science* 47, 231–234.

Momont, P.A., Pruitt, R.J., Emerick, R.J. and Pritchard, R.H. (1994) Controlled release chromic oxide and alkaline peroxide lignin marker methods. *Journal of Range Management* 47, 418–423.

Moore, J.A., Poor, M.H. and Swingle, R.S. (1990) Influence of roughage source on kinetics of digestion and passage, and on calculated extents of ruminal digestion in beef steers fed 65% concentrate diets. *Journal of Animal Science* 68, 3412–3420.

Moore, J.A., Pond, K.R., Poore, M.H. and Goodwin, T.G. (1992) Influence of model and marker on digesta kinetic estimates for sheep. *Journal of Animal Science* 70, 3528–3540.

Morse, D., Head, H.H., Wilcox, C.J., Van Horn, H.H., Hissem, C.D. and Harris, B. (1992) Effects of concentration of dietary phosphorus on amount and route of excretion. *Journal of Dairy Science* 75, 3039–3049.

Mroz, Z., Bakker, G.C.M., Jongbloed, A.W., Dekker, R.A., Jongbloed, R. and Van Beers, A. (1996) Apparent digestibility of nutrients in diets with different energy density, as estimated by direct and marker methods for pigs with or without ileo-cecal cannulas. *Journal of Animal Science* 74, 403–412.

Newman, J.A., Thompson, W.A., Penning, P.D. and Mayes, R.W. (1995) Least-squares estimation of diet composition from *n*-alkanes in herbage and faeces using matrix mathematics. *Australian Journal of Agricultural Research* 46, 793–805.

Ohajuruka, O.A., Wu, Z. and Palmquist, D.L. (1991) Ruminal metabolism, fiber, and protein digestion by lactating cows fed calcium soap or animal-vegetable fat. *Journal of Dairy Science* 74, 2601–2609.

Penning, P.D. and Johnson, R.H. (1983) The use of internal markers to estimate herbage digestibility and intake. 2. Indigestible acid detergent fibre. *Journal of Agricultural Science, Cambridge* 100, 133–138.

Perez, J.F., Balcells, J., Guada, J.A. and Castrillo, C. (1996) Determination of rumen microbial-nitrogen production in sheep: a comparison of urinary purine excretion with methods using ^{15}N and purine bases as markers of microbial-nitrogen entering the duodenum. *British Journal of Nutrition* 75, 699–709.

Piasentier, E., Bovolenta, S., Malossini, F. and Susmel, P. (1995) Comparison of *n*-alkanes or chromium oxide methods for estimation of herbage intake by sheep. *Small Ruminant Research* 18, 27–32.

Pond, K.R., Ellis, W.C. and Matis, J.K. (1984) Development and application of compartmental models for estimating various parameters of digesta flow in animals. *Texas Agricultural Experimental Station, Animal Science Technical Report no. 84/2.* Texas A&M Agricultural University, Texas.

Pond, K.R., Luginbuhl, J.-M., Burns, J.C., Fisher, D.S. and Buntinx, S.E. (1990) Estimating intake using rare-earth markers and controlled release devices. In: *Proceedings of the 45th Southern Pasture and Forage Crop Improvement Conference*, June 12–14, 1989. Little Rock, Arkansas, p. 73.

Quigley, J.D. and Schwab, C.G. (1988) Comparison of D-alanine and diaminopimelic acid as bacterial markers in young calves. *Journal of Animal Science* 66, 758–763.

Quiroz, R.A., Pond, K.R., Tolley, E.A. and Johnson, W.L. (1988) Selection among nonlinear models for rate of passage studies in ruminants. *Journal of Animal Science* 66, 2977–2986.

Raats, J.G. and Clarke, B.K. (1992) Remote control collection of oesophageal fistula samples in goats. *Small Ruminant Research* 7, 245–251.

Raats, J.G., Cockcroft, S.G., Clarke, B.K., King, D.A. and Stead, J.W.A. (1993) Surgical procedure and closing device for large oesophageal fistulae in goats. *Small Ruminant Research* 11, 65–70.

Rahnema, S.H. and Theurer, B. (1986) Comparison of various amino acids for estimation of microbial nitrogen in digesta. *Journal of Animal Science* 63, 603–612.

Reese, G.R., Reese, A.A., Mathison, G.W., Okine, E.K. and McDonald, A.D. (1995) The Poisson process as a model for compartment digesta flow in ruminants. *Journal of Animal Science* 73, 177–190.

Remillard, R.L., Johnson, D.E., Lewis, L.D. and Nockels, C.F. (1990) Starch digestion and digesta kinetics in the small intestine of steers fed on a maize grain and maize silage mixture. *Animal Feed Science and Technology* 30, 79–89.

Sadik, M.S., Huber, J.T., King, K., Wanderley, R., De Young, D., Ai-Dehneh, A. and Dudas, C. (1990) Comparison of nitrogen-15 and diaminopimelic acid for estimating bacterial protein synthesis of lactating cows fed diets of varying protein degradability. *Journal of Dairy Science* 73, 694–702.

Salt, C.A., Mayes, R.W., Colgrove, P.M. and Lamb, C.S. (1994) The effect of season and diet composition on the radiocaesium intake by sheep grazing on heather moorland. *Journal of Applied Ecology* 31, 125–136.

Schneider, B.H. and Flatt, W.P. (1975) *The Evaluation of Feeds Through Digestibility Experiments.* University of Georgia Press, Athens, Georgia, pp. 168–178.

Schönhusen, U., Voigt, J., Kreienbring, F. and Teuscher, F. (1995) Bewertung verschiedener Marker für die Messung der mikrobiellen Stikstoffpassage am Duodenum der Milchkuh. *Archives of Animal Nutrition* 48, 147–158.

Siddons, R.C., Paradine, J., Beever, D.E. and Cornell, P.R. (1985) Ytterbium acetate as a particulate-phase digesta-flow marker. *British Journal of Nutrition* 54, 509–519.

Sinclair, L.A., Garnsworth, P.C., Newbold, J.R. and Buttery, P.J. (1993) Effect of synchronizing the rate of dietary energy and nitrogen release on rumen fermentation and microbial protein synthesis in sheep. *Journal of Agricultural Science, Cambridge* 120, 251–263.

Smith, L.W. (1989) A review of the use of intrinsically ^{14}C and rare earth-labeled neutral detergent fiber to estimate particle digestion and passage. *Journal of Animal Science* 67, 2123–2128.

Sunvold, G.D. and Cochran, R.C. (1991) Evaluation of acid detergent lignin, alkaline peroxide lignin, acid insoluble ash, and acid indigestible acid detergent fiber as internal markers for prediction of alfalfa, bromegrass, and prairie hay digestibility by beef steers. *Journal of Animal Science* 69, 4951–4955.

Susmel, P., Stefanon, B., Spanghero, M. and Mills, C.R. (1996) Ability of mathematical models to predict faecal output with a pulse dose of indigestible marker. *British Journal of Nutrition* 75, 521–532.

Tamminga, S., Robinson, P.H., Meijs, S. and Boer, H. (1989) Feed components as internal markers in digestion studies with dairy cows. *Animal Feed Science and Technology* 27, 49–57.

Tan, T.N., Weston, R.H. and Hogan, J.P. (1971) Use of [103]Ru-labelled tris (1,10-phenanthroline) ruthenium (II) chloride as a marker in digestion studies with sheep. *International Journal of Applied Radiation and Isotopes* 22, 301–308.

Teeter, R.G., Owens, F.N. and Mader, T.L. (1984) Ytterbium chloride as a marker for particulate matter in the rumen. *Journal of Animal Science* 58, 465–473.

Thewis, A., Rodriguez Paz, F., Francois, E. and Bartiaux-Thill, N. (1989) Utilization of lignin according to Christian as an internal marker for assessing digestibility of temperate grasses with or without supplementation in adult rams. *XVI International Grassland Congress*. Nice, France, pp. 835–836.

Todd, L.K., Sauer, W.C., Christopherson, R.J., Coleman, R.J. and Caine, W.R. (1995a) The effect of feeding different forms of alfalfa on nutrient digestibility and voluntary intake in horses. *Journal of Animal Physiology and Nutrition* 73, 1–8.

Todd, L.K., Sauer, W.C., Christopherson, R.J., Coleman, R.J. and Caine, W.R. (1995b) The effect of level of feed intake on nutrient and energy digestibilities and rate of feed passage in horses. *Journal of Animal Physiology and Animal Nutrition* 73, 140–148.

Udén, P., Colucci, P.E. and Van Soest, P.J. (1980) Investigation of chromium, cerium and cobalt as markers in digesta. Rate of passage studies. *Journal of the Science of Food and Agriculture* 31, 625–632.

Van Bruchem, J., Kamphuis, F., Janssen, I., Lammers-Wienhoven, S.C.W., Bangma, G.A. and Van den Hoek, J. (1990) Tritiated hay and chromium-mordanted neutral-detergent fibre as particulate markers for digesta kinetics in the reticulo-rumen. *Netherlands Journal of Agricultural Science* 38, 1–8.

Van den Hoek, J., Ten Have, M.H.J., Gerber, G.B. and Kirchmann, R. (1985) The transfer of tritium-labelled organic material from grass into cow's milk. *Radiation Research* 103, 105–113.

Van Keulen, J. and Young, B.A. (1977) Evaluation of acid-insoluble ash as a natural marker in ruminant digestibility studies. *Journal of Animal Science* 44, 282–287.

Van Soest, P.J. (1963) Use of detergents in the analysis of fibrous feeds. II. A rapid method for the determination of fiber and lignin. *Journal of the Association of Official Agricultural Chemists* 46, 829–835.

Vulich, S.A., O'Riordan, E.G. and Hanrahan, J.P. (1991) Use of *n*-alkanes for the estimation of herbage intake in sheep: accuracy and precision of the estimates. *Journal of Agricultural Science, Cambridge* 116, 319–323.

Worley, R.R. (1987) Some physical aspects of digestion of forages by steers and binding of ytterbium and hafnium as digesta particles markers. PhD thesis, Texas A&M University, College Station, USA.

Young, B.A., Turner, B.V., Dixon, A.E., Winugroho, M., Abidin, Z., Exley, D.M. and Young, S.B. (1991) Evaluation of radiolabelled microspheres as digesta markers. In: *Isotope Aided Studies on Sheep and Goat Production in the Tropics*. Proceedings of the final research co-ordination meeting on improving sheep and goat productivity with the aid of nuclear techniques organized by the joint FAO/IAEA Division of Nuclear Techniques in Food and Agriculture, 20–24 February 1989. Perth, Australia.

Chapter 13

Methods for Measuring Ileal Amino Acid Digestibility in Pigs

W.C. Sauer[1], M.Z. Fan[2], R. Mosenthin[3] and W. Drochner[3]

[1]*Department of Agricultural, Food and Nutritional Science, University of Alberta, Edmonton, Alberta, Canada;* [2]*Department of Animal and Poultry Science, University of Guelph, Guelph, Ontario, Canada;* [3]*Institute of Animal Nutrition, Hohenheim University, Stuttgart, Germany*

Introduction

The nutritive value of protein in feedstuffs for monogastric animals is determined not only by the amino acid composition but also by the bioavailability of the amino acids, in particular, the limiting amino acids.

The bioavailability of amino acids is defined as the proportion of the total dietary amino acids not combined with compounds which interfere with digestion, absorption or utilization for the purpose of maintenance or growth of new tissue (Agriculture Research Council, 1981). Defined as such, availability is an abstract concept which cannot be really measured but only estimated.

The animal growth and digestibility assays are the two major evaluation systems for assessing the bioavailability of amino acids in feedstuffs for pigs. The process of utilization of dietary amino acids in pigs is presented in Fig. 13.1.

The animal growth assay (the slope–ratio assay) is the most direct approach for the estimation of amino acid availability in protein in feedstuffs since it provides a combined estimation of digestibility and post-absorptive utilization of amino acids at the tissue level (e.g. Batterham, 1979). However, many other factors, including amino acid balance, dietary protein level, energy level, chronology of appearance of absorbed amino acids at the tissue level, genotype and physiological stage, can influence protein retention and therefore affect the results (e.g. Adeola, 1996). In addition, the assay is expensive, time-consuming and provides an estimate of the availability of only one amino acid per assay (e.g. Austic, 1983; Henry, 1985; Sibbald, 1987). Availability values of amino acids, particularly of lysine, have been estimated by the growth assay for various protein supplements in growing pigs (Knabe, 1991; Batterham, 1992).

Amino acid digestibility should not be confused with amino acid availability. Amino acid digestibility is defined as the difference between the amount of amino acids in the diet and in ileal digesta or in faeces, divided by the amount in the diet (Low, 1982a; Sauer and Ozimek, 1986). As illustrated in Fig. 13.1, digestibility is probably the most important single determinant of amino acid availability. A large number of studies have been carried out on

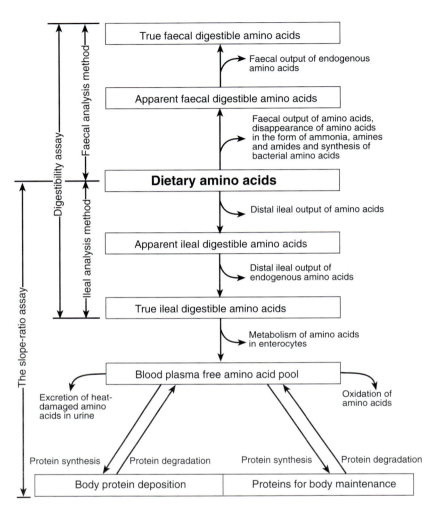

Fig. 13.1. Schematic representation of amino acid utilization in growing pigs (Fan, 1994).

the topic of amino acid digestibility in pigs during the last three decades. Evidence indicates that ileal rather than faecal amino acid digestibility values provide a more reliable estimation of protein digestion, peptide and amino acid absorption, and usually predict amino acid availability values in feedstuffs for pigs, as was discussed by Low (1982a), Austic (1983), Tanksley and Knabe (1984), Sauer and Ozimek (1986) and Sibbald (1987). Nevertheless, special caution should be exercised in interpreting amino acid digestibility values in feedstuffs which have been heat-treated. As some essential amino acids including lysine, threonine,

methionine and tryptophan are susceptible to the effect of heat, they may be partly damaged and absorbed in a form which renders these unavailable to the animal for protein synthesis. In this case, ileal amino acid digestibility values usually over-estimate amino acid availability values (e.g. Batterham *et al.*, 1990a,b; Wiseman *et al.*, 1991).

Apparent ileal amino acid digestibility values in a wide variety of feedstuffs have been reported. It is easy to recognize that there are large differences in ileal amino acid digestibility values between feed-stuffs. However, it comes as somewhat of a surprise to note considerable variation in ileal amino acid digestibility values among samples of the same feedstuff (in name) (Sauer *et al.*, 1990). Some factors responsible for differences between feedstuffs have been discussed previously (e.g. Sauer and Ozimek, 1986; Knabe *et al.*, 1989). The objective of this chapter was narrowed down to discuss the major factors that influence the variation within rather than between feedstuffs, with emphasis on methodology for determining ileal amino acid digestibility values.

Determination of Amino Acid Digestibility

Several *in vivo* assays for determining amino acid digestibility in feedstuffs for pigs have been developed during the last two decades. Considerable efforts have been made to compare the validity of the different amino acid digestibility assays. Evaluation of different digestibility assays has been addressed by Sauer and Ozimek (1986) and Sibbald (1987). In the first part of this chapter, the principles of different digestibility assays will be introduced. Faecal versus ileal amino acid digestibility assays are discussed thereafter. Apparent ileal versus true ileal amino acid digestibility assay are also discussed.

Principles of digestibility assays

Apparent ileal and faecal amino acid digestibility values are determined from studies in which a diet is fed and the corresponding ileal digesta or faeces are collected. Samples of the diet and ileal digesta or faeces are analysed for the contents of amino acids and other items. There are two techniques available, namely: the total collection and the indicator technique. With the total collection technique, the intake of the diet and the output of ileal digesta or faeces have to be measured accurately and the digestibility values are calculated according to Equation 13.1.

$$D_A = ((A_I - A_D)/A_I) \times 100 \qquad (13.1)$$

where D_A is the apparent ileal or faecal digestibility values of amino acids in the assay diets (%), A_I is the amount of amino acids consumed (g) and A_D is the amount of amino acids excreted in ileal digesta or faeces (g).

However, the indicator technique avoids the necessity of total collection of ileal digesta or faeces and the measurement of feed consumption. With the indicator technique, an indigestible marker (e.g. Cr_2O_3) is included in the assay diet and representative samples of diet and ileal digesta or faeces are taken; the digestibility values are calculated according to Equation 13.2.

$$D_D = 100\% - ((I_D \times A_F)/(I_F \times A_D)) \times 100\% \qquad (13.2)$$

where D_D is the apparent digestibility value of amino acids in the assay diet (%), I_D is the indicator concentration in the assay diet (g kg^{-1}), A_F is the amino acid concentration in ileal digesta or faeces (g kg^{-1}), I_F is the indicator concentration in ileal digesta or faeces (g kg^{-1}) and A_D is the amino acid concentration in the assay diet (g kg^{-1}).

Apparent amino acid digestibility values do not take into account amino acids in ileal digesta or in faeces of endogenous origin. True amino acid digestibility values are calculated on the basis of apparent digestibility values and the estimated amount of endogenous amino acids in ileal digesta or faeces according to Equation 13.3.

$$D_T = D_A + (A_E/A_D) \times 100\% \qquad (13.3)$$

where D_T is the true ileal or faecal amino acid digestibility value in the assay diet (%), D_A is the same definition as described for Equation 13.1, A_E is the amount of endogenous amino acids recovered in ileal digesta or faeces (g kg^{-1} dry matter diet) and A_D is the amino acid concentration in the assay diet (g kg^{-1} dry matter diet).

Faecal versus ileal amino acid digestibility values

Amino acid digestibility values can be determined according to the ileal or faecal analysis method, as defined previously in Equations 13.1 and 13.2. The faecal analysis method, developed by Kuiken and Lyman (1948), has been used extensively in studies with pigs (e.g. Eggum, 1973). These studies, in particular those by Eggum (1973), opened the field of research on the topic of amino acid digestibility.

The ileal analysis method should be considered an improvement over the faecal analysis method. The original studies by Zebrowska (1973) showed that both intact and enzymatically hydrolysed casein infused into the distal part of the ileum of pigs fed a protein-free diet was fermented and absorbed; however, the absorbed material was excreted in urine rapidly and almost completely. When casein was given orally, the levels of free amino acids in portal blood were high. Other reports (e.g. Wünsche et al., 1982) showed that protein or amino acids infused into the large intestine make little or no contribution to the protein status of the pig. Some contribution could occur under dietary conditions when nitrogen per se is limiting for the synthesis of the dispensable amino acids, thereby sparing the utilization of the indispensable amino acids.

A series of events occur when undigested protein, from both dietary and endogenous origin (including peptides and amino acids not absorbed before reaching the end of the small intestine), enters the large intestine. A certain proportion of dietary protein passes through the large intestine and is excreted in faeces; the remainder is fermented by the microflora. Nitrogen will be either absorbed, primarily in the form of ammonia (a small proportion in the form of amines and amides), or incorporated into microbial protein. Some of the microbial protein will be fermented and the nitrogen absorbed, primarily in the form of ammonia. The remainder will be excreted in faeces. The fate of endogenous protein is likely to be similar to that of dietary protein. Additional evidence of bacterial fermentation in the large intestine is shown by the large amount of bacterial nitrogen present in faeces. Mason (1984) showed that bacterial nitrogen can amount to 62–76% of total nitrogen in faeces. The factors that affect

microbial activity in the large intestine, including the amount of available fermentable carbohydrates, were discussed previously by Mason (1984) and Sauer and Ozimek (1986).

Evidence that the ileal rather than faecal analysis method should be used for determining amino acid digestibility values was provided by Dierick et al. (1988) in studies in which the performance of pigs was related to digestibility measurements. There was a higher correlation between average daily gain and ileal rather than faecal protein digestibility ($r = 0.76$ versus $r = 0.34$). In the same order, for feed conversion efficiency (kg feed consumed kg^{-1} carcass gain), the correlation coefficients were -0.87 and -0.65, respectively. These results further support the view that nitrogen absorbed in the large intestine does not contribute significantly to protein synthesis.

Amino acid digestibility values obtained with the faecal analysis method are, for most amino acids in most feedstuffs, higher than those determined with the ileal analysis method. However, net synthesis of methionine and lysine has been reported in the large intestine in several studies (Zebrowska, 1978; Low, 1980; Sauer et al., 1982; Tanksley and Knabe, 1982). Therefore, depending on the amino acid and on the feedstuff, digestibility values obtained by the faecal analysis method overestimate (which is usually the case) or underestimate those obtained by the ileal analysis method. Lysine, the sulphur-containing amino acids, threonine and tryptophan can be considered as the most important amino acids in practical diet formulation, as these are often the first, second or third limiting amino acids. Of these amino acids, cysteine, threonine and tryptophan usually disappear to a large extent in the large intestine (Zebrowska, 1978; Low, 1980; Sauer et al., 1982; Tanksley and Knabe, 1982).

Apparent versus true ileal amino acid digestibility values

Many studies have shown that proteins in the body are in a dynamic state and that there is intensive protein turnover at the cellular level (Waterlow *et al.*, 1978). The gastrointestinal tract has a very strong nitrogen (including endogenous protein and non-protein nitrogen) recycling mechanism. Considerable amounts of endogenous protein are produced via secretions (saliva, bile juice, pancreatic juice and intestinal juice) and desquamated mucosal cells. For example, the production of endogenous protein was estimated to be 113.1 g day^{-1} for pigs with a body weight of 45 kg (Low, 1982b). Studies by Krawielitzki *et al.* (1990) in pigs, with an initial body weight of 30 kg, showed a minimum production of endogenous protein of 100.6 g day^{-1}. However, the direct determination of the production of endogenous protein is difficult and, in most cases, the results are possibly underestimated as the entry and the digestion/absorption of endogenous protein occur simultaneously in most regions of the gut. Many factors including dietary conditions, physiological state and differences in the method of determination may affect the estimation. Endogenous protein enters the lumen of the gastrointestinal tract and mixes with exogenous protein. It has been reported that about 70% of endogenous protein was digested and reabsorbed at the distal end of the ileum in pigs (Souffrant *et al.*, 1986; Krawielitzki *et al.*, 1990). The reabsorbed endogenous amino acids may rebalance the dietary pattern of amino acids, especially under conditions of amino acid deficiency. However, the amount of non-reabsorbable endogenous amino acids recovered in ileal digesta has complicated the determination of amino acid digestibility values in feedstuffs for pigs. In principle, true amino acid digestibility, as defined previously in Equation 13.3, should be the preferred criterion in digestibility measurements. As apparent ileal rather than faecal amino acid digestibility values are determined, the estimation of the recovery of non-reabsorbable endogenous amino acids is usually carried out in digesta collected from the distal ileum. The estimation of

endogenous amino acid levels in ileal digesta has been the focus in research for many years. Several techniques have been used including the feeding of protein-free diets, the regression analysis technique (Carlson and Bayley, 1970; Taverner *et al.*, 1981; Furuya and Kaji, 1989; Fan *et al.*, 1995; Fan and Sauer, 1997) and the ^{15}N isotope dilution technique (Krawielitzki and Smulikowaka, 1977; Souffrant *et al.*, 1981; De Lange *et al.*, 1989). Furthermore, the homoarginine labelling technique (Hagemeister and Erbersdobler, 1985) and [^{15}N]amino acid isotope dilution technique (Lien *et al.*, 1993) have been reported for estimation. Comparative evaluation of these techniques was given by Souffrant (1991) and Sauer and De Lange (1992). Each of these techniques is subject to certain limitations and criticisms. Furthermore, evidence at present suggests that the regulation of endogenous protein secretions, digestion and reabsorption is a highly complex matter depending on many factors. It thus seems prudent now to use apparent rather than true ileal amino acid digestibility values (Sauer and Ozimek, 1986; Low, 1990; Knabe, 1991).

With regard to the relationship between apparent and true ileal amino acid digestibility, true ileal digestibility values are higher than their corresponding apparent values as expressed in Equation 13.3. Recent studies (Fan *et al.*, 1995) showed that apparent ileal amino acid digestibility values are quadratic functions of the dietary amino acid content, whereas true ileal amino acid digestibility values are relatively constant and independent of the dietary amino acid content (Fig. 13.2). As is illustrated using methionine as an example, apparent ileal amino acid digestibility values initially increase sharply then gradually reach their plateau values. Upon reaching the plateau values, apparent ileal amino acid digestibility values become independent of the dietary amino acid content; then, apparent ileal amino acid digestibility values can be related to their corresponding true digestibility values.

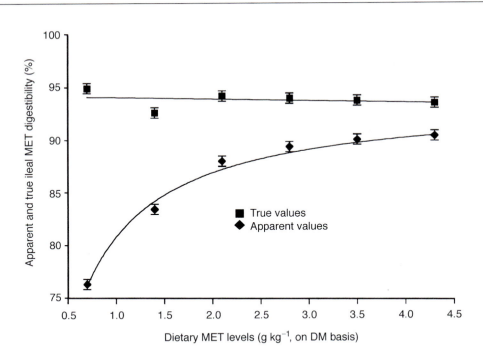

Fig. 13.2. The relationships between the apparent and true ileal methionine (MET) digestibility values (Y: %, means ± SE) and dietary MET content (X: g kg^{-1}, on dry matter basis, Fan *et al.*, 1995).

Variation in Apparent Ileal Amino Acid Digestibility Values

There is an abundance of information in the literature on apparent ileal amino acid digestibility values in feedstuffs. In addition to differences in ileal amino acid digestibility values between feedstuffs, there are large differences in ileal amino acid digestibility values among different samples of the same feedstuff (in name). This variation is different depending on the type of feedstuff.

Cereal grains

Cereal grains may contribute a considerable proportion of crude protein to swine diets. The apparent ileal amino acid digestibility values in different samples of cereal grains (e.g. barley, maize and wheat) have been reported. Sauer and Ozimek (1986) and Knabe (1991) summarized the

apparent ileal amino acid digestibility values of various cereal grains.

There are substantial differences in ileal amino acid digestibility values among samples of the same cereal grain as reflected by large standard deviations. For example, as summarized by Sauer and Ozimek (1986) for the essential amino acids, the differences were relatively large for lysine, methionine and threonine within barley and wheat, ranging from 64.9 to 79.0%, 72.1 to 88.0% and 64.4 to 76.0%, respectively in barley and from 62.3 to 81.0%, 79.4 to 92.4% and 61.9 to 78.4%, respectively in wheat. Some of the differences in ileal amino acid digestibility values may be attributed to differences in processing conditions and other factors including variety of grain, fertilizer application and environmental conditions, which were discussed by Sauer and Ozimek (1986). Furthermore, there were relatively small differences in ileal amino acid digestibility values between different cereal grains compared with differences within the same cereal grain. For instance, based on values compiled by Sauer and Ozimek (1986), the digestibility values ranged from 72.3 to 74.5%, 79.8 to 84.6% and 69.0 to 73.7% for lysine, methionine and threonine, respectively between barley and wheat. The rather larger within than between variation in cereal grains indicates that methodological rather than other factors may be responsible for a large proportion of this variation.

Protein supplements

Many studies have been carried out to determine amino acid digestibility values in protein supplements. These values were summarized by Sauer and Ozimek (1986), Knabe *et al.* (1989) and Knabe (1991). There were large differences in ileal amino acid digestibility values among samples of the same protein supplement, although the range of variation in protein supplements is smaller compared with cereal grains. The variation in ileal amino acid digestibility values within the same protein supplement was larger in cottonseed meal, fish meal, meat and bone meal and ground-nut meal, and smaller in blood meal (except for isoleucine), canola meal, casein, soybean meal and sunflower meal. For example, the amino acids that showed a relatively large variation in ileal digestibility values were lysine, methionine and threonine within different soybean meal samples, ranging from 80.1 to 90.7%, 74.5 to 96.7% and 70.7 to 82.2%, respectively. However, isoleucine digestibility values in blood meal and tryptophan in meat and bone meal showed the largest differences, ranging from 60 to 80% and 35 to 65%, respectively (Sauer and Ozimek, 1986; Knabe *et al.*, 1989).

In addition to differences in processing conditions, differences in amino acid digestibility values between samples of the same protein supplement (e.g. meals from oil seeds, meat and bone meal and fish meal) may also arise from other factors. For example, differences in digestibility values in canola meal may result from different levels of fibre (e.g. Fan *et al.*, 1996).

Last but not least, differences in amino acid digestibility values for the same feed-stuff, as reported by different research groups, may result from differences in methodology, which will affect, in particular, the limiting amino acids.

Legume seeds

Legume seeds, such as peas, field beans and lupins, which can provide a rich protein and energy source for swine diets, are increasingly used, especially peas. The evaluation of the nutritive value in pigs for these ingredients is receiving much attention. The apparent ileal amino acid digestibility values in legume seeds, mainly in peas, were summarized by Gatel (1992). There were also considerable differences in ileal amino acid digestibility values among different pea samples. Of the essential and semi-essential amino acids, the differences were relatively large for cysteine, methionine, threonine and tryptophan, ranging from 44.0 to 85.0%, 58.0 to 80.7%, 56.8 to 92.1% and 46.6 to 78.0%, respectively. As discussed by Gatel (1992), differences in processing conditions, anti-nutritional factors and other factors associated with variety and growing conditions were only in part responsible for the large variation.

Methodological Sources of Variation

As indicated previously, there are large differences in the apparent ileal digestibility values of amino acids among samples of the same feedstuff. These differences decrease the sensitivity and reliability of apparent ileal amino acid digestibility values for assessing amino acid availability between different feed-stuffs and cause inaccuracy in diet formulation for swine.

In addition, this variation may misrepresent the real variation among samples of the same feedstuff, as methodological factors are most probably responsible for a large proportion, whereas inherent factors may only elicit relatively minor variations.

Therefore, the variation in apparent ileal digestibility values of amino acids within the same feedstuff may be simply a reflection of experimental error.

Furthermore, precise apparent ileal digestibility values of amino acids are also essential to calculate the corresponding true digestibility values whenever the amount of endogenous amino acids recovered at the distal ileum can be estimated reliably.

Factors responsible for inherent variation in apparent ileal digestibility values of amino acids among samples of the same feedstuff were discussed previously by Sauer and Ozimek (1986) and Knabe (1991); some of the factors have not been identified yet. The major responsible methodological factors, those including dietary amino acid levels and methods of determination, will be addressed.

The effect of dietary amino acid level

As was illustrated by Eggum (1973) in studies with rats, the apparent faecal crude protein digestibility in soybean meal increased curvilinearly with increasing dietary crude protein content. Similarly, it is expected that apparent ileal amino acid digestibility values will increase curvilinearly with increasing amino acid contents in the assay diet. Therefore, values for apparent ileal amino acid digestibility are only meaningful and valid under strictly standardized conditions, at least with respect to the amino acid content in the assay diet. Examination of the literature reveals that, in many instances, this has not been the case. The determination and comparison of apparent ileal digestibility values of amino acids were performed at various dietary amino acid levels as indicated by differences in dietary crude protein content. For example, the crude protein contents in maize starch-based soybean meal diets were 210, 140 and 120 g kg^{-1}, respectively, in studies by Holmes et al. (1974), Jørgensen et al. (1984) and Knabe et al. (1989). Differences in crude protein and amino acid content in the assay diets may explain, in part, the

variation in apparent ileal amino acid digestibility values among different samples of the same feedstuff (e.g. Sauer and Ozimek, 1986).

Studies reported by Fan et al. (1994) with maize starch-based soybean meal diets showed that there were large increases ($P < 0.01$) in apparent ileal digestibility values of crude protein and all amino acids when the dietary crude protein content was increased from 40 to 240 g kg^{-1}. For crude protein, the increase in digestibility was 26.7%. Of the indispensable amino acids, the increases in digestibility ranged from 11.8 (phenylalanine) to 30.9% (threonine). Of the dispensable amino acids, the increases ranged from 7.1 (glutamic acid) to 47.7% (glycine). The increases in apparent ileal digestibility values of amino acids were greatest at the lower crude protein levels; the increases became negligible at the higher crude protein levels as endogenous protein accounts for a smaller proportion of protein in ileal digesta (Fan et al., 1994). Differences in apparent ileal digestibility values of crude protein and amino acids in relation to their dietary contents were also reported by Furuya and Kaji (1989).

The determination of the quadratic relationships between amino acid digestibility values and the amino acid content and the plateau digestibility values were analysed according to a segmented quadratic with plateau model (Fan et al., 1994). The quadratic relationships between the ileal digestibility values and dietary content and the corresponding plateau ileal digestibility values are presented in Table 13.1. The quadratic with plateau relationships between the ileal digestibility values and dietary content are illustrated in Fig. 13.3 for leucine, lysine, methionine and threonine. A similar pattern was observed for the other amino acids. Initially, the apparent ileal crude protein and amino acid digestibility values increased sharply; thereafter, the increases became smaller and reached their plateau values, after which there were no further increases and the digestibility values became independent of the dietary amino acid levels. The

Table 13.1. The quadratic with plateau relationship between apparent ileal crude protein and amino acid digestibility values and dietary contents (Fan *et al.*, 1994).

Items	Regression equations[a–c]	Plateau values[d]	R^2
Crude protein	$Y = 41.6 + 0.38X - 0.0009X^2$	83.1 ± 2.2	0.99
Amino acids			
Indispensable			
Arginine	$Y = 68.0 + 3.16X - 0.103X^2$	92.1 ± 1.5	0.99
Histidine	$Y = 67.8 + 7.04X - 0.590X^2$	88.8 ± 1.6	0.99
Isoleucine	$Y = 64.7 + 4.18X - 0.190X^2$	87.6 ± 1.3	0.99
Leucine	$Y = 65.7 + 2.42X - 0.069X^2$	86.9 ± 1.3	0.99
Lysine	$Y = 66.5 + 3.28X - 0.129X^2$	87.4 ± 1.4	0.99
Methionine	$Y = 67.1 + 14.99X - 2.433X^2$	90.1 ± 1.1	0.99
Phenylalanine	$Y = 71.8 + 3.06X - 0.133X^2$	89.4 ± 1.5	0.99
Threonine	$Y = 30.0 + 12.39X - 0.786X^2$	78.9 ± 1.9	0.99
Valine	$Y = 58.5 + 4.87X - 0.223X^2$	85.2 ± 1.5	0.99
Dispensable			
Alanine	$Y = 47.8 + 7.59X - 0.422X^2$	82.0 ± 1.8	0.99
Aspartic acid	$Y = 61.2 + 2.12X - 0.048X^2$	84.8 ± 1.3	0.99
Cysteine	$Y = 40.9 + 25.34X - 4.073X^2$	80.3 ± 1.8	0.99
Glutamic acid	$Y = 71.1 + 1.04X - 0.017X^2$	87.3 ± 1.2	0.99
Glycine	$Y = 2.0 + 16.46X - 0.915X^2$	76.0 ± 1.8	0.99
Serine	$Y = 46.3 + 6.95X - 0.320X^2$	84.2 ± 1.6	0.99
Tyrosine	$Y = 65.2 + 5.71X - 0.345X^2$	88.7 ± 1.1	0.99

[a] Y = apparent ileal crude protein or amino acid digestibility values (%).
[b] X = crude protein or amino acid content (g kg^{-1}, on dry matter basis).
[c] The intercept, linear and quadratic slopes of the equations are significant ($P < 0.01$, $n = 36$).
[d] The plateau digestibility values of apparent ileal crude protein and amino acids up to which the quadratic regression equations are valid and their 95% confidence intervals.

lower end points of 95% confidence intervals of the plateau digestibility values are defined to be the initial plateau digestibility values. The dietary crude protein and amino acid contents, corresponding to the initial plateau digestibility values, are referred to as the dietary threshold levels. The initial plateau ileal digestibility values and the corresponding threshold levels of crude protein and amino acids are presented in Table 13.2.

As illustrated in Fig. 13.4 for crude protein, methionine, threonine and tyrosine, the apparent ileal digestibility values of crude protein and amino acids did not reach their initial plateau values simultaneously at the same dietary crude protein content. This shows that the dietary amino acid content affects apparent ileal amino acid digestibility values, irrespective of the dietary crude protein content. Therefore, to obtain the plateau values, the level of inclusion of a feedstuff

in the assay diet should be such that the amino acid contents in the assay diet are equal to or exceed the corresponding threshold levels. This consideration is especially important for the determination of the digestibility values of the limiting amino acids (Fan *et al.*, 1994).

On the other hand, although the dietary threshold levels of crude protein and amino acids are not warranted to be constant under other experimental conditions, these values remain valuable for reference. Dietary factors that influence amino acid recoveries at the distal ileum, including source of fibre and level (e.g. Sauer *et al.*, 1977a,b; Taverner *et al.*, 1981) and anti-nutritional factors (e.g. Begbie and Pusztai, 1989), can alter the ratio of exogenous to endogenous amino acids, thereby affecting the threshold levels.

Differences in dietary amino acid levels are responsible for the variation in ileal amino acid digestibility values within

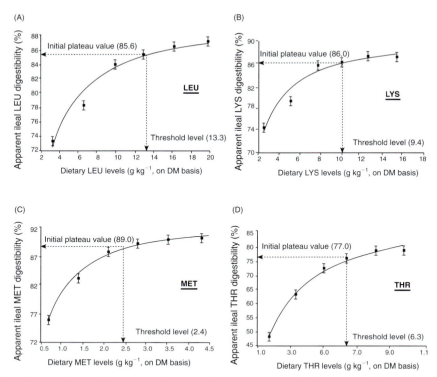

Fig. 13.3. The quadratic with plateau relationships between apparent ileal amino acid digestibility values
(Y: %, means ± SE) and dietary amino acid contents (X: g kg^{-1}, on dry matter basis). (A) Leucine (LEU); (B)
lysine (LYS); (C) methionine (MET); (D) threonine (THR) (Fan *et al.*, 1994).

the same feedstuff. As discussed previously, there is considerable variation in apparent ileal digestibility values of amino acids within each cereal grain. Of the essential amino acids, the variation is especially large for lysine and threonine. The determination of apparent ileal digestibility values of amino acids in low-protein feedstuffs is routinely carried out with the direct method in which the test feedstuff provides the sole amino acids in the assay diet. However, the total contents of crude protein and the majority of the amino acids in cereal grains are usually below the threshold levels (Table 13.3). As summarized in Table 13.3 for barley, wheat and maize, there are large differences in the contents of crude protein and amino acids in the assay diets within the same cereal grain (compiled from various research groups) which arise mainly from differences in the inclusion level and the crude protein

and amino acid contents. As a result, small differences in dietary contents of crude protein and amino acids below the threshold levels will result in relatively large variations in the digestibility values of amino acids, especially those amino acids present at low levels in cereal grains (lysine, threonine and tryptophan) and/or amino acids of which the ileal endogenous recovery is relatively high (e.g. threonine), as illustrated in Fig. 13.3.

The ranges of crude protein and amino acid contents in the assay diets for determining apparent ileal digestibility values of crude protein and amino acids in protein supplements are summarized for soybean meal, canola meal and sunflower meal, which were compiled from different research groups (Table 13.4). Similarly for other protein supplements, there are differences in the dietary contents of crude protein and amino acids for the determination

Table 13.2. The initial plateau ileal digestibility values of crude protein and amino acids and the threshold levels of dietary crude protein and amino acids (Fan *et al.*, 1994).

Items	Initial plateau[a]	Threshold level[b]	Corresponding protein levels[c]
Crude protein	80.9	171	154
Amino acids			
Indispensable			
Arginine	90.6	11.5	154
Histidine	87.2	4.3	161
Isoleucine	86.2	8.3	164
Leucine	85.6	13.3	163
Lysine	86.0	9.4	147
Methionine	89.0	2.4	137
Phenylalanine	87.9	8.2	147
Threonine	77.0	6.3	155
Valine	83.7	8.4	165
Dispensable			
Alanine	80.2	6.9	154
Aspartic acid	83.5	17.1	140
Cysteine	78.5	2.4	143
Glutamic acid	86.2	23.1	110
Glycine	71.2	6.7	160
Serine	82.6	8.7	157
Tyrosine	87.6	6.2	163

[a]Lower end points of 95% confidence intervals at the estimated plateau ileal digestibility values.
[b]g kg^{-1} (dry matter basis).
[c]The dietary levels of crude protein (g kg^{-1}, on dry matter basis) corresponding to the threshold levels of each amino acid.

of ileal amino acid digestibility values among different samples of the same protein supplement. Differences in dietary contents of crude protein and amino acids are partly responsible for the large variation in ileal amino acid digestibility values within the same feedstuff, especially for the limiting amino acids. For example, the relatively large variation that was reported for the digestibility of methionine among samples of soybean meal may result, in part, from the fact that methionine is the limiting amino acid in soybean meal. A relatively small change in the methionine content in the diet may therefore cause a relatively large change in its digestibility value. Nevertheless, differences in analytical techniques for measuring methionine may also have contributed to this variation.

With respect to peas, there was a relatively large variation in the apparent ileal digestibility values of methionine, cysteine and tryptophan compared with the other amino acids. The sulphur-containing amino acids and tryptophan are the first and second limiting amino acids, respectively in peas. Therefore, small differences in dietary contents of these amino acids may have been responsible for a large proportion of the variation in digestibility values.

The effect of methods for determination

The determination of apparent ileal digestibility values of amino acids in cereal grains is usually carried out by the direct method, partly due to the fact that most cereal grains are very palatable. However, as discussed previously, the ileal digestibility values of amino acids in cereal grains determined with the direct method are influenced by their amino acid content in the assay diet. Therefore, it is questionable whether the direct method is valid for determining ileal amino acid digestibility values in cereal grains (Sauer *et al.*, 1989).

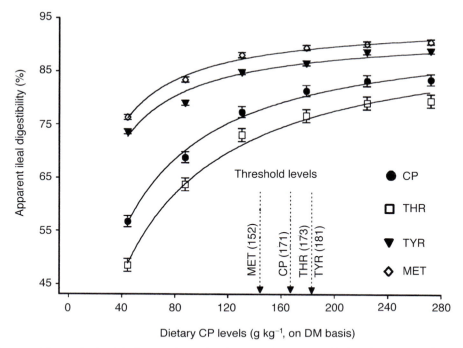

Fig. 13.4. The quadratic with plateau relationships between the apparent ileal crude protein and amino acid digestibility values (Y: %, means ± SE) and the dietary crude protein content (X: g kg^{-1}, on dry matter basis). CP, crude protein; THR, threonine; TYR, tyrosine; and MET, methionine (Fan *et al.*, 1994).

Table 13.3. The range of crude protein and amino acid contents (g kg^{-1}, on dry matter basis) in the assay diets for the determination of apparent ileal crude protein and amino acid digestibility values in cereal grains.

Cereal grains	Barley[b–f,h–k] (n=12)	Wheat[a–f,i–k] (n=15)	Maize[b,e–g,j] (n=5)	Threshold level[l] (n=1)
Crude protein	105–149	121–193	82–125	171
Amino acids				
Indispensable				
Arginine	4.8–7.4	5.4–7.1	3.6–4.5	11.5
Histidine	2.3–3.3	2.5–3.6	2.3–2.5	4.3
Isoleucine	3.7–5.2	4.6–5.5	3.3–3.5	8.3
Leucine	6.8–9.8	8.3–10.2	10.9–13.1	13.3
Lysine	3.9–4.6	3.1–4.6	2.3–3.4	9.4
Phenylalanine	4.5–8.2	5.5–6.8	3.8–5.2	8.2
Threonine	3.4–4.7	3.1–4.5	2.7–3.6	6.3
Valine	5.0–7.1	5.6–6.5	4.5–4.6	8.4
Dispensable				
Alanine	4.0–5.4	3.8–5.2	5.2–7.6	6.9
Aspartic acid	6.1–8.1	5.4–8.0	5.1–7.2	17.1
Glutamic acid	24.4–40.6	31.1–51.7	13.9–20.9	23.1
Glycine	3.1–5.8	4.1–4.8	2.6–4.0	6.7
Serine	3.8–6.0	5.0–6.3	3.8–5.1	8.7
Tyrosine	2.1–4.4	3.1–3.3	3.1–4.0	6.2

[a]Ivan and Farrell (1976); [b]Sauer *et al.* (1977a,b); [c]Sauer *et al.* (1981); [d]Just *et al.* (1985); [e]Lin *et al.* (1987); [f]Green *et al.* (1987); [g]Van Leeuwen *et al.* (1987); [h]Imbeah *et al.* (1988); [i]De Lange *et al.* (1990); [j]Furuya and Kaji (1991); [k]Fan *et al.* (1993); [l]Fan *et al.* (1994).

Table 13.4. The range of crude protein and amino acid contents (g kg^{-1}, on dry matter basis) in the assay diets for the determination of apparent ileal crude protein and amino acid digestibility values in protein supplements.

Protein supplements	Soybean meal[a–m] (n=15)	Canola meal[c,i,k–m,o] (n=7)	Sunflower meal[e,g,j,k] (n=6)	Threshold level[n] (n=1)
Crude protein	120–193	157–202	111–196	171
Amino acids				
Indispensable				
Arginine	9.6–13.4	8.2–13.3	9.4–15.6	11.5
Histidine	3.2–5.1	4.8–6.9	3.1–4.5	4.3
Isoleucine	5.7–9.0	6.8–8.7	4.6–7.9	8.3
Leucine	9.8–14.5	12.6–13.9	6.7–12.0	13.3
Lysine	7.9–11.4	9.2–11.1	4.3–6.9	9.4
Methionine	1.8–2.6	3.2–5.0	2.7–4.2	2.4
Phenylalanine	5.6–9.6	6.9–8.4	4.9–8.2	8.2
Threonine	4.6–7.8	8.1–9.4	3.8–6.9	6.3
Valine	9.4–9.7	8.9–10.9	5.2–9.6	8.4
Dispensable				
Alanine	4.9–8.4	8.0–8.9	4.6–8.1	6.9
Aspartic acid	14.3–17.9	13.4–16.1	10.1–17.3	17.1
Cysteine	1.8–2.6	3.0–5.3	1.9–3.1	2.4
Glutamic acid	23.7–32.2	30.6–36.5	21.5–38.9	23.1
Glycine	4.6–8.1	8.9–10.0	6.0–11.0	6.7
Serine	6.0–9.1	7.9–8.5	4.5–8.7	8.7
Tyrosine	4.7–5.6	3.7–4.9	3.0–4.9	6.2

[a]Holmes *et al.* (1974); [b]Tanksley *et al.* (1981); [c]Sauer *et al.* (1982); [d]Rudolph *et al.* (1983); [e]Jørgensen *et al.* (1984); [f]La Rue *et al.* (1985); [g]Just *et al.* (1985); [h]Chang *et al.* (1987); [i]Imbeah *et al.* (1988); [j]Green and Kiener (1989); [k]Knabe *et al.* (1989); [l]De Lange *et al.* (1990); [m]Fan *et al.* (1993); [n]Fan *et al.* (1994); [o]Fan *et al.* (1996).

With respect to protein supplements and legume seeds, most measurements of apparent ileal digestibility values are made with the direct method, whereas in the case of some protein supplements or legume seeds, some of which are of poor palatability and/or have a high content of anti-nutritional factors, the determination is often carried out with the difference method (Sauer *et al.*, 1989).

The likelihood exists that the improper use of determination methods may also be partly responsible for the considerable variation in apparent ileal digestibility values of amino acids within the same feedstuff. Few studies have been carried out to compare methods.

Some of the methods for determination of nutrient digestibility in assay diets and assay feed ingredients have been described by Schneider and Flatt (1975). The principles of three methods to determine nutrient digestibility in feed ingredients for ruminants were described briefly by Giger and Sauvant (1983).

Indicators (e.g. Cr$_2$O$_3$) are widely used in nutrient digestibility measurements, as reviewed by Kotb and Luckey (1972) and Van Soest *et al.* (1983), since they obviate the need to measure the quantity of assay diet input or ileal digesta or faeces output (see Chapter 12). The digestibility values in the assay diet are usually calculated by the indicator technique (Equations 13.2 or 13.4) rather than by total collection (Equation 13.1).

$$D_D = A_D - ((I_D \times A_F)/I_F) \qquad (13.4)$$

where D_D is the apparent digestible content of a nutrient in the assay diet (g kg^{-1}), A_D is the nutrient concentration in the assay diet (g kg^{-1}), I_D is the indicator concentration in the assay diet (g kg^{-1}), A_F is the nutrient concentration in ileal digesta or faeces (g kg^{-1}) and I_F is the indicator concentration in ileal digesta or faeces (g kg^{-1}).

The use of methods for the determination of nutrient digestibility values in an assay feed ingredient is dependent on the level of inclusion of the ingredient incorporated into the assay diet. There are three methods for determination (Fan and Sauer, 1995a,b).

1. Direct method: the assay diet is formulated in such a manner that the assay ingredient provides the sole dietary nutrient in question. Therefore, the nutrient digestibility in the assay feed ingredient is equal to the corresponding value in the assay diet and can be calculated from Equation 13.5.

$$D_A = (D_D \times 100\%)/(A_A \times S_I) \qquad (13.5)$$

where D_A is the apparent digestibility of a nutrient in the assay feed ingredient (%), D_D is the apparent digestible content of a nutrient in the assay diet (g kg^{-1}), A_A is the nutrient concentration in the assay feed ingredient (g kg^{-1}) and S_I is the inclusion level of the assay feed ingredient in the assay diet (%).

2. Difference method: this method involves the formulation of both a basal and an assay diet. The basal diet contains the basal feed ingredient which provides the sole assay nutrient in the diet, whereas the assay diet consists of a mixture of the basal and the assay feed ingredient. If there is no interaction in nutrient digestibility between the basal and the assay feed ingredient, their relationship in the assay diet can be expressed according to Equation 13.6.

$$D_D = D_B \times S_B + D_A \times S_A \qquad (13.6)$$

where D_D is the apparent digestibility of a nutrient in the assay diet (%), D_B is the apparent digestibility of a nutrient in the basal feed ingredient (%), S_B is the contribution level (%) of a nutrient from the basal feed ingredient to the assay diet, D_A is the apparent digestibility of a nutrient in the assay feed ingredient (%) and S_A is the contribution level (%) of a nutrient from the assay feed ingredient to the assay diet.

The apparent nutrient digestibility in the basal feed ingredient is determined from the basal diet according to the direct method from Equation 13.5. The nutrient digestibility in the assay feed ingredient can be determined by difference according to Equation 13.7 which is derived from Equation 13.6.

$$D_A = (D_D - D_B \times S_B)/S_A \qquad (13.7)$$

3. The regression method: this method evaluates the basal and the assay feed ingredient simultaneously. If both the basal and the assay feed ingredient provide the sole assay nutrient in the assay diets and if there is no interaction between the two feed ingredients, the ingredients can be mixed at various graded levels and more than two assay diets are, therefore, formulated. The relationship between amino acid digestibility in the assay diets (D_{Di}) and the contribution levels (S_{Ai} and S_{Bi}) of the nutrient from the basal and the assay feed ingredient to the assay diets can be expressed according to Equation 13.8. The relationship between S_{Ai} and S_{Bi} is expressed according to Equation 13.9.

$$D_{Di} = D_B \times S_{Bi} + D_A \times S_{Ai} \qquad (13.8)$$

$$S_{Bi} + S_{Ai} = 100\% \qquad (13.9)$$

where D_{Di} is the apparent digestibility of a nutrient in the ith assay diet (%), D_A is the apparent digestibility of a nutrient in the assay feed ingredient (%), S_{Ai} is the contribution level (%) of a nutrient from the assay feed ingredient to the ith assay diet, D_B is the apparent digestibility of a nutrient in the basal feed ingredient (%) and S_{Bi} is the contribution level (%) of a nutrient from the basal feed ingredient to the ith assay diet. When replacing S_{Ai} by $S_{Ai} = 100\% - S_{Bi}$, Equation 13.8 can also be written in the form of Equation 13.10.

$$D_{Di} = D_B \times S_{Bi} + D_A \times (1 - S_{Bi})$$
$$= D_A + (D_B - D_A) \times S_{Bi} \qquad (13.10)$$

According to the previous definitions, D_A and D_B are the digestibility coefficients estimated for the assay and basal feed ingredients. We define $A = D_A$, $B = D_B - D_A$, so Equation 13.11 can be derived from Equation 13.10.

$$D_{Di} = A + B \times S_{Bi} \qquad (13.11)$$

Equation 13.11 is actually a simple linear regression model in which D_{Di} is the dependent and S_{Bi} the independent variable. The regression coefficients of A and B can be obtained by fitting the simple linear regression model.

$$D_A = A \qquad (13.12)$$

$$D_B = D_A + B = A + B \qquad (13.13)$$

The assay nutrient digestibility values (D_A and D_B) in the basal and the assay feed ingredients can be determined from the regression coefficients shown in Equations 13.12 and 13.13, respectively.

Studies were carried out to determine the effect of the aforementioned methods on apparent ileal digestibility values of amino acids (Fan and Sauer, 1995a,b). Barley, canola meal and peas were chosen to be the representative feed ingredients for cereal grains, protein supplements and legume seeds, respectively.

Cereal grains
Five barrows, average initial body weight 35 kg, were surgically fitted with a simple T-cannula at the distal ileum and fed five diets according to a 5×5 Latin square design. Five maize starch-based diets were formulated. Diet 5 contained 900 g kg^{-1} barley providing the sole source of amino acids. In diets 2, 3 and 4, barley and canola meal were the only amino acid sources and were included at three levels, 225, 450 and 675 g kg^{-1}, respectively for barley and 366, 305 and 244 g kg^{-1}, respectively for canola meal. Diet 1 contained 427 g kg^{-1} canola meal providing the sole source of amino acids. Except for diet 5, all other diets were formulated to contain 160 g kg^{-1} crude protein. Chromic oxide was included in the diets as the indicator for calculating ileal amino acid digestibility values in the assay diets (Fan and Sauer, 1995a).

The apparent ileal digestibility values of crude protein and amino acids in barley were determined according to Equation 13.7 at three levels of inclusion of barley (diets 2, 3 and 4). There were increases ($P < 0.05$) in the ileal digestibility values of crude protein and the majority of amino acids in barley as the level of inclusion was increased from 225 (diet 2) to 675 g kg^{-1}

(diet 4). With an increasing level of inclusion of barley, there were large increases in the contribution levels of crude protein and amino acids from barley to the assay diets. For crude protein, the increase in contributions ranged from 14.2 to 42.6%. Of the indispensable amino acids, the increases in contributions were smallest for lysine, ranging from 9.5 to 32.1%, and largest for phenylalanine, ranging from 18.5 to 50.6%. Of the dispensable amino acids, the increases were smallest for tyrosine, ranging from 9.9 to 33.1%, and largest for glutamic acid, ranging from 18.0 to 49.6%. The accuracy of determination of ileal nutrient digestibility values by the difference method is dependent on the contribution levels of crude protein and amino acids from the assay feedstuff to the contents of the assay diets. The higher the contribution level, the more accurate the estimation of ileal digestibility values (Fan and Sauer, 1995a). This was reflected by decreases in the standard error of the means of ileal digestibility values in response to the increase in inclusion level of barley in the assay diets. A similar observation was reported by Van Leeuwen *et al.* (1987) in studies with maize soybean meal diets.

To estimate the ileal digestibility values of crude protein and amino acids in the assay ingredient (barley) by the regression method, the linear relationships between the apparent ileal digestibility values of crude protein and amino acids in the assay diets and the contribution levels of crude protein and amino acids from the basal feed ingredient (canola meal) to the assay diets were established according to Equation 13.11 from diets 2, 3, 4 and 5. The regression equations are presented in Table 13.5. The principle of the regression method is illustrated in Fig. 13.5 for lysine. The ileal digestibility values of crude protein and amino acids in barley by the regression method were obtained from the equations presented in Table 13.5 according to Equations 13.12 and 13.13. The digestibility values are presented in Table 13.6. However, the ileal digestibility values of aspartic acid, isoleucine, leucine,

Table 13.5. The linear relationships between the apparent ileal digestibility values and the contribution levels of crude protein and amino acids for the determination of apparent ileal digestibility values of amino acids in barley with the regression method (Fan and Sauer, 1995a).

Items	Regression equations[a,b]	r^2	$S_{y.x}$ [c]	P [d]	
Crude protein[e]	$Y = 57.7 + 6.6X$	0.52	3.39	0.001	0.05
Amino acids					
Indispensable					
Arginine[e]	$Y = 68.4 + 11.1X$	0.69	2.49	0.001	0.01
Histidine[e]	$Y = 70.5 + 8.2X$	0.48	2.71	0.001	0.05
Isoleucine	$Y = 64.5 + 2.6X$	0.01	3.81	0.001	0.66
Leucine	$Y = 67.6 + 1.5X$	0.01	3.75	0.001	0.78
Lysine[e]	$Y = 59.3 + 12.5X$	0.72	3.54	0.001	0.01
Phenylalanine	$Y = 68.6 + 0.6X$	0.01	4.41	0.001	0.91
Threonine	$Y = 62.3 + 1.9X$	0.01	3.68	0.001	0.52
Valine	$Y = 63.9 + 1.5X$	0.01	3.94	0.001	0.79
Dispensable					
Alanine[e]	$Y = 53.9 + 12.7X$	0.74	4.04	0.001	0.05
Aspartic acid	$Y = 60.1 + 1.9X$	0.01	3.75	0.001	0.75
Glutamic acid[e]	$Y = 72.2 + 7.4X$	0.55	3.02	0.001	0.03
Glycine[e]	$Y = 43.5 + 18.5X$	0.76	5.51	0.001	0.01
Serine	$Y = 61.8 + 1.3X$	0.01	3.45	0.001	0.79
Tyrosine[e]	$Y = 58.2 + 6.3X$	0.54	3.54	0.001	0.04

[a] Y = apparent ileal digestibility values of crude protein or amino acids (%) in the assay diets.
[b] X = the contribution levels of crude protein or amino acids from the basal feed ingredient (canola meal) to the content of the assay diets.
[c] Standard error of estimate of the regression equation.
[d] The probabilities of significance for the intercept and the slope of the regression equation.
[e] The linear regression equation is significant ($P < 0.05$, $n = 20$).

phenylalanine, serine, threonine and valine could not be estimated. This resulted from the fact that the differences in ileal digestibility values of these amino acids between the assay and the basal feed ingredients were not large enough to create linear variations (Table 13.5).

The apparent ileal digestibility values of crude protein and amino acids in barley were also determined by the direct method according to Equation 13.5 from diet 1. The digestibility values are compared in Table 13.6.

Among the three methods, the regression method is in principle the most accurate. The apparent ileal digestibility values of crude protein and amino acids in barley estimated by the regression method are considered to be the most precise values for evaluating the results obtained by the other two methods. As shown in Table 13.6, the ileal digestibility values in barley estimated by the regression method

were not different ($P > 0.05$) from values determined by the difference method at the barley inclusion level of 675 g kg^{-1} (diet 4). However, determined by the difference method, the ileal digestibility values of amino acids in barley were underestimated at the lower inclusion levels (225 and 450 g kg^{-1}). This shows that the difference method is only reliable when the inclusion levels of the assay amino acids from the test feedstuff in the diets are high. Furthermore, the ileal digestibility values of crude protein and amino acids determined by the difference and regression method were usually higher ($P < 0.05$ or 0.10) than those determined by the direct method. This shows that the direct method is not a valid approach for the determination of amino acid digestibility values in feedstuffs with a low protein content. On the other hand, for some low-protein feedstuffs that have a limited level of inclusion in the assay diets because of poor

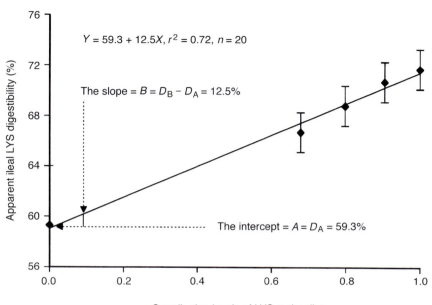

Fig. 13.5. Estimation of the apparent ileal digestibility of lysine (LYS) in the assay feed ingredient (barley) by linearly regressing the ileal digestibility values (*Y*: %, means ± SE) of lysine in the assay diets against the contribution levels (*X*) of lysine from the basal feed ingredient (canola meal) to its content in the assay diets (Fan and Sauer, 1995a).

palatability, such as rye, wheat bran and forage plants, the determination is often carried out by the difference rather than by the direct method. Kreienbring *et al.* (1988) reported that the apparent ileal digestibility values of amino acids in forage plants determined by the difference method varied considerably, indicated by large standard deviations. As the amino acid contents in these forage plants were low and the inclusion levels in the assay diets were also low, the large variation probably resulted from the magnifying effect induced by the calculation process of the difference method. This indicates that the difference method may not be suitable for these low-protein feedstuffs. The regression method is most suited.

In summary, for the determination of apparent ileal digestibility values of amino acids in feedstuffs with a low protein content, the regression method is the most accurate approach. The difference method, with a high inclusion level of a test feedstuff, is also a valid approach. The direct method, which underestimates the ileal digestibility values of amino acids, is not valid for these feedstuffs.

Protein supplements
Information with respect to the effect of methods of determination on the apparent ileal amino acid digestibility values in protein supplements was also obtained with canola meal (Fan and Sauer, 1995a).

With respect to the difference method, the apparent ileal digestibility values of crude protein and amino acids in canola meal were determined according to Equation 13.7 at three levels of inclusion (diets 2, 3 and 4). It seemed somehow contradictory, at first, to note that the ileal digestibility values of crude protein and amino acids in canola meal calculated by the difference method at the low level of inclusion (244 g kg^{-1}) were higher (P < 0.05 or 0.10) than those at the higher levels of inclusion (305 and 366 g kg^{-1}). The ileal digestibility values of amino acids in canola meal were calculated by the

Table 13.6. Determination of the apparent ileal digestibility values[1] (%) of crude protein and amino acids in barley by the direct, the difference and the regression methods (Fan and Sauer, 1995a).

	Methods of determination		
Items	Direct method	Difference method[2]	Regression method
No. of observations	5	5	20
Crude protein	56.6 ± 1.88	58.9 ± 3.36	57.7 ± 2.83
Amino acids			
Indispensable			
Arginine[3]	64.7 ± 1.93	69.8 ± 3.15	68.4 ± 2.39
Histidine	69.5 ± 2.68	71.9 ± 3.56	70.5 ± 2.27
Isoleucine	61.1 ± 3.29	66.9 ± 4.80	—
Leucine	66.6 ± 2.80	70.3 ± 3.79	—
Lysine[3]	54.1 ± 4.18	61.3 ± 4.93	59.3 ± 4.65
Phenylalanine	69.6 ± 3.41	72.1 ± 4.28	—
Threonine	53.3 ± 3.12[a]	62.4 ± 3.90[b]	—
Valine	62.6 ± 2.96	67.2 ± 3.94	—
Dispensable			
Alanine	48.8 ± 2.96[a]	57.3 ± 3.39[b]	53.9 ± 2.81[b]
Aspartic acid	50.5 ± 3.83[a]	62.1 ± 4.68[b]	—
Glutamic acid	75.1 ± 2.52	73.9 ± 2.10	72.2 ± 2.89
Glycine	31.7 ± 3.41[a]	48.1 ± 5.64[b]	34.5 ± 5.08[b]
Serine	58.4 ± 3.19[a]	64.8 ± 2.67[b]	—
Tyrosine[3]	51.5 ± 3.88	61.2 ± 5.62	58.2 ± 3.43

[1]Mean and standard error of the mean.
[2]Digestibility values calculated from diet 4 (675 g kg^{-1} inclusion of barley).
[3]Means in the same row show a trend to increase ($P < 0.10$, by one-tailed Student's t-test).
[a,b]Means in the same row with different superscript letters differ ($P < 0.05$).

difference method using barley as the basal feed ingredient. However, Fan and Sauer (1995a) showed that the ileal digestibility values of amino acids in barley, calculated by the direct method, were underestimated. Therefore, the ileal digestibility values of amino acids in canola meal determined by the difference method were probably overestimated at the low inclusion level of canola meal (244 g kg^{-1}). Furthermore, there were no differences ($P > 0.05$) in the ileal digestibility values of amino acids in canola meal between the inclusion levels of 305 and 366 g kg^{-1} as determined by the difference method. The inclusion of barley was lower at the higher inclusion levels of canola meal (305 and 366 g kg^{-1}). Therefore, the overestimation of ileal digestibility values of amino acids in canola meal determined by the difference method was eliminated at the higher inclusion levels (305 and 366 g kg^{-1}). There were decreases in the standard errors

of the means of ileal digestibility values of amino acids when the inclusion level of canola meal was increased from 244 to 366 g kg^{-1}. This shows once more that the accuracy of the difference method depends on the inclusion level of the assay feed ingredient (canola meal) in the assay diet. The higher the inclusion level, the more accurate the estimation of ileal digestibility values of amino acids by the difference method.

For estimating the apparent ileal digestibility values of crude protein and amino acids in canola meal by the regression method, the linear relationships between apparent ileal digestibility values (diets 2, 3, 4 and 5) and the contribution levels of crude protein and amino acids from the basal feed ingredient (barley) to the diets were analysed according to the model described in Equation 13.11. The regression equations are presented in Table 13.7. Unexpectedly, linear relationships could not

Table 13.7. The linear relationships between the apparent ileal digestibility values and the contribution levels of crude protein and amino acids for the determination of apparent ileal digestibility values of amino acids in canola meal with the regression method (Fan and Sauer, 1995a).

Items	Regression equations[a,b]	r^2	$S_{y.x}$ [c]	P[d]	
Crude protein[e]	$Y = 64.3 + 6.6X$	0.52	3.39	0.001	0.05
Amino acids					
Indispensable					
Arginine[e]	$Y = 79.5 + 11.1X$	0.69	2.49	0.001	0.01
Histidine[e]	$Y = 78.7 + 8.2X$	0.48	2.71	0.001	0.05
Isoleucine	$Y = 67.1 + 2.6X$	0.01	3.81	0.001	0.66
Leucine	$Y = 69.1 + 1.5X$	0.01	3.75	0.001	0.78
Lysine[e]	$Y = 71.8 + 12.5X$	0.72	3.54	0.001	0.01
Phenylalanine	$Y = 69.2 + 0.6X$	0.01	4.41	0.001	0.91
Threonine	$Y = 64.2 + 1.9X$	0.01	3.68	0.001	0.52
Valine	$Y = 65.4 + 1.5X$	0.01	3.94	0.001	0.79
Dispensable					
Alanine[e]	$Y = 66.6 + 12.7X$	0.74	4.04	0.001	0.05
Aspartic acid	$Y = 62.0 + 1.9X$	0.01	3.75	0.001	0.75
Glutamic acid[e]	$Y = 79.6 + 7.4X$	0.55	3.02	0.001	0.03
Glycine[e]	$Y = 62.0 + 18.5X$	0.76	5.51	0.001	0.01
Serine	$Y = 63.1 + 1.3X$	0.01	3.45	0.001	0.79
Tyrosine[e]	$Y = 64.5 + 6.3X$	0.54	3.54	0.001	0.04

[a] Y = apparent ileal digestibility values of crude protein or amino acids (%) in the assay diets.
[b] X = the contribution levels of crude protein or amino acids from the basal feed ingredient (barley) to the content of the assay diets.
[c] Standard error of estimate of the regression equation.
[d] The probabilities of significance for the intercept and the slope of the regression equation.
[e] The linear regression equation is significant ($P < 0.05$, $n = 20$).

be established ($P > 0.05$) for aspartic acid, isoleucine, leucine, phenylalanine, serine, threonine and valine. This was due to the fact that the differences in apparent ileal digestibility values for these amino acids between the assay (canola meal) and the basal feed ingredient (barley) were not large enough to create linear variations (Table 13.7). The principle of estimating apparent ileal amino acid digestibility values in the assay feed ingredient (canola meal) by the regression method is illustrated in Fig. 13.6 for arginine. The ileal digestibility values of crude protein and some amino acids in canola meal were estimated by the regression method according to Equations 13.12 and 13.13. The ileal digestibility values of amino acids in canola meal estimated by the regression method are presented in Table 13.8. However, as mentioned previously, the ileal digestibility values of several amino acids in canola meal could not be estimated (Table 13.8).

The apparent ileal digestibility values of crude protein and amino acids in canola meal were determined by the direct method (Equation 13.5) from diet 5, and the digestibility values are presented in Table 13.8.

As shown in Table 13.8, the apparent ileal digestibility values of crude protein and amino acids in canola meal estimated by the regression method were not different ($P > 0.05$) from those determined by the direct method and were very close to ($P > 0.05$) the values determined by the difference method at the higher inclusion levels of canola meal (305 and 366 g kg^{-1}). These values were usually lower than those determined by the difference method at the low inclusion level of canola meal (244 g kg^{-1}). These results show that the regression and direct methods are valid for determining the apparent ileal digestibility values of amino acids in protein supplements. With respect to the difference

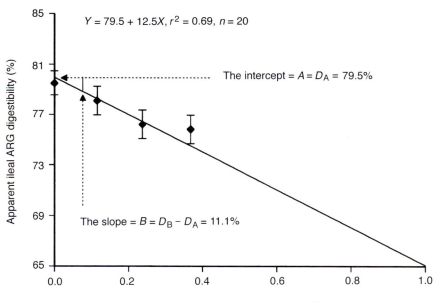

Fig. 13.6. Estimation of the apparent ileal digestibility of arginine (ARG) in the assay feed ingredient (canola meal) by linearly regressing the ileal digestibility values (*Y*: %, means ± SE) of arginine in assay diets against the contribution levels (*X*) of arginine from the basal feed ingredient (barley) to its content in the assay diets (Fan and Sauer, 1995a).

Table 13.8. Determination of the apparent ileal digestibility values[a] (%) of crude protein and amino acids in canola meal by the direct, the difference and the regression methods (Fan and Sauer, 1995a).

	Methods of determination		
Items	Direct method	Difference method[b]	Regression method
No. of observations	5	5	20
Crude protein	66.0 ± 0.85	62.5 ± 1.44	64.3 ± 1.46
Amino acids			
Indispensable			
Arginine	80.8 ± 1.19	79.4 ± 1.14	79.5 ± 0.95
Histidine	80.0 ± 0.78	77.4 ± 1.19	78.7 ± 1.09
Isoleucine	69.3 ± 0.77	65.3 ± 1.58	—
Leucine	70.8 ± 1.15	67.7 ± 1.68	—
Lysine	73.7 ± 0.79	70.7 ± 1.10	71.8 ± 1.38
Phenylalanine	70.8 ± 1.18	67.9 ± 1.90	—
Threonine	63.1 ± 0.88	60.7 ± 1.64	—
Valine	67.5 ± 0.84	63.8 ± 1.72	—
Dispensable			
Alanine	68.9 ± 0.60	65.2 ± 1.95	66.6 ± 1.55
Aspartic acid	64.1 ± 1.04	61.2 ± 1.65	—
Glutamic acid	80.3 ± 1.17	75.8 ± 1.42	79.6 ± 1.19
Glycine	63.4 ± 1.95	63.7 ± 1.28	62.0 ± 1.89
Serine	65.0 ± 0.64	62.0 ± 1.65	—
Tyrosine	66.0 ± 0.81	64.5 ± 1.53	64.5 ± 1.49

[a]Mean and standard error of the mean.
[b]Digestibility values calculated from diet 2 (366 g kg^{-1} inclusion of canola meal).

method, the apparent ileal digestibility values of amino acids in the test protein supplement (canola meal) were over-estimated ($P < 0.05$ or 0.10) when a low-protein feedstuff (barley) was the basal feed ingredient and when the inclusion of the test protein supplement (canola meal) was low in the assay diet; however, this over-estimation was eliminated through including a high level of the protein supplement (canola meal). Therefore, it is recommended that a protein supplement rather than a low-protein feedstuff (e.g. cereal grains) is the basal feed ingredient when the difference method is used. On the other hand, in the case of some protein supplements of poor palatability (e.g. feather meal and blood meal), the ileal digestibility values of amino acids should be determined by the difference rather than by the direct method (e.g. Knabe *et al.*, 1989; Sauer *et al.*, 1989). Because of the low level of inclusion of these protein supplements in the assay diets, the ileal digestibility values of amino acids determined by the difference method may not be reliable, especially for the limiting amino acids. For example, Knabe *et al.* (1989) reported that the ileal digestibility values of isoleucine calculated by the difference method for three samples of blood meal were 60, 70 and 80%, respectively. As pointed out by these authors, these values do not represent the variation in ileal digestibility values of isoleucine and may simply be a reflection of experimental error. Blood meal provided only 15% of the isoleucine content in the assay diets. Therefore, the regression rather than the direct or difference method is only suitable for these protein supplements.

In conclusion, the regression method is, in principle, the most accurate approach for determining apparent ileal digestibility values of amino acids in protein supplements. In order to apply the regression method successfully for all amino acids, the basal and the assay feed ingredient should be paired in such a way that differences in ileal digestibility values of amino acids between the two feed ingredients are large enough to create linear variations.

With respect to the difference method, it is recommended that a protein supplement rather than a low-protein feedstuff (e.g. cereal grains) is the basal feed ingredient and that the inclusion level of the test protein supplement is high in the assay diet. However, for some protein supplements of poor palatability, the regression rather than the direct or the difference method should be used.

Legume seeds

In further studies with peas (Fan and Sauer, 1995b), five barrows, as described previously, were fed five maize starch-based diets according to a 5×5 Latin square design. Diet 1 contained 885 g kg^{-1} wheat providing the sole source of amino acids. In diets 2, 3 and 4, peas were included at three levels at the expense of maize starch, 168, 336 and 504 g kg^{-1}, respectively. Diet 5 contained 671 g kg^{-1} peas providing the sole source of amino acids. All diets were formulated to contain 160 g kg^{-1} crude protein.

The apparent ileal digestibility values of crude protein and amino acids in peas were determined by the difference method (Equation 13.7) at three inclusion levels (diets 2, 3, and 4). There were no differences ($P > 0.05$) in ileal digestibility values of crude protein and amino acids in peas determined by the difference method between the three inclusion levels. Although the ileal digestibility values appeared to be higher at the high (504 g kg^{-1}) rather than at the low inclusion level (168 g kg^{-1}) for some amino acids, the differences were not significant ($P > 0.05$), for example, for histidine, methionine and serine. The level of inclusion of peas did not affect the digestibility values of crude protein and amino acids when these were determined by the difference method from diets 2, 3, and 4. Furthermore, these results also showed that increases in trypsin inhibitor activity up to 2.32 TIU mg^{-1} of diet, resulting from increasing the inclusion of peas in the diets, did not affect the ileal digestibility values of crude protein and amino acids when these were determined by the difference method. In addition, there were decreases in the standard errors of the means of the ileal digestibility values of crude protein and amino acids when the inclusion level of peas was increased from 168 to 504 g kg^{-1}. This shows that the accuracy of the determination of apparent ileal amino acid digestibility values by the difference method is dependent on the inclusion level of the assay feed ingredient (peas) in the assay diet.

For estimating the apparent ileal digestibility values of crude protein and amino acids in the assay feed ingredient (peas) by the regression method, the linear relationships between the apparent ileal digestibility values in the diets (diets 2, 3, 4 and 5) and the contribution levels of crude protein and amino acids from the basal feed ingredient (wheat) to the diets were analysed according to Equation 13.11. The regression equations are presented in Table 13.9. However, linear relationships were not significant ($P > 0.05$) for crude protein, alanine, glycine, histidine, threonine and valine (Table 13.8). This was due to the fact that the differences in apparent ileal digestibility values of crude protein and these amino acids between the assay (peas) and the basal feed ingredient (wheat) were not large enough to create linear variations. The principle for determining apparent ileal amino acid digestibility values in the assay feed ingredient (peas) by the regression method is illustrated in Fig. 13.7 with cysteine as an example. The apparent ileal digestibility values of the majority of the amino acids in peas were determined by the regression method according to Equations 13.12 and 13.13 (Table 13.10). On the other hand, the presence of linear relationships for the majority of amino acids between the assay (peas) and the basal feed ingredient (wheat)

Table 13.9. The linear relationships between the apparent ileal digestibility values and the contribution levels of crude protein and amino acids for the determination of apparent ileal digestibility values of amino acids in peas with the regression method (Fan and Sauer, 1995b).

Items	Regression equations[a,b]	r^2	$S_{y.x}$[c]
Crude protein[d]	$Y = 74.9 + 2.9X$	0.09	2.98
Amino acids			
Indispensable			
Arginine[d]	$Y = 89.4 + 7.9X$	0.46	1.95
Histidine	$Y = 79.9 + 0.9X$	0.01	2.58
Isoleucine[d]	$Y = 74.9 + 7.0X$	0.23	3.68
Leucine[d]	$Y = 74.8 + 8.0X$	0.33	3.39
Lysine[d]	$Y = 82.5 + 17.7X$	0.65	2.51
Methionine[d]	$Y = 64.9 + 14.6X$	0.56	4.24
Phenylalanine[d]	$Y = 76.2 + 7.9X$	0.42	2.77
Threonine	$Y = 67.2 + 1.0X$	0.01	4.11
Valine	$Y = 72.5 + 5.8X$	0.14	4.12
Dispensable			
Alanine	$Y = 70.1 + 2.1X$	0.01	4.86
Aspartic acid[d]	$Y = 77.6 + 8.6X$	0.23	3.61
Cysteine[d]	$Y = 56.5 + 26.1X$	0.85	3.53
Glutamic acid[d]	$Y = 83.9 + 7.3X$	0.58	2.07
Glycine	$Y = 65.8 + 4.0X$	0.03	6.71
Serine[d]	$Y = 71.9 + 7.7X$	0.42	3.45
Tyrosine[d]	$Y = 69.0 + 7.2X$	0.26	3.61

[a] Y = apparent ileal digestibility values of cude protein or amino acids (%) in the assay diets.
[b] X = the contribution levels of crude protein or amino acids from the basal feed ingredient (wheat) to the content of the assay diets.
[c] Standard error of estimate of the regression equation.
[d] The linear regression equation is significant ($P < 0.05$, $n = 20$).

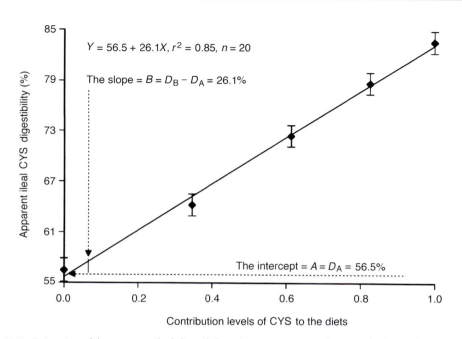

Fig. 13.7. Estimation of the apparent ileal digestibility of cysteine (CYS) in the assay feed ingredient (peas) by linearly regressing the ileal digestibility values (*Y*: %, means ± SE) of cysteine in assay diets against the contribution levels (*X*) of cysteine from the basal feed ingredient (wheat) to its content in the assay diets (Fan and Sauer, 1995b).

proves that there are no interactions in apparent ileal digestibility values of amino acids between these two ingredients.

The apparent ileal digestibility values of crude protein and amino acids in peas were determined by the direct method (Equation 13.5) from diet 5. The digestibility values are presented in Table 13.10.

As shown in Table 13.10, there were no differences (*P* > 0.05) between the direct, difference and the regression methods for the determination of apparent ileal digestibility values of amino acids in peas. However, measured with the difference method, the inclusion level of the test feedstuff in the assay diet should be high in order to obtain more precise digestibility values.

In conclusion, these results show that the regression method is, in principle, the most accurate approach for determining apparent ileal digestibility values of amino acids in legume seeds. The direct and difference methods are also suitable for these feedstuffs. With respect to the difference method, it is recommended that the inclusion level of the test feedstuff in the assay diet is high in order that the apparent ileal digestibility values of amino acids in the test feedstuff can be determined more precisely.

Conclusions

The ileal rather than faecal analysis method should be used for determining amino acid digestibility; values determined with this method reflect the digestive utilization of amino acids in feed ingredients by pigs. Ileal amino acid digestibility values provide an estimate of amino acid availability values and should be used in feed evaluation.

Apparent ileal amino acid digestibility values from the literature, determined with the ileal analysis method, were reviewed and showed considerable variation among different samples of the same feedstuff. The variation in ileal amino acid digestibility values within the same feedstuff was

Table 13.10. Determination of the apparent ileal digestibility values[a] (%) of crude protein and amino acids in peas by the direct, the difference and the regression methods (Fan and Sauer, 1995b).

Items	Methods of determination		
	Direct method	Difference method[b]	Regression method
No. of observations	5	5	20
Crude protein	75.9 ± 1.20	75.1 ± 1.20	—
Amino acids			
Indispensable			
Arginine	89.8 ± 0.81	90.9 ± 0.57	89.4 ± 0.67
Histidine	80.1 ± 1.08	81.3 ± 1.12	—
Isoleucine	75.2 ± 1.05	76.9 ± 2.13	74.9 ± 1.36
Leucine	74.9 ± 1.38	77.0 ± 1.68	74.8 ± 1.27
Lysine	83.5 ± 1.20	83.8 ± 0.70	82.5 ± 0.85
Methionine	66.3 ± 1.43	65.3 ± 1.58	64.9 ± 1.67
Phenylalanine	76.1 ± 1.55	78.5 ± 1.23	76.2 ± 1.04
Threonine	68.0 ± 1.80	69.8 ± 1.54	—
Valine	72.8 ± 1.29	74.5 ± 1.82	—
Dispensable			
Alanine	71.0 ± 1.45	70.5 ± 1.88	—
Aspartic acid	78.1 ± 0.85	79.6 ± 1.45	77.6 ± 1.25
Cysteine	57.3 ± 1.27	56.3 ± 1.91	56.5 ± 1.39
Glutamic acid	84.1 ± 0.88	88.4 ± 1.23	83.9 ± 0.83
Glycine	67.4 ± 1.67	64.7 ± 3.28	—
Serine	72.7 ± 1.21	72.1 ± 0.65	71.9 ± 1.00
Tyrosine	69.5 ± 1.91	70.2 ± 1.50	69.0 ± 1.35

[a]Mean and standard error of the mean.
[b]Digestibility values calculated from diet 4 (504 g kg^{-1} inclusion of peas).

reviewed for cereal grains, protein supplements and legume seeds. In addition to different processing conditions and inherent factors among samples of the same feedstuff, a large proportion of the differences can be attributed to approaches in methodology.

Differences in dietary amino acid levels are likely to be the largest single contributor to the variation of ileal amino acid digestibility values within the same feedstuff. Dietary amino acid levels quadratically affect ileal amino acid digestibility values. In order to remove the effect of dietary amino acid levels, the plateau apparent ileal amino acid digestibility values should be determined.

Finally, methods of determination can also result in differences in ileal amino acid digestibility values within the same feedstuff. In order to eliminate this variation, methods of determination specifically suited for different feedstuffs are recommended. For cereal grains, the regression and the difference method rather than the direct method should be used. For most protein supplements, the direct, the difference and the regression methods are all suited for the determination. However, for feedstuffs including some protein supplements and by-products that can only be included at low levels in the assay diets, the regression rather than the direct or the difference method should be used.

References

Adeola, O. (1996) Bioavailability of tryptophan in soybean meal for 10-kg pigs using the slope–ratio assay. *Journal of Animal Science* 74, 2411–2419.

Agriculture Research Council (1981) *The Nutrient Requirements of Pigs*. Commonwealth Agricultural Bureau, Slough, UK.

Austic, R.E. (1983) The availability of amino acids as an attribute of feeds. In: Robards, G.E. and Packham, R.G. (eds) *Feed Information and Animal Production – Proceedings of the 2nd Symposium of the International Network of Feed Information Centres*. Commonwealth Agricultural Bureau, Slough, UK, pp. 175–189.

Batterham, E.S. (1992) Availability and utilization of amino acids for growing pigs. *Nutrition Research and Reviews* 5, 1–18.

Batterham, E.S., Murison, R.D. and Lewis, C.E. (1979) Availability of lysine in protein concentrates as determined by the slope–ratio assay with growing pigs and rats and by chemical techniques. *British Journal of Nutrition* 41, 383–391.

Batterham, E.S., Anderson, L.M., Baigent, D.R., Darnell, R.E. and Taverner, M.R. (1990a) A comparison of the availability and ileal digestibility of lysine in cottonseed and soybean meals for grower/finisher pigs. *British Journal of Nutrition* 64, 663–677.

Batterham, E.S., Anderson, L.M., Baigent, D.R., Beech, S.A. and Elliott, R. (1990b) Utilization of ileal digestible amino acids by pigs: lysine. *British Journal of Nutrition* 64, 679–690.

Begbie, R. and Pusztai, A. (1989) The resistance to proteolytic breakdown of plant (seed) proteins and their effects on nutrient utilization and gut metabolism. In: Friedman, M. (ed.) *Absorption and Utilization of Amino Acids*, Vol. III. CRC Press Inc., Boca Raton, Florida, pp. 243–263.

Carlson, K.H. and Bayley, H.S. (1970) Nitrogen and amino acids in the feces of young pigs receiving a protein-free diet and diets containing graded levels of soybean meal or casein. *Journal of Nutrition* 100, 1353–1361.

Chang, C.J., Tanksley, T.D., Jr, Knabe, D.A. and Zebrowska, T. (1987) Effects of different heat treatments during processing on nutrient digestibility of soybean meal in growing swine. *Journal of Animal Science* 65, 1273–1282.

De Lange, C.F.M., Sauer, W.C. and Souffrant, W.B. (1989) The effect of protein status of the pig on the recovery and amino acid composition of endogenous protein in digesta collected from the distal ileum. *Journal of Animal Science* 67, 755–762.

De Lange, C.F.M., Souffrant, W.B. and Sauer, W.C. (1990) Real ileal protein and amino acid digestibilities in feedstuffs for growing pigs as determined with the ^{15}N-isotope dilution technique. *Journal of Animal Science* 68, 409–418.

Dierick, N., Vervaeke, I., Decuypere, J., van der Heyde, H. and Henderickx, H.K. (1988) Correlation of ileal and fecal digested protein and organic matter to production performance in growing pigs. *Wissenschaftliche Zeitschrift WPU, Rostock. N-Reihe* 37, 50–51.

Eggum, B.O. (1973) A study of certain factors influencing protein utilization in feedstuffs in rats and pigs. PhD thesis. Copenhagen, Denmark.

Fan, M.Z. (1994) Methodological considerations for the determination of amino acid digestibility in pigs. PhD dissertation, University of Alberta, Edmonton, Alberta, Canada.

Fan, M.Z. and Sauer, W.C. (1995a) Determination of apparent ileal amino acid digestibility in barley and canola meal for pigs with the direct, difference, and regression methods. *Journal of Animal Science* 73, 2364–2374.

Fan, M.Z. and Sauer, W.C. (1995b) Determination of apparent ileal amino acid digestibility in peas for pigs with the direct, difference, and regression methods. *Livestock Production Science* 44, 61–72.

Fan, M.Z. and Sauer, W.C. (1997) Determination of true ileal amino acid digestibility in feedstuffs for pigs with the linear relationships between distal ileal output and dietary inputs of amino acids. *Journal of the Science of Food and Agriculture* 73, 189–199.

Fan, M.Z., Sauer, W.C. and Li, S. (1993) The additivity of the digestible energy and apparent ileal digestible amino acid supply in barley, wheat and canola meal or soybean meal diets for growing pigs. *Journal of Animal Physiology and Animal Nutrition* 70, 72–81.

Fan, M.Z., Sauer, W.C., Hardin, R.T. and Lien, K.A. (1994) Determination of apparent ileal amino acid digestibility in pigs: effect of dietary amino acid level. *Journal of Animal Science* 72, 2851–2859.

Fan, M.Z., Sauer, W.C. and McBurney, M.I. (1995) Estimation by regression analysis of endogenous amino acid levels in digesta collected from the distal ileum of pigs. *Journal of Animal Science* 73, 2319–2328.

Fan, M.Z., Sauer, W.C. and Gabert, V.M. (1996) Variability of apparent ileal amino acid digestibility in canola meal for growing–finishing pigs. *Canadian Journal of Animal Science* 76, 563–569.

Furuya, S. and Kaji, Y. (1989) Estimation of the true ileal digestibility of amino acids and nitrogen from their apparent values for growing pigs. *Animal Feed Science and Technology* 26, 271–285.

Gatel, F. (1992) Protein quality of legume seeds for monogastrics animals. In: *Proceedings of the First European Conference on Grain Legumes*. Angers, France, pp. 461–473.

Giger, S. and Sauvant, D. (1983) Comparison of various methods to determine digestibility coefficients of concentrates and by products by ruminants. In: Robards, G.E. and Packham, R.G. (eds) *Feed Information and Animal Production – Proceedings of the 2nd Symposium of the International Network of Feed Information Centres*. Commonwealth Agricultural Bureau, Slough, UK, pp. 243–248.

Green, S. and Kiener, T. (1989) Digestibilities of nitrogen and amino acids in soybean, sunflower, meat and rapeseed meals measured with pigs and poultry. *Animal Production* 48, 157–179.

Green, S., Bertrand, S.L., Duron, M.J.C. and Mailard, R.A. (1987) Digestibility of amino acids in maize, wheat and barley meal measured in pigs with ileo-rectal anastomosis and isolation of the large intestine. *Journal of the Science of Food and Agriculture* 41, 29–43.

Hagemeister, H. and Erbersdobler, H. (1985) Chemical labelling of dietary protein by transformation of lysine to homoarginine: a new technique to follow intestinal digestion and absorption. *Proceedings of Nutrition Society* 44, 133A.

Henry, Y. (1985) Principles of protein evaluation in pig feeding. *World Review of Animal Production* 21, 48–59.

Holmes, J.H.G., Bayley, H.S., Leadbeater, P.A. and Horney, F.D. (1974) Digestion of protein in the small intestine and large intestine of the pig. *British Journal of Nutrition* 32, 479–489.

Imbeah, M., Sauer, W.C. and Mosenthin, R. (1988) The prediction of the digestible amino acid supply in barley–soybean meal or canola meal diets and pancreatic enzyme secretion in pigs. *Journal of Animal Science* 66, 1409–1417.

Ivan, M. and Farrell, D.J. (1976) Nutritional evaluation of wheat. 5. Disappearance of components in digesta of pigs prepared with two re-entrant cannulae. *Animal Production* 23, 111–119.

Jørgensen, H., Sauer, W.C. and Thacker, P.A. (1984) Amino acid availabilities in soybean meal, sunflower meal, fish meal and meat and bone meal fed to growing pigs. *Journal of Animal Science* 58, 926–934.

Just, A., Jørgensen, H. and Fernandez, J.A. (1985) Correlation of protein deposition in growing pigs to ileal and faecal digestible crude protein and amino acids. *Livestock Production Science* 12, 145–159.

Knabe, D.A. (1991) Bioavailability of amino acids in feedstuffs for swine. In: Miller, E.R., Ullrey, A.E. and Lewis, A.J. (eds) *Swine Nutrition*. Butterworth-Heinemann, Boston, pp. 327–339.

Knabe, D.A., LaRue, D.C., Gregg, E.J., Martinez, G.M. and Tanksley, T.D., Jr (1989) Apparent digestibility of nitrogen and amino acids in protein feedstuffs by growing pigs. *Journal of Animal Science* 67, 441–458.

Kotb, A.R. and Luckey, T.D. (1972) Markers in nutrition. *Nutrition Abstracts and Reviews* 42, 813–849.

Krawielitzki, K. and Smulikowaka, S. (1977) Versuche zur Bestimmung des endogenen und exogenen fäkalen N-Anteiles monogastrischer Tierarten. *Archives Tierernährung* 27, 39–47.

Krawielitzki, K., Zebrowska, T., Schadereit, R., Kowalczyk, J., Hennig, U., Wünsche, J. and Herrmann, U. (1990) Determination of nitrogen absorption and nitrogen secretion in different sections of the pig's intestine by digesta exchange between ^{15}N labelled and unlabelled animals. *Archives of Animal Nutrition* 40, 25–37.

Kreienbring, F., Wünsche, J. and Kesting, U. (1988) Studies on the apparent preacecal and fecal crude protein digestibility and the absorption of amino acids from forage plants in fattening pigs. *Archives of Animal Nutrition* 38, 573–582.

Kuiken, K.A. and Lyman, C.M. (1948) Availability of amino acids in some foods. *Journal of Nutrition* 36, 359–368.

LaRue, D.C., Knabe, D.A. and Tanksley, T.D., Jr (1985) Commercially processed glandless cottonseed meal for starter, grower and finisher swine. *Journal of Animal Science* 60, 495–502.

Lien, K.A., Sauer, W.C., Dugan, M.E.R. and Mosenthin, R. (1993) Evaluation of the ^{15}N-isotope dilution technique for determining the recovery of endogenous protein in ileal digesta of pigs: effect of the pattern of blood sampling, precursor pools, and isotope dilution technique. *Journal of Animal Science* 75, 159–169.

Lin, F.D., Knabe, D.A. and Tanksley, T.D., Jr (1987) Apparent digestibility of amino acids, gross energy and starch in corn, sorghum, wheat, barley, oat groats and wheat middlings for growing pigs. *Journal of Animal Science* 64, 1655–1667.

Low, A.G. (1980) Nutrient absorption in pigs. *Journal of the Science of Food and Agriculture* 31, 1087–1130.

Low, A.G. (1982a) Digestibility and availability of amino acids from feedstuffs for pigs: a review. *Livestock Production Science* 9, 511–520.

Low, A.G. (1982b) Endogenous nitrogen evaluation from absorption studies. In: *Physiology Digestive chez le Porc. Les Colloques de l'INRA* Vol. 12. Jouy-en-Josas, pp. 189–198.

Low, A.G. (1990) Protein evaluation in pigs and poultry. In: Wiseman, J. and Cole, D.J.A. (eds) *Feedstuff Evaluation*. Butterworth, London, pp. 91–114.

Mason, V.C. (1984) Metabolism of nitrogenous compounds in the large gut. *Proceedings of the Nutrition Society* 43, 45–53.

Rudolph, B.C., Boggs, L.S., Knabe, D.A., Tanksley, T.D., Jr and Anderson, S.A. (1983) Digestibility of nitrogen and amino acids in soybean products for pigs. *Journal of Animal Science* 57, 373–386.

Sauer, W.C. and De Lange, C.F.M. (1992) Novel methods for determining protein and amino acid digestibilities in feedstuffs. In: Nissen, S. (ed.) *Modern Methods in Protein Nutrition and Metabolism*. Academic Press Inc., California, pp. 87–120.

Sauer, W.C. and Ozimek, L. (1986) Digestibility of amino acids in swine: results and their practical application. A review. *Livestock Production Science* 15, 367–387.

Sauer, W.C., Stothers, S.C. and Parker, R. (1977a) Apparent and true availabilities of amino acids in wheat and milling by-products for growing pigs. *Canadian Journal of Animal Science* 57, 775–784.

Sauer, W.C., Stothers, S.C. and Philips, G.D. (1977b) Apparent availabilities of amino acids in corn, wheat and barley for growing pigs. *Canadian Journal of Animal Science* 57, 585–597.

Sauer, W.C., Kennelly, J.J. and Aherne, F.X. (1981) The availabilities of amino acids in barley and wheat for growing pigs. *Canadian Journal of Animal Science* 61, 793–802.

Sauer, W.C., Cichon, R. and Misir, R. (1982) Amino acid availability and protein quality of canola and rapeseed meal for pigs and rats. *Journal of Animal Science* 54, 292–301.

Sauer, W.C., Dugan, M., De Lange, C.F.M., Imbeah, M. and Mosenthin, R. (1989) Considerations in methodology for the determination of amino acid digestibilities in feedstuffs for pigs. In: Friedman, M. (ed.) *Absorption and Utilization of Amino Acids*. Vol. III. CRC Press, Boca Raton, Florida, pp. 217–230.

Sauer, W.C., Imbeah, M. and Dugan, M. (1990) Amino acid digestibility in swine. In: *Proceedings of 26th Nutrition Conference for Feed Manufacturers*. Guelph, Ontario, pp. 1–15.

Schneider, B.H. and Flatt, W.P. (1975) *The Evaluation of Feeds Through Digestibility Experiments*. University of Georgia Press, Athens, Georgia.

Sibbald, I.R. (1987) Estimation of bioavailable amino acids in feedingstuffs for poultry and pigs: a review with emphasis on balance experiments. *Canadian Journal of Animal Science* 67, 221–300.

Souffrant, W.B. (1991) Endogenous nitrogen losses during digestion in pigs. In: Verstegen, M.W.A., Huisman, J. and den Hartog, L.A. (eds) *Digestive Physiology in Pigs – Proceedings of the 5th International Symposium on Digestive Physiology in Pigs*. EAAP Publication No. 54. Wageningen (Doorwerth), The Netherlands, pp. 147–166.

Souffrant, W.B., Köhler, R. and Gebhardt, G. (1981) Untersuchungen zur Bestimmung der Endogenen N-Sekretion im Dünndarm bei Schweinen. *Archives of Animal Nutrition* 31, 35–43.

Souffrant, W.B., Darcy-Vrillon, B., Corring, T., Laplace, J.P., Köhler, R., Gebhardt, G. and Rérat, A. (1986) Recycling of endogenous nitrogen in the pig (preliminary results of a collaborative study). *Archives of Animal Nutrition* 36, 269–274.

Tanksley, T.D., Jr and Knabe, D.A. (1982) Amino acid digestibility of some high protein feedstuffs and possible use in formulating swine diets. *Feedstuffs* 54, 16–21.

Tanksley, T.D., Jr, Knabe, D.A., Purser, K. and Zebrowska, T. (1981) Apparent digestibility of amino acids and nitrogen in three cottonseed meals and one soybean meal. *Journal of Animal Science* 52, 769–777.

Taverner, M.R., Hume, I.D. and Farrell, D.J. (1981) Availability to pigs of amino acids in cereal grains. 1. Endogenous levels of amino acids in ileal digesta and feces of pigs given cereal diets. *British Journal of Nutrition* 46, 149–158.

Van Leeuwen, P., Sauer, W.C., Huisman, J., van Weerden, E.J., van Kleef, D. and den Hartog, L.A. (1987) Methodological aspects for the determination of amino acid digestibilities in pigs fitted with ileo-cecal re-entrant cannulas. *Journal of Animal Physiology and Animal Nutrition* 58, 122–133.

Van Soest, P.J., Uden, P. and Wrick, K.F. (1983) Critique and evaluation of markers for use in nutrition of humans and farm and laboratory animals. *Nutrition Reports International* 27, 17–28.

Waterlow, J.C., Garlick, P.J. and Millward, D.J. (1978) *Protein Turnover in Mammalian Tissues and in The Whole Body.* North-Holland Publishing Co., Amsterdam.

Wiseman, J., Jaggert, S., Cole, D.J.A. and Haresign, W. (1991) Digestion and utilization of amino acids of heat-treated fish meal by growing/finishing pigs. *Animal Production* 53, 215–224.

Wünsche, J., Hennig, U., Meinl, M., Kreienbring, F. and Bock, H.D. (1982) Investigation of the absorption and utilization of amino acids infused into cecum of growing pigs. I. N-balance measurement with regard to the utilization of lysine and isoleucine and requirement of growing pigs. *Archives of Animal Nutrition* 32, 337–348.

Zebrowska, T. (1973) Digestion and absorption of nitrogenous compounds in the large intestine of pigs. *Roczniki Nauk Rolniczych* B95, 85–90.

Zebrowska, T., Buraczewska, L., Pastuszewska, B., Chamberlain, A.G. and Buraczewski, S. (1978) Effect of diet and method of collection on amino acid composition of ileal digesta and digestibility of nitrogen and amino acids in pigs. *Roczniki Nauk Rolniczych* B99, 75–83.

Chapter 14
Rapid Metabolizable Energy Assays

J.M. McNab
Roslin Institute (Edinburgh), Roslin, Midlothian, UK

Introduction

The economic importance of energy in the formulation of least-cost diets for poultry and the increasing poor profitability of commercial poultry production are sustaining interest in the metabolizable energy (ME) values of diets and constituent raw materials. The need to formulate diets with accurate ME values and to make judgements on the effects of treatments, such as conditioning or the addition of enzymes, is re-emphasizing the need to have a reliable means of deriving ME. From time to time, it is debated whether a net energy (NE) system might be a better basis on which to judge the energy status of poultry diets, but whatever system is finally adopted energy balance experiments are almost certain to form the means whereby both ME and NE values are derived.

Over the past two decades, two factors have stimulated research in energy derivations. The first was the introduction of rapid bioassays for ME in the late 1970s and their development during the 1980s; the second was the adoption of energy declarations, with the associated chemical control equation, into the animal feed trade

in Europe in 1986. The latter event focused particularly on the accuracy, repeatability and suitability of different methods as a means of measuring ME.

Not surprisingly in view of its commercial relevance, the topic has been widely reviewed. Sibbald (1979) described the evolution of his method and later produced a very detailed review (Sibbald, 1982); at various times, others have assessed progress (Farrell, 1981; McNab and Fisher, 1982; McNab, 1990). Since 1975, an enormous number of publications have appeared on this subject; for example, 13 years ago Sibbald (1986) listed 561 references related to this area of research, only five of which pre-dated 1975. Since then, the pace has slowed somewhat but without any consensus on what constitutes the ideal procedure to derive ME.

Most recently, emphasis seems to have fallen on repeatability of ME values, across laboratories, across time, across ages and across species, and of variations in dietary ME data. The introduction of energy declarations and of a control equation encourages this, because it is presumed that each system is based on a well-defined and reproducible characteristic, namely the ME of the feed. Attempts to test or verify the validity of equations obviously founder if consistent values cannot be produced. Extension of this philosophy to dietary ingredients also requires the establishment of appropriate prediction equations which relate ME to chemical composition or, perhaps, to some other quality control parameter (e.g. in the case of wheat, density). Here, progress is greatly facilitated if data from different laboratories can be combined, and this results in variations in techniques being highlighted, especially if they are seen to lead to different biases. It might have been hoped that the introduction of an effective rapid bioassay based on robust scientific principles would have resulted in its standardization and universal adoption. There appear to have been two main reasons why this has not happened; firstly, rapid assays almost invariably require birds to be starved, and this has proved controversial; secondly, it is clear that some laboratories experience problems in adopting published techniques, and this has resulted in the introduction of a number of major and minor modifications. Consequently, there are probably more different methods being used to derive ME now than at any time in the past, and the prospect of establishing a single standardized assay is probably as remote as it has ever been.

Definition of ME

Although ME is frequently believed to be a property of a diet, it is actually a characteristic of the animal to which the diet is fed. ME measurements relate to complete diets, and values for dietary components or ingredients must, in most cases, be obtained by comparing data from two or more appropriate diets (so-called substitution or replacement methods). In such derivations, the assumption that ME values amongst feedstuffs are additive is essential, and very little progress can be made if this is not upheld. Energy is, of course, a useful currency for describing mass conversion of the components of the food in the bird. There is another set of problems, similar to those

discussed here for ME, in determining the 'metabolizability' of any nutrient; lipid, protein or carbohydrate. For many purposes, and especially for prediction, it would be invaluable if both ME values and digestibility coefficients for the main chemical components were measured concurrently, but this is only done on rare occasions.

The terminology used in the topic of ME is relatively free from dispute and ambiguity. The widely used convention, mainly in agreement with Sibbald (1982, 1986) will be followed here. The term ME is used in a general sense rather than to mean bioavailable energy (Sibbald, 1982), and the expression endogenous energy loss (EEL) is usually defined, not as a biological entity, but as an empirical quantity, i.e. the energy loss from a starved bird. This is convenient and need not be confusing. The almost invariable convention of ignoring gaseous losses resulting from fermentation is also followed.

Some years ago, Pesti and Edwards (1983) proposed that ME nomenclature should be changed quite radically to reflect the methods which had been used in the evaluation experiments. The approach must have been considered to be unhelpful and unnecessary because it has not been adopted; however, their proposition that more care should be taken in relating experimental observations to well-defined biological elements should be mandatory. In this context, there is probably not enough discipline exercised by editors of scientific journals. ME values are not measured or observed but are the results of derivations from a number of measurements. Because too little basic information is reported, it is often impossible to make critical comparisons between different experiments. By tabulating results in more detail, greater use could be made of existing data and allow outcomes of experiments in different laboratories to be combined.

Classical Methods for Deriving ME

Two approaches traditionally have been followed to generate ME values and these still find favour in many laboratories today. In the substitution method (Hill and Anderson, 1958), the dietary ingredient to be assayed is substituted for an ingredient of known ME value (invariably glucose) in a basal diet to yield a test diet. Simply by comparing the energy balances (gross energy eaten–gross energy excreted) of both basal and test diets and with a knowledge of the ME value of glucose, the ME of the test diet can be calculated. In the replacement method (Sibbald and Slinger, 1963), the ingredient for which the ME is required is exchanged for a known amount of basal diet to form the test diet. By deriving the ME values of basal and test diets, it is a simple matter to calculate the ME of the ingredient. Both these assays were assumed to result in identical values for the test ingredient, but this may not be correct.

Although these two approaches have led to the derivation of values which have long been referred to in terms of ME, they should perhaps more correctly be described as apparent ME (AME). The energy metabolized is now considered 'apparent' because only part of the energy excreted after the food is consumed has emanated directly from the food, i.e. only part consists of undigested and unmetabolized residues. Part of what is excreted has come directly from the bird and has come to be known as the endogenous energy loss (EEL). Part of the EEL is of faecal origin and is generally considered to consist of gut tissue, bile excretions and unabsorbed enzymes; part is urinary and consists primarily of products of nitrogen metabolism.

Throughout the years, the AME system has generally served the scientific community well and played an invaluable role in the development of poultry nutrition. Occasionally, however, concern has been expressed on reliability and, although the reasons put forward generally centred around interactions between dietary ingredients, Sibbald (1982, 1986) has argued persuasively that most of the anomalies which had been associated with AME derivations could be attributed to the effects of EEL. He devised a novel bioassay in which EEL was determined directly and

proposed that, in future, the energy status of both diets and their ingredients should be expressed in terms of their true ME (TME).

Nitrogen Correction

It would be misleading to present the debate as simply one between AME and TME. For many years, it has been common practice to 'correct' AME values derived from balance experiments to take into account any changes in the nitrogen status of the birds during the period of the trial. The rationale for this adjustment arises from the knowledge that the catabolism of protein stored in the body results in the need to dispose of the nitrogen it contained. In poultry, this nitrogen is excreted mainly as uric acid which contains energy; for each gram of nitrogen excreted as uric acid, 34.4 kJ of energy are lost from the body and appear in the urine (droppings). However, a bird which is storing protein (e.g. a broiler) is spared the energy cost of excreting so much nitrogen, and less uric acid, and hence energy, appears in the droppings. Thus the same diet (or ingredient of a diet), when eaten by different birds, may have a different AME value because of differences in the amounts of the ingested protein different birds have retained. To make ME values independent of the conditions under which they were derived, it has become usual to adjust them to what they might have been under standard conditions. The most frequently, although not exclusively, used standard is one where the birds are in nitrogen equilibrium (i.e. where nitrogen retention is zero). The principle of nitrogen correction has often been criticized because a diet (and feedstuff) is penalized as an energy source when it is promoting the retention of protein, often the objective of animal production. However, because the function of any ME system is to describe the energy status of diets and ingredients and not their ability to retain nitrogen, correction to nitrogen equilibrium is justifiable. In any case, failure to make a correction is tantamount to correcting to the nitrogen retention prevailing in the assay. Just as AME values are corrected to nitrogen equilibrium (AME_N), so too should TME values (TME_N).

McNab and Fisher (1982) suggested that the following three observations were required from a bioassay designed to derive ME values: (i) a knowledge of energy balance at (ii) a known food intake and (iii) an appropriate measure of EEL. For correction to nitrogen equilibrium, nitrogen balance must also be known. The choice of bioassay should then be determined largely by how well it provides these essential pieces of information; other factors which may influence choice will be speed, cost and, perhaps, convenience. Three general types of energy balance assays have been identified as follows.

1. Traditional assays which involve preliminary feeding periods to establish a state of 'digestive equilibrium'. Differences between the amounts of dry matter in the digestive tract at the beginning and end of the assay period ('end effects') are controlled by taking precautions to ensure they are the same. In most cases, complete diets must be fed, and substitution or replacement methods, which have been described earlier, must be used to study ingredients.

2. Rapid assays, using starvation both before and after allowing the birds free access to the diet to control any end effects. Again, complete diets must be fed and substitution/replacement methods used to derive values for ingredients in most cases.

3. Rapid assays, as above, but using tube feeding to place the test material directly into the birds' crops. These methods almost invariably avoid any need for replacement/substitution, most diets or ingredients being fed as received.

Whilst many individual variations are found within these three general approaches to deriving ME values, the classification provides a convenient framework within which to debate the many procedural details.

Energy Balance and Food Intake

Food presentation and the accurate measurement of energy intake are arguably the most demanding aspects of ME resolution. When birds are given access to food *ad libitum*, a practice which still seems to be the most widely accepted and free from criticism, great care needs to be taken to prevent food spillage (loss), to minimize any separation of the dietary components, to correct for any changes in the moisture content of the food during the course of the assay and to take (analyse) representative samples of both food and droppings. These are all difficult to control in a consistent way, but specially designed systems have been described and used with apparent success (Terpstra and Janssen, 1975).

Such free-feeding methods are used in type 1 assays which, overall, probably account for the most frequent approach to ME derivation in poultry. Farrell (1978) proposed that the advantage of a rapid assay of the type 2 variety could be gained by training birds to consume sufficiently large intakes of food in the 1 h immediately following a 23 h starvation period. In this assay, it is recommended that equal quantities of a basal diet and test ingredient are combined, and pelleting was also advocated in order to ensure that high food intakes were maintained across a range of raw materials. Soon after its introduction, a number of laboratories reported serious difficulties in achieving satisfactory food intakes but, notwithstanding this, the assay has had its adherents, although its popularity does seem to have waned over the last 10 years. Apart from speed (which has implications for cost) and a reduction in the amount of raw materials required, the technique offers few, if any, advantages over type 1 assays in terms of the precise measurement of food intake or energy balance. Furthermore, the need to pellet precludes the application of this approach to studies concerned with the effects of pelleting on ME values.

It should be beyond debate that the introduction of the food into the crops of birds by tube, as is effected in type 3 assays, is the most precise means of measuring energy intake, because both food spillage and changes in dietary dry matter content are avoided. However, because the dose sizes are reduced and much lower than those seen in *ad libitum* feeding regimes, there may be difficulties in achieving and feeding representative samples. The only legitimate objections to the technique are the obvious limits on the amount of food consumed and, perhaps, attitudes to a procedure frequently referred to as 'force feeding'. Long experience in our laboratory is that, with practice, the entire activity is very rapid (15–20 s per bird to feed 50 g of most feedstuffs) and there is little evidence of more stress beyond that induced by simple handling. Skill is required, however, and experience is essential, although this is readily achieved by most operators. The use of slurry feeding as a means of reducing stress has been proposed and apparently has been reported successfully from a few laboratories, but it is our experience that slurry feeding prolongs the processes, reduces the accuracy of determining food intake and invariably further restricts the quantity of dry matter introduced to the crop. Finely divided, hygroscopic or very bulky ingredients can present problems but, with experience and patience, these can all generally be overcome. In our laboratory, glucose monohydrate is fed routinely; this can cause complications, and granulation is carried out to reduce the difficulty in feeding a hygroscopic powder.

The collection of droppings is another simple task which can be difficult to do well in routine experiments. When trays placed under the cages are used to collect droppings, far and away the most common practice, problems can be caused by the adherence of the droppings to the birds' plummage, contamination with scurf and feathers, changes resulting from fermentation and perhaps losses during removal and transfer from the trays to containers. Losses may also result from the birds excreting away from the tray, and there is the possibility of droppings being contaminated with regurgitated food. This

can be surprisingly difficult to detect and, even when observed, almost impossible to compensate for in a meaningful way. It is relatively easy to draw up a list of sensible precautions to take to ensure good laboratory practices; frequent collections (say, 8 or 12 hourly) are the sorts of devices that are often judged beneficial but, as most tend to be labour intensive, they often erode the advantages of a low-cost bioassay. Alternatives to collection trays (e.g. plastic bags attached to O-rings sutured round the anus) have been promoted from time to time but have never proved popular, and it has to be concluded that the use of trays is unavoidable in routine experiments.

Minimizing End Effects

In assessing the reliability from type 3 assays, it is important to keep in mind that, because inputs are small, any imprecision or uncertainty in the measurement of the intakes or outputs will have a potentially greater effect on the ME value derived. In the ideal system, only droppings stemming from the recorded intake should be debited against that intake. In type 1 assays, where it is customary to carry out the balance over several days and food intakes are often several hundred grams, discrepancies or differences in gut-fills at the beginning and end of the experiment are considered to cancel each other out. Although this is widely accepted, it is not entirely satisfactory because changes in the intakes of rapidly growing birds or responses to unpalatable ingredients are more likely to result in systematic bias than random error. With the much lower intakes found in types 2 and 3 assays, great care must be taken to ensure that the digestive tract is empty of residues at both the beginning and the end of the balance period. Factors which are likely to influence the amount of digesta remaining in the gastrointestinal tract are the nature of the previous diet, the period for which it was removed, the nature of the test feedstuff and the amount given, the length of the collection period, water intake and the random nature of caecal evacuation. Sibbald (1976) originally proposed an initial starvation period of 24 h followed by a collection window of 24 h (24 h + 24 h assay), but latterly recommended 24 h + 48 h for regular use. In our laboratory, 48 h + 48 h is used routinely, with 48 h + 72 h for some raw materials (high-protein or particularly bulky ingredients). The longer periods are clearly more stressful, and factors such as bird size and the administration of glucose come into consideration (McNab and Blair, 1988).

It has been demonstrated unequivocally that 12 h starvation before feeding is insufficient to clear the digestive tract of the residues of the previous diet. Although in some cases extension beyond 24 h has been argued to exert only a small effect on TME values, a direct investigation in our laboratory has shown measurable differences between the energy content of the residues remaining after 24 (20.25 kJ) and 48 h (2.06 kJ) starvation (McNab and Blair, 1988). This finding and the logic of equalizing the pre- and post-feeding starvation periods encourage the application of a 48 h + 48 h assay and the adjustment of other factors to cope with any increased stress. In general, we find clearance rates are quite variable between feedstuffs and the amounts fed and it seems sensible that a constant diet comprising highly digestible components should be used for the maintenance of the birds. To some extent, however, a correction is made for any carry-over of energy from the previous diet in calculating the TME value of a feedstuff, because it seems reasonable to expect that a comparable error will occur in both the fed and negative control birds (those used to derive EEL).

The time required to ensure complete residue clearance from the digestive tract, especially when single ingredients are fed in type 3 assays, is a complex and largely unresolved issue. Our experience with 50 g intakes leads us to believe that 48 h is insufficient for some ingredients. Lower intakes obviously alleviate the problem, but probably at the cost of both reduced

accuracy and increased influence of endogenous factors. It is our view that complete residue clearance is harder to achieve with high-protein, and especially finely divided, animal products; materials of low density, which are packed very tightly in the crop, can also cause problems, where wetting of the feedstuff in the crop may be a complicating factor.

Palatability may also be involved because, for example, when blood meal-fed birds were given water, distaste appeared to be experienced and regurgitation occurred. The sudden introduction of some ingredients may induce gut stasis; attempts to evaluate coffee residues by tube feeding had to be abandoned because the material did not pass from the crop. Less severe but similar responses have been experienced with quinoa. At the present time, it is only possible to advise caution, particularly with unfamiliar ingredients, to look out for the excretion after the end of the balance period and to be wary about accepting unexpected results without further careful scrutiny. While routinely extending the balance period to 72 h could provide an empirical solution to at least some of these problems, it would be at the cost of increased stress on the birds. Longer periods where no food is given also result in higher endogenous:exogenous energy ratios, and the relative importance of the error introduced by correcting for EEL assumes greater importance.

The significance of these factors in type 2 assays is difficult to judge. With higher intakes, such as 70–80 g, collection periods shorter than 48 h may be insufficient for certain feedstuffs. On the other hand, the use of complete diets and allowing the birds access to them for 1 h, may reduce any problems in comparison with tube feeding single ingredients. It seems reasonable to presume that, because the crop will be unlikely to become so tightly packed with dry food under the conditions prevailing, water intake and the passage rate of food residues might be more normal.

The impact of water consumption in these assays is another neglected research area and one where firm conclusions are not possible. In our laboratory, it has been observed consistently that, despite the ready availability of water, tube-fed birds were rarely seen to be drinking. Furthermore, because 90% of water consumption by poultry is believed to be a direct consequence of eating, it could be that the lack of access to food has a marked effect on the stimulus to drink. Whether atypically low and variable water intakes explain erratic and slow food passage rates, and consequently residue clearance, must remain uncertain, but some rather simple evaluations in our laboratory (McNab and Blair, 1988) have resulted in the routine administration of water (50 ml per bird, by tube) during the balance period about 24 h after feeding. This practice also provides the opportunity to palpate the crop and mix any food residues still there with the water. Only rarely (e.g. with blood meal) has it led to losses of food from the crop. However, it does seem reasonable to expect that it will change the relationship between the amounts of food given and the clearance rates. More work is required to clarify the effects of water consumption on ME values over a range of ingredients and diets.

Endogenous Energy Loss (EEL)

Knowledge of the EEL is a prerequisite for the determination of TME and it patently has an effect on the value attributed to AME. That there are both difficulties and uncertainties associated with its quantification is undisputed. Three methods have been used to derive EEL: starving birds; giving birds a completely metabolizable energy source (e.g. glucose); or by extrapolating to zero intake a line relating energy excretion to its consumption.

Starvation has been the most widely used means of deriving EEL. However, during starvation, individual birds void quite variable amounts of energy. Values ranging from 33 to 82 kJ 24 h^{-1} (Farrell, 1978) and from 25 to 69 kJ 24 h^{-1} (Sibbald 1979) have been reported for the second

24 h period of 48 h of starvation (24 h + 24 h assay). In our laboratory, a somewhat wider range has been found, presumably a consequence of the greater maintenance demands associated with the 48 h + 48 h assay. Individual values ranged from 47 to 238 kJ 48 h^{-1} (24–119 kJ 24 h^{-1}) and the average coefficient of variation within an experiment (six replicates) was 36.8%.

No consistent variation can be explained by bird weight or by body weight changes and, although there have been quite reasonable claims that the size of the EEL is related to the temperature of the environment, we have not been able to observe any differences in the EEL from birds fed 50 g of glucose and housed at either 5 or 35°C. In our laboratory, with a 48 h + 48 h bioassay and using the birds approximately every 4 weeks, we have found a substantial reduction in EEL and conspicuously less between-bird variation when droppings are collected from birds fed glucose (50 g) rather than from starved counterparts. There are some sound scientific reasons to believe that body composition and basal metabolic rate influence EEL, but the significance of these in ME evaluations has still to be clarified.

Collaborative studies with a type 1 bioassay, designed to establish a standard method throughout Europe, have shown its reliability as a means of deriving the AME_N values of diets (Bourdillon *et al.*, 1990). However, when these data were used to derive AME_N values of two of the components of the diets, wheat and soybean meals, by a replacement approach, the results proved conspicuously less robust. This example illustrates the difficulty, if not impossibility, of deriving meaningful ME values for raw materials, as opposed to diets, using type 1 assays, even when great care is taken by experienced people.

The simplicity and speed of type 3 assays mean that many more can be carried out in a given time, and this leads to an increase in the amount of information available to practising nutritionists. For the evaluation of ingredients, which can be assayed directly rather than after dietary substitution/replacement, they must be the methods of choice for the future. To fulfil this objective, no effort should be spared to resolve the uncertainty surrounding the size of the EEL. At the present time, there seems good grounds for suspecting that many values quoted and used in the derivation of TME values are overestimates and that under the practical conditions of *ad libitum* feeding, EEL_N lies somewhere between 0 and 20 kJ 24 h^{-1} for a mature bird. With our 48 h + 48 h regime, giving 25 g of glucose at the start of the balance, we most frequently find an EEL_N of around 20 kJ 24 h^{-1}. Applying this value to birds eating 100 g day^{-1}, it can be readily calculated that the difference between TME_N and AME_N is only 0.20 kJ g^{-1}. In other words, an ingredient with a TME_N value of 15.0 kJ g^{-1} would have an AME_N value of 14.8 kJ g^{-1}, only 1.3% lower. The effect is, of course, greater with raw materials of low ME content, but can still be considered small. If the conditions adopted for food presentation can be confirmed to affect EEL, as has been suggested by a number of people, then the differences between AME_N and TME_N may be even smaller and it is doubtful if biological assays would be capable of their detection. With food intakes greater than 100 g the differences would be reduced further and this may explain why efforts to detect them have largely been unsuccessful.

Conclusions

Despite the enormous amount of research devoted to the development of a universally acceptable rapid bioassay to derive the ME values of diets and feedstuffs, attempts have foundered for two reasons. Firstly, rapid assays almost invariably require birds to be starved and this has led to the introduction of the controversial concept of EELs. Secondly, problems have been experienced in some laboratories when tube feeding birds, and this has led to the introduction of many technique modifications. Although the prospect of establishing a single standard method seems remote, this chapter reviews the advantages and disadvantages associated with three general approaches to the derivation of ME in poultry.

References

Bourdillon, A., Carré, B., Conan, L., Duperray, J., Huyghebaert, G., Leclercq, B., Lessire, M., McNab, J. and Wiseman, J. (1990) European reference method for the *in vivo* determination of metabolisable energy with adult cockerels: reproducibility, effect of food intake and comparison with individual laboratory methods. *British Poultry Science* 31, 557–565.

Farrell, D.J. (1978) Rapid determination of metabolisable energy of foods using cockerels. *British Poultry Science* 19, 303–308.

Farrell, D.J. (1981) An assessment of quick bioassays for determining the true metabolisable energy and apparent metabolisable energy of poultry feedstuffs. *World's Poultry Science Journal* 37, 72–83.

Hill, F.W. and Anderson, D.L. (1958) Comparison of metabolisable and productive energy determinations with growing chicks. *Journal of Nutrition* 64, 587–603.

McNab, J.M. (1990) Apparent and true metabolisable energy of poultry diets. In: Wiseman, J. and Cole, D.J.A. (eds) *Feedstuff Evaluation*. Butterworths, London, pp. 41–54.

McNab, J.M. and Blair, J.C. (1988) Modified assay for true and apparent metabolisable energy based on tube feeding. *British Poultry Science* 29, 697–707.

McNab, J.M. and Fisher, C. (1982) The choice between apparent and true metabolisable energy systems – recent evidence. *Proceedings of the 3rd European Symposium on Poultry Nutrition*, The European Federation of Branches of World's Poultry Science Association, pp. 45–55.

Pesti, G.M. and Edwards, H.M. (1983) Metabolisable energy nomenclature for poultry feedstuffs. *Poultry Science* 62, 1275–1280.

Sibbald, I.R. (1976) A bioassay for true metabolisable energy in feedingstuffs. *Poultry Science* 55, 303–308.

Sibbald, I.R. (1979) Metabolisable energy evaluation of poultry diets. In: Haresign, W. and Lewis, D. (eds) *Recent Advances in Animal Nutrition – 1979*. Butterworths, London, pp. 35–49.

Sibbald, I.R. (1982) Measurement of bioavailable energy in poultry feedingstuffs: a review. *Canadian Journal of Animal Science* 62, 983–1048.

Sibbald, I.R. (1986) The T.M.E. system of feed evaluation: methodology, feed composition data and bibliography. *Research Branch Contribution 86–4E*. Animal Research Centre, Agriculture, Canada.

Sibbald, I.R. and Slinger, S.J. (1963) A biological assay for metabolisable energy in poultry feed ingredients together with findings which demonstrate some of the problems associated with the evaluation of fats. *Poultry Science* 42, 313–325.

Terpstra, K. and Janssen, W.M.M.A. (1975) Methods for the determination of metabolisable energy and digestibility coefficients of poultry feeds. *Spelderholt Report 101.75*. Spelderholt Institute for Poultry Research, Beekbergen, The Netherlands.

Part III

Intake and Utilization

Chapter 15
Physiological and Metabolic Aspects of Feed Intake Control

J.M. Forbes

Centre for Animal Sciences, School of Biology, University of Leeds, Leeds, UK

Introduction

The great majority of farm animals are fed *ad libitum*, that is, with free access to food for most of the time. High levels of voluntary intake are required for efficient production because, in general, the more an animal eats the more it produces and the more efficient it becomes. To a considerable extent intake is driven by nutrient requirements, and an approximate estimate of how much food an animal will eat can be calculated from what quantities of energy, protein and nutrients it requires for maintenance and production. However, there are numerous factors which can interfere with the concordance between requirements and intake, and some of these will become clear in this chapter. Briefly, it is unlikely that the nutrients in the food(s) on offer will be present in the same ratio as required by the animal; perhaps protein content will be too low in relation to energy and the animal is then faced with the decision as to whether to increase its intake in order to satisfy its protein requirements, thereby taking in an excess of energy, or whether to reduce its intake in order to avoid overconsumption of energy;

in the latter case, the quantity and/or quality of product will be reduced due to lack of dietary protein. The bulk of the food is another major determinant of the level of intake actually achieved, especially in ruminant animals (see also Chapter 16).

It is generally considered that intake is controlled by a series of negative feedback signals from the digestive tract, liver and other organs in response to the presence of nutrients. In addition, animals learn the metabolic consequences of eating foods with particular sensory properties (appearance, flavour, texture) and can then use 'feed-forward' to choose preferentially or avoid foods which they have experienced previously. The whole system can be viewed as a cascade, depicted in Fig. 15.1. Briefly, potentially ingestible material is selected by sight and/or smell and a decision is made regarding whether or not to eat it. Once in the mouth, the food can be swallowed or rejected, depending on its taste and texture. After swallowing, the animal is committed to dealing with the food, in terms of digestion, absorption and metabolism, although if it is strongly toxic it may well be vomited (see Chapter 18). Following absorption, most of the products of digestion go to the liver

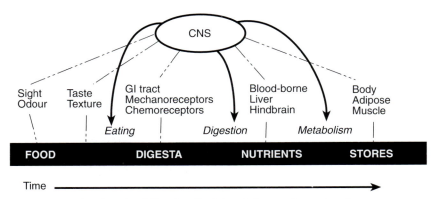

Fig. 15.1. Satiety cascade (after Blundell and Halford, 1994). See text for explanation.

and thence to the general circulation. There are several types of receptor in the stomach, intestines and liver which can inform the central nervous system (CNS) about the volume, osmolality, pH and concentration of some specific types of chemical in digesta and portal blood. Once in the general circulation, the metabolites are available for supporting the various metabolic activities. Any major imbalance between entry of a material into the circulation and its rate of removal is postulated to cause 'metabolic discomfort' which will become associated with the sensory properties of the recently eaten food and tend to induce avoidance of that food when it is next encountered by the animal. Such learned associations are particularly well illustrated in situations in which animals have a choice between two or more foods with different flavours and different patterns of nutrient supply. Of course, the whole system is coordinated by the CNS in a diverse set of pathways that includes the hindbrain and the hypothalamus as important components. The complexities of feeding behaviour, as observed in spontaneously feeding animals (see Chapter 17), are unlikely to be fully explained, therefore, only by a knowledge of physiology and metabolism, however complete that might become.

Each of the aspects outlined in this Introduction will be considered in turn. Further information on all aspects covered in this chapter can be found in Forbes (1995).

Mechanisms of Intake Control

Central nervous system

The brain collects information from the special senses and receptors in the digestive tract wall and metabolizing tissues. This information is integrated and used to determine what food to eat and whether feeding should start or stop. Extensive studies, mostly with laboratory animals, have been carried out to determine the nature of the anatomical sites and neural transmitters involved, and the relatively few studies with farm animals provide confirmation that they are, in general, similar to rats. Electrolytic lesions of the ventromedial hypothalamus cause overeating and obesity while in the lateral hypothalamus they cause undereating, often to the extent that animals die if not kept alive by force feeding. These are not the only parts of the brain involved in intake control, however, and the paraventricular nuclei of the hypothalamus, just ventral to the ventromedial nuclei, are particularly sensitive to the effects of transmitter chemicals, including noradrenaline and neural peptide Y (NPY) (Parrott *et al.*, 1986). Figure 15.2 shows the effect of several doses of NPY injected into the lateral ventricles of the brain in pigs trained to work for food by pressing a panel in the wall of their pen (operant conditioning); with a dose of 100 µg, the pigs worked to obtain 60 rewards of food

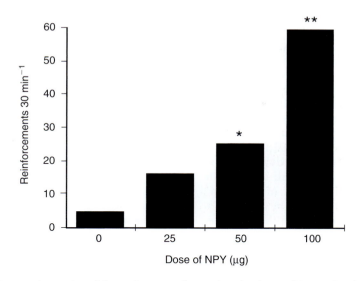

Fig. 15.2. Increase in number of times pigs press a button for a food reward in 30 min when injected intracerebroventricularly with increasing doses of neuropeptide Y (NPY) (Parrott *et al.*, 1986).

during a 30 min test, compared with four when saline was injected (Parrott *et al.*, 1986).

Even if it were thought sensible to use such substances to enhance food intake under commercial conditions, there are two limitations: firstly, how are they to be administered into the brain? Secondly, is it likely that licences will be granted for their use in animals whose products are to be consumed by humans? It is not likely that central nervous active substances will be used commercially to enhance voluntary intake for these reasons and also because, if the animals are already well fed and managed so that the rate of production of meat, milk or eggs is already optimal, then to stimulate intake would only lead to more deposition of fat, which is not required in modern animal production.

While the hypothalamus and surrounding parts of the forebrain are likely to be the seat of intake control, there are centres in the hindbrain, such as the nucleus of the solitary tract, which receive information from receptors in the visceral organs such as the stomach and liver. Also in this area are neurons directly sensitive to shortage (but not to excess) of energy-yielding substrates. It is likely, also, that the hypothalamus itself can sense energy availability, and it originally was thought that the sensor for glucose in Mayer's 'glucostatic' hypothesis of intake control was the ventromedial hypothalamus. However, it is a vital task of the rest of the body to protect the CNS from harmful fluctuations in its environment, including its nutrient supply, and it is unlikely that under- or oversupply of nutrients from the ingestion of food would remain unsensed by the rest of the body until the CNS itself was faced with it. As we will see below, there are numerous mechanisms whereby the brain is forewarned of events that might lead to nutrient imbalance in order that the CNS can take action to prevent a serious lack of nutrients that might threaten its own proper functioning.

Learning
As stated above, animals developed the ability to learn to associate the sensory properties of a food with the metabolic consequences of eating that food at a very early stage in evolution; indeed it might be said that such capability accompanied the origin of the chemical and visual senses. We will see later how such learned associations are used in diet selection.

As an example of learning, consider the effect of injections of cholecystokinin (CCK, see below) on the preference by chickens for foods of different colours (Covasa and Forbes, 1994). CCK given intraperitoneally (i.p.) is known to depress food intake, and the aim of the experiment, the results of which are shown in Fig. 15.3, was to determine whether this reduction was due to a pleasantly satiating effect or to an unpleasantly nauseating effect of CCK. On days 1, 4 and 7, half of the birds were injected with 100 µg of CCK i.p., sufficient to depress intake by about 20% over the next 2 h; for 2 h after the injection, the normal food was replaced with food of the same composition but coloured green for one-quarter of the birds and red for the other quarter. The other half of the birds were injected with saline and again a quarter given green food, a quarter red for the next 2 h. On days 2, 5 and 8, each bird was given the alternate injection with the alternate colour and on days 3, 6 and 9 were made mildly hungry by fasting for 1 h and then individually given a choice between green and red food. The colour approached was noted and, as shown in Fig. 15.3, they became progressively averse to the colour of food associated with CCK; it is clear that the effects of the hormone are unpleasant and that the birds had become conditioned to believe that their discomfort was due to food of a particular colour – which colour it was is not important. For the next 11 days, no injections were made but the preference test was repeated from time to time; the aversion was lost within a few days. Then, for each bird, injections were paired with the opposite colours to those used in the first phase of the experiment and aversion rapidly developed, again followed by return to no preference within a few days of stopping the injections. Thus, colour preference can be easily manipulated and the same is true for the association between food flavour and the consequences of eating that is more readily evident in mammals.

It is known that the intake depression caused by giving CCK i.p. can be prevented

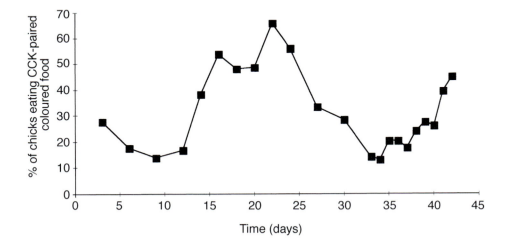

Fig. 15.3. Proportion of chicks showing preference for food of the colour paired with injections of CCK (Covasa and Forbes, 1994). From days 1 to 9, injections of CCK were paired with one colour of food and injections of saline with another colour; preference steadily moved away from the CCK-paired colour. From days 10 to 20, no injections were given; the aversion quickly disappeared. From days 21 to 33, CCK and saline injections were paired with the opposite colours to those used on days 1 to 9; aversion to the new colour was established progressively. From day 34, no injections were given and the aversion gradually disappeared.

by section of the vagus nerves (i.e. CCK stimulates abdominal receptors which transmit information to the CNS via the vagal pathway), and when the above experiment was repeated with chickens vagotomized at the level of the proventriculus, no significant colour preferences or aversions became established.

Another example of learned association, this time for ruminant animals, is the way in which lambs learn to avoid flavours associated with a deficiency or an excess of nitrogen in the diet (Villalba and Provenza, 1997). Lambs were conditioned with wheat straw (deficient in nitrogen) flavoured with two distinctive flavours. On alternate days, flavours were switched and with one of the flavours lambs received capsules containing different amounts of urea, ranging from 0.12 (insufficient) to 0.92 (excessive) g N day^{-1}. When, after 8 days of conditioning, they were given a choice between straws with each flavour, they preferred the flavours associated with urea at lower doses but avoided the flavour associated with urea at the highest dose. Thus, their preference was for the flavour they had learnt to associate with optimal nutrition, i.e. the most 'metabolic comfort'.

We can conclude then that animals learn to associate the metabolic consequences of eating a food with that food's sensory properties, and will discuss later in this chapter how this ability is used in diet selection and might be important in the control of voluntary food intake.

Gastrointestinal receptors

The ingestion of food causes changes in the degree of fill and the chemical composition of digesta which can be sensed by stretch receptors and chemoreceptors in the wall of the digestive tract.

Simple-stomached animals

Although it is not usually considered that stomach fill is a predominant factor limiting intake in pigs or poultry, extremes of distension can certainly limit intake, and stretch of stomach and intestine wall may contribute to satiety. Inflation of a surgically implanted balloon in the crop (a storage sac at the base of the oesophagus) depresses intake in chickens, while consumption increases when material of low or zero digestibility is added to a food, but not to the extent of maintaining the same rate of supply of nutrients to the animals as a more concentrated food – this is often ascribed to the bulky nature of the food stimulating stretch receptors in one or more parts of the digestive tract.

For example, duodenal infusion of glucose solutions inhibits feeding in chickens (Shurlock and Forbes, 1981a) but potassium chloride and sorbitol solutions, which are not absorbed, had a more prolonged effect, suggesting that it is the physical presence rather than the chemical nature that is important. This information is used by the brain, along with that from many other abdominal receptors, to determine whether feeding should stop or proceed.

As stated above, CCK is secreted by the wall of the duodenum in response to the passage of digesta, particularly fat and protein, and stimulates receptors locally which relay their information to the CNS where it results in a decrease in food intake. It has been suggested that it is by this means that food intake is controlled, but it is clear rather that this is only one of a large number of negative feedback signals involved (see below).

Ruminants

PHYSICAL LIMITS. Despite the fact that the rumen has such a large capacity, the slow rate of digestion of forage feeds means that rumen capacity can be limiting to intake (see Chapter 16). There are stretch receptors in the rumen wall, especially in the anterior dorsal part, and these signal the degree of distension to the brain via the vagus nerves (Leek and Harding, 1975). It is unlikely that forage intake is controlled only by distension, however, otherwise ruminants would take a succession of small meals as space became available by digestion and onward passage of digesta. In fact, they eat discrete meals with relatively long inter-meal intervals unless the rate of eating is so slow, due to the scarcity of pasture, that they must eat all day to obtain a reasonable level of intake (Chapter 17). This implies that there are other chemical and metabolic factors involved in intake control in ruminants, as in simple-stomached animals.

CHEMICAL FACTORS. The stretch receptors in the rumen wall are also sensitive to chemicals, including the acids produced by rumen fermentation. Figure 15.4 shows the effects of infusion into the rumen of sodium acetate or propionate, and of distension, on the intake of hay or silage by lactating cows prepared with rumen fistulas (Anil *et al.*, 1993). It is now clear that some of the effect of introduction of salts into the rumen is due to their osmotic properties, and it has been demonstrated that sodium chloride and other substances which increase the osmotic pressure of rumen fluid without providing nutrients can markedly depress intake when given into the rumen (Carter and Grovum, 1990). The relative importance of changes in osmotic pressure of rumen fluid in the control of feed intake by ruminants is not yet clear, however, and mole for mole

sodium acetate depresses intake more than sodium chloride when infused into the rimen.

Liver

The liver is the first organ which has a more or less complete picture of the nutrients yielded by a meal as the venous drainage of the digestive tract is funnelled into it. The liver is the first site after absorption which is able to monitor the results of eating a meal, although lipids are absorbed into the lymphatic system and might not, therefore, be able to exert their full effect on the liver before being utilized by some other tissues.

It was shown in dogs in 1963 that infusion of glucose into the hepatic portal vein depressed intake to a much greater extent than infusion of the same amount into the general circulation via the jugular vein. Subsequently, a great deal of evidence has accumulated that there are receptors in the liver sensitive to glucose and to other metabolites that are oxidized in the liver (Forbes, 1988); the mechanism is probably an activation of the sodium pump which changes the transmembrane potential of the hepatocytes resulting in a change in the

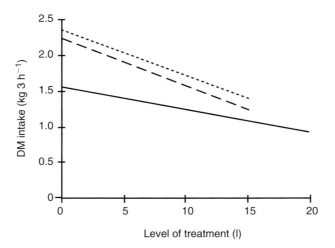

Fig. 15.4. Intake of grass silage by lactating dairy cows with a balloon inflated to different volumes (——, level of treatment = litres) for 3 h or infused with sodium acetate (....) or sodium propionate (----) at different rates (level of treatment = mol 3 h^{-1}) (Anil *et al.*, 1993).

rate of impulses generated in afferent fibres of the autonomic nerves terminating in the liver. In ruminants, glucose normally is synthesized from propionate and branched-chain amino acids, rather than being oxidized, and it is not surprising that infusions of glucose have little or no effect on feeding behaviour.

The importance of the liver innervation in communication of its metabolic status to the CNS has been shown by sectioning the branches of the vagal and sympathetic nerves entering the liver. The clear intake-depressing effect of glucose infused into the avian equivalent of the portal vein (the coccygeo-mesenteric vein) is also partly prevented by bilateral section of the vagus nerves as they pass over the surface of the proventriculus (stomach) (Shurlock and Forbes, 1981b).

Ruminant animals rely on liver uptake of propionate and its use for glucose synthesis. Figure 15.5 shows that infusion of sodium propionate into the hepatic portal vein of sheep depresses food intake relative to a control infusion of sodium chloride, while infusion of propionate into

the general circulation via the jugular vein had no effect (Anil and Forbes, 1980). Denervation of the liver prevents the effect of portal vein infusion of propionate, as does temporary blockade of impulses travelling towards the brain in the splanchnic nerves (Anil and Forbes, 1988), clearly demonstrating that the liver transmits its metabolic information to the CNS via the nervous system rather than in the blood.

One problem in the acceptance of the importance of the liver in the control of food intake has been the lack of a significant effect of liver denervation on daily food intake. It would be expected that, if the role of the liver was central, intake would increase in the absence of the negative feedback information to the CNS. However, there are clear changes in feeding behaviour after liver denervation in several species (rabbit, sheep, chicken) in which the meals become much larger but less frequent. This is what would be expected if there were other mechanisms, in addition to liver sensitivity, involved in the control of intake; the absence of signals from the

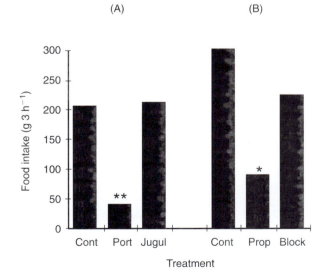

(A)   (B)

Fig. 15.5. Intake of pelleted food by sheep infused with (A) saline (Cont) or sodium propionate into the mesenteric (Prop) or jugular (Jugul) veins (Anil and Forbes, 1980); (B) saline (Cont) or sodium propionate into the mesenteric vein without (Prop) or with (Block) anaesthetic blockade of the splanchnic nerves (Anil and Forbes, 1988).

liver indicating an increase in nutrient absorption during a meal would allow larger meals to be eaten but the subsequently higher than normal levels of nutrients in the intestines and/or blood would trigger other types of receptor and maintain abnormally long inter-meal intervals, thus leading to a maintenance of normal daily intakes.

Another limitation to the acceptance of an important role for the liver is the lack of evidence of nerve endings in the parenchyma of the liver; although such anatomical evidence has been obtained for the guinea-pig, it has not been forthcoming for other species, despite careful searching with light and electron microscopy. However, Berthoud *et al.* (1992) recently have found nerve endings only in the porta hepatis in the rat (entrance of the portal vein in to the liver) and not in the parenchyma. It seems, therefore, that in most species the supply of metabolites is monitored at the entry to the liver rather than throughout the whole liver. This would account for the lack of effect of infusions of propionate deep into the liver: Leuvenink *et al.* (1997) found that while infusion of propionate into the mesenteric or hepatic portal vein of sheep both stimulated insulin secretion, only the former caused a reduction in food intake, which explains why Anil and Forbes (1980) found intake to be depressed when they infused sodium propionate into the mesenteric vein of sheep, while de Jong *et al.* (1981) observed no significant depression in intake when similar rates of infusion were given deep into the portal area in goats. Hitherto this had been ascribed to some mysterious difference between the two species!

Infusions into the general circulation

Mayer envisaged that the CNS monitored the concentration of glucose in the blood; when it was below a certain threshold, feeding started while when it was above a threshold the meal was terminated. Several pieces of evidence suggested that the receptors responsible were in the ventromedial nuclei of the hypothalamus but, while there might be hypothalamic sensitivity to blood glucose concentration, significant fluctuations in this concentration would mean that the body had failed in its task of maintaining a relative constancy of nutrient supply to the brain. Subsequent to Mayer's 'glucostatic theory' has been the realization that there are receptors in intestines and liver that normally prevent over- or undereating, and the focus of attention has moved away from the concentration of glucose in the general circulation as a major factor in the control of intake. However, an acute deficiency of oxidizable substrate supply to the brain is sensed, both by the hypothalamus and, more importantly, by the hindbrain, as evidenced by increased feeding when these parts of the CNS are treated locally with 2-deoxyglucose (2DG) which blocks glucose transport into cells and therefore mimics underfeeding.

If, despite the controls already reviewed in the digestive tract and liver, blood concentrations of important metabolites are excessively high or low, then they may be sensed and used as emergency signals to prevent extreme over- or undereating.

Adipose tissue

Metabolites in blood must be either utilized or stored by tissues, such as adipose and muscle, or else excreted by the kidneys. In the adult animal, by far the greater proportion of glucose and fatty acid uptake, once maintenance requirements have been met, is by adipose tissue. The relative constancy of body weight suggests that there is a signal from adipose tissue which is integrated with those other signals already mentioned and which alters feeding behaviour in a subtle manner to adjust for any changes in body fat content. This is not to say that there is a fixed 'set-point' for body fat content because there is greater fatness in animals fed on diets with high energy concentrations than in those fed low-energy foods. Rather, body fat content and food intake settle at levels at which the positive and negative effects on feeding are in balance.

Kennedy's 'lipostatic' theory of intake control envisaged the monitoring of the state of the adipose stores by the brain so that an excess of fat could be countered by a reduction in food intake, and depletion of body energy reserves could be compensated by an increase in intake. The existence of a humoral factor was shown by joining pairs of rats in parabiotic union and destroying the ventromedial hypothalamus of one by electrolytic lesions. The lesioned rat overate and became obese, while the unlesioned partner lost weight, presumably due to a reduction in its food intake (Hervey, 1959). The parabiotic union provides a slow exchange of blood between the partners, presumably allowing sufficient of the 'feedback from fat factor' to reach the unlesioned animal from the obese one but insufficient to allow enough of the excess nutrients being taken in by the latter to provide sufficient nutrition to maintain the former. The nature of the humoral factor was unknown but it was speculated that it might be a steroid hormone. However, more recent evidence has implicated insulin, and it now seems clear that the most important feedback signal from adipose tissue to the CNS is leptin.

Insulin

In the 1970s, it was shown that insulin infused at a low rate into the ventricular cavities of the brain, from which it can quickly reach the hypothalamus, caused reduced food intake in monkeys. Plasma insulin levels rise as an animal gets fatter (Vandeermeerschen-Doize *et al.*, 1983), due to progressive insulin resistance, providing a link between body fatness and intake control. However, treatment of animals with exogenous insulin has often been observed to cause an increase in intake, probably in response to the increase in rate of fat deposition and growth, suggesting that an insulin-mediated control of intake by fatness is not a primary means of control of intake.

In the short term, it has been suggested that the rise in insulin secretion during spontaneous meals is responsible for their termination.

Leptin

In 1994, the nature of the deficit of one of the genetically obese strains of mice was elucidated with the discovery of ob-protein (leptin). Recent evidence shows that there is a similar hormone in sheep (Dyer *et al.*, 1997), pigs (Barb *et al.*, 1998) and chickens (Taouis *et al.*, 1998).

Leptin is a hormone, secreted by adipose cells in proportion to their size, which circulates in the bloodstream and influences receptors in the brain. It appears to interact with the insulin and NPY systems and thus to be part of an important control system for food intake in relation to fatness and metabolism. At the time of writing, there has been little published on this subject concerning farm animals, but its discovery seems likely to prove very important in view of the reduced food intake in fat animals. However, it is not easy to see how knowledge of the leptin system could be made use of commercially in farm animals: if intake is being limited by this feedback signal from excessive adipose stores, then neutralizing leptin (e.g. with specific antibodies) would allow food intake to increase but the extra nutrients would be used for fat synthesis which is not usually required. If, on the other hand, the animal is eating insufficient to support its metabolic needs, then adipose tissue will have been depleted and its production of leptin will be very low, rendering neutralization ineffective.

If it is required to reduce voluntary intake as, for example, in pregnant sows and broiler breeder stock, then treatment with leptin (or an analogue or secretagogue) would limit intake but likely effects on reproduction would have to be contended with (Houseknecht *et al.*, 1998).

Integration of factors

Although it has sometimes been stated that only one factor controls intake in any given set of circumstances, this does not seem to be a tenable point of view. Consider, for example, sheep offered a poor-quality forage, whose intake is thought to be limited by rumen capacity, in which progressively increasing the digestibility of the feed leads to progressive increases in feed intake (see Forbes, 1995). Eventually, metabolic control of intake limits the amount eaten to less than that which the animal is physically capable of putting in its rumen, so we say that intake is no longer physically limited. It does not seem feasible that the stretch receptors in the rumen are no longer subject to any stimulation, nor does it seem likely that the CNS suddenly ignores the signals from the stretch receptors. Rather, it seems most likely that the stretch signals are integrated with the metabolic signals, and there is evidence that this integration is by simple addition. Figure 15.6 shows that the effects of distending a balloon in the rumen are additive with those of infusing sodium

acetate and sodium propionate (Mbanya *et al.*, 1993) and there is also evidence for such additivity in sheep and of glucose and lysine given into the liver of chickens.

The implications are that voluntary intake is not controlled only by physical factors, even in ruminants, and that it is the sum total of the strengths of signals received by the brain from many types of receptors in many parts of the body which determines how much an animal eats. Thus we have an explanation for the fact that lactating cows have a greater amount of digesta in the rumen than non-lactating cows even when they are both fed on a forage whose intake traditionally would be supposed to be limited physically (Forbes, 1986). The fact that the lactating cow has a much greater demand for nutrients to support lactation causes a more rapid removal of chemical and metabolic feedback factors from blood, liver and digestive tract, thus providing a weaker set of signals from metabolic receptors which gives the

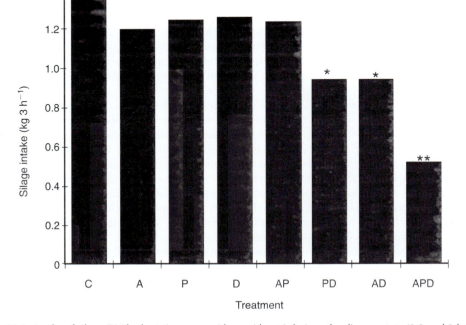

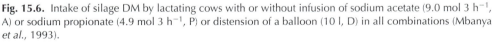

Fig. 15.6. Intake of silage DM by lactating cows with or without infusion of sodium acetate (9.0 mol 3 h^{-1}, A) or sodium propionate (4.9 mol 3 h^{-1}, P) or distension of a balloon (10 l, D) in all combinations (Mbanya *et al.*, 1993).

animal the opportunity to fill her rumen to a greater extent before the *total* of all the signals reaches a satiating level.

Diet Selection

So far we have considered only those situations in which animals have a single food available so that they have no opportunity to alter the nutritive value of the food other than by eating more or less food. This is a very artificial situation for most species which evolved in rich environments in which a wide variety of food types was available. Although it might be thought that a grazing animal might by chance eat such a mixture of plant species so that it would be unlikely to over- or undereat any particular nutrient, there is ample evidence that farm animals can make directed decisions about which foods to eat in order to match more closely their requirements for various nutrients.

One of the clearest demonstrations of 'nutritional wisdom' is the ability of the growing pig to select between foods with protein contents higher and lower than that required, so as to provide sufficient protein for growth without overconsumption. Kyriazakis and colleagues (1990) have shown that choice-fed growing pigs select a diet containing very close to 205 g protein kg^{-1} which is very similar to the optimum for growth under the conditions of the experiment. They avoid an excess protein intake as much as they avoid a deficiency, presumably as both make them feel metabolically uncomfortable and they learn to avoid such discomfort by appropriate diet selection. Note that if the two foods were exactly similar in flavour, colour and texture, the animals could not learn the association with metabolic consequences.

Growing broiler chickens demonstrate a clear ability to select a protein intake appropriate to their requirements and, like growing pigs, choose progressively less protein, relative to energy, as they get older, to match the declining requirements for protein relative to energy (Shariatmadari and Forbes, 1993). Figure 15.7 shows that

when given a choice between two foods, both of which have a higher concentration of protein (protein:energy ratio) than that required for optimum growth, broilers eat almost all of the lower protein food, i.e. they avoid eating excess protein. Conversely, with two low-protein foods, birds eat more of the higher protein food. When they can make a balanced diet from foods of two protein contents they do so, and the chosen protein:energy ratio declines as the birds grow with time as the dietary protein concentration for optimum growth is known to decline. In the case of the birds offered foods containing 280 and 65 g protein kg^{-1}, the mixture chosen provided 226 g of protein kg^{-1} at 27 days and 183 g kg^{-1} at 63 days after hatching, contents quite close to those found to be optimum for growth in experiments with single foods.

Thus, growing pigs and poultry show considerable 'nutritional wisdom' and there is evidence that ruminants also do (e.g. Kyriazakis and Oldham, 1993). However, in addition to optimizing nutritional balance, they also choose sufficient fibrous food to stabilize rumen fermentation and prevent rapid changes in fermentation and unstable pH. For example, sheep changed from long hay to a diet free of long fibre immediately started to eat chopped polyethylene fibre which they previously ignored (Campion and Leek, 1997). The polythene intake was reduced when a polyethylene fibre pompom was introduced via a rumen fistula. This suggests that ruminants have evolved a 'fibre appetite' in order to reduce the risk of disorders due to low intake of inert fibre and that this might be a result of the reduction of ruminal sensory input to the brain normally provided by fibrous reticulo-ruminal contents.

Specific appetites

Protein supplies many amino acids, and the above-mentioned ability to balance protein and energy intakes independently is not a clear example of a specific appetite. However, poultry have been shown to

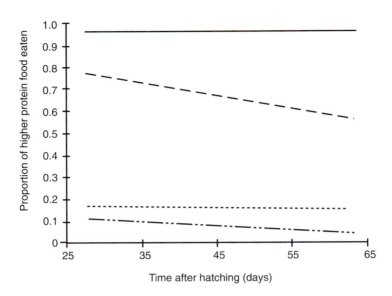

Fig. 15.7. Proportion of high- and low-protein foods taken by chickens from 27 to 63 days after hatching (Shariatmadari and Forbes, 1993). ——: choice between foods containing 225 and 65 g kg^{-1};–––: 280 and 65 g kg^{-1}; ·····: 280 and 225 g kg^{-1}; –·–: 320 and 280 g kg^{-1}. For discussion, see text.

select for lysine, methionine, thiamine (vitamin B1), vitamin B6, ascorbic acid (vitamin C), calcium and zinc (see Forbes, 1995). Pigs show appetites for several specific nutrients, while ruminants have a well-developed appetite for sodium. Figure 15.8 shows the ascorbic acid intake chosen by young broiler chicks by selecting between an unsupplemented food and one supplemented with 200 mg kg^{-1} ascorbic acid (Kutlu and Forbes, 1993). When kept in heat-stressing conditions, which are known to increase the metabolic requirement for ascorbic acid, the chicks voluntarily take in almost twice as much of the vitamin as when in a thermoneutral environment.

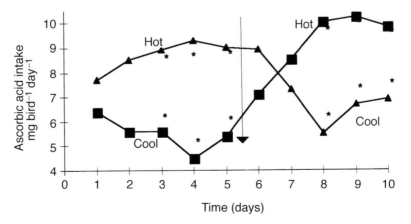

Fig. 15.8. Intake of ascorbic acid (vitamin C) by young chicks given a choice between two foods, coloured differently, containing 0 or 250 mg g^{-1} ascorbic acid. Cool: thermoneutral zone; Hot: 35°C for 10 h day^{-1}. *, significantly different from random choice between foods (Kutlu and Forbes, 1993).

They can distinguish between the two foods only by their colour and learn to associate this with their metabolic feelings after consuming the foods.

Optimizing Voluntary Intake

In practice, marginal deficiencies of a nutrient result in an increase in intake but severe shortage of an essential nutrient causes intake to decline (Fig. 15.9) (Forbes, 1995), causing a reduction in rate of growth, milk production or egg production. Alleviation of the deficiency is followed very quickly by a return to normal levels of intake and production. Also, most nutrients are toxic when present at very high levels in the diet so that intake and performance are also reduced when a gross excess of a nutrient is present.

These general effects of diet composition also affect the intake of ruminant animals. However, with the forage feeds typically available to ruminants, there is another factor which often imposes a limit to intake before an animal can satisfy its appetite for energy or essential nutrients, and this is the bulk of the food. Although the ruminant has a very capacious set of stomachs (up to 150 litres in the cow), the slow rate of digestion entails each particle of food remaining in the rumen for a very long time, typically 20–50 h; the more fibrous the forage, the slower its digestion. Rumen fill, acting through stretch receptors in the rumen wall, is therefore likely to be a dominant factor in the intake of forages. Any factor which decreases this residence time will increase voluntary intake; such factors include reducing the particle size of the food itself, increasing the activity of the rumen microflora by providing additional amounts of nutrients which limit their metabolism, and replacing some of the forage by rapidly digested concentrate supplements.

Conclusions

Voluntary food intake is influenced by many factors including negative feedbacks

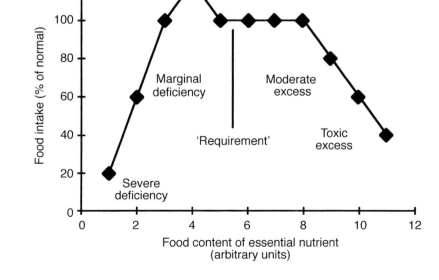

Fig. 15.9. General relationship between concentration of an essential nutrient in food and rate of voluntary food intake (Forbes, 1995).

from the consequences of eating a meal. If the nutrients present are in the same ratio as required, then food intake will be optimal, i.e. it will meet the animal's requirements. However, few single foods will meet these constraints for few animals for a short part of their productive life. Animals are therefore usually being offered an imbalanced diet, and the extent of the imbalance will determine the extent of the difference between the amount of food required and the amount actually eaten. What the animal learns from eating a food will also contribute to how much it eats on subsequent occasions, i.e. will play a part in the control of voluntary intake.

Where a choice between *n* foods is available, the animal is in theory able to control its intake of *n* constituents, e.g. energy and protein when *n* = 2, but this ability when *n* is >2 has been little explored in farm animals. Choice feeding is difficult to implement in practice and animals sometimes make nutritionally unwise choices, the reasons for which are not always clear (Forbes and Kyriazakis, 1995).

To provide for the animals' needs in farming practice, the composition of the food is usually changed at regular intervals during growth, lactation or egg-laying, to match the changes in requirements. With ruminants, a basal forage is usually offered *ad libitum*, with supplementary foods of compositions and in amounts judged to balance the diet.

There is no single factor responsible for the control of voluntary food intake. Rather, a multitude of influences are coordinated by the CNS and the animal eats that amount and mixture of food that it learns give the minimum of discomfort.

References

Anil, M.H. and Forbes, J.M. (1980) Feeding in sheep during intraportal infusions of short-chain fatty acids and the effect of liver denervation. *Journal of Physiology* 298, 407–414.

Anil, M.H. and Forbes, J.M. (1988) The roles of hepatic nerves in the reduction of food intake as a consequence of intraportal sodium propionate administration in sheep. *Quarterly Journal of Experimental Physiology* 73, 539–546.

Anil, M.H., Mbanya, J.N., Symonds, H.W. and Forbes, J.M. (1993) Responses to the voluntary intake of hay or silage by lactating cows to intraruminal infusions of sodium acetate or sodium propionate, the tonicity of rumen fluid or rumen distension. *British Journal of Nutrition* 69, 699–712.

Barb, C.R., Yan, X., Azain, M.J., Kraeling, R.R., Rampacek, G.B. and Ramsay, T.G. (1998) Recombinant porcine leptin reduces feed intake and stimulates growth hormone secretion in swine. *Domestic Animal Endocrinology* 15, 77–86.

Berthoud, H.R., Kressel, M. and Neuhuber, W.L. (1992) An anterograde tracing study of the vagal innervation of rat liver, portal vein and biliary system. *Anatomy and Embryology* 186, 431–442.

Blundell, J.E. and Halford, J.C.G. (1994) Regulation of nutrient supply: the brain and appetite control. *Proceedings of the Nutrition Society* 53, 407–418.

Campion, D.P. and Leek, B.F. (1997) Investigation of a 'fibre appetite' in sheep fed a 'long fibre-free' diet. *Applied Animal Behaviour Science* 52, 79–86.

Carter, R.R. and Grovum, W.L. (1990) A review of the physiological significance of hypertonic body fluids on feed intake and ruminal function: salivation, motility and microbes. *Journal of Animal Science* 68, 2811–2832.

Covasa, M. and Forbes, J.M. (1994) Exogenous cholecystokinin octapeptide in broiler chickens: satiety, conditioned colour aversion and vagal mediation. *Physiology and Behavior* 56, 39–49.

de Jong, A., Steffens, A.B. and de Ruiter, L. (1981) Effects of portal volatile fatty acid infusions on meal patterns and blood composition in goats. *Physiology and Behavior* 27, 683–689.

Dyer, C.J., Simmons, J.M., Matteri, R.L. and Keisler, D.H. (1997) cDNA cloning and tissue-specific gene expression of ovine leptin, npy-y1 receptor, and npy-y2 receptor. *Domestic Animal Endocrinology* 14, 295–303.

Forbes, J.M. (1986) Effects of sex hormones, pregnancy and lactation on digestion, metabolism and voluntary food intake. In: Milligan, L.P., Grovum, W.L. and Dobson, A. (eds) *Control of Digestion and Metabolism in the Ruminant*. Prentice-Hall, Englewood Cliffs, New Jersey, pp. 420–435.

Forbes, J.M. (1988) Metabolic aspects of the regulation of voluntary food intake and appetite. *Nutrition Research Reviews* 1, 145–168.

Forbes, J.M. (1995) *Voluntary Food Intake and Diet Selection in Farm Animals.* CAB International, Wallingford, UK.

Forbes, J.M. and Kyriazakis, I. (1995) Food preferences in farm animals: Why don't they always choose wisely? *Proceedings of the Nutrition Society* 54, 429–440.

Hervey, G.R. (1959) The effects of lesions in the hypothalamus in parabiotic rats. *Journal of Physiology* 145, 336.

Houseknecht, K.L., Baile, C.A., Matteri, R.L. and Spurlock, M.E. (1998) The biology of leptin: a review. *Journal of Animal Science* 76, 1405–1420.

Kutlu, H.R. and Forbes, J.M. (1993) Self-selection of ascorbic acid in coloured foods by heat-stressed broiler chicks. *Physiology and Behavior* 53, 103–110.

Kyriazakis, I. and Oldham, J.D. (1993) Diet selection in sheep: the ability of growing lambs to select a diet that meets their crude protein (nitrogen × 6.25) requirements. *British Journal of Nutrition* 69, 617–629.

Kyriazakis, I., Emmans, G.C. and Whittemore, C.T. (1990) Diet selection in pigs: choices made by growing pigs given foods of different protein concentrations. *Animal Production* 51, 189–199.

Leek, B.F. and Harding, R.H. (1975) Sensory nervous receptors in the ruminant stomach and the reflex control of reticulo-ruminal motility. In: McDonald, I.W. and Waner, A.C.I. (eds) *Digestion and Metabolism in the Ruminant.* England Publishing Units, Armidale, New South Wales, pp. 60–76.

Leuvenink, H.G.D., Bleumer, E.J.B., Bongers, L.J.G.M., Van Bruchem, J. and Van der Heide, D. (1997) Effect of short-term propionate infusion on feed intake and blood parameters in sheep. *American Journal of Physiology* 272, E997–E1001.

Mbanya, J.N., Anil, M.H. and Forbes, J.M. (1993) The voluntary intake of hay and silage by lactating cows in response to ruminal infusion of acetate or propionate, or both, with and without distension of the rumen by a balloon. *British Journal of Nutrition* 69, 713–720.

Parrott, R.F., Heavens, R.P. and Baldwin, B.A. (1986) Stimulation of feeding in the satiated pig by intracerebroventricular injection of neuropeptide Y. *Physiology and Behavior* 36, 523–525.

Shariatmadari, F. and Forbes, J.M. (1993) Growth and food intake responses to diets of different protein contents and a choice between diets containing two levels of protein in broiler and layer strains of chicken. *British Poultry Science* 34, 959–970.

Shurlock, T.G.H. and Forbes, J.M. (1981a) Factors affecting food intake in the domestic chicken: the effect of infusions of nutritive and non-nutritive substances into the crop and duodenum. *British Poultry Science* 22, 323–331.

Shurlock, T.G.H. and Forbes, J.M. (1981b) Evidence for hepatic glucostatic regulation of food intake in the domestic chicken and its interaction with gastrointestinal control. *British Poultry Science* 22, 333–346.

Taouis, M., Chen, J.W., Daviaud, C., Dupont, J., Derouet, M. and Simon, J. (1998) Cloning the chicken leptin gene. *Gene* 208, 239–242.

Vandeermeerschen-Doize, F., Bouchat, J.C., Bouckoms-Vandermeir, M.A. and Paquay, R. (1983) Effects of long-term *ad libitum* feeding on plasma lipid components and blood glucose, β-hydroxybutyrate and insulin concentrations in lean adult sheep. *Reproduction, Nutrition, Développement* 23, 51–63.

Villalba, J.J. and Provenza, F.D. (1997) Preference for flavoured foods by lambs conditioned with intraruminal administration of nitrogen. *British Journal of Nutrition* 78, 545–561.

Chapter 16

Feed Intake in Ruminants: Kinetic Aspects

W.C. Ellis[1], D. Poppi[2] and J.H. Matis[3]

[1]*Department of Animal Science and* [3]*Department of Statistics,*
Texas A&M University, College Station, Texas, USA;
[2]*Department of Agriculture, The University of Queensland,*
Brisbane, Queensland, Australia

Introduction

As for other mammals, feed intake in ruminants is regulated by a milieu of signals, and the level of feed intake achieved is that which maximizes benefits versus costs. The thesis of this chapter is that provision of indispensable amino acids required by the ruminant's tissues is the most basic nutritional benefit and regulates feed intake. Assuming that feed intake is not otherwise constrained, the rate of feed intake is proposed as that which provides the flux of net amino acids required by the ruminant's tissues. Feed intake may be constrained by metabolic or physical transformations of the feed by the ruminant's nutrient acquisition system. This chapter focuses on the dynamics of the physical and metabolic processes of the ruminant's nutrient acquisition system, processes that are proposed to both be driven by and contribute to the nutritional balance of amino acids at the ruminant's tissue level.

Ruminant Nutrition

Digestion dynamics

The ruminant has evolved a digestive system that maximizes efficiency of energy acquisition from its evolutionary environment. Characteristic features of this digestive system are its dynamic interactions with attributes of the feed resulting in the growth and maintenance of a significant microbial ecosystem whose end- and by-products are the primary source of nutrients for the ruminant's tissues. Efficiency of energy acquisition via the microbial ecosystem is maximized via interactions that extend the residence time of feed residues in the reticulo-rumen. Mean residence time, $N/\overline{\lambda}_e$, is slowed by an N order of age-dependent escape of feed residues, $\overline{\lambda}_e$, that is considerably less than the growth rate of the microbial ecosystem. As a consequence, sufficient residence time is available for the metabolically significant microbial ecosystem to be sustained from the flux of energy derived from hydrolysable structural carbohydrates (HF) that are hydrolysed at a relatively slow rate, k_h, i.e. HFk_h.

Protracted residence times, $N/\bar{\lambda}_e$, or, conversely, slower $\bar{\lambda}_e$, increase efficiency of energy capture in the ruminal mixing pool of digestion because efficiency of energy capture is determined by $k_h/(k_h + \bar{\lambda}_e)$. Maximizing efficiency of energy acquisition has survival value for ruminants whose metabolizable nutrient requirements are primarily for metabolizable energy (ME), i.e. maintenance and reproduction (Table 16.1). However, more productive ruminants have proportionally greater requirements for metabolizable protein (MP) (Table 16.1), i.e. protein that is derived from the sum of ruminal efflux microbial crude protein (MCP) and undegraded escape feed protein. As in any organism, the efficiency of MCP synthesis is a function of the rate of protein synthesis above that required for non-growth processes and protein losses of the microbial ecosystem (maintenance). The absolute growth rate of the rumen microbial ecosystem is constrained via the relatively slow flux of monomers derived from hydrolysis of structural carbohydrates, i.e. HFk_h. Consequently, large proportions of fermented monomers are utilized for maintenance of the microbial ecosystem with relatively small proportional yields of net microbial synthesis per unit yield of volatile fatty acids (VFAs). Other factors being equal, increasing flux of fermentable monomers via increasing either feed intake or dietary proportions of more rapidly hydrolysing carbohydrates will result in increasing proportions of digested MCP per unit of VFA produced. These effects can be demonstrated most clearly via results obtained from continuous flow culture systems (Isaacson *et al.*, 1978; Dijkstra *et al.*, 1998; Baker and Dijkstra, 1999).

The importance of dietary composition in regulating the dynamics of ruminal digestion and determining ruminal efflux yield of amino acids and VFAs is illustrated schematically in Fig. 16.1. Dietary concentration of potentially undigested neutral detergent fibre (UF) is important in that it represents mass whose ruminal efflux is entirely by physical means. A major determinant of residence time of feed residues in the ruminal digesta is the competition of ingested feed residues with the mass, or load, of feed residues in the mass action turnover pool. A lag-rumination pool contributes additional residence time (Ellis *et al.*, 1994). The effective mean age-dependent escape rate of UF from the two pools is $^2UF\bar{\lambda}_e$, with $\bar{\lambda}_e$ representing the dilution of UF influx rate by the load of UF

Table 16.1. Protein and energy required for various metabolic processes in the ruminant.

Metabolic process	g of MCP/Mj of ME
1. Ruminal anaerobic metabolism yield:	
Slow ruminal digesta turnover, 1 day^{-1}	8[a]
Fast ruminal digesta turnover, 1.4 day^{-1}	15[b]
2. Aerobic tissue requirement, 1/3 mature steer:	
Ruminant maintenance, 400 kg	81[c]
Specific growth rate, 0.0025 day^{-1}	110[c]
Specific growth rate, 0.0050 day^{-1}	80[c]
3. Aerobic tissue requirement, 1/3 mature pig:	
Maintenance, 200 kg	79
Specific growth rate, 0.003 day^{-1}	117
Specific growth rate, 0.006 day^{-1}	96

[a]Assuming a yield of 0.10 microbial CP 1 kJ^{-1} of fermented energy and a yield of 0.1 microbial CP that is 0.9 true protein and is 0.8 truly digested and 0.6 of fermented OM is converted to volatile fatty acids at 0.8 kJ kg^{-1} or 2.59 g metabolizable protein and 18 kJ ME 100 g^{-1} digestible dietary OM.
[b]Assuming a yield of 0.24 microbial CP 1 kJ^{-1} of fermented energy and a yield of 0.24 microbial CP that is 0.8 true protein and is 0.8 truly digested and 0.4 of fermented OM is converted to volatile fatty acids at 0.8 kJ g^{-1} or 5.529 g of metabolizable protein and 12 kJ ME 100 g^{-1} digested dietary OM.
[c]National Research Council (1996).

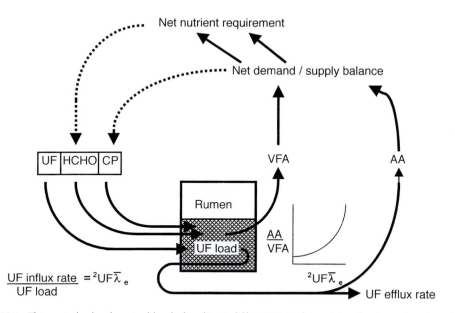

Fig. 16.1. The central role of ruminal load of undigested fibre (UF) in determining the dynamics of ruminant digestion. UF turnover, $^2UF\bar{\lambda}_e$, is an equilibrium between the influx forces of an amino acid requirement-driven feed intake and the inertial forces constraining escape of UF from the ruminal digesta mixing pools. $^2UF\bar{\lambda}_e$ regulates flux of hydrolysed carbohydrates (HCHO) and CP, and thereby the metabolic rate of the rumen microbial ecosystem and thus the flux proportions of energy, VFAs and amino acid (AA) to the ruminant's tissues. The feed intake rate finally achieved is determined iteratively as that which provides the requirements for AA or that which is constrained by insufficient ruminal efflux of AA.

in the rumen digesta. Physiologically, $^2UF\bar{\lambda}_e$ may be viewed as an equilibrium rate between the opposing forces of a nutrient requirement-driven intake of feed containing UF versus the inertial force of the mass of UF in the ruminal digesta mixing pools. These physical effects of UF determine the flux of nutrients derived from potentially hydrolysable entities such as carbohydrates and crude protein (CP) and, consequently, the ruminal efflux proportions of amino acids and energy change with level of intake. Because the processes illustrated in Fig. 16.1 involve interactions among driving and driven processes, estimation of intake involves an iterative cycling of the processes portrayed in Fig. 16.1. Biologically, the level of intake is suggested to involve similar iterative successive approximations of processes to arrive at a level which either supplies the net amino acid requirements or is constrained by either the physical or metabolic capacity

of the nutrient acquisition system or imbalances in the flux of metabolizable nutrients.

Sequential ecosystems

The nutrition of ruminants should be viewed as the nutrition of two sequential ecosystems. The nutrition of the initial ecosystem, that of the rumen micro-organisms, is derived via anaerobic metabolism of monomers derived from hydrolysed polymers of plant tissues. The nutrition of the second ecosystem, the ruminant's tissues, is derived primarily directly from metabolism of absorbed VFAs and indirectly from amino acids produced from intestinal digestion of ruminal efflux microbial protein. The two ecosystems have distinctively different metabolic and nutritional characteristics, differences that have important nutritional implications for the ruminant ecosystem. Hungate (1966) has emphasized the potential thermodynamic limitations of the ruminant's dependence upon a sequential food chain of anaerobic and aerobic metabolisms. As indicated in Table 16.1, the anaerobic rumen fermentation yields a gross disproportion of energy to MP relative to the energy and protein requirements of the ruminant's aerobic metabolism.

Ruminal efflux of amino acids synthesized in the rumen from purified, low-protein rations containing cellulose, starch and urea appears to supply adequate MP for maintenance and limited milk production. However, the flux of amino acids derived from microbial protein is insufficient for more productive ruminants. Rationing systems are required to formulate rations based on ruminal escape protein and yield of ruminal efflux protein. Ruminal efflux of microbial protein and escaping dietary protein are intimately related to ruminal kinetics.

Additionally, Hungate (1966) suggested that the propensity of ruminants to deposit fat may be the consequence of excessive proportions of energy relative to amino acids in the ruminal efflux. Possible effects of nutrient supply on body composition are clearly evident but prove difficult to modify favourably (Poppi, 1990). The consequences of such obligatory excesses of energy upon body compositon seem not to have been considered. If such excesses of energy are causal of excessive fat deposition or, conversely, limited protein deposition, systems for estimating nutrient requirements based on body composition will overestimate energy and underestimate protein requirements.

The first thesis for this chapter is that ruminants consume feed to provide for their tissue requirements for amino acids unless intake is otherwise constrained. A second thesis is that level of intake *per se* alters the dynamics of ruminal turnover and thereby the metabolic dynamics and the ruminal efflux yield of protein and energy. The cyclic sequence of diet–digestive–metabolic interactions illustrated in Fig. 16.1 is given as a framework for examining the literature.

Metabolizable nutrient supply versus demand

Support for the thesis that ruminants regulate intake to provide the net amino acids required by their tissue metabolism was investigated in a collation of data from the literature. This collation involved 29 reports involving non-lactating cattle and sheep and 23 reports involving lactating dairy cows. A total of 240 treatment means were represented. Reports were selected that provided data concerning dietary intake and faecal output of organic matter (OM) and CP and ruminal efflux of OM, microbial protein and undegraded intake protein. To standardize data across reports, daily intake of truly digested OM (TDOMI) was computed assuming that faecal nitrogen consisted of unhydrolysed feed protein and ruminal efflux microbial protein and that microbial protein comprised 0.12 of the faecal OM. Daily MP effluxing the rumen was calculated as the sum of microbial protein (0.85 true protein nitrogen of microbial nitrogen $\times$ 6.25) and undegraded intake protein (total non-ammonia nitrogen minus microbial nitrogen each multiplied by 6.25) which was assumed 0.9 truly digestible. Fermented carbohydrates were computed as the difference between intake and ruminal efflux of neutral detergent fibre (NDF) and non-structural carbohydrates. The OM of non-structural carbohydrates, NSC, was computed as OM minus the sum of NDF, CP and lipids. When not reported, dietary lipids were assumed to represent 20 g kg^{-1} of dietary OM and to be 0.5 hydrolysable.

Feed intake versus balance of metabolizable nutrients

Feed intake is commonly expressed as TDOMI. However, TDOMI represents a mixture of potential nutrients of which only the first limiting nutrient will limit intake. Simple calculations given in Table 16.2 illustrate variations in intake of TDOM that would be expected to occur if MP first limited feed intake. It is clear that wide variations in TDOMI may occur in

Table 16.2. Estimation of a nutrient requirement-driven feed intake requires knowledge of the ruminant's tissue requirement for and the flux rate of the specific nutrient that first limits intake. Truly digestible OM is not a specific nutrient so does not drive intake. Example calculations below assume that MP is the first limiting nutrient so that expected intake of TDOM = MP requirement × (TDOM/MP).

Assumed MP requirement Daily MP, g kg^{-1} BW	Flux of TDOM:flux of MP g g^{-1}	Expected TDOM intake Daily g TDOM kg^{-1} BW
4	7	28
3	7	21
4	6	24
3	6	18

response to small differences in animal attributes (requirement for MP) in combination with different feed attributes (proportions of DOM:MP). These considerations clearly demonstrate that feed intake cannot be estimated reliably without knowledge of the productive potential of the ruminant (requirement) and the ruminal efflux proportions of TDOMI to the nutritional entity that first limits feed intake.

Plots of intake of observed TDOMI kg^{-1} BW versus observed ruminal efflux of MP kg^{-1} BW (TDOMI:MP) indicated a conspicuous positive relationship with considerable scatter. Nine reports contained three or more treatment means having values for TDOMI or MP that varied by at least 15%. Data from these reports are plotted in Fig. 16.2 together with the linear regressions via report. Regression coefficients varied from 2.4 to 40 g TDOMI g^{-1} of MP. With two exceptions, the regression lines converged in the order of 1.5 g MP kg^{-1} BW. The two exceptions were data reported by Cruickshank *et al.* (1987) for rapidly growing, early weaned lambs, and Hannah *et al.* (1990) for cattle fed forages of low OM digestibility (0.48) and CP content (24 g kg^{-1}). The linear regression for the data of Hannah *et al.* (1990) encompassed values reported by Gunter *et al.* (1990) for diets with similar nutritive attributes to those reported by Hannah *et al.* (1990).

Based on nitrogen balance data given in these reports, the apparent convergence point of 1.5 g MP slightly exceeded zero nitrogen balance for the ruminants involved. The large responses in TDOMI:MP (regression coefficient in the order of 40 g

TDOMI g^{-1} of MP) observed in the report of Hannah *et al.* (1990) were responses to supplemental undegraded protein being used to spare tissue losses of protein (MP intake of 0.8 g kg^{-1} BW). The large response for lambs was probably due to simple body weight being an inadequate scaling parameter to correct for differences in body weight across species. Consistency was not improved via use of BW$^{0.75}$. Other than for these two exceptions, the TDOMI versus MP response ranged from 4 to 10 TDOMI g^{-1} MP. Thus, variations in intake responses of TDOMI to MP largely reflect differences in TDOMI:MP supply versus TDOMI:MP requirements by the different experimental animals (see example calculations in Table 16.2).

Positive responses in TDOMI intake to flux of MP such as those in Fig. 16.1 are similar to numerous reports of associations between feed intake and various expressions of CP concentrations and intake. Like all such empirical relationships, it is difficult to interpret whether the intake relationship to CP was due to the nutritional effects on the rumen microbial ecosystem or to that of the ruminant's tissues. Egan (1977) observed linear responses in feed intake in response to a wide range of levels of casein infused post-ruminally. The range of casein infused (2–9 g of digested amino acids per MJ of digestible energy) spanned that expected to be required by both the microbial and mammalian ecosystems. Thus the linear responses observed by Egan (1977), and those in Fig. 16.2, appear due specifically to enhanced flux of amino acids to the ruminant's tissues.

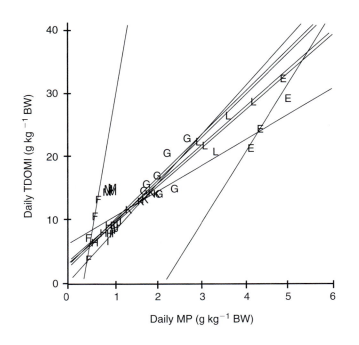

Fig. 16.2. Linear regressions for treatment means of TDOMI versus MP within experiments (A,B, … M). With the exceptions of two experiments (F and E), all regressions converge at approximately 1.4 g of MP kg^{-1} BW or approximately 1.5 times the estimated MP requirements for maintenance. Divergences in the slope above this convergence point are interpreted to reflect differences among experiments in digestive yield of proportions of TDOM and MP and differences among animals in their productive requirement for MP (see Table 16.2).

Feed intake versus energy balance

In the individual reports of Beever *et al.* (1985, 1986), intake of ryegrass by cattle progressively exceeded that of clover when TDOMI exceed an intake in the order of 13 g TDOM kg^{-1} BW. Cammell *et al.* (1986) observed that metabolizable energy (ME) from clover versus ryegrass was used with progressively greater efficiency for energy retention as intake of ME exceeded 1.65 that of a maintenance requirement of 50 MJ day^{-1}. Consumption of ryegrass versus clover reported by Beever *et al.* (1985, 1986) was 1.21-fold greater at the highest level of consumption of clover. This ratio of 1.21 was comparable with the observed ratio for the partial efficiencies of ME utilization from clover versus ryegrass (1.19, Table 5 of Cammell *et al.*, 1986). Thus, differences in TDOMI of ryegrass versus clover were equivalent to differences in net availability

of ME required to provide the flux of net energy accreted as body protein and fat.

Feed intake versus balance of metabolizable amino acids

Feed intake appears related to the net efficiency of metabolizable amino acid utilization in an analogous manner to that inferred above for net energy. In the data of Hill (1991), TDOMI from grazed pastures was unrelated to flux of MP associated with supplemental proteins that differed in both ruminal degradability and amino acid composition (Ellis *et al.*, 1995; and Figures 3 and 5 of Ellis *et al.*, 1999). However, intake was positively related to the chemical score of MP expressed as the balance of amino acid in the supplemental protein relative to that in whole egg protein. Intake of grazed pasture was positively correlated with flux of net protein estimated as the chemical score of the mixture of amino acids derived from rumen escape protein of forage and supplemental protein and from microbial true protein. TDOMI was positively related to estimated flux of duodenal methionine and lysine (Figure 5 of Ellis *et al.*, 1999) but not to the flux of any other amino acid. Equivalent intake responses to flux of either supplemental lysine or methionine are consistent with rumen microbial protein being equally deficient in lysine and methionine when used for the net protein requirements of body weight gain (Storm and Oskrov, 1985).

Response to the balance of amino acid supply is as expected for a metabolism having a fastidious amino acid requirement such as that of mammalian tissue. Such responses to balance of amino acids would not be expected for a metabolism having a relatively non-fastidious requirement such as the rumen microbial ecosystem.

Collectively, these results suggest that feed intake is regulated to provide the net energy and net amino acid requirements of the ruminant's aerobic metabolism. The major uncertainty involved in predicting the level of feed intake by ruminants resides in predicting the yield of metabolizable nutrients derived from the ruminant's nutrient acquisition system.

The Ruminant's Nutrient Acquisition System

For simplicity, most models of ruminal digestion assume steady-state flux, i.e. perfect and instantaneous mixing of a constant input rate with a constant mass of resident feed residues from which efflux is constant via escape and hydrolysis of potentially hydrolysable entities. Obviously, such constancy does not prevail in the ruminant because of its consumption of meals that are irregular in their frequency, level and, for the grazing animal, chemical and physical composition. Effects of meal consumption have important implications in short-term (hourly) regulation of feed intake (Aitchson *et al.*, 1986) and microbial

metabolism (Baker and Dijkstra, 1999). However, this chapter will focus on the regulation of feed intake over longer terms, i.e. a daily mean of observations during 1–2 weeks. Therefore, emphasis is placed on the mean daily flux of feed residues over days and we make the assumption that such longer term responses reflect the corresponding mean for shorter term, rapidly fluctuating influx, flux and efflux.

Flux of unhydrolysable entities

Matis (1972) proposed that flux through the ruminant's gastrointestinal tract may be modelled either as flux through a single age-dependent mixing pool or sequential flux through two sequential pools having age-dependent or sequential age-dependent and age-independent residence time distributions. Either model yields identical estimates of total residence time and total pool size (Ellis *et al.*, 1994, 1999). Graphical illustrations of age-dependent distributions of residence time are given in Fig. 16.3.

Different processes constrain escape of feed residues from each of the two sequential mixing pools. To be descriptive of these processes, the two sequential pools are proposed to be referred to as the lag-rumination and mass action turnover pools, respectively. Because of the imperfect mixing of ruminal digesta, these two pools are commingled and cannot be fully resolved by sampling ruminal digesta. Resolution of the two pools requires sampling of ruminal efflux to reveal their functional differentiation. Fitting either a single age-dependent mixing pool or a sequential age-dependent, age-independent mixing pool model yields identical profiles of marker efflux from the rumen, as illustrated in Fig. 16.3. The two-pool model is preferred in order to identify separately the two different causal biological processes. However, equal statistical fit is possible for either model provided with adequate quality data (Figure 10 of Ellis *et al.*, 1994).

Both the lag-rumination and mass action turnover pools primarily (≥95%) reside in ruminal digesta (Wylie, 1987;

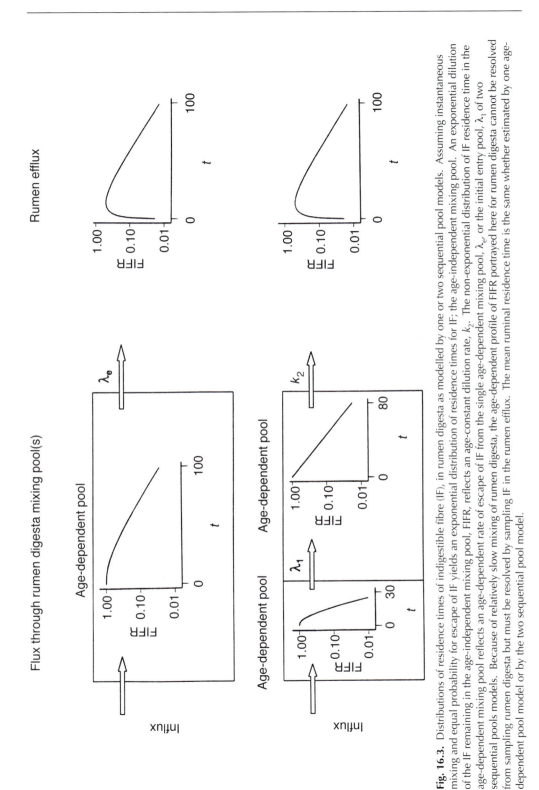

Fig. 16.3. Distributions of residence times of indigestible fibre (IF), in rumen digesta as modelled by one or two sequential pool models. Assuming instantaneous mixing and equal probability for escape of IF yields an exponential distribution of residence times for IF; the age-independent mixing pool. An exponential dilution of the IF remaining in the age-independent mixing pool, FIFR, reflects an age-constant dilution rate, k_2. The non-exponential distribution of IF residence time in the age-dependent mixing pool reflects an age-dependent rate of escape of IF from the single age-dependent mixing pool, λ_e, or the initial entry pool, λ_1 of two sequential pools models. Because of relatively slow mixing of rumen digesta, the age-dependent profile of FIFR portrayed here for rumen digesta cannot be resolved from sampling rumen digesta but must be resolved by sampling IF in the rumen efflux. The mean ruminal residence time is the same whether estimated by one age-dependent pool model or by the two sequential pool model.

Ellis *et al.*, 1999). Therefore, ruminal residence time can be estimated from marker profiles in the faeces by fitting either model that also contains a time delay parameter to estimate post-ruminal transit time, τ. Problems associated with deviations from the steady-state assumptions and representative sampling are less for faecal as compared with abomasal or duodenal digesta sampling. Thus fitting models to marker profiles in the faeces results in greater precision for resolving residence time due to non-mixing, post-ruminal transit time, the lag-rumination and the mass action turnover pools (Figure 10 of Ellis *et al.*, 1994). A summary of gastrointestinal residence times resolved from fitting age-dependent, age-independent models with a time delay to marker profiles in the faeces is summarized in Fig. 16.4.

The post-ruminal transit time and the mean residence time in the lag-rumination pool are relatively unaffected by dietary level of indigestible NDF and are relatively constant at approximately 10 h each in cattle (Fig. 16.4). In contrast, the mean residence time in the mass action turnover pool appears to be related positively and linearly to dietary concentration of indigestible fibre.

Models involving assumptions of age-dependent distribution of residence time, yield estimates of ruminal residence time and digesta load that are longer and larger, respectively, than that modelled by a single mixing pool such as the models of Orskov and McDonald (1979), Forbes (1980) and the Cornell Net Protein Net Carbohydrate System (Russell *et al.*, 1992). The additional age-dependent residence time due to the lag-rumination pool affords an additional mechanism for maximizing efficiency of hydrolysing slowly but potentially hydrolysable structural carbohydrates. The need for this additional residence time for reconciling observed versus model estimates

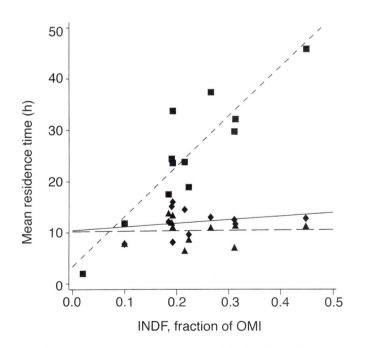

Fig. 16.4. Relationships between mean transit time as estimated for first detectable appearance of marker in faeces (♦ and ——), mean residence time in the lag-rumination pool (▲ and – – –) and the mass action turnover pool (■ and ---) estimated from marker profiles in the faeces of cattle consuming a variety of forages.

of fibre digestion has been emphasized by Huhtanen and Vanhatalo (1997). This additional residence time due to the lag-rumination pool also imposes an additional load of digesta mass.

Digestion and flux in sequential mixing pools

Estimating flux from a mixing pool requires an integrating of the rates of escape and hydrolysis of individual entities. This is illustrated for potentially hydrolysable neutral detergent fibre (HF), which is assumed hydrolysed via an age-independent rate (HFk_h). The fractional extent of hydrolysis of HF (HFH), from an age-independent mixing pool is simply the proportion $HFk_h/(HFk_h + HFk_2)$. However, this expression is not applicable to an age-dependent mixing pool. If the objective of the integration is relatively long, e.g. daily means, the age-dependent escape rate λ_1 or λ_e, (Fig. 16.3) can be converted to a mean age-dependent rate ($HF\bar{\lambda}_1$ for two compartment and $HF\bar{\lambda}_1$ for two pool models; Ellis et al., 1994, 1999). Extent of hydrolysis of HF in single age-dependent mixing pool is computed as:

$$HFH = HFk_h/(HF\bar{\lambda}_e + HFk_h) \qquad (16.1)$$

HF unhydrolysed via flux through a sequence of two mixing pools, ^2HFU, is the product of their fractional escape from each pool, e.g.

^2HFU = fraction of HFU escaping pool 1 × fraction of HFU escaping pool 2   (16.2)

The extent of hydrolysis of HF via flux through two sequential pools, ^2HFH, is then computed as:

$$^2HFH = 1-((HF\bar{\lambda}_1/(HF\bar{\lambda}_1 + HFk_h)) \\ \times (HFk_e/(HFk_e + HFk_h))) \qquad (16.3)$$

Estimates of HFH or ^2HFH via one age-dependent or two sequential pools are similar. The two pool model is preferred because of its delineation of the two pools that contribute residence time. Resolving

and accurately estimating model parameters of rumen flux requires adequate number and critical timing in sampling ruminal efflux, timing that differs for one and two pool models (Fig. 10 of Ellis et al., 1994).

Because potentially hydrolysable and potentially unhydrolysed entities are constituents of the same insoluble feed fragment, $HF\bar{\lambda}_1$ and $UE\bar{\lambda}_1$ are equal until HF is hydrolysed and no longer chemically associated with UF. Escape rate for UF from a specific meal must be estimated by markers specifically applied (Ellis et al., 1994) to a single meal of UF and indelibly associated with UF during its residence time in the rumen. Indelibility of marker and UF during postruminal flux is not required to estimate ruminal residence time. The validity of rare earths as markers of UF flux in the rumen has been established (Table 16.3 of Faichney et al., 1989 and Fig. 7 of Ellis et al., 1994).

Because UF can disappear from the rumen only via escape, level of dietary UF has the major impact on ruminal load. The contribution of potentially hydrolysable entities to ruminal digesta load is related to the ratio of their HFk_h / $HF\bar{\lambda}_1$ (or $HF\bar{\lambda}_e$ for a single age-dependent mixing pool). Thus entities such as HF that is hydrolysed at rates less than that of $HF\bar{\lambda}_e$ are major contributors to ruminal digesta load.

Regulation of Ruminal Residence Time

Metabolically, the rumen microbial ecosystem should be viewed as an open flow fermentation system whose kinetics may be regulated by physical or metabolic mechanisms. Physical mechanisms involve entities that either are intrinsically indigestible or are potentially digestible but are undigested due to insufficient mean residence time, i.e. ruminal escape.

Physical regulation of residence time

Mechanisms for physical regulation involve the coordinated motility of the reticulo-

Table 16.3. Ruminal dynamics of unhydrolysable fibre (UF) and crude protein (CP) in sheep consuming cottonseed hull (CSH) or CSH and cottonseed meal (CSM) diets (adapted from Wylie, 1987).

Item	Diet		CSH + CSM
	CSH	CSH + CSM	CSH
Dietary composition: g kg^{-1} DM			
CP	52	123	24
UF	518	362	7
Daily ruminal influx, g kg^{-1} BW			
DM	8.6	33.7	3.9
UF	16.2	22.3	1.4
Ruminal digesta load, g kg^{-1} BW			
UF	14.5	23.4	1.6
Daily mean ruminal escape rate, $\bar{\lambda}_e$			
UF	0.34	0.54	1.6
CSH-rare earth	0.31	0.50	1.6
CoEDTA-Co	0.46	1.06	2.3
Ruminal efflux composition, g g^{-1} DM			
Efflux CP/efflux DM	0.08	0.14	1.8
Ruminal influx/efflux ratios, g g^{-1}			
Influx of CP/efflux of CP	0.577	1.20	2.1
Influx of DM/efflux of CP	9.77	9.78	1.0

rumen that invokes physical competition among feed residues for escape from the mass action turnover pool. Physical regulation also occurs via interactions of these mixing forces with the un-mixing forces of buoyancy. Buoyancy is derived from the innate buoyancy of feed residues on initial ingestion and fermentation-derived buoyancy that large feed residues acquire as the result of age-dependent processes of colonization and metabolism of feed residues by the rumen microbial ecosystem (Sutherland, 1986; Ellis *et al.*, 1991). It is the physical buoyancy that sorts 'recent' residues into flow paths for ruminative mastication and 'aged' feed residues into the mass action turnover pool. These flow paths for the lag-rumination pool are easier to conceive than to measure explicitly. Such flow paths may not be mimicked via insertion of feed fragments into the ruminal digesta accessible via rumen cannulae (Vega and Poppi, 1997).

The rather invariant nature of resident time observed for the lag-rumination pool (Fig. 16.4) suggests that variation in resistance to mastication is small relative to factors affecting their escape (Figure 13 of Ellis *et al.*, 1999). Diets of stem versus leaf fragments (Poppi *et al.*, 1981) may be an extreme exception.

Regulation of residence time by physical forces is in part self-regulating in that increasing levels of NDF result in increased load of NDF and proportional increases in competition for escape from the mass action turnover pool. This self-regulating mechanism is proposed as a mechanism for maximizing the extent of digestion of HF. For example, fermentation-based buoyancy would tend to constrain escape until potentially digestible entities were largely expended. Thus, the combination of physical factors in the lag-rumination pool combined with the mass action turnover pool constrain HF$\bar{\lambda}_e$ of forages until HF is digested to the order of 0.85 in forage-fed ruminants (Figure 18 of Ellis *et al.*, 1999).

Metabolic regulation of residence time

Moir and Harris (1962) clearly demonstrated that the level of dietary protein (30–110 g kg^{-1} DM) was positively and curvilinearly related both to concentrations of rumen bacteria and to the rate of intraruminal hydrolysis of cotton. The data of Moir and Harris (1962) together with those summarized in Fig. 16.5 indicate that levels of CP in the order of 80 g kg^{-1} DM are required to maximize apparent dry matter digestion in the rumen (Buentello and Ellis, 1969). Protein supplementation of forages containing <80 g CP kg^{-1} results in increased rate of digestion of structural carbohydrates and increased voluntary intake (Buentello and Ellis, 1969).

The effects of the level of dietary CP on ruminal dynamics are illustrated in Table 16.3. Increasing the level of dietary CP from 52–123 g kg^{-1} was associated with essentially equal increases in voluntary intake of UF (1.4-fold), ruminal digesta load of UF (1.6-fold) and the CP content of ruminal efflux DM (1.8-fold). Voluntary intake of DM per unit of ruminal efflux of CP was essentially identical for the two diets (9.77 versus 9.78 g DM intake g^{-1} of ruminal efflux CP), strongly implying that intake was being regulated by the quantity of ruminal efflux CP. Voluntary intake of DM and CP and ruminal efflux rate of CP was significantly negatively related to plasma levels of 3-methylhistidine and to

increases in plasma methionine and lysine, but no other amino acid (Wylie, 1987).

The voluntary intake responses to dietary CP in Table 16.3 were interpreted to be the result of a nutrient requirement-driven intake to defray nutritional deficiencies at the ruminant's tissue level of the first limiting nutrient, as evidenced by reductions in plasma 3-methylhistidine. Feed intake was not constrained by physical capacity to harbour or process UF.

Results of protein supplementation of growing calves grazing bermuda or annual ryegrass pastures are summarized in Table 16.4. Compared with results with less digestible roughage in Table 16.3, cattle consuming these more digestible diets exhibited much smaller ruminal loads of UF and more rapid ruminal escape rates for UF. In spite of large differences in ruminal load and escape rates for UF, the voluntary influx of OM relative to ruminal efflux of non-ammonia CP did not differ significantly for bermudagrass versus ryegrass (11.83 versus 9.24 g influx OM g^{-1} efflux non-ammonia CP). If allowances are made for differences in ash, the relationships between dietary influx and ruminal efflux are

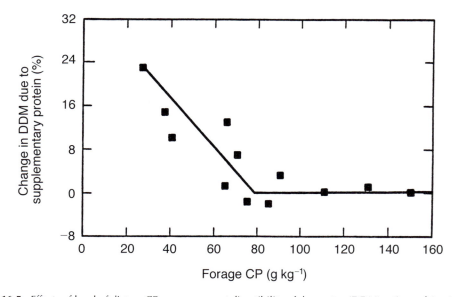

Fig. 16.5. Effects of level of dietary CP upon apparent digestibility of dry matter (DDM) estimated *in vitro* as forage with supplemental casein hydrolysate as compared with DDM observed when the same forage was fed to lambs without CP supplementation.

Table 16.4. Ruminal dynamics of unhydrolysable fibre (UF) and crude protein (CP) in cattle grazing semi-tropical (bermuda) or temperate (ryegrass) forage pasture (adapted from Hill, 1991).

	Diet		Ryegrass
Item	Bermuda	Ryegrass	Bermuda
Dietary composition, g kg^{-1} OM			
CP	76	250	33
UF	340	117	3
Daily ruminal influx, g kg^{-1} BW			
OM	14.1	23.7	1.7
UF	4.8	2.8	0.6
Ruminal digesta load, g kg^{-1} BW			
UF	9.2	2.5	0.3
Daily mean ruminal escape rates, $\bar{\lambda}_e$			
UF-rare earth,	0.65	1.34	2.1
CoEDTA-Co	1.3	4.8	3.7
Rumen microorganisms-organic bound ^{35}S	0.41	0.53	1.3
Ruminal efflux composition, g g^{-1} OM			
Total CP	0.169	0.205	1.2
Non-ammonia CP	0.156	0.187	1.2
Microbial CP	0.084	0.111	1.3
Ruminal influx/ruminal efflux ratios, g g^{-1}			
Influx of CP/efflux of CP	0.73	1.90	2.6
Influx of OM/efflux of non-ammonia CP	9.24	11.83	1.3
Influx of OM/efflux of microbial CP	17.27	19.90	1.2

essentially equal for all four widely different diets summarized in Tables 16.3 and 16.4 which were in the order of 10 g feed intake g^{-1} of ruminal efflux of CP. Unfortunately, ruminal microbial protein was not measured for the less digestible diet (Table 16.3). For the more digestible diets (Table 16.4), ruminal influx of OM per efflux of microbial CP was relatively constant at 17.27 and 19.9 and supports the generalization that the rate of rumen microbial synthesis first limited the ruminal efflux rate of OM. If the levels of ruminal load and efflux rate of UF are taken as some indication of an upper limit to the physical capacity for ruminal flux, physical factors did not appear to constrain intake of the diets in Table 16.4.

For cattle fed the more digestible diets (Table 16.4), the mean effective escape rates of UF from the sequence of the lag-rumination and mass action turnover pools, ^{2}UF$\bar{\lambda}_e$, were inversely related to mean ruminal digesta loads of UF of from 2.5 to 9.2 g UF kg^{-1} BW. In contrast, ^{2}UF$\bar{\lambda}_e$ was directly proportional to ruminal digesta

loads of UF in sheep having ruminal digesta loads of 14.5 and 22.3 g UF kg^{-1} BW (Table 16.3). When consuming the more digestible diets, ruminal digesta load of UF increased from 2.5 to 9.2 g kg^{-1} BW and ^{2}UF$\bar{\lambda}_e$ decreased by 0.48-fold (from 1.34 to 0.65 day^{-1}). In contrast, in sheep fed the less digestible diets, ^{2}UF$\bar{\lambda}_e$ increased 0.77-fold (0.54–0.34 day^{-1}) when ruminal digesta load was increased from 6.2 to 22.3 g UF kg^{-1} BW. These responses suggest that ^{2}UF$\bar{\lambda}_e$ is regulated primarily by a nutrient requirement-driven intake when diets are low in UF and contribute a relatively small ruminal load of UF (<9 g UF kg^{-1} BW as for bermudagrass in Table 16.4). As ruminal load of UF increases with consumption of diets higher in UF, the inertia of larger ruminal loads become more dominant and less opportunity exists for metabolic regulation via an MP requirement-driven intake.

Efficiency of microbial growth would respond to flux rate of hydrolysable entities if the escape rates of the microorganisms were associated with ^{2}UF$\bar{\lambda}_e$. However, the escape rate for microbial protein was less responsive to flux rate of UF than was $^2UF\overline{\lambda}_e$ (1.4 versus 2.1, Table 16.3). Differential escape rates for different feed residues and for microbial protein exemplified in Table 16.4 will complicate more mechanistic interpretations of physical and metabolic regulation of flux of specific feed and microbial entities.

These interpretations suggest that the ruminal microbial ecosystem may be considered a continuous flow system whose mean residence time may be regulated in response to intake level and composition of diet that is driven to provide for the ruminant's requirements at the tissue level.

Dietary–Digestive–Metabolic Interactions

More extensive *in vivo* data are needed to verify or refute and extend the above interpretations of the nutrient acquisition system as both a regulating and a regulated open flow system. Such data were collated from the literature. The following assumptions were utilized to standardize the available literature and acquire the maximal number of observations relevant to kinetic measurements.

1. NDF is the major feed entity contributing mass and volume of feed residues to ruminal digesta and, until hydrolysed, the rates of ruminal escape of potentially hydrolysable fibre (HF), $^2HF\overline{\lambda}_e$ and potentially unhydrolysable fibre (UF), $^2UF\overline{\lambda}_e$ are equal.
2. The rate of ruminal escape of HF is estimated equally either as the mean age-dependent rate, $HF\overline{\lambda}_e$, or as the mean effective escape rate from two sequential pools, $^2HF\overline{\lambda}$. Specifically bound rare earths (Ellis *et al.*, 1994) and tris-(1,10-phenanthroline)-ruthenium(II) chloride were considered indelible markers of the ruminal flux of UF.
3. Where only age-independent escape was estimated by a single-pool exponential distributed residence time model (k_e), the mean residence time in the lag-rumination pool was assumed to be 10 h and the mean

effective rate of escape from the two sequential pools, $^2UF\overline{\lambda}_e$, was calculated as $1/(10 + 1/k_2)$.
4. In order to incorporate data involving the lactating ruminant, data obtained via the rumen evacuation procedure were used. The mean ruminal residence time calculated by this procedure assumes that all ruminal residence time is represented by mass action turnover and therefore does not include mean residence due to the lag-rumination pool. Therefore, $^2UF\overline{\lambda}$ was calculated as for 3 above. Values were recalculated from the raw data in one report where an incorrect mathematical expression was cited by the authors.
5. Rumen digesta load of undigested NDF (UNDFL) was computed as ruminal efflux of NDF/$^2UF\overline{\lambda}_e$. As calculated, UNDFL represents indigestible NDF plus potentially hydrolysable NDF that escapes the rumen. The actual load of digesta NDF, as estimated via rumen evacuation methods, will exceed UNDFL due to the quantity of potentially digestible NDF that will be hydrolysed.

Animal Bymicrobial Metabolic Regulation of Ruminal Residence Time

Output from an open flow mixing system such as the rumen, may be conceived as the product of UNDFL and $^2UF\overline{\lambda}_e$ so that:

$$UNDF\ intake\ rate = UNDFL \times {}^2UF\overline{\lambda}_e$$
$$= UNDFL\ output\ rate \qquad (16.4)$$

Flux through the open flow mixing system may be altered via changes in either UNDFL or $^2UF\overline{\lambda}_e$. If only passive, mass action effects regulated UNDFL and $^2UF\overline{\lambda}_e$, these two variables should be exponentially related. Earlier investigations of the relationship between UNDFL and escape from the mass action turnover pool indicated that this relationship contained more curvilinearity than could be attributed to an exponential relationship (Ellis *et al.*, 1999). The relationship between UNDFL and the effective escape from the sequence of the two pools, $^2UF\overline{\lambda}_e$, is shown in Fig. 16.6.

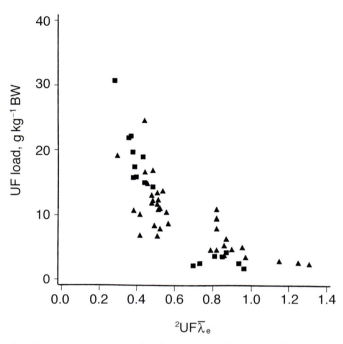

Fig. 16.6. Relationships between rumen load of undigested neutral detergent fibre (UF) and mean effective escape rate from the sequence of lag-rumination and mass turnover pools, $^2UF\bar{\lambda}_e$, in lactating (■) and non-lactating (▲) cattle and sheep fed a variety of diets. Note that when UF load is less than approximately 6 g of UF kg^{-1} BW UF, load is relatively constant at approximately 2–3 kg^{-1} BW, in contrast to a positive relationship when UF loads exceeded 6 g UF kg^{-1} BW.

Rather than a continuous relationship between the two variables, a transition point in the order of 6 g UNDFL kg^{-1} BW appeared evident. This value is consistent with the interpretation of data in Tables 16.2 and 16.3 suggesting a transition point no greater than 9 g UF kg^{-1} BW in a data set involving only four levels of ruminal load of UF. Relationships between dietary UF concentrations, UF load and ruminal efflux rate of UF are plotted in Fig. 16.7. Dietary levels of UF in excess of approximately 0.25 g g^{-1} OMI (Fig. 16.7C) resulted in ruminal digesta loads of UF >6 g kg^{-1} BW (Fig. 16.7A) and what appeared to be minimal $^2UF\bar{\lambda}_e$ in the order of 0.35 day^{-1} (Fig. 16.7B). Conversely, dietary levels <0.2 g UF g^{-1} OMI (Fig. 16.7C) resulted in digesta loads of UF <6 g kg^{-1} BW (Fig. 16.7A) and were associated with relatively large, >0.7 day^{-1}, and variable $^2UF\bar{\lambda}_e$ (Fig. 16.7B).

Thus when UNDFL was <6 g UNDFL kg^{-1} of BW, ruminal flux of UF was dominated by changes in $^2UF\bar{\lambda}_e$ whereas ruminal flux of UF was dominated by changes in UNDFL when UNDFL exceeded 6 g UNDFL kg^{-1} BW. The data in Fig. 16.7 exclude data from animals receiving diets containing <0.1 CP because variations in these lower levels of CP were associated with variations in UF flux and load as indicated in Table 16.3. This relationship suggested that variations in $^2UF\bar{\lambda}_e$ and ruminal efflux would respond to ruminal efflux of MP, and this is examined in Fig. 16.8.

When UF load was >6 g kg^{-1} BW, flux of MP kg^{-1} BW was positively related to changes in UF load and unrelated to changes in $^2UF\bar{\lambda}_e$. In contrast, when UF load was <6 g kg^{-1} BW, increased flux of MP kg^{-1} BW was positively related to changes in $^2UF\bar{\lambda}_e$ and unrelated to UF load. Although UF load may be accomplished via hypertrophy of the rumen in lactating ruminants, differential responses by

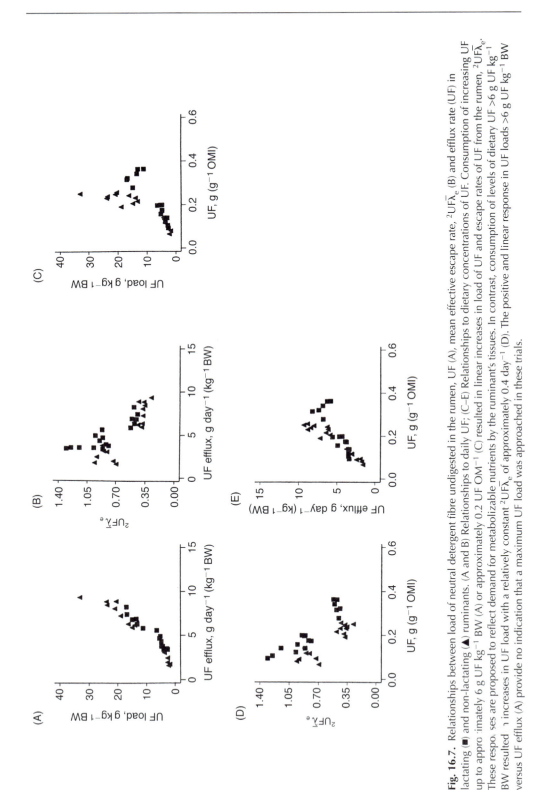

Fig. 16.7. Relationships between load of neutral detergent fibre undigested in the rumen, UF (A), mean effective escape rate, $^2\overline{UFX}_e$ (B) and efflux rate (UF) in lactating (■) and non-lactating (▲) ruminants. (A and B) Relationships to daily UF; (C–E) Relationships to dietary concentrations of UF. Consumption of increasing UF up to approximately 6 g UF kg^{-1} BW (A) or approximately 0.2 UF OM^{-1} (C) resulted in linear increases in load of UF and escape rates of UF from the rumen, $^2\overline{UFX}_e$. These responses are proposed to reflect demand for metabolizable nutrients by the ruminant's tissues. In contrast, consumption of levels of dietary UF >6 g UF kg^{-1} BW resulted in increases in UF load with a relatively constant $^2\overline{UFX}_e$ of approximately 0.4 day^{-1} (D). The positive and linear response in UF loads >6 g UF kg^{-1} BW versus UF efflux (A) provide no indication that a maximum UF load was approached in these trials.

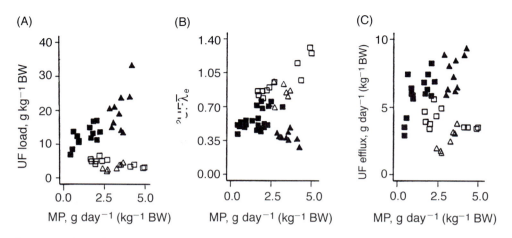

Fig. 16.8. Relationships between daily flux of metabolizable protein (MP) and mean load of neutral detergent fibre undigested in the rumen, UF (A), mean effective escape rate, $^2\mathrm{UF}\bar{\lambda}_e$ (B) and efflux rate (C). Load, escape and efflux rates are for UF loads ≤6 g kg^{-1} BW for lactating (□) and non-lactating ruminants (△) or ≥6 g kg^{-1} BW for lactating (■) and non-lactating ruminants (▲). Note the inverse relationships between ruminal efflux rate of metabolizable protein (MP) and rumen UF load (A), mean effective escape rate (B) and ruminal efflux rate (C) depending upon rumen loads of UF. These differential responses are interpreted to reflect interactions between achieved ruminal load of UF and the drive to acquire the MP requirements of the ruminant's tissues.

lactating and non-lactating ruminants were not evident. The relationships in Figs 16.7 and 16.8 were interpreted to indicate that ruminants regulate ruminal flux of UF primarily via $^2\mathrm{UF}\bar{\lambda}_e$ when consuming diets of 0.2 or less of UF and via increasing UF load when consuming diets of greater UF content.

The relationships illustrated in Fig. 16.8 are consistent with UF intake and ruminal dynamics being driven by an unfulfilled requirement for MP (Fig. 16.1). With concomitant increases in flux of HF and HCHO, the efficiency of microbial growth rate might be expected to be increased due to the combination of increased flux of hydrolysable carbohydrates and to increased turnover or the microbial ecosystem associated with increased $^2\mathrm{UF}\bar{\lambda}_e$.

Physical limitations to ruminal efflux of UF

As indicated in Equation 16.4, the physical capacity of the rumen to process UF is determined by both capacity to harbour

(UNDFL) and to process feed residues for efflux (UF efflux). The relationships between ruminal load and efflux of UF above a UNDFL of 6 g kg^{-1} BW in Fig. 16.7C appear linear throughout the range of the data. Some evidence for a non-linear approach to a physical limit to processing UF would be expected if such a physical limit for ruminal efflux of UF was approached by the range of the current data. Thus, together with other evidence to be reviewed, it is concluded that processes other than physical limitations appear to constrain ruminal efflux of UF and, thereby, feed intake.

Microbial metabolic regulation of residence time

Mechanisms have been suggested whereby ruminal residence time of feed residues might be related to the degree of microbial colonization of feed residues and/or by rate of hydrolysis and metabolism of derived monomers. One example of this is the relatively complete hydrolysis of HF observed in forages whose HFk_h differ (Ellis *et al.*, 1991, 1994, and Figure 18 of Ellis *et al.*, 1999). Biological mechanisms involving buoyancy and the self-regulation nature of physical regulation have been proposed whereby HFk_h may regulate ^{2}UF$\overline{\lambda}_e$ (Ellis *et al.*, 1991). Another example is the relatively constant degree of colonization of ruminal efflux (16.3 g microbial CP g^{-1} ruminal efflux OM; Table 16.4; and Tables 5 and 9 of Ellis *et al.*, 1999). This level of microbial CP in the ruminal efflux OM approximates that attained on forage residues subsequent to an *in situ* incubation for ruminal residence times comparable with those reviewed in Fig. 16.4 and elsewhere (Van Milgen *et al.*, 1993; Figure 20 of Ellis *et al.*, 1994).

In contrast to earlier proposals of a constant microbial CP in the ruminal efflux OM, significant trends occur in microbial CP concentrations of ruminal efflux OM for the current data set. These trends appeared most related to the dietary level of fermentable carbohydrate and protein in the diet and may be due to obscuring differences in dilution of microbial CP by different non-microbial protein OM components. The dynamic and complex interactions that determine intraruminal synthesis of microbial protein are of paramount significance. However, a less direct but less complex approach involves estimating ruminal efflux yield of microbial protein and inferring the causal intraruminal process.

Ruminal efflux yield of microbial protein

Relationships between ruminal dynamics and efficiency of ruminal efflux yield of microbial protein, MCPE (g of ruminal efflux of MCP g^{-1} of ruminally hydrolysed carbohydrate) were investigated. These relationships were of necessity restricted to data supporting the calculation of ruminally hydrolysed carbohydrates. The difference in NDF intake and NDF effluxing the rumen was assumed to represent hydrolysed structural carbohydrates.

Relationships involving MCPE versus various candidate independent variables are shown in Fig. 16.9. None of the candidate independent variables alone exhibited impressive correlations, including flux of hydrolysed carbohydrates (Fig. 16.9D), rate of hydrolysis of component carbohydrates HF and NSC (Figs 16.9B and C) or effective escape rate from the two ruminal pools, UF$\overline{\lambda}_e$ (Fig. 16.9A). These candidate independent variables are utilized in various models to predict MCPE and/or yield. In contrast, the proportions of ruminally hydrolysed protein to ruminally hydrolysed total carbohydrates (RHP:HCHO) were more highly correlated with MCPE than that observed for other candidate independent variables. This improvement in correlation was due in part to ruminally hydrolysed total carbohydrates (g of HCHO day^{-1}) being common to both the dependent (g of ruminal efflux MCP g^{-1} of hydrolysed HCHO) and the independent variable (g of RHP g^{-1} of HCHO). However, the relationship MCPE versus (RHP:HCHO) has considerable biological logic as an expression of flux proportions of two different types of precursors, molecular precursors and ME. The linear nature of MCPE versus (RHP:HCHO) observed in Fig. 16.9F suggests that RHP provided molecular precursor(s) that first limited efficiency of ruminal microbial protein synthesis throughout the range of 0–0.9 (RHP:HCHO). The regression equation was MCPE = 0.06 + 0.46 × (RHP:HCHO). It is interesting that, statistically, a ratio of 0.46 of (RHP:HCHO) was applicable throughout the entire range of the data up to the maximal observed efficiency value of 0.56 g of MCP g^{-1} of HCHO.

Dijkstra *et al.* (1998) reported expected maximal growth yields within the rumen of 0.45 and 0.65 g of microbial DM g^{-1} of hydrolysed CHO in the absence or presence of 'pre-formed monomers', respectively. It is clear that a response to pre-formed precursors would be expected even though the precise molecular precursors are unidentified here. It should also be noted that values for MCPE summarized here are for ruminal efflux yield of MCP g^{-1} of ruminally hydrolysed CHO. If rumen microbial DM is assumed to contain

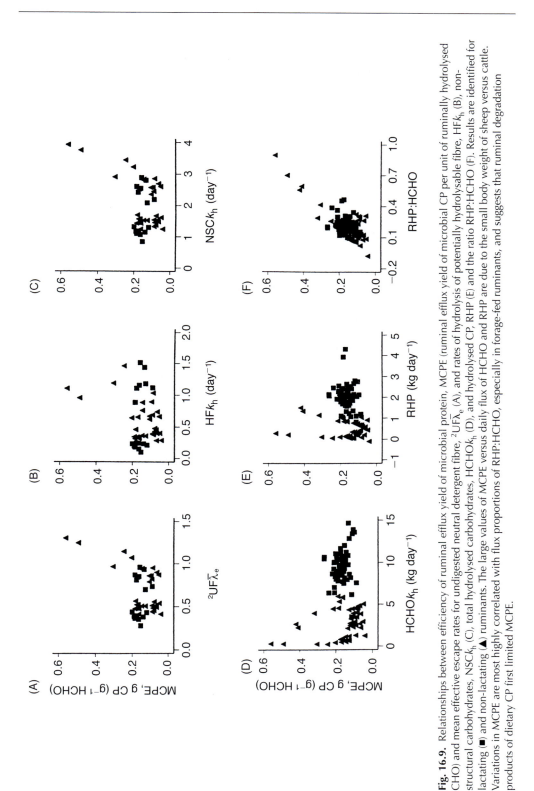

Fig. 16.9. Relationships between efficiency of ruminal efflux yield of microbial protein, MCPE (ruminal efflux yield of microbial CP per unit of ruminally hydrolysed CHO) and mean effective escape rates for undigested neutral detergent fibre, $^2UF\bar{\lambda}_e$ (A), and rates of hydrolysis of potentially hydrolysable fibre, HFk_h (B), non-structural carbohydrates, NSCk_h (C), total hydrolysed carbohydrates, HCHOk_h (D), and hydrolysed CP, RHP (E) and the ratio RHP:HCHO (F). Results are identified for lactating (■) and non-lactating (▲) ruminants. The large values of MCPE versus daily flux of HCHO and RHP are due to the small body weight of sheep versus cattle. Variations in MCPE are most highly correlated with flux proportions of RHP:HCHO, especially in forage-fed ruminants, and suggests that ruminal degradation products of dietary CP first limited MCPE.

0.65 CP (including that of nucleic acids) and 0.5 of ruminally synthesized MCP is recycled in the rumen (Wells and Russell, 1996), the maximal value for MCPE reported in Fig. 16.9 (0.56) would be equivalent to 1.7 g of intraruminally synthesized DM g^{-1} of HCHO. Clearly, either systematic errors are involved with estimation of ruminal efflux yield of MCP or indispensible molecular precursors for microbial growth must be recycled very efficiently in the rumen. Regardless of these apparent discrepancies, it is clear that efficiency of ruminal efflux yield of intraruminal microbial growth is first limited severely by some molecular precursors associated with ruminal hydrolysis of CP.

Combining the expression of efficiency of ruminal efflux yield of microbial growth, MCPE, with the observed intraruminal flux of hydrolysed entities yields the ruminal efflux yield of MCP, MCPY (kg day^{-1}). Figure 16.10 displays relationships between MCPY and flux of candidate independent variables. Intraruminal flux of HCHO, NSC, CP and RHP were all highly correlated with MCPY. All of these variables are positively and highly correlated with RHP, so it seems probable that the nutritional variable first limiting MCPY is RHP.

The significance of these relationships involving RHP is not so much because they are a reliable predictor of MCPE or MCPY but rather because of their statistical support of the biological inference that some product of ruminal hydrolysis of protein and/or amino acid metabolism first limits efficiency of ruminal efflux yield of microbial protein. The results can be interpreted further in terms of current knowledge of ruminal proteolysis, peptidolysis and amino acid utilization. Candidates for indispensable precursor include degradation products of proteins and the accompanying nucleic acids. Microbial synthesis presumably involves *de novo* synthesis of the nucleosides and nucleotides rather than utilizing any expected degradation products of nucleic acids.

A nutritional requirement by a number of species of rumen bacteria has been demonstrated for molecular precursors such as peptides, amino acids, branched-chained and aromatic fatty acids. However, it is generally assumed that requirements for such molecular precursors is relatively simple, relatively small and adequately provided for *in vivo* from degraded intake protein (Hume *et al.*, 1970) and the extensive lysis and metabolism of a large proportion of the microbial population (Wells and Russell, 1996). Because of the kinetics of hydrolysis and metabolism of proteins, it is suggested that ruminal hydrolysis and degradation of low levels of dietary protein may not provide even the small requirements for a limiting precursor.

The hydrolysis of dietary proteins by the rumen microbial ecosystem (Wallace, 1991) is characterized as a multistep process consisting of: (i) initial hydrolysis of dietary proteins to relatively large peptides by a wide spectrum of endo-peptidases; (ii) hydrolysis of large peptides to tri- and dipeptides by a single, molecularly specific dipeptidyl dipeptidase; (iii) hydrolysis of tri- and dipeptides to amino acids by a single, molecularly specific dipeptidase; (iv) microbial uptake of amino acids; or (v) their rapid oxidative deamination to carbon dioxide, ammonia and fatty acids that are transported into the microbial cell and used for synthesis of amino acids and lipids. The rate-limiting step in this process is thought to be hydrolysis by the endopeptidases, enzymes that differ widely in their mode of classification based on cleavage site and which are produced by the majority of feed-adherent bacterial species.

In comparison with the initial cleavage to peptides, rates of peptidylosis and amino acid deamination are more rapid so that extremely low concentrations of these intermediate products exist in the rumen. Many species of rumen bacteria are capable of deaminating amino acids but most do so at relatively slow rates, possibly reflecting the energetic inefficiency for these as a source of energy for microbial growth. However, several bacterial species have been identified that have high affinities for fermenting amino acids and are suggested

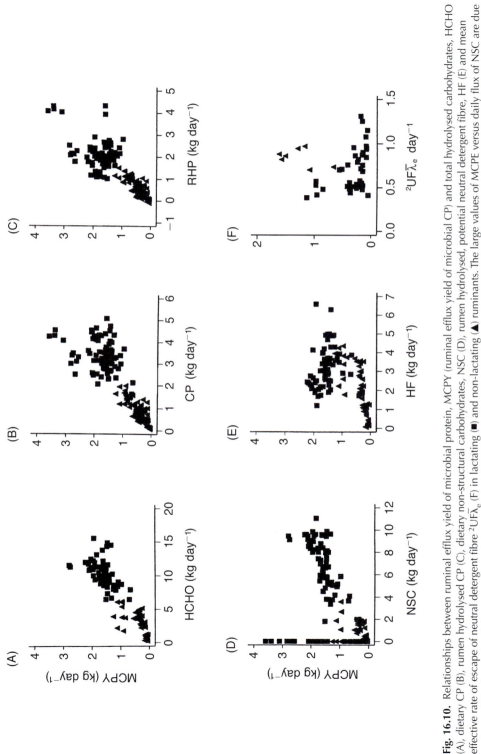

Fig. 16.10. Relationships between ruminal efflux yield of microbial CP, MCPY (ruminal efflux yield of microbial CP) and total hydrolysed carbohydrates, HCHO (A), dietary CP (B), rumen hydrolysed CP (C), dietary non-structural carbohydrates, NSC (D), rumen hydrolysed, potential neutral detergent fibre, HF (E) and mean effective rate of escape of neutral detergent fibre $^2UF\bar{\lambda}_e$ (F) in lactating (■) and non-lactating (▲) ruminants. The large values of NSC are due to the small body weight of sheep versus cattle.

to account for the major proportion of amino acids fermented *in vivo* (Krause and Russell, 1996).

The relatively high levels of RHP apparently required for MCP synthesis may be a reflection of limiting concentrations of the precursor(s) relative to its utilization affinity. The concentration of such indispensable precursors could differ markedly due to slight changes in the dynamics of their rates of genesis and utilization (Wallace, 1991). It is therefore not reasonable to expect a consistent relationship between the ruminal concentration of the first limiting molecular intermediate and the quantity of protein hydrolysed. Consistent with this proposal is the fact that the significance of a relationship involving RHP was only evident when data from forage legume diets were included, i.e. diets that provided extremely large concentrations of dietary protein (0.20–0.36) that were hydrolysed extensively (0.8–1) (Figs 16.9 and 16.10).

These considerations suggest the probability that low concentrations of peptides, amino acids or fatty acids derived from amino acids first limit rumen efflux yield of microbial protein from the usual levels of dietary protein. Assuming that the first limiting nutrient is a peptide or amino acid, an obvious approach for improving MCPE would be to limit the rate of removal of this indispensable intermediate.

Manipulating protein hydrolysis and fermentation

The feasibility of specifically inhibiting the rate of fermentation of amino acids as a method for improving efficiency of ruminant protein utilization has been demonstrated. Chalupa *et al.* (1983) demonstrated that the diaryliodonium compounds, and specifically diphenyldiodonium chloride (DIC), reduced accumulation of ammonia from dietary protein *in vitro*, increased ruminal efflux of CP and reduced the dietary requirements of the ruminant for CP. Although DIC specifically inhibits oxidative deamination of isoleucine, the

rate of hydrolysis of protein is also slowed (Ramirez Piñeres *et al.*, 1997). Considerations unrelated to its efficacy limited further development of DIC.

Another compound (LY292253, LY29) has been identified that is equally as effective in limiting the accumulation of ammonia from dietary proteins when incubated *in vitro* with rumen microorganisms. *In vivo*, both LY29 and DIC increased flux of trichloroacetic acid-soluble and insoluble, Lowry-reactive protein to the duodenum of steers grazing pastures or receiving a diet containing grain at 80 g kg^{-1} (Ysunda *et al.*, 1995). Common effects of both LY29 and DIC (Table 16.5) were to increase ruminal efflux of OM and protein by approximately 140% of that of the control animals. Unfortunately, efflux specifically of microbial protein and free amino acids were not measured in these studies. However, subsequent studies have established that LY29 does not inhibit initial hydrolysis of proteins or peptides but inhibits deamination by mixed rumen bacteria *in vitro* (Floret *et al.*, 1999). Also, LY29 was without effect on rumen protozoa but inhibited growth of several ruminal bacterial species including all species of bacteria identified as having a high affinity for amino acid fermentation (Krause and Russell, 1996).

The *in vivo* responses to LY29 and DIC summarized in Table 16.5 are similar to those reported by Ishaque *et al.* (1971) for lambs that, as evidenced by rumen VFA profiles, appeared to adapt different microbial populations during transition to grain-based diets. Lambs exhibiting rumen VFA profiles characterized by large proportions of propionate also exhibited greater ruminal efflux of OM, CP and diaminopimelic acid. Ruminal efflux was increased in the order of 150–180% for animals fed the same diet but having an adapted microbial ecosystem characterized by smaller proportions of propionate (Table 16.6).

Although not replicated by subsequent experimentation (J.A.F. Rook, personal communication), the results of Ishaque *et al.* (1971) are suggested to represent an

Table 16.5. Mean responses to LY29[a,c] and DIC[b] expressed as fraction of control diet.

Response variable	LY29 Trial			DIC	
	Bermuda	Ryegrass	Mixed diet	Rye	Mean
Dietary OM intake	1.47	1.14	1.15	1.87	1.41
Duodenal flow					
OM	1.31	1.33	1.42	1.51	1.39
Ammonia	0.77	1.25	1.43	ND	1.22
TCA-insoluble protein	1.62	2.05	1.26	1.58	1.32
TCA-soluble protein	1.62	1.13	1.65	1.50	1.48
Total protein	1.41	1.65	1.61	1.54	1.55

[a]Response to LY29 = response to 500 mg/response to 0 mg of LY29.
[b]Response to DIC = response to 80 mg of DIC/response to 0 mg of DIC.
[c]Response to LY29 to dose, $P = 0.07$.

infrequently adapted rumen microbial ecosystem that is capable of more efficient microbial protein synthesis. It is speculated that the more efficient ecosystem observed by Ishaque *et al.* (1971) may have excluded those bacterial species having a high affinity for fermenting amino acids. That such a more efficient microbial ecosystem may occur frequently is suggested further by the results of Dove and Milne (1994). Dove and

Table 16.6. Mean ($n = 6$) ruminal metabolic characteristics and digesta flow in two groups of lambs that, based on the proportion of propionate in their rumen, appear to have adapted different microbial ecosystems while receiving equal and limited amounts of an 83 g CP kg^{-1} diet (summarized from Ishaque *et al.*, 1971).

Item	Group		Group 2/ Group 1
	1	2	
DM intake, g day^{-1}	900	900	
Rumen characteristics			
pH	6.06	6.10	1.01
Ammonia, mg (100 ml)$^{-1}$	27.9	11.3	0.40
Total volatile fatty acids, mEq (100 ml)$^{-1}$	101.8	132.0	1.30
Propionate, molar %	14.9	33.2	2.23
Duodenal digesta			
DM flow, g day^{-1}	186.0	291.0	1.56
Nitrogen, fraction of DM	0.037	0.042	1.14
Nitrogen, g day^{-1}	6.9	12.5	1.82
Cellulose, dig	0.76	0.54	0.71
DAPA[a], g 100 g^{-1} DM	0.108	0.162	1.50
DAPA[a], g day^{-1}	0.201	0.472	2.35
Duodenal N flow/N intake	0.57	1.04	1.82
Ruminal digestion (recalculated from data)			
Estimated truly fermented DM[b], g day^{-1}	712	629	0.46
Estimated g BCP g^{-1} TFDM[c]	0.03	0.075	0.40
Composition of ruminal efflux: g g^{-1} duodenal DM			
Non-ammonia nitrogen	0.23	0.25	0.90
Microbial protein nitrogen	0.125	0.144	0.87

[a]DAPA = diaminopimelic acid.
[b]Estimated as ((DM intake × apparent ruminal indigestibility of energy) − (DAPA flow/0.005 g DAPA g^{-1} microbial DM)).
[c]Estimated as ((DAPA flow, g day^{-1}/0.01 g DAPA g^{-1} microbial crude protein)/(estimated truly digested DM)).

Milne observed that prediction of MCPY as a function of abomosal OM flux differed between experiments but yielded a common regression to ruminal hydrolysed OM when molar proportions of propionate were included in a multiple regression model.

Results with LY29 and DIC and those of Ishaque *et al.* (1971) suggest considerable potential for increasing the efficiency of ruminal microbial protein synthesis and, thereby, the level and efficiency of ruminant productivity via favourably modifying the rates of ruminal amino acid deamination. Growth rate hysteresis recently has been suggested as a possible cause of variations in MCPE (Baker and Dijkstra, 1999). Growth rate hysteresis represents inefficiencies in microbial growth as the consequence of asynchronous flux of precursors for the energetically expensive synthesis of macromolecules such as rRNA and RNA polymerase. Protein synthesis *per se* is preceded by the synthesis of poly-nucleosides, and lack of synchrony of this rate with the subsequent synthesis of polypeptides will contribute energetic inefficiency associated with the degradation of excessive polynucleotides. Occurrence of growth rate hysteresis as conceived by Baker and Dijkstra (1999) could be accentuated via the rapid fluctuations in the short-term dynamics associated with infrequent meals.

The increased ruminal efflux of microbial protein associated with inhibitors of amino acid deamination suggests that the intermediates of ruminal protein degradation are free amino acids rather than peptides or products of amino acid fermentation.

Ionophores

Ionophores such as monensin appear to affect microbial utilization of protein and inhibit microbial species having an affinity for amino acid fermentation (Krause and Russell, 1996). We have demonstrated consistent responses to supplemental protein and monensin in liveweight gain by grazing calves which is attributed to increased grazed intake (Hill, 1991). A synergistic effect of supplemental protein and monensin was demonstrated by increases in liveweight gain from 207 g of supplemental protein plus 200 mg of monensin to a level otherwise obtained for 320 g of supplemental protein without monensin.

We have interpreted these responses to monensin in grazing ruminants to be associated with the growth inhibition of some but not all species of amino acid-fermenting bacteria (Krause and Russell, 1996). Responses in calves grazing annual ryegrass were similar whether supplemented with monensin plus grain or protein. Thus, responses due to monensin were interpreted as due to effects of monensin on reducing amino acid deamination of this high CP forage and improved synchrony with energy genesis from the more slowly hydrolysing supplemental starch. In contrast, semi-tropical forage contained 1.0–1.3 g CP kg^{-1} and benefited from supplemental protein whose ruminally degraded amino acids were fermented less rapidly due to the effects of monensin. The relatively large liveweight gain responses, 1.3 and 1.6 times the mineral controls, from ryegrass and bermudagrass respectively, are proposed to reflect the extensive degradation of proteins of growing foliage (0.85+) that contributed to a deficiency of amino acids as first limiting grazed forage intake and liveweight gains. It is further proposed that the productive potential of growing ruminants commonly is limited by deficiencies of net amino acids when grazing actively growing forages. This generalization is illustrated most dramatically by the responses in empty body weight gain of early weaned lambs to abomasally infused amino acids when the lambs grazed white clover pastures that contained 3.8 g CP kg^{-1} (Frazer *et al.*, 1991).

Voluntary Intake

Evidence reviewed to this point suggests that the metabolic flux of indispensable amino acids required by mammalian tissues is generally first limiting at the ruminant's tissue level. Thus the flux of ME:MP surplus to the ME required for indispensable metabolic requirements (such as vital activities and tissue protein synthesis) may be considered incidental in regulating intake. This priority for dietary CP is manifested in feed selection trials where mammals in general and ruminants in particular exhibit preferences for combinations of protein that tend to maximize productivity (Kyriazakis and Oldham, 1997).

Voluntary intake commonly is related to the dietary level of CP in a curvilinear manner, as shown in Fig. 16.11. Figure 16.11 summarizes the relationship between voluntary intake by lambs of various forage *Sorghum* sp. varieties and cultivars of different maturities with and without supplemental levels of a purified soybean protein (Buentello and Ellis, 1969). When fitted to a Michaelis–Menten type response function, voluntary intake appears related to dietary concentration of CP in a manner analogous to Michaelis–Menten kinetics, i.e. rapid increases in response rate that diminish as supply of substrate approaches and saturates the responding mechanism(s) and achieves its maximal rate. Based on the Michaelis–Menten function estimated from levels of CP ranging from 40–190 g kg^{-1} DM, maximum intake was not achieved even when projected levels of CP exceeded 1000 g kg^{-1} DM.

Clearly, voluntary intake of forage responds to dietary levels of CP that considerable exceed those commonly investigated, just as MCPE responds to levels of CP and RHP. The projected response in voluntary intake beyond the range of dietary CP in Fig. 16.11 is consistent with implications that the amino acid requirement of the ruminant's tissues may never be met via normal feeding practices

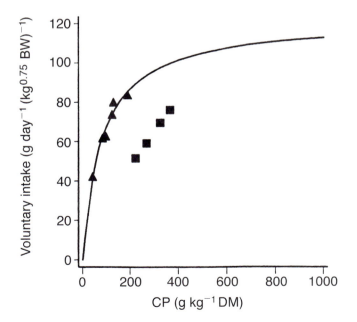

Fig. 16.11. Relationships between voluntary intake by lambs of forage *Sorghum* sp. varieties (▲, Buentello and Ellis, 1986) with and without supplemental purified protein, expected voluntary intake based on Michaelis–Menten kinetics (——) and the voluntary intake of grazed forages by early weaned lambs (■, Cruickshank *et al.*, 1992).

due to inefficiencies in ruminal amino acid digestion reviewed here. Also shown in Fig. 16.11 is the voluntary intake by early weaned lambs of highly digestible, grazed grass and legume pastures (Cruickshank *et al.*, 1992). In the case of these early weaned lambs, intake responses were linear throughout the range of 224–366 g CP kg^{-1} diet. Indicative of their growth rate potential for lean muscle growth, these early weaned lambs exhibited very rapid liveweight gains, and this consequential large requirement for MP is proposed as the cause of the linear responses in voluntary intake over the range in dietary CP. Relationships between voluntary intake and ruminal efflux of TDOM and MP were also linear (Fig. 16.12). The ruminal efflux proportions of TDOM:MP increased slightly with level of dietary CP and ranged from 5 to 6.4. This proportion is within the range (4–10) of proportions of intake of ruminal efflux of TDOM/MP observed in Fig. 16.2. The observed range in proportions of ruminal efflux yield of TDOM and MP was proposed to be the consequence of differences in feed compositional attributes determining ruminal efflux of TDOM and MP and of an MP requirement driving feed

intake of such variable TDOMI:MP as illustrated in Table 16.2.

Uncertainties about the amino acid requirements, or even the MP requirements, of the experimental ruminants in the current data set do not permit testing of the hypothesis of an MP requirement-driven intake. However, it should be biologically evident that voluntary intake, or the processes constraining intake, cannot be estimated reliably without quantitative knowledge of the feed's ruminal efflux yield of the metabolizable nutrient that first limits the ruminant's genetic potential for maintenance and production. Further, the disparate proportions of TDOMI:MP supplied versus those required all support the suggestion that flux of indispensable molecules, i.e. amino acids, rather than energy may severely constrain feed intake by ruminants.

Lippke (1980) investigated various ruminant responses to a variety of forages and reported that liveweight performance could be best described by a multiple regression equation having negative coefficients for indigestible NDF and positive coefficients for CP. The observed liveweight gain could be described by

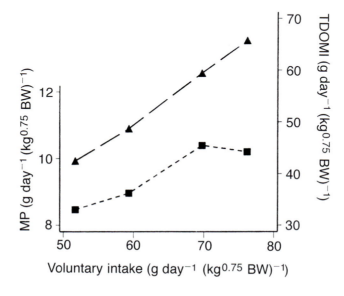

Fig. 16.12. Relationships between voluntary intake of grazed pasture by early weaned lambs and their ruminal efflux yield of MP (■) and TDOMI (▲).

these two dietary entities with greater precision than could voluntary intake or digestibility. Such empirical observations are consistent with the negative effects of UF upon digesta kinetics, the positive effects of CP upon nutrient acquisition of MP and the general insufficiency of MP for ruminant tissues in the metabolizable nutrients which exit the rumen. The superior empirical description of liveweight gain by this model and failure reliably to predict intake and digestion reflect the complexity of dietary–digestive–metabolic interactions described in this chapter.

Conclusions

The anaerobic metabolism of the rumen microbial anaerobic fermentation yields deficient proportions of metabolizable amino acids relative to the amino acid and energy requirements of the aerobic metabolism of ruminants' tissues. Nutritionally, feed intake appears to be regulated in an attempt to provide the flux of amino acids required by the animal's genetic potential. However, voluntary intake by ruminants appears constrained by the metabolic capacity of its nutrient acquisition system. Such constraints appear related to inefficient utilization of amino acids for microbial growth in addition to thermodynamic limitations inherent in anaerobic metabolism. These constraints are accentuated further by levels of undigested entities in the diet that increase ruminal residence time and, thereby, ruminal efflux yield of metabolizable amino acids. Reflecting such constraints, voluntary intake of forages by ruminants appears not to be maximized even by levels of dietary protein well beyond those which they normally contain.

Acknowledgement

This chapter is based, in part, upon work supported by the Texas Advanced Research (Technology) Program under Grant No. 517–0170–1997.

References

Aitchison, E., Gill, M., France, J. and Dhanoa, M.S. (1986) Comparison of methods to describe the kinetics of digestion and passage of fibre in sheep. *Journal of the Science of Food and Agriculture* 37, 1065–1072.

Baker, S.K. and Dijkstra, J. (1999) Dynamic aspects of the microbial ecosystem of the reticulo-rumen. In: Jung, H.J.G. and Fahey, G.C., Jr (eds) *Vth International Symposium on the Nutrition of Herbivores*. American Society of Animal Science, Savoy, Illinois, pp. 261–311.

Beever, D.E., Thompson, D.J., Ulyatt, M.J., Cammell, S.B. and Spooner, M.C. (1985) The digestion of fresh perennial ryegrass (*Lolium perenne* L. cv. Melle) and white clover *(Trifolium repens* L. cv. Blanca) by growing cattle fed indoors. *British Journal of Nutrition* 54, 761–775.

Beever, D.E., Losada, H.R., Cammell, S.B., Evans, R.T. and Haines, M.T. (1986) Effect of forage species on nutrient digestion and supply in grazing cattle. *British Journal of Nutrition* 56, 209–225.

Buentello, J.L. and Ellis, W.C. (1969) Protein levels for maximizing voluntary intake and digestibility. *Proceedings of the Texas Nutrition Conference*, pp. 167–174.

Cammell, S.B., Thomson, D.J., Beever, D.E., Haines, M.J., Dhanoa, M.S. and Spooner, M.C. (1986) The efficiency of energy utilization in growing cattle consuming fresh perennial ryegrass (*Lolium perenne* cv. Melle) or white clover (*Trifolium repens* cv. Blanca). *British Journal of Nutrition* 55, 669–680.

Chalupa, W., Patterson, J.A. and Parish, R.C. (1983) Effects of the 4,4″-dimethyldiphenyliodonium chloride on performance of growing cattle. *Journal of Animal Science* 57, 201–205.

Cruickshank, G.J., Poppi, D.P. and Sykes, A.R. (1992) The intake, digestion and protein degradation of grazed herbage by early-weaned lambs. *British Journal of Nutrition* 68, 349–364.

Dove, H. and Milne, J.A. (1994) Digesta flow and rumen microbial protein production in ewes grazing perennial ryegrass. *Australian Journal of Agricultural Research* 45, 1229–1249.

Dijkstra, J., France, J. and Davies, D.R. (1998) Different mathematical approaches to estimating microbial protein supply in ruminants. *Journal of Dairy Science* 81, 3370–3384.

Egan, A.R. (1977) Nutritional status and intake regulation in sheep. VIII. Relationships between the voluntary intake of herbage by sheep and the protein/energy ratio in the digestion products. *Australian Journal of Agricultural Research* 28, 907–915.

Ellis, W.C. and Hill, T.H. (1995) Importance of dietary amino acids in the nutrition of grazing ruminants. *Annales de Zootechnie* 44 (Suppl. 1), 231.

Ellis, W.C., Kennedy, P. and Matis, J.H. (1991) Passage and digestion of plant tissues fragments in herbivores. In: Ho, Y.W., Wong, H.K., Abdullah, N. and Tajuddin, Z.A. (eds) *Proceedings of the 3rd International Symposium of Nutrition of Herbivores.* Malaysian Society of Animal Production, Vinlin Press, Kuala Lumpur, pp. 227–236.

Ellis, W.C., Matis, J.H., Hill, T.M. and Murphy, M.R. (1994) Methodology for estimating digestion and passage kinetics of forages. In: Fahey, G.C. (ed.) *Forage Quality, Evaluation, and Utilization.* University of Nebraska, Lincoln, Nebraska, pp. 682–756.

Ellis, W.C., Poppi, D.P., Matis, J.H., Lippke, H., Hill, T.M. and Rouquette, F.M. (1999) Dietary–digestive interactions determining the nutritive potential of ruminant diets. In: Jung, H.J.G. and Fahey, G.C., Jr (eds) *Vth International Symposium on the Nutrition of Herbivores.* American Society of Animal Science, Savoy, Illinois, pp. 423–481.

Faichney, G.J., Poncet, C. and Boston, R.C. (1989) Passage of internal and external markers of particulate matter though the rumen of sheep. *Reproduction and Nutrition in Development* 29, 325–339.

Floret, F., Chaudhary, L.C., Ellis, W.C., El Hassan, S., McKain, N., Newbold, C.J. and Wallace, R.J. (1999) Influence of 1-[(E)-2-(2-methyl-4-nitrophenyl)diaz-1-enyl]pyrrolidine-2-carboxylic acid and diphenyliodonium chloride on ruminal protein metabolism and ruminal microorganisms. *Applied and Environmental Microbiology* 65, 3258–3260.

Forbes, J.M. (1980) A model of the short-term control of feeding in the ruminant: effects of changing the animal or feed characteristics. *Appetite* 1, 21–41.

Fraser, D.L., Poppi, D.P. and Fraser, T.J. (1991) The effect of protein or amino acid supplementation on growth and body composition of lambs grazing white clover. *Proceedings of the 3rd International Symposium on the Nutrition of Herbivores.* Malaysian Society of Animal Production, Vinlin Press, Kuala Lumpur, p. 22.

Gunter, S.A., Krysl, L.J., Judkins, M.B., Broesder, J.T. and Barton, R.K. (1990) Influence of branched-chain fatty acid supplementation on voluntary intake, site and extent of digestion, ruminal fermentation, digesta kinetics and microbial protein synthesis in beef heifers consuming grass hay. *Journal of Animal Science* 68, 2885–2892.

Hannah, S.M., Cochran, R.C., Vanzant, E.S. and Harmon, D.L. (1990) Influence of protein supplementation on site and extent of digestion, forage intake, and nutrient flow characteristics in steers consuming dormant blue stem-range forage. *Journal of Animal Science* 69, 2624–2633.

Hill, T.M. (1991) Effects of source of supplemental nutrients on forage intake, digestive kinetics and protein supply to the small intestine of grazing calves. PhD dissertation, Texas A&M University, College Station, Texas.

Huhtanen, P. and Vanhatalo, A. (1997) Ruminal and total plant cell-wall digestibility estimated by a combined *in situ* method utilizing mathematical models. *British Journal of Nutrition* 78, 583–598.

Hume, I.D., Moir, R.J. and Somers, M. (1970) Synthesis of microbial protein in the rumen. *Australian Journal of Agricultural Research* 21, 283–296.

Hungate, R.E. (1966) *The Rumen and its Microbes.* Academic Press, New York.

Ishaque, M., Thomas, P.C. and Rook, J.A.F. (1971) Consequences to the host of changes in rumen microbial activity. *Nature* 231, 253–256.

Isaacson, H.R., Hinds, F.C., Bryant, M.P. and Owens, F. (1975) Efficiency of energy utilization by mixed rumen bacteria in continuous culture. *Journal of Dairy Science* 58, 1645–1659.

Krause, D.O. and Russell, J.B. (1996) An rRNA approach for assessing the role of obligate amino acid-fermenting bacteria in ruminal amino acid deamination. *Applied and Environmental Microbiology* 62, 815–821.

Kyriazakis, I. and Oldham, J.D. (1997) Food intake and diet selection in sheep: the effect of manipulating the rates of digestion of carbohydrates and protein of the foods offered as a choice. *British Journal of Nutrition* 77, 243–254.

Lippke, H. (1980) Forage characteristics related to intake, digestibility and gain by ruminants. *Journal of Animal Science* 50, 952–961.

Matis, J.H. (1972) Gamma time-dependency in Blaxter's compartmental model. *Biometrics* 28, 597–602.

Moir, R.J. and Harris, L.E. (1962) Ruminal flora studies in the sheep. X. Influence of nitrogen intake upon ruminal function. *Journal of Nutrition* 77, 285–298.

Orskov, E.R. and McDonald, I. (1979) The estimation of protein degradability in the rumen from incubation measurements weighted according to rate of passage. *Journal of Agricultural Science, Cambridge* 92, 499–503.

Poppi, D.P. (1990) Manipulation of nutrient supply to animals at pasture: opportunities and consequences. *Proceedings of the 5th Asian Australasian Association of Animal Production.* Taipei, Taiwan, Lincoln University, Canterbury, New Zealand, Vol. 1, 40–79.

Poppi, D.P., Minson, D.J. and Ternouth, J.H. (1981) Studies of cattle and sheep eating leaf and stem fractions of grasses *Digitaria decumbens,* chloris gayana III. The retention time in the rumen of large feed particles. *Australian Journal of Agricultural Research* 32, 123–137.

Ramirez Piñeres, M.A., Ellis, W.C., Wu, G. and Ricke, S.C. (1997) Effects of diphenyliodonium chloride on proteolysis and leucine metabolism by rumen microorganisms. *Animal Feed Science and Technology* 65, 139–149.

Russell, J.B., O'Connor, J.D., Fox, D.G., Van Soest, P.J. and Sniffen, C.J. (1992) A net carbohydrate and protein system for evaluating cattle diets: I. Ruminal fermentation. *Journal of Animal Science* 70, 3551–3561.

Storm, E. and Orskov, E.R. (1983) The nutritive value of rumen micro-organisms in ruminants. 4. The limiting amino acid of microbial protein in growing sheep determined by a new approach. *British Journal of Nutrition* 50, 486–492.

Sutherland, T.M. (1986) Particle separation in the forestomach of sheep. In: Dobson, A. and Dobson, M.H. (eds) *Aspects of Digestive Physiology in Ruminants.* Cornell University Press, Ithaca, New York, pp. 43–73.

Van Milgen, J., Berger, L.L. and Murphy, M.R. (1993) An integrated, dynamic model of feed hydration and digestion, and subsequent bacterial mass accumulation in the rumen. *British Journal of Nutrition* 70, 471–483.

Vega, A. and Poppi, D.P. (1997) Extent of digestion and rumen condition as factors affecting passage of liquid and digesta particles in sheep. *Journal of Agricultural Science, Cambridge* 128, 207–215.

Wallace, R.J. (1991) Rumen proteolysis and its control. In: Jouany, J.P. (ed.) *Microbial Metabolism and Ruminant Digestion.* INRA Editions, Paris, pp. 131–150.

Wells, J.E. and Russell, J.B. (1996) Why do many bacteria die and lyse so quickly? *Journal of Dairy Science* 79, 1487–1495.

Wylie, M.J. (1987) The flow of feed residues through the gastrointestinal tract of ruminants. PhD dissertation, Texas A&M University, College Station, Texas.

Ysunza, F., Ellis, W.C., Richardson, L. and Thomas, E.E. (1995) Effects of LY292253 upon intake and digesta flow in cattle. *Journal of Animal Science* 73 (Suppl. 1), 273.

Chapter 17
Feeding Behaviour

R.J. Grant[1] and J.L. Albright[2]

[1]*Department of Animal Science, University of Nebraska, Lincoln, Nebraska, USA;*
[2]*Department of Animal Sciences, Purdue University,*
West Lafayette, Indiana, USA

Introduction

Adequate consumption of feed ensures survival and productivity of the animal, so an understanding of factors affecting feeding behaviour of farm animals is critical. Feeding is the predominant behaviour of ruminants and is illustrated by the fact that feeding activity has priority over rumination whenever the causal factors of the two activities conflict (Metz, 1975). Well-designed management systems accommodate normal feeding behaviour to improve animal comfort and well-being. For example, accessibility of feed during times of the day when cows want to eat, e.g. when leaving the milking parlour, promotes greater feeding activity in dairy cattle (Menzi and Chase, 1994). Likewise, proper animal grouping strategies within dairy herds will reduce competition for feed at the bunk or manger and improve feed intake. For feedlot cattle, pre-conditioning diets fed prior to entering the feed yard may aid the animal in overcoming neophobia, or fear of new diets (Launchbaugh, 1995). This feeding behaviour apparently is innate and usually develops when cattle are first exposed to feedlot diets even though the diet is not toxic. In contrast, recent research with pigs indicates that palatability, not novelty, of a feed may be responsible for feed intake responses to certain feeds such as spray-dried plasma and dried skimmed milk (Ermer *et al.*, 1994).

This chapter will focus primarily on the feeding behaviour of cattle in confinement systems, specifically dairy cattle. Feeding behaviour of grazing cattle has been reviewed (Albright, 1993, 1997). Water undoubtedly is the most important nutrient, and drinking behaviour and water intake have been reviewed by Murphy (1992). Some information regarding the feeding behaviour of feedlot cattle and other ruminants will be presented in this chapter, but more detailed discussions of eating activity in beef cattle may be found in Hicks *et al.* (1989). Research on feeding and drinking behaviour in pigs was summarized by Bigelow and Houpt (1988). Forbes (1995) published a review which focused on techniques to monitor feeding behaviour and analysis of feeding data for cattle, pigs, sheep, goats and poultry.

For any dairy enterprise, the feeding management system must promote intense feeding behaviour by the milking herd.

Researchers at Michigan State University (Dado and Allen, 1994) observed that higher producing, older cows consumed more feed, ate larger meals more quickly, ruminated longer and more efficiently, and drank more water than lower producing, younger cows. To achieve this intensity of feeding behaviour, the cow's environment must be such that it ensures cow comfort, non-disrupted feeding activity and normal social behaviour. Intense feeding behaviour results in maximum dry matter intake, optimal milk production and reproduction, and improved herd health (Grant and Albright, 1997). This chapter will focus especially on social dominance and competition for feed, grouping strategies that influence feeding behaviour, feeding system design, and feed attributes such as palatability that influence feed preference and intake. Dry matter intake is the major factor that influences milk production and change in body condition score during lactation. Promoting intense feeding behaviour to maximize feed intake will be a central theme of this chapter.

Feeding Behaviour and Feed Intake

Daily feed intake comprises the number of meals consumed daily, the length of each meal and the rate of eating. By adjusting the number of daily meals and the average meal size (length × rate of eating), the ruminant animal can adjust daily dry matter intake. High-producing dairy cows allowed continuous access to totally mixed rations (TMR) ate 9–14 meals day^{-1}, while lower-producing cows consumed only 7–9 meals daily (Grant and Albright, 1995). Even though the definition of what constituted a meal differed substantially among researchers, the eating patterns of high-producing cows differ considerably from those of lower producing cows.

Feedlot cattle spend approximately 6–10% of their day eating, seemingly less with higher concentrate diets, and they are relatively unaffected by temperature or time of year (Hicks *et al.*, 1989). Additionally, cattle appear to eat more

rapidly with fewer meals as they become heavier and their feed intake declines. Typically, feedlot cattle have three major periods of feeding activity, closely associated with sunrise, sunset and the middle of the night. In general, beef and dairy cattle are crepuscular or, in other words, they are most active at sunrise and sunset (Albright, 1993, 1997).

Although not a focus of this chapter, it is interesting to note that pigs housed in groups ate more quickly, had higher feed intake per meal, but less meals per day, less eating time per day and a lower daily feed intake than pigs penned individually (de Haer and Merks, 1992). Typically, two peaks of feeding activity occurred during the day, especially in group housing: one in the morning and one in the beginning of the afternoon. With pigs, a distinction can be made between meals which contribute a major portion of the daily feed consumption and meals of minor importance (de Haer and Merks, 1992). In group housing systems, 69% of the daily meals accounted for 87% of daily feed intake and 83% of daily feeding time. In individual housing, 39% of meals accounted for 90% of daily feed intake and 79% of feeding time.

Feeding behaviour in non-competitive environments

In the specific case of lactating dairy cattle, understanding how to optimize feeding behaviour within a given feeding and grouping environment will be crucial to making profitable dairy management recommendations. Albright (1993) extensively reviewed feeding behaviour for competitive and non-competitive feeding situations. Research summarized indicated that dairy cattle will spend between 248 and 392 min day^{-1} eating, 464 to 579 min day^{-1} ruminating and have 10–17 rumination bouts day^{-1}. Meals were consumed most frequently at the beginning and the end of the daylight period. Housing appeared to have an effect on feeding behaviour. Cows in box stalls fed hay spent 6 h eating and 8 h ruminating daily, whereas cows in stanchions spent 3 h eating and 8 h ruminating each day.

The most intensive research on feeding behaviour in dairy cattle since the review by Albright (1993) was reported by Dado and Allen (1993, 1994). Twelve Holstein cows (six primiparous) averaging 63 days in milk were offered a common diet and monitored for 21-day periods with a continuous data acquisition system (Dado and Allen, 1993) to measure feed and water intake and subsequent chewing activity. It is important to note that this was a non-competitive feeding environment with animals housed in individual tie stalls. Milk production was correlated positively with dry matter and water intake within and across parities. For multiparous cows, milk production was correlated positively with meal size ($r = 0.78$) and length of eating bouts ($r = 0.75$), but was unrelated to number of meals and eating rate, a relationship also observed for non-lactating cows (Metz, 1975). For primiparous cows, milk production was related positively to number of meals ($r = 0.55$) and eating rate ($r = 0.87$) but unrelated to meal size. In summary, high-producing dairy cows attained greater feed intake by increasing meal size and spending less time eating and ruminating per unit of feed intake.

These observations of Dado and Allen (1994) suggest that different mechanisms may be controlling individual meals and total daily feed intake between cows of different parity, ruminal capacity and body size. Behavioural traits of the highly productive dairy cow include aggressive eating habits and consumption of large amounts of high-quality feed. For example, the dry matter intake achieved by Beecher Arlinda Ellen ranged from 4.4 to 6.7% of body weight during the lactation in which she produced a world record 25,248 kg of milk in 1 year (Albright, 1981).

Table 17.1 summarizes the milk production and feeding behaviour data from the research of Dado and Allen (1993, 1994). The data presented in the table illustrate that higher producing cows ate more total feed, ate larger meals more quickly, ruminated longer and more efficiently, and

drank more water than lower producing, primiparous cows.

Primiparous cows eat more slowly than older cows (Grant and Albright, 1995). In addition, primiparous cows have a slower rate of increase in dry matter intake during the first 5 weeks of lactation (Kertz *et al.*, 1991). The increased time needed by younger cows to chew and process feed should be an important consideration for group feeding strategies designed to enhance feeding activity and promote feed intake. Greater feed availability and reduced competition at feeding should increase feed intake for primiparous cows, especially in early lactation.

Two major questions raised by intensive feeding behaviour research include: (i) what gives the highly productive cow the ability to process more feed per unit of chewing time?; and (ii) do behavioural relationships observed by Dado and Allen (1994) differ markedly for animals housed and fed under competitive feeding situations? For instance, cows fed in tie stalls had more eating bouts than those in free stalls (cubicles), but total eating times were similar (Grant and Albright, 1995).

Social Dominance and Competition for Feed

When dairy cows are grouped, their social behaviour modifies feeding activity and productivity. Cattle are social creatures and readily form dominance hierarchies, particularly at the feed bunk (Friend and Polan, 1974). Social dominance correlates strongly with age, body size, horns and seniority in the herd (Grant and Albright, 1995; Albright, 1997) and plays a pivotal role in any existing, or newly formed, group of cattle. Social hierarchies and the competition for feed and water affect feeding behaviour. A highly competitive time at the feed bunk or manger coincides with return of cows from milking and when fresh feed is offered (Friend and Polan, 1974). Early research with small groups of cows indicated that the maximum effect of dominance hierarchies and competition

Table 17.1. Summary statistics for milk production and feeding behaviour of six primiparous and six multiparous lactating Holstein cows measured for 10 days[a,b].

Variable	Primiparous		Multiparous		All cows	
	$\bar{x}$	(%) CV	$\bar{x}$	(%) CV	$\bar{x}$	(%) CV
Milk production, kg day^{-1c}	28.7	15.5	37.5	13.7	33.1	19.7
DMI, kg day^{-1c}	20.0	13.6	24.8	11.3	22.8	16.1
NDF intake, kg day^{-1c}	6.2	13.8	7.6	11.4	7.0	16.1
Meal size, kg						
DM	1.8	17.0	2.5	29.8	2.2	30.6
NDF	0.56	17.3	0.75	29.7	0.67	30.5
Eating bouts per day	11.3	17.3	10.8	25.4	11.0	22.1
Eating bout length, min	25.9	22.2	31.1	33.4	28.8	31.3
Eating time						
min day^{-1}	284	16.5	314	16.8	301	17.3
min kg^{-1} of DM	15.9	23.7	13.6	14.1	14.6	21.0
min kg^{-1} of NDF	51.1	22.4	44.3	14.4	47.2	20.1
Eating chews per day	18,276	22.8	19,256	16.9	18,832	19.6
Eating chew rate, chews min^{-1}	62.7	7.4	60.8	8.7	61.6	8.3
Ruminating bouts per day	15.4	17.5	12.9	13.3	14.0	17.8
Ruminating bout length, min^c	29.7	15.9	36.0	19.9	33.3	20.9
Ruminating time						
min day^{-1}	453	18.3	460	14.8	457	16.3
min kg^{-1} of DM	22.9	21.1	18.7	18.9	20.5	22.5
min kg^{-1} of NDF	74.1	20.8	60.9	19.0	66.6	22.3
Ruminating chews per day	29,645	21.5	28,946	17.6	29,248	19.3
Ruminating chew rate, chew min^{-1}	64.4	10.7	61.8	7.2	62.9	9.1
Total chewing time						
min day^{-1}	738	13.9	774	11.4	758	12.6
min kg^{-1} of DM^c	37.2	15.9	31.4	13.6	33.9	17.1
min kg^{-1} of NDF^c	120.7	15.6	102.0	13.8	110.1	17.0
Total chews per day	47,921	19.1	48,201	14.3	48,080	16.4
Water intake, l day^{-1c}	63.2	19.5	89.5	15.0	77.6	23.8
Drinking bout size, l	5.4	33.2	7.2	43.8	6.4	43.1
Drinking bouts per day	13.0	35.9	14.9	41.9	14.0	40.2
Drinking time, min day^{-1}	17.7	37.4	19.1	20.0	18.5	28.7
Drinking time, l min^{-1}	3.9	31.0	4.6	11.0	4.3	22.4

[a]Statistics calculated from daily total or daily mean for each cow and day combination.
[b]Table from Dado and Allen (1994).
[c]Means differ between parities ($P < 0.05$).

lasted for 30–45 min after delivery of fresh feed. This experimental observation suggests that, relative to group size, bunk space must not be limited, or that feed availability should not be limited to avoid reductions in feed intake for non-combative and the more submissive cows.

Bunk space and feeding behaviour

Grant and Albright (1995) recently reviewed the literature pertaining to competition,

bunk space and feeding behaviour. When a competitive situation exists at the feed bunk, dominant cows typically spend more total time eating than cows of lower social rank, resulting in greater feed intake. Recently, Swedish researchers (Olofsson, 1994) evaluated the effect of increasing competition per TMR feeding station from one to four cows. As competition per feeder increased, cows exhibited shorter average eating times and accelerated eating rates. Similarly, visits to the feeding station increased in direct proportion to greater aggression during feeding. However, feed intake was unchanged. In contrast, when cows were fed limited amounts of feed, dominant cows consumed 14% more feed than submissive cows. This divergence increased to 23% as competition increased from one to four cows per feeding station. Thus, under conditions of limited feed availability, competition escalates and feed intake of submissive cows suffers.

A major consideration when managing dairy cattle is the proper amount of feeding space allowed per animal to ensure that feeding behaviour is not affected adversely. When lactating dairy cows are fed at a feed bunk or manger, the critical length of bunk space per cow, below which excessive competition occurs, varies with the group size and amount and availability of feed. However, manger divisions that protect the head may allow submissive cows to eat longer, even in competitive situations (Bouissou, 1970). Several early reports established that little change occurred in feeding behaviour when bunk space was reduced from 0.61 to 0.31 m per cow (Albright, 1993). A reduction in bunk space from 0.49 to 0.09 m per cow to increase competition strengthened the correlation between dry matter intake and the dominance value of the individual cow. Albright (1993) postulated that a gradual reduction in bunk or manger space for an established group of cows may be better tolerated than adaptation of a new group to limited manger space.

The early research on feeding space and behaviour evaluated small groups of cows (50–60 or fewer) at low to moderate levels of milk production. Application of these results to modern dairies requires observations of larger groups of cows at

higher levels of milk production and feed intake. The traditional rule of thumb of 0.61 linear metres of bunk space per cow is the minimal amount of space required for all cows to eat at one time. However, the advent of TMR and proper feed bunk management raises questions regarding the adequacy of this relationship. Table 17.2 summarizes the relationship between feed bunk space and feeding activity as summarized from the scientific literature (Grant and Albright, 1997).

Menzi and Chase (1994) conducted a field study using two commercial dairy herds in New York state to examine feeding behaviour and bunk use for high-producing herds. Both herds were producing in excess of 10,600 kg of milk yearly, were milked three times daily, used 6-row drive-through free stall barns, and were fed a TMR two (Herd 1) or three (Herd 2) times daily, with 88–90 cows in each group. The groups of cows observed for each farm had the highest feed intake and milk production per cow, and therefore should have exerted the greatest feeding pressure on the bunk. Cows in these groups averaged 40 kg of milk day^{-1} with a dry matter intake of at least 24 kg day^{-1}. A video camera was mounted above and slightly behind the feeding area to provide the best view of feeding activity. Each herd was videotaped for a 24-h period during August when high temperatures were 27°C and low temperatures were near 16°C. Using the videotape, a feed bunk usage score was developed where 0 represented no animals at the feed bunk and 10 indicated that the bunk space was entirely occupied with no additional room for animals to eat. The feeding behaviour data from these two herds are shown in Fig. 17.1.

Table 17.2. Bunk space and feeding behaviour of lactating dairy cows[a].

Bunk space	Effect on dry matter intake
<0.20 m	Reduced eating time and dry matter intake
0.20–0.51 m	Increased competition with variable effect on dry matter intake
>0.51–0.61 m	No measurable effect on dry matter intake

[a]Data summarized from Albright (1993), Friend and Polan (1974), Friend *et al.* (1977), Manson and Appleby (1990) and Menzi and Chase (1994).

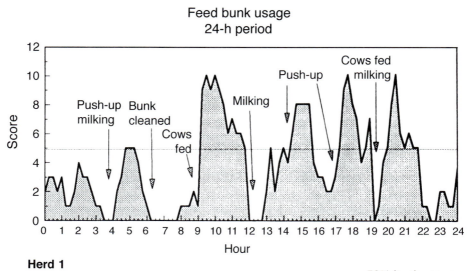

Herd 1

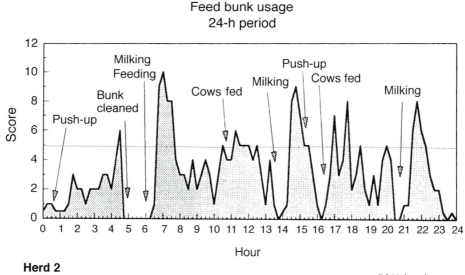

Herd 2

Fig. 17.1. Impact of management factors on feed bunk usage in two commercial dairy herds (adapted from Menzi and Chase, 1994).

Observations of other management activities are noted also in Fig. 17.1. These activities include milking, feeding, feed push-up and bunk cleaning. In these herds, cows increased bunk usage after feeding, when feed was pushed up, or when return-ing from the parlour. Feed bunk management that provided fresh feed throughout a 24-h period, within reach of the cows, promoted numerous, smaller meals throughout the day.

Accessibility of feed may be more important than the actual amount of nutrients provided, within reason (Albright, 1993; Grant and Albright, 1995). Cow space, cow density and distribution of feed and water facilities all influence feed intake. Feed intake generally will improve when cows are allowed access to feed when they want to eat, such as leaving the milking parlour. Feed restriction can occur under a number of conditions. Apart from simply providing inadequate amounts of feed daily, other common, but less obvious, causes include excessive time spent in holding areas, time spent in exercise lots without access to feed and water, unstable, highly fermented silage, poor ventilation, slippery floors, inadequate or poorly maintained free stalls, rough feeding mangers, and overcrowding that results in inadequate stall or bunk space (Grant and Albright, 1995).

Menzi and Chase (1994) concluded that 0.37–0.40 m of bunk space per cow did not necessarily restrict feed intake. Periods of full bunk use were few during a 24-h period. Herd 1 exhibited four periods when the feed bunk was fully occupied. These periods were brief, lasting only approximately 15 min. Herd 2 had only one brief point of restricted bunk space and two periods of nearly full utilization of feeding space. In both herds, peak feed bunk usage was typically followed by a rapid decline in feeding activity, particularly in Herd 2. Although current recommendations for linear feed bunk space are 0.61 m per cow, research results and on-farm observations of high-producing herds with large group sizes indicate that 0.21 m per cow is near the critical bunk space. One should consider, however, the difference between minimum bunk space that can be tolerated in existing facilities with excellent management and desired bunk space in newly designed facilities. Barns tend to become overcrowded with time, and underdesigning a barn with regard to bunk space may not be advisable. The actual optimal bunk space will be a function of feed availability throughout 24 h, relative to when cows want to eat, and the degree of crowding and competition placed on the cows by grouping strategy.

Future research must focus on the relationships among feeding management, bunk space and barn design with feeding behaviour and feed intake of higher milk-yielding dairy cattle.

Bunk space for dairy heifers

Much less is known about the need for feeding space and the feeding behaviour of dairy heifers at various ages and body sizes. Maintaining adequate growth of a group of heifers, and also of the individual heifers within a group, depends on the housing and feeding system, and their impact on comfort and feeding behaviour. To achieve growth rates that allow parturition at 24 months of age requires that bunk space should not limit feed intake. Previous recommendations were based on heifers with much slower rates of gain than currently desired. Beef cattle research indicates that an animal within a group is able to maintain adequate growth rate, or even exceed it, when allowed 0.15 and 0.13 m of feed bunk length per animal under conditions of restricted feed intake with daily gains of 1.45 and 1.07 kg day^{-1} (Gunter *et al.*, 1996).

Recent research (Longenbach *et al.*, 1997) evaluated the amount of feed bunk space required by dairy heifers at various ages grown at uniformly rapid rates of gain to achieve adequate size and body weight for parturition by 24 months of age. Three groups of heifers were defined by an average age of 4, 11.5 and 17 months. Bunk space of 0.15, 0.31 and 0.47 m per heifer was evaluated. Heifers were fed a TMR at restricted intakes to achieve an average daily gain of either 0.82 kg (4 and 11.5 months of age) or 0.91 kg day^{-1} (17 months of age). The authors concluded that, based on the observed feeding and growth responses for each group, the following feed bunk space recommendations are optimal for rapidly growing Holstein heifers being fed a TMR in either a free stall or loose housing system: 0.15 m for 4–8 months of age, 0.31 m for 11.5–15.5 months of age, and 0.47 m for 17–21 months of age.

Grouping Strategy, Competition and Feeding Behaviour

Behaviour of cows in a group represents the interaction of several driving forces. For newly commingled cows, aggression is dominant but, as soon as the social order is established, the feeding drive becomes dominant (Albright, 1993).

Group size and feeding behaviour of dairy cattle

Traditionally, dairy cows have been managed in relatively small groups (30–100 cows). Improvements in milking and feeding systems have allowed group sizes to increase up to 200 or more cows. It is unknown if a breakdown in the social structure of the herd occurs when groups of cows become too large. Traditional thinking has been that smaller groups help to reduce stress on cows, maintain social structure of the group, allow for better traffic patterns and increase effectiveness of feeding and breeding programmes (Grant and Albright, 1997). Even if social structure weakens with large groups, does it have a significant impact on cow behaviour, comfort and feed intake?

Social dominance is observed in cows when certain individuals initiate and win encounters. These encounters most frequently are head-to-head attacks (60%), followed by attack in the neck region (~10%), with attacks on the side or flank regions being least frequent (Albright, 1978). In a group of a size that allows adequate opportunity for social interaction, the dominance hierarchy can be so stable that a single day's observations can determine the order. French researchers in the 1970s (Bouissou, 1970) found that establishment of dominance–submissive relationships is extremely rapid; about half of the relationships were determined during the first hour. With 20 groups of four previously unacquainted heifers, establishment of dominance–submissive relationships took place without fighting and even without physical contact between animals,

although 35% of relationships were determined after a fight. Despite the rapidity of establishment of these dominance hierarchies, the relationships were very stable, and only approximately 4% of the relationships were reversed.

For group sizes larger than 100 cows, the ability to recognize all group mates may diminish. In larger groups, small subgroups may form, as in a poultry flock (Albright, 1978). Within a large group, however, cows should be given the opportunity to know one another. Some behaviourists have suggested that stress could arise due to failure to establish a stable dominance hierarchy. A question deserving further research is the relative importance, in groups of 100–200 or more cows, of subgroups versus interaction with the entire group. The relative importance may be a function of the living space allowed per group and the level of competition for feed, water, space or stalls.

To evaluate the effect of group size on dairy cattle behaviour, Albright (unpublished data, 1995; FASS, 1998) observed various group sizes of lactating dairy cattle ranging from small (50–99), to medium (100–150 and 150–199) to large (≥200) on commercial dairies in Arizona, New Mexico and Texas (Fig. 17.2). Cows within a group were scanned for feeding and other behavioural activities each hour. The overall observations of this research indicated that there is not a problem with variation in size of group *per se*. Rather, a number of daily management decisions, such as overcrowding with insufficient headlocks or inadequate manger space per cow, play a larger role in determining overall cow well-being. For example, with 120 headlocks and 150 cows trying to feed, there were 12 fights per min following feed delivery. An hour later there were eight fights per min. Irregular or infrequent feeding, and excessive walking to and from the milking parlour, also appeared to have a substantial negative impact on cow behaviour and overall well-being. Importantly, even with larger group sizes, typical behaviour patterns were observed for social facilitation, leadership–followship and congregating at the gate nearest to the milking parlour.

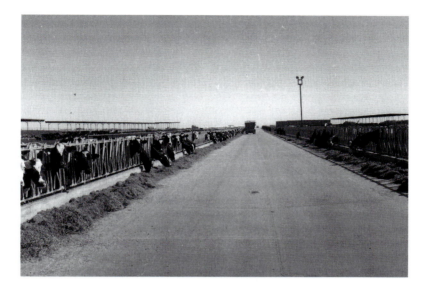

Fig. 17.2. Feeding activity in large group of dairy cows following delivery of fresh feed.

Grouping of primiparous cows

When practical, heifers within several weeks of parturition should be grouped separately and adapted to the early postpartum environment (Grant and Albright, 1995). Cows that undergo abrupt environmental and social changes during the periparturient period often exhibit aberrant feeding behaviour and are more susceptible to metabolic disorders (Grant and Albright, 1995).

Primiparous cows can benefit from separate grouping (Fig. 17.3). Phelps (1992) reported the response to grouping older dairy cows separately from younger, smaller primiparous cows. When separated, primiparous cows produced significantly more milk. Competition with older cows resulted in less feed intake and milk production for the primiparous animals. The difference in performance was proportional to the difference in body size between young and mature cows. Other research summarized by Grant and Albright (1997) showed that when heifers were separated from older cows, eating time increased by 11.4%, meals per day increased by 8.5%, silage dry matter intake increased by 11.8%, lying time increased by 8.8% and lying periods increased by 19% day^{-1}.

Due to constraints of limited cattle numbers and facilities at most research farms, very few data exist regarding the interaction between group size and feeding activity. Data from lambs, however, indicated that as the number of lambs per pen increased, feed consumption per visit to a feeding station increased linearly. However, total feed consumption was greatest for an intermediate number of lambs. One possible explanation for these observations could be that social facilitation increased feeding activity to a point, and then excessive competition resulted in a subsequent decline in feed intake. Similarly, some researchers have observed that beef cattle eat less when fed individually versus when group-fed, perhaps because of increased anxiety due to isolation and lack of social facilitation from group mates (Kidwell *et al.*, 1954).

Feeding Area Design and Feeding Behaviour

Facility design plays an important role in facilitating aggressive feeding behaviour. In

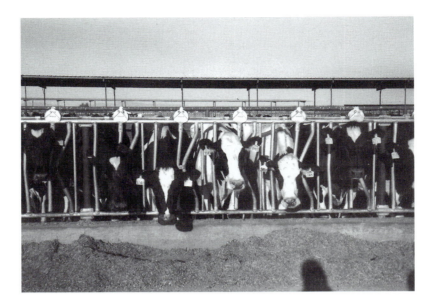

Fig. 17.3. Separate grouping of primiparous dairy cows results in greater feed intake.

field observations of ten dairy herds in Nebraska during the summer of 1997 (Grant and Albright, 1997), in most cases, farms with the highest dry matter intake and productivity had alleys of sufficient width so that two cows could walk comfortably in opposite directions behind the row of cows standing and eating at the feed line. With insufficient space, either from poor barn design or overcrowding a group of cows, normal movement of cows in the alley behind the feed manger disrupted eating activity, precipitated fights and interfered with intense, focused feeding activity. Many free stall barns designed today in the USA provide floor space of approximately 3.7–5.1 m² per cow, excluding free stall and drinking areas. The alley between the feeding line and the first row of free stalls should be at least 4.3 m wide to allow comfortable cow movement and avoid interference with aggressive, focused feeding activity.

Feed bunk or manger design

Many dairies use fenceline feeding systems in which cows eat with their heads in a natural grazing position. Evidence exists that cows eating with their heads in a downward position secrete 17% more saliva than cows eating with their heads held horizontally, which could result in better ruminal function (Albright, 1993).

Concrete mangers that have been renovated with epoxy finishes, wood or tiles aid feed consumption. Over time, lower pH silages can etch and pit concrete, which exposes the cow's tongue and mouth to rough and sharp edges.

Cows exhibit more rooting behaviour in shallow, elevated feed bunks or troughs. Albright (1993) observed lactating dairy cows once weekly for feed tossing behaviour when they were fed TMR. Approximately 10% of the cows observed participated in this behaviour. The amount of feed wasted was 0–5% each week. Feed tossing was especially prevalent in summer during heavy fly concentrations, but occurred in winter as well. When given the choice of eating from an elevated bunk with the floor either 28 or 76 cm from ground level, or from the same trough at ground level, cows chose the lower level. Also, the group fed at ground level exhibited no feed tossing behaviour. It appears that the optimally constructed feed bunk or manger is at a height that allows cows to consume feed in a natural grazing position. Although rare, feed tossing behaviour can still occur with cows in self-locking stanchions with their heads in the head down position (Fig. 17.4).

Data summarized by Albright (1993) indicated that the floor of the feed trough should be level or slope no more than 1% along the length of the feed bunk. When mangers have slopes of >3–5%, cows shift and move in the direction of the slope. This movement is continual and interferes with feeding activity.

Feed barrier design: restraint with headlocks

As part of a regional dairy management research project in the USA, scientists at Purdue University and Utah State University evaluated the effect of extended lock-up times on cow behaviour, well-being and productivity. Self-locking stanchions (headlocks) are used commonly in commercial dairies (Fig. 17.5) to restrain cattle for various management tasks such as: (i) artificial insemination; (ii) pregnancy checking; (iii) monitoring herd health; and (iv) top-dressing a supplement (Fig. 17.6). This system of restraining animals in the feeding area can be abused, and thus compromise cow comfort, when cows are allowed to remain in the headlocks beyond the period of time actually necessary for the management routine.

To investigate the effect of restraint using self-locking stanchions, 64 Holstein cows from peak to end of lactation were restrained in these stanchions for approximately 4 h day^{-1} for four periods in a modified switchback design (Bolinger *et al.*, 1997). Milk production, somatic cell count and total daily feed intake were unaffected by the restraint. Behaviourally, cows that were locked up spent significantly more time lying down after release from restraint. For cows that were locked in stanchions, eating frequency over 24 h was significantly reduced, but dry matter intake was not affected. Total rumination frequency

over 24 h was not affected, but restrained cows ruminated less during the following day. Grooming was significantly increased during all times that cows were not locked up, and was considered to be a behavioural need. Grooming was also one of the first behaviours performed following release. Acts of aggression were elevated during all periods following restraint. Although the proper use of self-locking stanchions for restraint does not seem substantially to affect the overall well-being of the cow, there appears to be some potential to impact feeding and ruminating behaviour adversely.

Feed barrier design: slope and pressure exerted during feeding

Feed barriers and mangers should provide free access to feed without risk of injury or discomfort. Feed mangers or barriers should also allow undisturbed feeding activity and minimize feed wastage. Additionally, cows can be restrained by some feed barriers such as self-locking stanchions. A relationship may exist between the layout of the feeding area, particularly feed barrier design, and the number of injuries for cattle. The barrier between the cows and their feed is often constructed in such a way that cows press hard against the barrier when attempting to reach their feed, thereby increasing the risk of injury or discomfort.

A well-designed feeding system should result in cows needing to exert the lowest pressure against the feeding barrier while consuming feed. Pressures of <500 N have no effect on the cow, pressures of 500–1000 N may cause harm, and pressures >1000 N may cause acute damage (Hansen and Pallesen, 1998). Hansen and Pallesen (1998) evaluated the effect of the pressure exerted by dairy cows on self-locking feeders on feeding activity and cow comfort. Measurements taken during both day and night showed that >80% of the pressure occurred within the first hour after feeding. Peaks in pressure applied to the feed barrier occurred when remaining

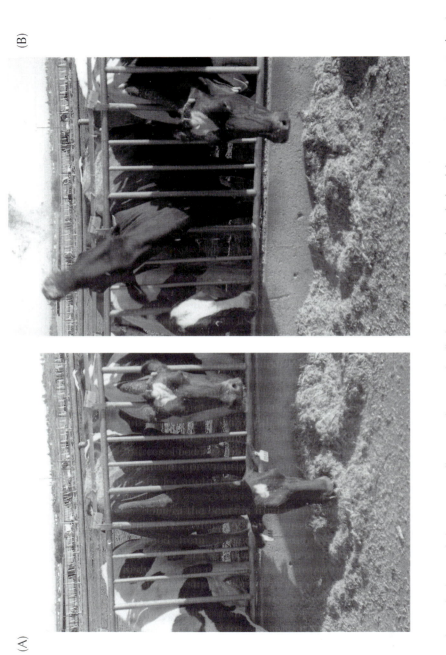

Fig. 17.4. Although rare, feed tossing behaviour can still occur with cows in headlocks and with their heads in the head down, grazing position. Feed tossing behaviour normally occurs in elevated feed bunks. Note the sequence of a cow taking a mouthful of feed (A) and tossing it over her head (B). Photographs from Albright (1997).

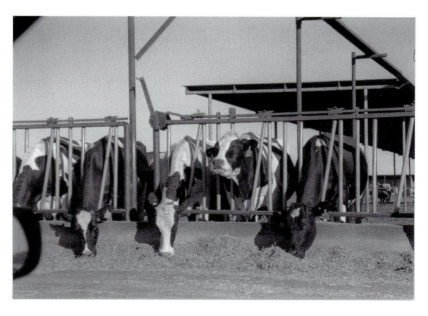

Fig. 17.5. Self-locking stanchions (headlocks) are used commonly on commercial dairy farms to restrain cattle for various management tasks.

feed in the manger was outside of the cow's reach. Almost no pressures >500 N were recorded during the first minutes of a meal, as the cow ate the feed within its reach. Pressure against the feed barrier gradually increased as the cow tried to consume the feed at the outer limits of its reach. Importantly, cows gave up trying to reach

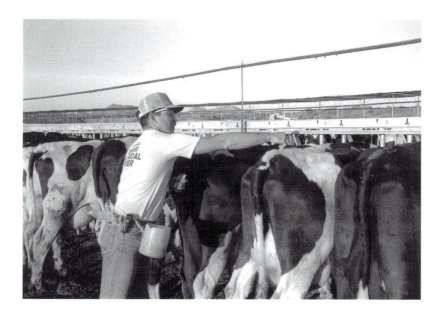

Fig. 17.6. Use of self-locking stanchions for cattle restraint during a herd management activity.

feed after about 14 min, and left the feed manger. This observation reinforces the importance of the observations of Menzi and Chase (1994) who noted a spike in feeding activity when feed was pushed up within easy reach of the cows.

When accumulated pressure distribution was analysed, the pressure on the feed barrier was >500 N for about 76 s, which could be harmful in the long term (Hansen and Pallesen, 1998). A pressure >1000 N lasted for 43 s, which can cause acute tissue trauma. The highest pressure was recorded when cows reached straight for the feed. The effect was more pronounced as manger width increased, and feed could be pushed more easily beyond the reach of the cows.

Hansen and Pallesen (1998) also evaluated the angle of the feed barrier, either vertical or with a 20° slope outward. The sloping feed barrier increased the cow's reach and reduced pressures exerted on the barrier by the cow. There was a 98.7% probability that pressure >500 N would be placed on the feed barrier when vertical versus tilted out at the 20° angle. This research indicated that cows willingly will place pressures of >2000 N against a feed barrier to reach as much feed as possible. At this amount of pressure, injury can easily occur, therefore feed should always be within reach of the cow (pushed up as needed). Mounting self-locking stanchions in a 20° sloped position increases the cow's reach by 0.14 m, with no increase in pressure, and enables a wider feeding area in front of the cow. Sloping a feed barrier can result in a maximum reach that is up to 25% greater than that obtained with a vertical feed barrier.

Palatability and Taste Preferences

Promoting feed intake is a critical element of most animal management systems. For example, in the early lactation dairy cow, any management factor that will stimulate dry matter intake can result in improved performance, body condition and health (Grant and Albright, 1995). Likewise, in the

feedlot, much of the management programme is directed toward controlling feed intake and avoiding situations in which the cattle 'go off feed' (Launchbaugh, 1995).

Palatability and dietary moisture content influence feed intake. Diets associated with maximum feed intake for lactating dairy cattle typically fall within the range of 50–85% dry matter. Research into the area of improving dietary palatability is warranted because of the tremendous need to promote feed intake in highly productive animals. Maximum feed intake is especially critical for the early lactation dairy cow, and the potential exists to enhance feed intake by exploiting preferences for various flavours and perhaps even odours.

Taste preferences and palatability

Exploiting cow preferences for various flavour additives may enhance feeding behaviour during the early lactation, transitional period in dairy cattle. Dairy cattle possess a sense of taste that can change with the diet (Albright, 1993). For example, cows eating silages have reduced sensitivity to sour taste and enhanced sensitivity to sweet taste (Albright, 1993). An experiment conducted at the University of Illinois evaluated dietary flavour additives for the early lactation dairy cow (Nombekela et al., 1994). These researchers tested the effects of various additives on preference ranking of TMR fed twice daily beginning 8 days post-partum. In one trial, taste preference ranking was sweet (sucrose at 15 g kg^{-1} DM) > control > bitter (urea at 10 g kg^{-1}) > salt (NaCl at 40 g kg^{-1}) > sour (HCl at 12.5 g kg^{-1}). Cows consumed 12.8% more dry matter for sweet than for the second place (control) diet. In trial 2, monosodium glutamate was preferred equally to a control diet > molasses > dehydrated lucerne > anise.

More recently, the same research group (Murphy et al., 1997) has examined the effect of dietary variety via sweetening on feed intake. Diets were: (i) a control TMR consisting of lucerne haylage, maize silage, and a maize and soybean meal concentrate; and (ii) a sweetened TMR in which a brown sugar food product constituted 1.5% of the dietary dry matter. The treatments were arranged as follows: (i) control TMR fed on both sides of a divided feed bunk; (ii) sweetened TMR fed on both sides of a divided feed bunk; and (iii) both rations fed on alternating (daily) sides of divided feed bunks in tie stalls. The observation periods were 2 weeks in duration. A choice of control or sweetened ration did not affect feed intake. However, the authors noted that the outcome of their experiment might have been affected by the composition of the control ration, its similarity to the sweetened ration, availability of both diets simultaneously when a choice was offered and use of a TMR rather than separate feeds or even simpler mixtures of feed ingredients. Another experiment in the same laboratory (Nombekela and Murphy, 1995) indicated a transient increase in consumption of a sucrose-supplemented diet during the first 2 weeks after parturition.

The acceptability of traditionally unpalatable feeds, such as animal protein by-products, has been improved by treatment with sugars. For example, non-enzymatically browning of meat and bone meal with xylose solutions has significantly increased feed intake in lactating Holstein dairy cows (Allen *et al.*, 1997). Twenty cows housed in a tie stall barn were allowed access to two individual feed containers of equal size and accessibility for each cow. Naive cows were allowed access for 30 min to 4.5 kg of two grain mixes, each containing 250 g kg^{-1} treated or untreated meat and bone meal, top-dressed onto a basal ration. Cows consumed 16% more of the grain mix containing the treated meat and bone meal on day 1, but nearly 62% more by day 8. Feed intake of the basal ration increased by 12.2% when the treated product was top-dressed versus the untreated product. The xylose-treated meat and bone meal was substantially more acceptable and resulted in greater feed intake when contained in a top-dressed supplement.

Olfaction and feed preference

When flavours are used to manipulate the senses of cattle, the intensity of the flavour is a function not only of taste, but also of olfaction. Olfaction and taste function together to create a given perception of a food (Arnold *et al.*, 1980). These two senses detect and then quantify chemosensory stimuli in feed and provide the information on which eating decisions are based. The sense of smell determines the presence of volatile substances, whereas taste detects sweet, sour, salty or bitter compounds in a feed ingredient. There is evidence that dietary preference and total feed intake are altered in bulbectomized and anosmic cats and poultry (Snapir and Robinzon, 1989). To date, little information is available concerning olfaction and feed preference in cattle due in large part to the lack of a good technique that can separate the effects of taste and olfaction.

Neophobia

Cattle associate sensory information about harmful phytochemicals (such as poisonous plants) with appropriate behaviour through instinct, learning as an individual, learning as part of a social group or combinations of these behaviours (Albright, 1993). Ruminants almost always sample only a small amount of a new feed when it is first offered. This cautious sampling, or even complete rejection of new feeds, is termed neophobia or 'fear of the unknown or new'. Neophobia, and not unpalatability, is the primary factor influencing feeding behaviour by naive or inexperienced herbivores (Launchbaugh, 1995). Neophobia typically is displayed as a period of low or rapidly accelerating feed intake prior to a stable maximum feed intake level. This behaviour pattern is innate and typically is exhibited when feedlot diets are first offered to animals even though the feeds are not inherently toxic (Launchbaugh, 1995). Neophobia tends to be more pronounced in experienced adult animals, individual animals not part of a social

group and animals with a prior history of ill-
ness following ingestion of novel feeds. The
effect of flavour enhancers on feed-related
neophobia is unclear; certainly no feed or
flavour has been discovered that is instantly
acceptable to all ruminants, except possibly
mother's milk (Launchbaugh, 1995).

Heat Stress and Feeding Behaviour

In addition to feeding management and
strategy, the environment can affect cow
comfort and feeding behaviour. Environmental   factors   include   temperature,
humidity, air movement and solar radiation.
Temperature is one of the primary factors
affecting the physiological requirements and
meal patterns of the dairy cow. Thermal
stress has decreased feed intake by 3–4 kg
day^{-1} in mid-lactation dairy cows (Grant
and Albright, 1995). Heat stress may slow
the rate of increase in dry matter intake post-
partum and exaggerate the pre-partum
decline in dry matter intake in dairy cows
(Grant and Albright, 1995).

Shaded cows in loose housing had
higher feed intake than cows without

shading (Fig. 17.7). Shaded and non-
shaded cows had greater eating activity at
night during conditions of heat stress.
Shading feed bunks located in outside lots
during heat stress conditions increased
feeding activity of periparturient cows by
63% versus unshaded feed bunk areas
during daylight hours (Grant and Albright,
1995).

Conclusions

Feeding   is   usually   the   predominant
behaviour in ruminants; rumination can
take precedence only when it has been
restricted abnormally. Dairy cattle consume
feed efficiently whether at a feed bunk or
grazing. However, the grouping strategy,
feeding system design and apparatus, and
attributes of the feed itself may all impact
the cow's ability to express aggressive
eating behaviour. Key components in determining feeding behaviour are the social
hierarchy, competition for feed, water,
space and feed availability within a group
of cattle. In fact, feed accessibility may be
the most important factor affecting an

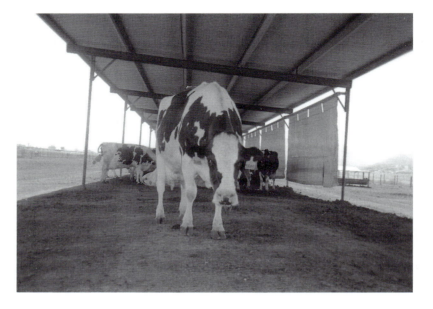

Fig. 17.7. Use of shading to reduce heat stress results in greater feed intake by lactating dairy cattle.

animal's ability to maximize feed intake. Feed should be available when cows desire to eat, e.g. at sunrise or after milking. Adequate bunk or manger space for adult and growing cattle helps to ensure that feeding behaviour and total feed intake are optimized.

Feeding behaviour has a tremendous impact on dry matter intake. Feeding behaviour and dry matter intake are controlled by gut fill and chemostatic mechanisms and modulated by feeding management and factors such as environment, health and social interactions. These factors that modulate feeding behaviour and intake can be optimized to promote intense feeding behaviour and maximum feed intake in dairy cattle.

References

Albright, J.L. (1978) Social considerations in grouping cows. In: Wilcox, C.J. and Van Horn, H.H. (eds) *Large Dairy Herd Management*. University Presses of Florida, Gainesville, Florida, pp. 757–779.

Albright, J.L. (1981) Behavior and management of high yielding dairy cows. *Dairy Science Handbook* 58, 217–230.

Albright, J.L. (1993) Feeding behavior in dairy cattle. *Journal of Dairy Science* 76, 485–498.

Albright, J.L. (1997) Feeding behaviour. In: Albright, J.L. and Arave, C.W. (eds) *The Behaviour of Cattle*. CAB International, Wallingford, UK, pp. 100–126.

Allen, D.M., Grant, R.J. and Kirstein, D. (1997) Impact of sulfite liquor-treatment of meat and bone meal on acceptability and dry matter intake by lactating dairy cows. *Journal of Dairy Science* 80 (Suppl. 1), 261.

Arnold, G.W., deBoer, E.S. and Boundy, C.A.P. (1980) The influence of odour and taste on the food preferences and food intake of sheep. *Australian Journal of Agricultural Research* 31, 571–587.

Bigelow, J.A. and Houpt, T.R. (1988) Feeding and drinking patterns in young pigs. *Physiology of Behavior* 43, 99–106.

Bolinger, D.J., Albright, J.L., Morrow-Tesch, J., Kenyon, S.J. and Cunningham, M.D. (1997) The effects of restraint using self-locking stanchions on dairy cows in relation to behavior, feed intake, physiological parameters, health, and milk yield. *Journal of Dairy Science* 80, 2411–2417.

Bouissou, M.F. (1970) Role du contact physique dans la manifestation des relations hierarchiques chez les bovins. Consequences pratiques. *Annals Zootechnica (Paris)* 19, 279–285.

Dado, R.G. and Allen, M.S. (1993) Continuous computer acquisition of feed and water intakes, chewing, reticular motility, and ruminal pH of cattle. *Journal of Dairy Science* 76, 1589–1600.

Dado, R.G. and Allen, M.S. (1994) Variation in and relationships among feeding, chewing, and drinking variables for lactating dairy cows. *Journal of Dairy Science* 77, 132–144.

deHaer, L.C.M. and Merks, J.W.M. (1992) Patterns of daily food intake in growing pigs. *Animal Production* 54, 95–104.

Ermer, P.M., Miller, P.S. and Lewis, A.J. (1994) Diet preference and meal patterns of weanling pigs offered diets containing either spray-dried porcine plasma or dried skim milk. *Journal of Animal Science* 72, 1548–1554.

FASS (Federation of Animal Science Societies) (1998) Guidelines for dairy cattle husbandry. In: Albright, J.L., Bickhert, W.G., Blauwiekel, R., Morrill, J.L., Olsen, K.E. and Stull, C.L. (eds) *Guide for the Care and Use of Agricultural Animals in Agricultural Research and Teaching*. 1st Revised edn. FASS Headquarters, Savoy, Illinois, pp. 37–46.

Forbes, J.M. (1995) Feeding behaviour. In: Forbes, J.M. (ed.) *Voluntary Food Intake and Diet Selection in Farm Animals*. CAB International, Wallingford, UK, pp. 11–37.

Friend, T.H. and Polan, C.E. (1974) Social rank, feeding behavior, and free stall utilization by dairy cattle. *Journal of Dairy Science* 57, 1214–1222.

Friend, T.H., Polan, C.E. and McGilliard, M.L. (1977) Free stall and feed bunk requirements relative to behavior, production and individual feed intake in dairy cows. *Journal of Dairy Science* 60, 108–118.

Grant, R.J. and Albright, J.L. (1995) Feeding behavior and management factors during the transition period in dairy cattle. *Journal of Animal Science* 73, 2791–2803.

Grant, R.J. and Albright, J.L. (1997) Dry matter intake as affected by cow groupings and behavior. In: *Proceedings of the 58th Minnesota Nutrition Conference*. University of Minnesota, Bloomington, Minnesota, pp. 93–103.

Gunter, S.A., Galyean, M.L. and Malcolm-Callis, K.J. (1996) Factors influencing the performance of feedlot steers limit-fed high-concentrate diets. *The Professional Animal Scientist* 12, 167–175.

Hansen, K. and Pallesen, C.N. (1998) Dairy cow pressure on self-locking feed barriers. In: Chastain, J.P. (ed.) *Proceedings of the Fourth International Dairy Housing Conference*. American Society of Agricultural Engineers, St Louis, Missouri, pp. 312–319.

Hicks, R.B., Owen, F.N. and Gill, D.R. (1989) Behavioral patterns of feedlot steers. *Oklahoma Agricultural Experiment Station MP 127*. Stillwater, Oklahoma, pp. 94–96.

Kertz, A.F., Reutzel, L.F. and Thomas, G.R. (1991) Dry matter intake from parturition to midlactation. *Journal of Dairy Science* 74, 2290–2295.

Kidwell, J.F., Bohman, V.R. and Hunter, J.E. (1954) Individual and group feeding of experimental beef cattle as influenced by hay maturity. *Journal of Animal Science* 13, 543–549.

Launchbaugh, K.L. (1995) Effects of neophobia and aversions on feed intake: why feedlot cattle sometimes refuse to eat nutritious feeds. In: *Symposium: Intake by Feedlot Cattle*. Oklahoma State University, Stillwater, Oklahoma, pp. 36–48.

Longenbach, J.I., Heinrichs, A.J. and Graves, R.E. (1997) Feed bunk space requirements for rapid rates of growth and performance of the dairy heifer. *Journal of Dairy Science* 80 (Suppl. 1), 202.

Manson, F.J. and Appleby, M.C. (1990) Spacing of dairy cows at a food trough. *Applied Animal Behavior Science* 26, 69–74.

Menzi, W. and Chase, L.E. (1994) Feeding behavior of cows housed in free stall barns. In: *Dairy Systems for the 21st Century*. American Society of Agricultural Engineers, St Joseph, Michigan, pp. 829–832.

Metz, J.H.M. (1975) Time patterns of feeding and rumination in domestic cattle. PhD dissertation, University of Wageningen, The Netherlands.

Murphy, M.R. (1992) Water metabolism of dairy cattle. *Journal of Dairy Science* 75, 326–333.

Murphy, M.R., Geijsel, A.W.P., Hall, E.C. and Shanks, R.D. (1997) Dietary variety via sweetening and voluntary feed intake of lactating dairy cows. *Journal of Dairy Science* 80, 894–897.

Nombekela, S.W. and Murphy, M.R. (1995) Sucrose supplementation and feed intake of dairy cows in early lactation. *Journal of Dairy Science* 78, 880–885.

Nombekela, S.W., Murphy, M.R., Gonyou, H.W. and Marden, J.I. (1994) Dietary preferences in early lactation as affected by tastes and some common feed flavors. *Journal of Dairy Science* 77, 2393–2399.

Olofsson, J. (1994) Competition for feed in loose housing systems. In: *Dairy Systems for the 21st Century*. American Society of Agricultural Engineers, St Joseph, Michigan, pp. 825–828.

Phelps, A. (1992) Vastly superior first lactations when heifers feed separately. *Feedstuffs* 11, 11–13.

Snapir, N. and Robinzon, B. (1989) Role of the basomedial hypothalamus in regulation of adiposity, food intake, and reproductive traits in the domestic fowl. *Poultry Science* 68, 948–957.

Chapter 18
Anti-nutritional Factors and Mycotoxins

J.P.F. D'Mello

Biotechnology Department,
The Scottish Agricultural College, Edinburgh, UK

Introduction

The secondary metabolism of plants and fungi results in the production of a diverse array of compounds with the capacity to induce anti-nutritional or toxic effects in farm animals. In addition, some products of primary metabolism of plants may also be associated with adverse effects in these animals. The term 'anti-nutritional factor' conventionally is reserved for those substances which reduce nutrient utilization or feed intake in animals. In practice, a wider definition is often adopted to include compounds causing anti-physiological effects such as impaired reproductive function or reduced immunocompetence. Additionally, manifestations of toxicity may accompany these anti-nutritional and anti-physiological effects. Furthermore, cereal plants, legumes and grasses may become infected with fungi during crop development or during storage of harvested or processed grain. Many of these fungi have the potential to synthesize toxic secondary metabolites known as mycotoxins. Although anti-nutritional factors and mycotoxins conventionally are considered to be distinct groups of compounds by virtue of their different

biological origins, there are many parallel features. Thus amino acids are common precursors for certain compounds in both groups. Furthermore, some anti-nutritional factors (ANFs) share common chemistry with mycotoxins, while other ANFs and mycotoxins induce similar deleterious responses in animals, precipitating effects on rumen function, feed intake, reproduction and immunocompetence.

Anti-nutritional Factors

Table 18.1 provides a list of the major ANFs which may occur in different plant species. The table is not designed to be exhaustive but illustrative of the diversity of compounds with anti-nutritional activity. These substances may be divided into two primary categories: a heat-labile group, comprising lectins, proteinase inhibitors and cyanogens which are sensitive to standard processing temperatures, and a heat-stable group including, among many others, antigenic proteins, condensed tannins, quinolizidine alkaloids, glucosinolates, the non-protein amino acids *S*-methylcysteine sulphoxide and mimosine, and phyto-oestrogens. A

Table 18.1. Diversity of anti-nutritional factors in plants.

Plant type	Plant species	Major anti-nutritional factors
Forage		
Legumes	*Medicago* spp.	Phyto-oestrogens
		Saponins
	Trifolium spp.	Phyto-oestrogens
	Lotus spp.	Condensed tannins
Grasses	*Brachiaria decumbens*	Saponins
	Panicum spp.	Saponins
Cruciferae	*Brassica* spp.	Glucosinolates
		S-methylcysteine sulphoxide
		Erucic acid
Browse		
Legumes	*Acacia* spp.	Condensed tannins
		Cyanogens
	Leucaena leucocephala	Mimosine
		Condensed tannins
Pine	*Pinus ponderosa*	Vasoactive lipids
Grain		
Legumes	*Glycine max*	Proteinase inhibitors
		Antigenic proteins
		Lectins
		Phyto-oestrogens
		Saponins
	Lupinus spp.	Quinolizidine alkaloids
		Saponins

number of the above compounds together with others such as saponins, vasoactive lipids, gossypol and cyanogens are associated with anti-physiological and toxic effects. It is generally accepted that the diversity and severity of adverse effects of ANFs are greater in tropical than in temperate legumes (Kumar and D'Mello, 1995).

Studies are continuing on virtually all aspects of the compounds listed in Table 18.1 and, as they do, newer concepts have evolved. Thus the adverse effects of soybeans (*Glycine max*) have long been associated with their content of proteinase inhibitors (Norton, 1991). However, recent data point to a significant role for antigenic proteins in the aetiology of post-weaning hypersensitivity reactions of piglets and calves fed on diets based on heated soybean products. Proteins with anti-nutritional activity have been the subject of considerable research at the fundamental level and in feeding trials, particularly with non- and pre-ruminant animals. Attention has focused on the anti-nutritional proteins

of soybeans. However, these proteins, in the form of lectins, proteinase inhibitors and specific antigens, are widely distributed and contribute significantly to the poor nutritional value of seeds from diverse tropical and temperate legume species (D'Mello, 1995). The condensed tannins, quinolizidine alkaloids, glucosinolates, non-protein amino acids, phyto-oestrogens, saponins and cyanogens are also ubiquitous, occurring in both grain and forage plants.

Lectins

Lectins are proteins with a characteristic affinity for certain sugar molecules or glycoproteins present in the membranes of different animal cells, including those of the intestinal mucosa. Lectins also react by this mechanism with red blood cells *in vitro*, causing agglutination. This reaction is used to recognize and detect lectins in raw materials. The alternative term, haemagglutinin, is thus often used to denote lectin activity. In contrast to most dietary proteins, lectins resist proteolytic degradation *in vivo,* and thus substantial quantities of ingested lectins may be recovered intact from the digestive tract and faeces of animals fed diets containing one of a number of legume seeds (D'Mello, 1995). The prime example of a lectin with potent anti-nutritional and toxic properties is concanavalin A, a component of the jack bean (*Canavalia ensiformis*). This lectin is composed of four identical subunits each containing two metal-binding sites and an additional site for a sugar residue. Due to its particular sugar specificity, concanavalin A binds mainly to the lower regions of the intestinal villi where membrane proteins of the less differentiated crypt cells have predominantly polymannose-type side chains. The lectin of the winged bean (*Psophocarpus tetragonolobus*), on the other hand, with its requirement for more complex sugar structures, binds largely to the upper part of the villi. Despite these differences, both lectin types confer profound anti-nutritional properties to diets containing raw jack beans and winged beans (D'Mello, 1995).

Proteinase inhibitors

The proteinase inhibitors are typical examples of heat-labile ANFs. They constitute a unique class of proteins with the ability to react in a highly specific manner with a number of proteolytic enzymes in the digestive secretions of animals. The proteinase inhibitors of soybeans are now well characterized, and the complete amino acid sequence of two of these (Kunitz and Bowman–Birk inhibitors) have been elucidated (Norton, 1991). They exert their effects in a strictly competitive manner and the complex formed between inhibitor and enzyme is devoid of catalytic activity. Proteinase inhibitors are widely distributed in the plant kingdom, particularly in leguminous seeds such as soybean, field beans (*Vicia faba*), winged beans, pigeon pea (*Cajanus cajan*) and cow pea (*Vigna unguiculata*).

Antigenic proteins

There is now unequivocal evidence that certain storage proteins of legume seeds are capable of crossing the epithelial barrier of the intestinal mucosa to elicit adverse effects on immune function in farm animals. In the case of the soybean, the antigenic proteins have been identified as glycinin and conglycinin. The latter is subdivided further into α, β and γ isotypes, with the β component representing the predominating protein. The antigenic proteins are characterized by their resistance to denaturation by conventional thermal processing procedures and to digestive attack in the alimentary canal of mammals.

Condensed tannins

Tannins belong to a class of compounds with a molecular weight in excess of 500 Da with a sufficiently large number of phenolic hydroxyl groups to form cross-linkages with proteins and other macro-molecules. Condensed tannins (CTs) are a subset of this group, being dimers or higher oligomers of variously substituted flavan-3-ols (Griffiths, 1991). It is widely accepted that CTs are the most abundant type of tannins in economically important plants, occurring in leguminous seeds and forages and certain cereal grains, particularly sorghum (*Sorghum bicolor*). On heating with strong acids, CTs polymerize further to yield small quantities of anthocyanidins, giving rise to the term 'proanthocyanidins' as an alternative generic name for CTs.

Quinolizidine alkaloids

The alkaloids of lupins (*Lupinus* spp.) are commonly bicyclic, tricyclic or tetracyclic derivatives of quinolizidine (Petterson *et al.,* 1991). The bicyclic alkaloids are exemplified by lupinine, the tricyclics by angustifoline and the tetracyclics by sparteine. In addition, lupanine, a derivative of sparteine, as well as hydroxylated compounds of lupanine occur regularly in most lupin species.

Glucosinolates

Glucosinolates are thioglucosides which are of particular significance in brassica vegetables and forage crops. Over 100 different glucosinolates have been identified and characterized (Duncan, 1991). They all share a common structure, being composed of a thioglucose group attached to an R-group. A wide range of R-groups has been identified. Removal of glucose from the glucosinolates by plant or microbial thioglucosidase (myrosinase) results in the release of a diverse array of aglycone moieties. The aglycone residues undergo further degradation to yield a number of toxic metabolites. The most common breakdown products are isothiocyanates and nitriles but, depending upon conditions such as pH, temperature and metallic ion concentrations, a number of other metabolites may also be produced.

Amino acids

In addition to the glucosinolates, forage and root brassica crops contain a non-protein amino acid in the form of S-methylcysteine sulphoxide (SMCO). Its structural resemblance with the indispensable amino acid, methionine, has been alluded to by D'Mello (1991a). The aromatic non-protein amino acid, mimosine, occurs in the foliage and seeds of the tropical legume ipil ipil or koa haole, commonly referred to as *Leucaena leucocephala*. Mimosine is widely regarded as an analogue of the physiologically important amino acid, tyrosine, and its neurotransmitter derivatives, dopamine and norepinephrine, found in the brain (D'Mello, 1994).

Phyto-oestrogens

The phyto-oestrogens are a diverse group of isoflavonoid compounds found primarily in legumes (Whitten *et al.*, 1997). Isoflavonoids have been classified into seven groups based on structural features including: isoflavone, isoflavan, isoflavanone, coumestan, pterocarpan, rotenoid and coumaronochromone (Whitten *et al.*, 1997). It is well recognized that soybeans contain relatively high concentrations of the glycosides of the isoflavones, daidzein, genistein and glycitein. In subterranean clover (*Trifolium subterraneum*) and in red clover (*T. pratense*), an important isoflavone is formononetin (Adams, 1995).

Other plant secondary compounds

A diverse array of other plant secondary metabolites have been associated with specific toxic effects in farm animals. These include steroidal saponins which occur as glycosides in certain pasture plants (e.g. *Brachiaria decumbens* and *Panicum* spp.), vasoactive lipids of western yellow pine (*Pinus ponderosa*), gossypol pigments of the cotton plant (*Gossypium* spp.) and HCN present as glycosides in a wide range of plants such as linseed (*Linum usitatissimum*), cassava (*Manihot esculenta*) and sorghum (*Sorghum* spp.).

Mycotoxins

The major toxigenic species of fungi and their respective toxic metabolites are presented in Table 18.2. These metabolites are known as mycotoxins, while the deleterious effects they precipitate are referred to as mycotoxicosis. The synthesis of a particular mycotoxin generally is restricted to a relatively small number of fungal species and may be species- or even strain-specific. A significant feature now emerging is the co-production of two or more mycotoxins by the same species of fungus which offers a different perspective to the interpretation of well-known cases of mycotoxicoses.

Aflatoxins

Over the past 30 years or so, attention has focused predominantly on the aflatoxins

Table 18.2. Toxigenic species of fungi and their principal mycotoxins.

Fungal species	Mycotoxins
Aspergillus flavus; A. parasiticus	Aflatoxins
A. flavus	Cyclopiazonic acid
A. ochraceus; Penicillium viridicatum; P. cyclopium	Ochratoxin A
P. citrinum; P. expansum	Citrinin
P. expansum	Patulin
P. citreo-viride	Citreoviridin
Fusarium culmorum; F. graminearum	Deoxynivalenol
F. sporotrichioides; F. poae	T-2 toxin
F. sporotrichioides; F. poae	Diacetoxyscirpenol
F. culmorum; F. graminearum; F. sporotrichioides	Zearalenone
F. moniliforme	Fumonisins; moniliformin; fusaric acid
Alternaria alternata	Tenuazonic acid; alternariol; alternariol methyl ether; altenuene
Acremonium coenophialum	Ergopeptine alkaloids
A. lolii	Lolitrem alkaloids
Claviceps purpurea	Ergot alkaloids
Phomopsis leptostromiformis	Phomopsins
Pithomyces chartarum	Sporidesmin A

produced by certain strains of *Aspergillus flavus* and *A. parasiticus* (Smith, 1997). The aflatoxins are a group of structurally related fluorescent heterocyclic compounds characterized by dihydrofuran or tetra-hydrofuran residues fused to a substituted coumarin moiety. This group comprises aflatoxin B_1, B_2, G_1 and G_2 (designated AFB_1, AFB_2, AFG_1 and AFG_2, respectively). In addition, aflatoxin M_1 has been identified in the milk of dairy cows consuming AFB_1-contaminated feeds. The aflatoxigenic *Aspergilli* are generally regarded as storage fungi, proliferating under conditions of relatively high moisture/humidity and temperature. Aflatoxin contamination is, therefore, almost exclusively confined to tropical feeds such as oilseed by-products derived from groundnuts (*Arachis hypogaea*), cottonseed and palm kernel. Aflatoxin contamination of maize is also a significant issue in warm humid regions where *A. flavus* may infect the crop prior to harvest and remain viable during storage.

Ochratoxins

Another species of *Aspergillus* (*A. ochraceus*) produces a different group of mycotoxins, represented by the ochratoxins, a property it shares with at least two species of *Penicillium* (Abramson, 1997). The ochratoxins are a family of structurally related compounds based on an iso-coumarin molecule linked to phenylalanine. Ochratoxin A (OA) and ochratoxin B are the only two forms to occur naturally as contaminants, with OA being the more ubiquitous, occurring predominantly in temperate cereals and in the tissues of animals fed on these grains.

Fusarium *mycotoxins*

Extensive data now exist to indicate the global scale of contamination of cereal grains and animal feed with *Fusarium* mycotoxins (D'Mello *et al.*, 1997). Of particular importance are the trichothecenes, zearalenone (ZEN) and the fumonisins. The trichothecenes are subdivided into four basic groups, with types A and B representing the most important members. Type A trichothecenes include T-2 toxin, HT-2 toxin, neosolaniol and diacetoxyscirpenol (DAS). Type B trichothecenes include deoxynivalenol (DON, also known as vomitoxin), nivalenol and fusarenon-X. All trichothecenes possess a basic tetracyclic sesquiterpene structure with a six-membered oxygen-containing ring and an epoxide group. The synthesis of the two types of mycotoxins is characteristic for a particular *Fusarium* species. However, a common feature of the secondary metabolism of these fungi is their ability to synthesize ZEN, a phenolic resorcyclic lactone which occurs as a co-contaminant with certain trichothecenes. The fumonisins are synthesized by another distinct group of *Fusarium* species. These mycotoxins are long-chain polyhydroxyl alkylamines containing two propane tricarballylic acid moieties attached to two adjacent carbon atoms. Three members of this group (fumonisin B_1, B_2 and B_3) may occur together in maize.

Endophyte alkaloids

The endophytic fungus *Acremonium coenophialum* occurs in close association with perennial tall fescue, while another related fungus, *A. lolii*, may be present in perennial ryegrass (Porter, 1997). The fungi provide the grass with defensive secondary compounds while the plant serves as a source of essential nutrients for the fungus. These secondary metabolites are also toxigenic towards animals. Ergopeptine alkaloids, mainly ergovaline, occur in *A. coenophialum*-infected tall fescue, while the indole isoprenoid lolitrem alkaloids, particularly lolitrem B, are found in *A. lolii*-infected perennial ryegrass.

Phomopsins

In Australia, lupin stubble is valued as fodder for sheep, but infection with the fungus *Phomopsis leptostromiformis* is a major limiting factor due to toxicity arising from the production of phomopsins by the fungus. Mature or senescing parts of the plant, including stems, pods and seeds, are particularly prone to infection. Of these mycotoxins, phomopsin A is considered to be the primary toxic agent. Phomopsin A is

a hexapeptide with the sequence Phe-Val-Ile-Pro-Ile-Asp, modified by oxidation, chlorination and methylation.

Sporidesmin

Pithomyces chartarum is an ubiquitous saprophyte of pastures with the capacity to synthesize sporidesmin A which represents an important group of diketopiperazine derivatives arising from the formation of a cyclic anhydride between two amino acids. A sulphur-containing ring imparts biological activity to the molecule (Flaoyen and Froslie, 1997).

Metabolism

Many ANFs and mycotoxins are metabolized in the digestive system and in the tissues of animals, resulting in detoxification or in promotion of adverse effects. A number of instances have been selected here to illustrate the diversity of metabolism and consequences for farm animal productivity.

Amino acids

The toxicity of SMCO in cattle and sheep arises after its fermentation by rumen bacteria to dimethyl disulphide oxide which is then reduced to dimethyl disulphide. It is the latter metabolite which precipitates the typical symptoms of haemolytic or kale anaemia in ruminants (D'Mello, 1994). On the other hand, metabolism of mimosine by ruminants depends upon geographical differences in rumen microbial ecology. During this metabolism, 3-hydroxy-4(1H)-pyridone (3,4-DHP) is synthesized; this itself is endowed with deleterious properties, but in addition another isomer, 2,3-DHP may be produced in the rumen. Some rumen bacteria are capable of detoxifying both forms of DHP to as yet unidentified compounds (D'Mello, 1991a). Despite these reactions, considerable quantities of mimosine and 3,4-DHP may escape metabolism to appear in the faeces. Furthermore, conjugated forms of DHP may also appear in the faeces and urine, while mimosine may itself undergo decarboxylation within the tissues of the ruminant to yield mimosinamine which is then excreted in the urine. Ruminants in Australia, the USA and Kenya are known to lack the requisite bacteria involved in the detoxification of the two DHP isomers. In other regions where *Leucaena* is indigenous (Central America) or is naturalized (Hawaii and Indonesia), ruminants possess the full complement of bacteria required for DHP degradation, which accounts for the absence of *Leucaena* toxicity in these countries.

Phyto-oestrogens

Phyto-oestrogens are actively metabolized in the rumen with the result that activity of these substances in the plant depends upon the extent of microbial transformations in the rumen (Adams, 1995). Genistein, for example, is degraded to non-oestrogenic compounds. Formononetin, however, is demethylated and reduced to the more oestrogenic compound, equol. Rumen microbes may require up to 10 days to adapt to phyto-oestrogens, so genistein may initially evoke oestrogenic effects.

Aflatoxins

The aflatoxins are actively metabolized in the rumen and in the tissues of animals, with serious implications for human health (Smith, 1997). In dairy animals, ruminal transformation of AFB_1 to AFM_1 results in the latter being secreted in the milk. AFM_1 has been ascribed with carcinogenic properties. Carcinogenicity of AFB_1, however, is greater, arising from the formation of a reactive epoxide which then permits covalent binding to cellular components such as DNA to yield genotoxic adducts.

Zearalenone

The ovine metabolism of ZEN has been proposed to involve the synthesis of at least five metabolites including zearalanone, α-zearalenol, β-zearalenol, α-zearalanol and β-zearalanol (Miles *et al.*, 1996). It should be noted that α-zearalanol is used as a growth promoter with the name zeranol. High levels of some of these forms may be excreted in the urine as glucuronides by grazing sheep.

Toxicology

Acute toxicity

The classical assessment of toxicity of any compound generally centres on consideration of LD_{50} data. In the case of ANFs, such indicators of acute toxicity are of limited practical relevance in field cases of toxicity (Table 18.3). This is not to imply that ANFs do not induce lethality. Thus, it has been demonstrated that the dietary administration of concanavalin A can result in high mortality in quail (D'Mello, 1995). In calves, a total oral sporedesmin dose of 3 mg kg^{-1} body weight can cause 100% mortality within 3–5 days (Flaoyen and Froslie, 1997). For mycotoxins, much emphasis has been directed at the acquisition of LD_{50} data (Table 18.4) following an incident in 1960 in the UK when 100,000 turkey poults died from acute necrosis of the liver and hyperplasia of the bile duct ('turkey X disease'), attributed to the consumption of groundnuts infected with *A. flavus*. This event marked a defining point in the history of mycotoxicoses, leading to the discovery of the aflatoxins. However, it is now recognized that LD_{50} values are subject to wide variation depending, for example, upon age, sex and size of animals. There are also species differences in sensitivity to a particular mycotoxin (Table 18.4). More significantly, it is acknowledged that features of chronic toxicity are of greater relevance in practical husbandry of farm animals. Thus, ZEN is associated with relatively low intrinsic toxicity as judged by LD_{50} values, but chronic investigations demonstrate that its oestrogenic property towards mammals is an over-riding feature. Similarly, in human

Table 18.3. Adverse effects of proteins and secondary substances from plants.

Plant components	Adverse effects
Lectins	Intestinal lesions
	Reduced nutrient absorption
Proteinase inhibitors	Reduced protein digestion
	Endogenous loss of amino acids
Antigenic proteins	Intestinal lesions
	Diarrhoea
	Immune hypersensitivity
Condensed tannins	Impaired rumen function
	Reduced liveweight gain and wool growth
Quinolizidine alkaloids	Reduced feed intake
	Teratogenic effects
Glucosinolates	Organ damage
	Goitrogenic effects
	Reduced feed intake
Amino acids	
S-methylcysteine sulphoxide	Haemolytic anaemia
	Organ damage
Mimosine	Shedding of fleece
	Reduced appetite
	Organ damage
	Death
Phyto-oestrogens	Reproductive dysfunction
Steroidal saponins	Hepatogenous photosensitization
Vasoactive lipids	Late-term abortion in cattle
Gossypol	Organ damage
	Cardiac failure
	Death
Cyanogens	Inhibition of cytochrome oxidase
	Central nervous system dysfunction
	Respiratory failure
	Cardiac arrest

health, the carcinogenic potential of myco-toxins is perceived to be more important than their respective LD_{50} values.

Chronic effects

A number of ANFs and mycotoxins are associated with well-defined syndromes identified from field cases of toxicity (Tables 18.3 and 18.4). Thus the aetiology of 'clover disease' in sheep has been linked with the intake of phyto-oestrogens, while in the case of DON, the effects on feed refusal and emesis in pigs are now considered to be characteristic for this *Fusarium* mycotoxin.

It is not intended to review all aspects of the chronic toxicity of the ANFs and

mycotoxins described above. A more salutary approach entails a comparison of these two groups of compounds with a view to discerning common features in their primary effects on farm animals.

Digestive dysfunction and nutrient malabsorption

Many ANFs modulate digestive function and nutrient metabolism, but there is increasing evidence that some mycotoxins may act in a similar manner. The classical view of lectins is that they exert their deleterious effects via reduced nutrient absorption following extensive structural and functional disruption of the intestinal microvilli (D'Mello, 1995). Thus, con-canavalin A enhances shedding of brush-border membranes and decreases villus

Table 18.4. Deleterious effects of mycotoxins in animals.

Mycotoxins	Deleterious effects
Aflatoxin B_1	Acute toxicity: LD_{50} values, 1–17.9 mg kg^{-1} BW (laboratory animals), 0.5 mg kg^{-1} BW (ducklings); hepatic lesions; teratogenic. Reduced feed efficiency, immune function and reproductive performance in ruminants
Aflatoxin M_1	Hepatotoxic
Ochratoxin A	LD_{50} <6 mg kg^{-1} BW (pigs); implicated in porcine nephropathy; teratogenic; carcinogenic to mice and rats
Deoxynivalenol	LD_{50} 70 mg kg^{-1} (mice); potent feed intake inhibitor in pigs; causes erosion of gastric mucosa; affects feed choice in mink; teratogenic; immunosuppressive. Ruminants tolerant
Diacetoxyscirpenol (DAS) and T-2 toxin	LD_{50} 23 and 5 mg kg^{-1} BW, respectively (mice); mouth lesions in poultry; in sows T-2 toxin can cause infertility and abortion. Growth depression in broiler chicks caused by DAS increased by high-fat diet. Implicated in field cases of mycotoxicoses in ruminants
Zearalenone	LD_{50} range: 2–10 g kg^{-1} BW; causes vulvovaginitis in gilts and anoestrus in cycling females; feminization in male pigs; reduced spermatogenesis; reduced milk production and hyperoestrogenism in cows; infertility in sheep
Fumonisins	Mortality in chicken embryos; onset of mortality in chickens aided by moniliformin; hepatic lesions in pigs and cattle; porcine pulmonary oedema; equine leukoencephalomalacia
Fusaric acid	Suppresses cell-mediated immunity; interactions with fumonisins and deoxynivalenol
Tenuazonic acid	LD_{50} values 125–225 mg kg^{-1} BW in mice
Ergopeptine alkaloids	Reduced growth, reproductive performance and milk production in ruminants; increased susceptibility to heat stress
Lolitrem alkaloids	Neurological effects: incoordination, staggering, shaking of head and collapse in ruminants
Phomopsins	Lupinosis in sheep: ill-thrift, liver damage, jaundice, photosensitization and death; reduced reproductive performance of ewes
Sporidesmin A	Facial eczema in sheep: liver damage, urinary lesions, photosensitization

length, thereby reducing surface area for absorption in the small intestine. With other lectins, the lamina propria of the intestine may become infiltrated with eosinophils and lymphocytes. Although the proteinase inhibitors depress proteolysis in the digestive tract, the adverse effects on growth are thought to occur via more complex mechanisms. It is envisaged that inactivation of trypsin elicits the release of cholecystokinin which stimulates pancreatic production of digestive enzymes, including trypsin and chymotrypsin. The net effect is the loss of endogenous protein rich in the sulphur-containing amino acids. It is this depletion of critical amino acids which reduces growth. A concomitant enlargement of the pancreas may also occur, particularly in broiler chickens (D'Mello, 1995).

One of the most striking effects on intestinal morphology and function occurs on feeding soybean antigens to sensitized mammals (D'Mello, 1991b). There is a marked degree of uniformity in these lesions, irrespective of animal species or of the source of the antigenic protein. Detailed analysis of the morphological aberrations show that while normal villi appear long and slender with tall columnar epithelial cells, those of sensitized calves and piglets are substantially shorter and broader with some evidence of disorganized enterocyte architecture. A consistent feature accompanying these changes is the marked increase in crypt depth following antigen stimulation in both calves and piglets. Villi from sensitized animals are distinguished by prominent infiltration with lymphocytes which may extend into the lamina propria.

The extensive morphological lesions which occur in the small intestine of sensitized animals significantly impair digestive and absorptive function by virtue of markedly reduced surface area in the gut, through abnormalities in the maturation of entero-cytes and through reductions in the secretion of key enzymes such as lactase. For example, xylose absorption, an indicator of absorptive competence, is substantially higher in milk-fed than in soybean-fed calves, with these differences diverging with age. Similar effects are seen in piglets with soybean hypersensitivity, except that absorptive competence is restored rela-tively early in the post-weaning period. Direct measurements of nutrient uptake confirm the abnormalities implied by the xylose tests. For example, sensitized calves show a decline in net nitrogen absorption efficiency to 0.25 as compared with 0.57 for unsensitized and 0.85 for casein-fed calves. Calves given a series of liquid feeds containing heated soybean products readily develop abnormalities in movement of digesta leading to diarrhoea.

The digestive tract is the primary focal point for the action of CTs. The ability of animals to tolerate CTs has received much attention following the findings that certain animals are capable of secreting proline-rich proteins (PRPs) in saliva, which may constitute a first line of defence against ingested CTs (see D'Mello, 1992). The open structure of these proteins induces a high affinity for CTs, and there are indications that the complex so formed is resistant to digestive attack. There are suggestions that the goat produces PRPs in significant amounts, whereas grazing ruminants lack these salivary proteins. Domestic goats are well recognized as mixed feeders, consum-ing appreciable quantities of CT-rich browse. If the synthesis of PRPs by goats is confirmed, then this may account for the higher digestibility of fibre in goats com-pared with sheep when both are offered leaves of *Acacia pendula* or *Prosopis cineraria*, whereas no species differences were observed when lucerne (*Medicago saliva*) represented the main item of feed (Kumar and D'Mello, 1995). The two

browse legumes, *A. pendula* and *P. cineraria* are known to contain CTs.

Consistent with the above account, cattle and sheep would be expected to be sensitive to CTs. Adverse effects may be seen in sheep when CTs such as those in lotus (*Lotus pedunculatus*) or in browse legumes such as *Acacia* species comprise a significant part of their diets. The evidence is now unequivocal (Table 18.5). Primary manifestations include impaired rumen function, resulting in depressed intake, wool growth and liveweight gain. The deleterious effects on rumen function have been ascribed to complexing of CTs with microbial extracellular enzymes. However, an overall deficit of rumen-degradable N in ruminants fed high-tannin forages and browse may also occur. This undersupply may reduce the digestibility of structural carbohydrates.

A number of mycotoxins adversely affect digestive morphology and rumen function (Table 18.4). At 4 mg kg^{-1} diet, DON may induce greater corrugations in the fundic region of the stomach of the pig and, at higher levels (19 mg kg^{-1}), the mycotoxin may cause erosions in the gastric mucosa. T-2 toxin also induces lesions in pigs, specifically on the mucosa of the pars oesophageal region, the incidence being dose-related. Chronic exposure to aflatoxin affects ruminal func-tion by decreasing cellulose fermentation, volatile fatty acid synthesis, protein degradation and motility.

Effects on nutrient partitioning and utilization
DELETERIOUS EFFECTS. The deleterious effects on nutrient utilization are best exemplified by the action of the non-protein amino acid, canavanine, present in the jack bean (*C. ensiformis*). Canavanine is structurally similar to arginine, an essential amino acid for poultry. When jack beans form a sub-stantial proportion of a broiler diet, the resulting depression in growth of chicks can be explained on the basis of a canavanine–arginine antagonism. Such an interaction involves increased degradation of arginine and possibly synthesis of aberrant tissue proteins resulting in

Table 18.5. Anti-nutritional effects of condensed tannins present in legumes (adapted from Kumar and D'Mello, 1995).

Legume	Animal	Anti-nutritional effect
Lotus corniculatus	Steer	Reduced DM digestibility *in sacco*, reduced VFA production *in vitro*
L. pedunculatus	Sheep	Inhibition of rumen carbohydrate digestion and reduced weight gain
Acacia aneura	Sheep	Reductions in: N digestibility, S absorption and wool yield
A. cyanophylla	Sheep	Negative N digestibility, reduced feed intake and body weight loss
A. nilotica (pods)	Sheep	Reductions in: N and NDF digestibility and growth
Calliandra calothyrsus	Goat	Reduced N digestibility *in sacco*
Prosopis cineraria	Sheep	Reductions in: digestibility of protein, iron absorption, feed intake and wool growth. Weight loss
Lespedeza cuneata	Sheep	Reductions in: ADF, NDF, N and cellulose digestibility. Depressed feed intake

increased protein turnover. The overall effect is a reduction in the efficiency of utilization of absorbed arginine (D'Mello, 1995). AFB_1 can cause reduced feed efficiency in ruminants (Table 18.4). This may imply a reduced efficiency of utilization of nutrients, but direct evidence is lacking.

BENEFICIAL EFFECTS. Despite the evidence presented in Table 18.5, CTs are generally attributed with beneficial properties in ruminant nutrition (Table 18.6). It is consistently maintained that CTs may confer protection from degradation of leaf proteins in the rumen. Fraction 1 (F1) leaf protein predominates in forage and its digestion in the small intestine, as opposed to fermentation in the rumen, would be advantageous to ruminants since F1 is of high biological value, presumed to exceed that of microbial protein. It has been suggested that a complex is formed between CTs and F1 protein through reversible hydrogen bonding which is stable at pH values between 4 and 7, but which readily dissociates on either side of this range. Consequently, it is envisaged that this complex escapes fermentation in the rumen where the pH ranges from 5 to 7, but dissociates on exposure to gastric (pH 2.5–3.5) and pancreatic (pH 8–9) secretions. The obvious implication is that CTs protect labile plant proteins in the rumen, thereby increasing the supply of high-quality protein in the duodenum. In terms of individual amino acids, it has been shown that *Lotus pedunculatus*, a tannin-containing legume, promoted a higher degree of protection for cysteine, methionine and phenylalanine than *L. corniculatus*, a cultivar low in CTs.

Another attribute of CTs recently proposed relates to amino acid utilization

Table 18.6. Putative benefits of secondary compounds of legumes in animal production.

Legume	Beneficial properties	Conditions/comments
Lotus pedunculatus	Protein protection in the rumen	30–40 g of CTs kg^{-1} DM of legume
	Cysteine, methionine and phenylalanine protection in the rumen	50 g of CTs kg^{-1} DM of legume
	Bloat suppression	30–40 g of CTs kg^{-1} DM
L. corniculatus	Increased utilization of cysteine for tissue synthetic reactions	27 g of extractable CTs and 8 g of bound CTs kg^{-1} DM
Hedysarum coronarium	Reduced gastrointestinal parasitism in lambs	100–120 g of CTs kg^{-1}
Acacia spp.	Anti-protozoal properties	Nature of compounds unknown

in ruminants. From their studies with sheep, Wang *et al.* (1994) concluded that CTs are able markedly to increase transulphuration of methionine to cysteine for body synthetic reactions. This may be important, since cysteine is a major component of wool protein. CTs have also been implicated in bloat suppression in cattle. Bloat is believed to be due primarily to the formation of a stable foam in which fermentation gases are entrapped. The active foaming agent is the soluble F1 fraction of leaf protein. Bloat in grazing ruminants is often associated with low-tannin pasture legumes such as lucerne and clover, but sainfoin, lotus and tropical browse legumes are considered to confer protection by virtue of their content of CTs. Using *in vitro* methods, it has been demonstrated that CTs from a variety of legumes reduced the compressive strength of protein foams in a dose-dependent manner, irrespective of differences in the chemical structures of these tannins.

Another attribute of high-tannin legumes has emerged from recent investigations with sheep infested with nematode parasites (Niezen *et al.*, 1995). In view of consumer apprehension about chemical residues in animal products, the potential use of such legumes as a substitute for conventional drugs would be consistent with efforts to promote sustainable practice in animal production. Preliminary indications are that the legume, sulla (*Hedysarum coronarium*) may confer beneficial effects in terms of performance of lambs infested with the nematode *Trichostrongylus colubriformis*, whereas lucerne was inferior in this respect. The effect is attributed to a direct action of CTs or some other component in sulla on the establishment or persistence of the parasite. However, it is conceded that the CTs in sulla may also have increased the post-ruminal supply of protein through protection in the rumen, and that this effect may have contributed to the improved performance of parasitized lambs.

A further benefit of plant secondary compounds may arise through an anti-protozoal action. It is maintained that more microbial and dietary protein becomes available to the ruminant when protozoa are excluded from the rumen. A number of tropical forages are endowed with defaunation properties, possibly arising from the secondary compounds they contribute. Although *Enterolobium* species are particularly effective, a number of *Acacia* species also show potential in this respect (Table 18.6).

Haemolytic anaemia

The adverse effects of SMCO in ruminants arises after its fermentation by rumen bacteria to dimethyl disulphide. The latter is a highly reactive metabolite which is believed to inactivate key proteins through blockage of sulphydryl groups. A severe haemolytic anaemia develops within 1–3 weeks in animals fed mainly or solely on *Brassica* forage. Early signs include loss of appetite, reduced milk production, the appearance of refractile, stainable granules (Heinz–Ehrlich bodies) within the erythrocytes and a decline in blood haemoglobin levels. Organ damage generally accompanies this condition. Spontaneous but incomplete recovery is observed in survivors continuing to graze the forage, but further fluctuations in blood haemoglobin concentrations may ensue. If the forage is withdrawn, blood chemistry is restored to normal within 3–4 weeks.

Hepatotoxicity

There is ample evidence that liver damage in farm animals may arise from intake of several ANFs and mycotoxins. Thus, haemolytic anaemia in sheep fed *Brassica* forage is attended by extensive liver damage in which the organ becomes swollen, pale and necrotic. Many hepatogenous photosensitization disorders are linked with the consumption of plants containing steroidal saponins (Flaoyen and Froslie, 1997). Plants such as *Narthecium ossifragum*, *Brachiaria decumbens* and various *Panicum* species have been implicated in these disorders. A common observation is the accretion of birefringent crystals in hepatocytes and in association with the bile duct. The crystals are composed of insoluble Ca^{2+} salts of sapogenin glucuronides derived from the saponins in the respective plants. These saponins are thought to be the hepatotoxin, and characteristic lesions include varying degrees of necrosis of hepatocytes, concentric lamellar periductal fibrosis and proliferation of the bile duct epithelium. Occlusion or obstruction of the biliary system causes the accumulation of the photosensitizing agent, phylloerythrin derived by the action of rumen microorganisms on chlorophyll. Retention of phylloerythrin may also arise from the inability of damaged hepatocytes to dispose of this compound into the biliary system. Any phylloerythrin reaching the skin, through inefficient hepatic and biliary elimination, is able to react with sunlight to cause photosensitization.

Lantana camara intoxication is another example of hepatogenous photosensitization disorders, in this instance caused by pentacyclic triterpene acids, primarily lantadene A and B. Incidence of *L. camara* intoxication has been reported almost exclusively in cattle in Australia, India, South Africa and the USA. Liver lesions include swelling and hydropic degeneration of hepatocytes, single cell necrosis of hepatocytes and bile duct damage leading to impaired disposal of phylloerythrin.

Abnormal liver function with photosensitization may also occur after consumption of certain mycotoxins. Thus, phomopsin A causes lupinosis which is essentially a hepatic disorder of sheep grazing lupin stubble. Manifestations include ill-thrift, jaundice, photosensitization and death. The mycotoxin interferes with microtubule-dependent intracellular transport mechanisms and acts as an antimitotic agent in the liver. Sporidesmin A is another mycotoxin with the capacity to induce liver lesions with photosensitization in ruminants. Effects include inflammation of the bile ducts, progressive obliterative cholangitis, obstructive jaundice and phylloerythrin accumulation.

The aflatoxins are well recognized for their potential to cause liver damage. Indeed, the high mortality of turkey poults in the 'turkey X disease' incident of 1960, referred to above, arose from acute necrosis of the liver and hyperplasia of the bile duct. Current disquiet about the aflatoxins centres on their capacity to induce liver cancer in humans.

Nephrotoxicity

In addition to photosensitization, certain plants will induce renal damage. Thus, *Narthecium ossifragum* may cause nephrotoxicity in cattle, sheep and goats, although current indications are that the agent is distinct from that involved in hepatogenous photosensitization (Flaoyen and Froslie, 1997). *Lantana* poisoning may be accompanied by kidney failure due to tubular degeneration and necrosis. Oxalates present in certain tropical grasses such as those in the genera *Cenchrus*, *Setaria*, *Pennisetum*, *Digitaria* and *Brachiaria* may cause chronic renal failure in grazing ruminants due to formation of oxalate crystals and urinary calculi (Marais, 1997).

Ochratoxin A frequently is implicated in porcine nephropathy (Abramson, 1997). Its action in the kidney may be exacerbated by the co-occurring mycotoxin, citrinin. Field cases of porcine nephropathy, associated with the consumption of moist cereal grains, have been reported in Denmark, where the condition is endemic. Affected kidneys are enlarged and pale while, internally, sections of the renal cortex show interstitial, peritubular and periglomerular fibrosis. Tubular function and efficiency may be impaired, consistent with tubular degeneration and atrophy. Balkan endemic nephropathy is a disorder of humans which has also been linked with OA and, in addition, there is evidence that an OA-related nephropathy may be widespread among Tunisians.

Neurotoxicity

Of the secondary compounds occurring in plants, the lathyrogenic non-protein amino acids, β-cyanoalanine, β-(*N*-oxalylamino) alanine and α, γ-diaminobutyric acid are notable for their neurotoxic properties. Whether this neurotoxicity accounts for the relatively low nutritional value of the seeds of *Lathyrus* and *Vicia* species remains to be established (D'Mello, 1995). On the other hand, at least two mycotoxins have been implicated definitively in field cases of toxicosis. The lolitrem alkaloids cause perennial ryegrass staggers in ruminants, a disorder characterized by neurological symptoms including incoordination, staggering, shaking of the head and collapse. Hepatic damage in sheep caused by phomopsin A can result in hyper-ammonaemia, which in turn may precipitate degenerative changes in the central nervous system. Spongy transformation of the brain in sheep affected by chronic lupinosis in the field has been described. Identical lesions in sheep were reproduced in experimental forms of acute and chronic lupinosis. A clear association was proposed between the extent of liver injury and the incidence of brain lesions. Evidence of spongy transformation included vacuolation of the white matrix of the brain stem. The vacuolation occurred with the highest frequency and severity in the cerebellar peduncles and around the nuclei present in the white matter of the cerebellum. Affected sheep may thus appear disorientated.

Immunocompetence

An immunological dimension has been attributed to the adverse effects of a wide range of ANFs and mycotoxins. However, the evidence is plausible for just a few of these compounds. Although soybean antigens are associated primarily with digestive aberrations, there is no doubt now that immunocompetence is also severely compromised in sensitized calves and piglets. The involvement of the immune system in antigen challenge arose from observations that the adverse effects in the calf occurred only after administration of successive feeds containing defatted and heated soybean products. This implied that the initial feeds sensitized the calf to the antigens, with overt digestive perturbations ensuing after subsequent feeds. Such a response is consistent with the classical pattern of antibody synthesis (D'Mello,

1991b). Confirmation of the involvement of the immune system in soybean hypersensitivity arose from direct observations linking elevated serum IgG concentrations with the specific antigens, i.e. glycinin and β-conglycinin. Although the evidence for the involvement of the immune system in calf and piglet soybean hypersensitivity is now unquestionable, it is still not clear which of the immune reactions precipitates the intestinal lesions. Tissue damage may be caused by release of lysosomal enzymes or an array of compounds such as histamine, kinins, leukotrienes and prostaglandins.

The immunotoxic effects of mycotoxins have been reviewed extensively (Pier, 1991; Pestka and Bondy, 1994). Most of the evidence is based largely on studies with laboratory animals or on *in vitro* measurements with lymphocytes subjected to mitogenic stimulation. It is apparent that, for example, oral administration of AFB_1 to chicks lowers peripheral blood lymphocyte proliferation to the mitogen and lectin, concanavalin A. Chicken macrophages treated with fumonisin B_1 develop morphological abnormalities, with reduced phagocytic potential (Pestka and Bondi, 1994). The implications for farm animal health in practical situations need to be addressed, particularly when feeds contain two or more mycotoxins as co-contaminants.

Reproductive dysfunction

The reproductive tract and associated endocrine systems are particularly sensitive to the action of secondary substances from plants and fungi and there are well-defined examples of field cases positively linked with these compounds. Thus, the aetiology of 'clover disease' in sheep has been correlated with the intake of the phyto-oestrogenic isoflavonoids. Although of less potency than endogenous steroidal oestrogens, isoflavonoids can exert significant effects due to their abundance in leguminous plants. In addition, they are capable of modulating the synthesis and action of oestrogen in a variety of pathways (Whitten *et al.*, 1997). The isoflavones competitively inhibit the binding of oestradiol to the oestrogen receptor, based upon common structural features. Equol is the major isoflavonoid in plasma of livestock and appears to be the oestrogenic agent in clover disease. A unifying feature of oestrogenic isoflavones is their capacity to stimulate proliferation of the female reproductive tract. Other indicators of reproductive derangements include precocious sexual development, and reduced ovulation rates. For example, ewes grazing on oestrogenic pastures around the time of mating, develop 'temporary infertility' characterized by low ovulation and conception rates (Adams, 1995). This form of infertility is reversed within 4–6 weeks of transfer of ewes to non-oestrogenic grazing. Temporary infertility may occur in the absence of overt symptoms, particularly in Merino ewes. Prolonged comsumption of oestrogenic pasture can induce permanent infertility in ewes. Reduced conception arises from a failure of the cervix to facilitate transport of spermatozoa following insemination. Irreversible changes of the cervix occur such that it resembles the histology and function of the uterus. Such changes are used in the diagnosis of permanent infertility from tissues obtained in abattoirs. Isoflavonoids may also impair male reproductive function by reducing testicular development and spermatogenesis.

Reproductive performance in cattle may be compromised through the ingestion of needles and buds from western yellow pine (*P. ponderosa*). The primary effect is late-term abortion in beef cattle (Ford *et al.*, 1997). There is evidence that this syndrome is a form of premature fetal-induced parturition rather than a non-specific abortion. Comparison of the steroid hormone status of *P. ponderosa*-fed and normal cows indicates similar patterns of periparturient endocrine changes. Thus, both groups display gradual increases in oestrogen concentrations which peak at parturition and decline thereafter. A major pre-partum difference between these groups, however, is a striking and progressive decline in blood flow to the gravid horn in cows fed *P. ponderosa* needles. The depression in blood flow specifically in the caruncular arterial bed results in reduced nutrient and O_2 supply at the placentome. The active agents causing these effects are thought to be the vasoactive lipids isolated from *P. ponderosa* needles.

The ergopeptine alkaloid mycotoxins present in endophyte-infected tall fescue are the causative agents of 'fescue summer toxicosis' or 'summer slump' in cattle. Effects include delayed onset of puberty and impaired function of the corpora lutea in heifers. The corpus luteum of affected heifers show increased numbers of large luteal cells, and ultrastructural examination of these cells reveal higher numbers of mitochondria, lipid droplets and secretory granules. Reduced calving rates may be associated with endocrine changes such as lower prolactin status. In ewes, delayed conception, attributed to embryonic mortality and delayed onset of oestrus rather than to failure in fertilization, is the primary effect of fescue toxicosis. The adverse effects in horses are associated almost entirely with reduced reproductive performance. Agalactia, extended gestation length, abortion and thickened placentas are common observations in affected mares. Placental abnormalities may include oedema, fibrosis and mucoid degeneration. It has been suggested that the effects in the placenta were the result of hypoxia caused by reduced blood flow to this organ. Foal losses have also been reported, 16% for fescue and <6% for other forages. Endophyte-infected tall fescue can, in addition, reduce testosterone secretion and testicular function in males, as indicated by studies on beef bulls.

Although lupinosis is essentially a disorder of the liver, reduced reproductive performance in ewes has been reported on administration of phomopsins (Barnes *et al.*, 1996). Ovulation rate is depressed, leading to markedly lower conception rates and numbers of lambs born.

A Critique

The occurrence of ANFs and mycotoxins as co-contaminants in raw materials and animal feed means that it is not always possible to attribute adverse effects to a particular compound. It will be clear from the foregoing account that both lectins and proteinase inhibitors are not only ubiquitous but may also occur together in the seed of the same leguminous plant. Studies with the winged bean illustrate the circuitous protocol employed in the identification of the primary ANFs in leguminous seeds (D'Mello, 1995). Thus, initial investigations focused on the activity of the trypsin inhibitors in the winged bean, but the weight loss and high mortality of experimental animals fed raw winged beans was indicative of some other factor. Further studies revealed the dominant role of lectins in the aetiology of winged bean toxicity. The soybean has long been recognized for its content of proteinase inhibitors, but recent studies indicate a significant role for lectins and antigenic globulins in the aetiology of post-weaning hypersensitivity in calves and piglets. In addition, the practical significance of the phyto-oestrogens in soybean have yet to be addressed with respect to farm animal productivity.

Another issue requiring elucidation centres on the protective role of CTs in the microbial fermentation of protein in the rumen. It is presumed that the CTs released post-ruminally do not exert any deleterious effects in the intestinal tract since pH conditions do not allow further reactions with dietary or endogenous proteins. However, it has been observed that the CTs of *P. cineraria* retain their capacity to precipitate pepsin at pH 2.0 and, consequently, an important digestive enzyme of gastric secretion may be inhibited (see Kumar and D'Mello, 1995). Furthermore, Waghorn *et al.* (1994) maintain that the benefits of protein protection may be offset, in part, by a reduction in the fractional absorption of essential as well as non-essential amino acids from the small intestine. A further question centres on the dissociation of the protein–CT complex at pH values below 4 and above 7. Since these pH criteria also occur in non-ruminants, the issue arises as to why such

a dissociation of the complex does not occur in these animals or, if it does, why adverse effects are observed in non-ruminants but not in ruminants (D'Mello, 1992).

There is now unequivocal evidence of co-contamination of animal feed with mycotoxins of diverse origins. Thus, it is conceivable that feeds based on groundnut cake and maize consistently may be contaminated with the aflatoxins and fumonisins. The additive or synergistic effects of these and other combinations only recently have become the focus of attention, providing improved understanding of well-established cases of mycotoxicoses. Thus, it is now recognized that the 'turkey X disease' incident of 1960, originally attributed to the aflatoxins, was compounded by the co-occurrence of cyclopiazonic acid, also produced by *A. flavus*. Fusaric acid is a common metabolite of several *Fusarium* species, co-occurring with ZEN, DON and the fumonisins. Although of minor intrinsic toxicity at levels found in feeds, fusaric acid can enhance the activity of other *Fusarium* mycotoxins. Fusaric acid can increase brain levels of serotonin in pigs, and a potential synergistic interaction with DON has been proposed in feed refusal and emesis in these animals.

Preventive and Remedial Measures

A selection of practical methods is presented here to illustrate the diversity of preventive and remedial measures available to the feed manufacturer and livestock producer. With the thermolabile ANFs such as lectins and proteinase inhibitors, heat processing has long been the method of choice for leguminous seeds containing these substances. The efficacy of moist-heating procedures as opposed to dry-heating methods has been established. Inactivation of soybean antigens, however, requires more rigorous processing involving hot aqueous ethanol extraction. It is suggested that detoxification is achieved by altering the protein structure of the antigens rather than by removal of osmotically active components such as sucrose and oligosaccharides. Inactivation is critically dependent upon alcohol concentrations and temperature. Maximum efficiency is achieved with proportions of 0.65–0.70 ethanol at 78°C. Ethanol extraction of soybean removes antigenicity and prevents gut inflammatory reactions in the calf, but other procedures, such as alkali treatment, are necessary for enhancing the nutritive value of soybean protein for early weaning of piglets. At least two soybean products are now available for commercial use in calf and piglet diets. The products are guaranteed free of antigens, but the nature of the processing techniques used remains undisclosed.

In the case of CTs, limited evidence suggests that dietary supplements such as polyethylene glycol 4000 (PEG-4000) or urea may be effective for ruminants fed on high-tannin browse legumes. CTs bind to PEG-4000 in preference to protein. Dietary protein thus becomes available for digestion and, in addition, activities of endogenous proteins and enzymes remain unaffected (Kumar and D'Mello, 1995). However, indiscriminate use of PEG-4000 may well compromise the bloat-retarding properties of CTs. An alternative approach based on urea supplementation has been found to be useful in farm conditions. Urea not only provides additional nitrogen, but it may also inactivate CTs.

Considerable amelioration, or even avoidance, of adverse effects in ruminants may be achieved by employing suitable grazing strategies. Current recommendations for the prevention of SMCO toxicity in sheep involve some control of *Brassica* intake, particularly in late winter when SMCO concentrations in the forage are maximal. In addition, further control of SMCO intake may be accomplished by feeding *Brassica* forage grown on low-sulphur soils which reduces SMCO levels in the crop. Mimosine toxicity in *Leucaena*-fed sheep may be averted by gradually increasing dietary concentrations of the legume over a 3-week period.

Management strategies are also advocated for reducing the adverse effects

of endophyte-infected grasses, since the introduction of endophyte-free cultivars is accompanied by agronomic disadvantages. Thus, managing grazing to maintain the grass in a vegetative state reduces toxicity by preventing consumption of seedheads which contain higher levels of the endophyte mycotoxins. Rotational grazing involving pastures free of endophyte-infected grasses, particularly in hot weather to offset heat stress, has been advanced as an additional measure.

With other mycotoxins, preventive rather than curative or management measures are necessary to ensure that performance and animal product safety are not compromised. When fungicides are used effectively to control fungal diseases of crop plants, then the risk of mycotoxin contamination of primary feeds may be minimized. However, in the case of certain *Fusarium* diseases of cereals, it is generally accepted that fungicide control is only partially effective and the potential exists for mycotoxin contamination of grain. One possible strategy, with environmental dividends, centres on plant selection and breeding. Experimental studies show that, for example, breeding maize plants that are resistant to colonization and ear rot caused by *A. flavus* generally results in lower contamination of grain with AFB_1. Similarly, exploitation of genetic resistance to *Fusarium* head blight in wheat can be used successfully to reduce DON levels in the grain. A similar approach is being advocated in the control of lupinosis, with the development of *Phomopsis*-resistant cultivars of lupin. It is salutary to note that plant selection and breeding have already proved to be commercially successful in reducing glucosinolate levels in rapeseed.

When mycotoxin contamination of primary feed ingredients has occurred, a number of damage-limitation and remedial options are available. Thus, removal of heavily contaminated outer layers of cereal kernels has been attempted in order to reduce DON. Dilution with feeds free of contamination may also be advocated within specified regulatory guidelines. In the case of aflatoxin-contaminated oilseeds destined for animal feed, however, specific detoxification procedures are commercially available in a number of countries. Ammoniation of contaminated oilseed meals appears to be the method of choice, involving treatment with either ammonium hydroxide or gaseous ammonia at high temperatures and pressure, as in commercial feed mills, or at ambient temperature and low pressure for small-scale operations. If the ammoniation reactions are allowed to proceed to completion, the detoxification process is irreversible and aflatoxin contamination is virtually eliminated. Providing that any residual ammonia is dissipated, diets containing de-contaminated meals are readily consumed by farm animals without adverse effects. Depending upon the efficacy of decontamination, residues of AFM_1 in the milk of dairy cows are substantially reduced or eliminated altogether. The use of phyllo-silicate clays (hydrated sodium calcium aluminosilicate) to complex with aflatoxins has also been attempted, resulting in reduced gut uptake and deposition of the mycotoxins in tissues and milk.

Future developments in preventive and remedial measures are likely to emerge from biotechnology. There is already practical evidence of the effectiveness of such strategies. Thus, *Leucaena* toxicity in cattle, arising from the two DHP products of mimosine metabolism, has been overcome in Australia by inoculating animals with bacteria capable of completely degrading these metabolites to non-toxic compounds (see D'Mello, 1992). Dosed animals feeding on *Leucaena* show markedly higher liveweight gains than untreated controls on the same legume. Excretion of DHP in urine of dosed steers declines rapidly to zero, whereas untreated steers on *Leucaena* continue to excrete DHP. The dispersal of bacteria to untreated animals occurs rapidly, and the isolation of active DHP-degrading bacteria from faeces of treated cattle indicates that inoculation of just a few animals in a herd may be all that is required to overcome *Leucaena* toxicity. This type of bioremediation may be applied to other ANFs and, indeed, to

mycotoxins. There is evidence of bacterial degradation of tannins, DON and ZEN.

Regulatory and Advisory Directives

The acute toxicity of certain secondary compounds, and in particular the carcinogenicity of mycotoxins, has led to the establishment of regulatory and advisory directives for primary feed ingredients and complete rations. Table 18.7 is designed to illustrate the type of directives in place in the UK, the European Union (EU) and in North America. Two plant secondary compounds, gossypol and HCN, are subject to statutory control. In addition, EU quality criteria have been published for glucosinolates in rapeseed. For CTs in lotus, Barry *et al.* (1986) recommended appropriate concentrations in the forage dry matter, to represent a balance between the beneficial effects for protein protection in the rumen and bloat suppression, and their negative effects in depressing microbial fermentation of structural carbohydrates. Extensive regulations also exist for the aflatoxins, but for OA and DON only advisory directives have been proposed, unsupported by legislative measures. Of particular concern is the absence of statutory regulations for the carcinogenic fumonisins.

Conclusions

Plants and fungi synthesize a wide range of substances with anti-nutritional and toxic effects in farm animals. Extensive rumen and tissue metabolism may occur in farm animals to initiate or enhance the potency of some of these compounds. Plant components with significant anti-nutritional activity include lectins, proteinase inhibitors, antigenic proteins, CTs, quinolizidine alkaloids, glucosinolates, non-protein amino acids and phyto-oestrogens. A number of these and other compounds such as saponins, vasoactive lipids, gossypol and HCN are associated with toxic and anti-physiological effects. These

Table 18.7. Examples of worldwide guidelines and regulations for plant and fungal secondary compounds.

Countries	Secondary compounds	Commodities	Maximum levels	Status
Worldwide	Condensed tannins (g kg^{-1} DM)	Pasture and browse plants	40	Advisory
EU	Total glucosinolates (µmol g^{-1})	Rapeseed	20–35	Statutory (for payment of subsidy)
UK	Free gossypol (mg kg^{-1})	Straight and complete feedstuffs except:	20	Statutory
		cottonseed cake or meal	1200	
		complete feedstuffs for cattle, sheep and goats	500	
		complete feedstuffs for poultry and calves	100	
UK	HCN (mg kg^{-1})	Straight and complete feedstuffs except:	50	Statutory
		linseed	250	
		linseed cake or meal, cassava products	350	
		complete feedstuffs for chicks	10	
EU	Aflatoxin B$_1$ (µg kg^{-1})	Straight feedstuffs except: groundnut, copra, palm kernel, cottonseed, babassu, maize and products derived from the processing thereof	50	Statutory
			20	
		Complete feedstuffs for cattle, sheep and goats (with the exception of complete feedstuffs for calves, lambs and kids)	50	
		Complete feedstuffs for pigs and poultry (except those for young animals)	20	
		Other complete feedstuffs	10	
	Aflatoxin M$_1$ (mg kg^{-1})	Milk/milk products	0.5	Statutory
	Ochratoxin A (µg kg^{-1})	Cereals and cereal products	4	Advisory
USA/ Canada	Deoxynivalenol (mg kg^{-1})	Animal feed	5–10	Advisory

effects include haemolytic anaemia, lesions in the liver, kidney and central nervous system and alterations in immune and endocrine function. The net result is a depression in food intake, growth and reproductive performance, but other effects such as diarrhoea and photosensitization may also occur with certain toxicants. The secondary metabolism of fungi results in the elaboration of deleterious substances known as mycotoxins. Compounds of significance include aflatoxins, ochratoxins, *Fusarium* mycotoxins, endophyte alkaloids, phomopsins and sporidesmins. Many of these mycotoxins also adversely affect digestive morphology and rumen function and act on other organs to cause hepatogenous photosensitization, nephropathy, neurotoxicity and reproductive dysfunction. There is increasing awareness that a number of plant and fungal toxicants may occur together to precipitate additive or even synergistic effects in farm animals. Consequently, major difficulties may be anticipated in future attempts to establish tolerance limits and regulatory guidelines for co-occurring anti-nutritional and toxic substances. Although chemical and physical methods are available for detoxification of some of these substances, there is increasing recognition of the role of biotechnological strategies in future efforts to enhance the quality and safety of animal feeds.

References

Abramson, D. (1997) Toxicants of the genus *Penicillium.* In: D'Mello, J.P.F. (ed.) *Handbook of Plant and Fungal Toxicants.* CRC Press, Boca Raton, Florida, pp. 303–317.

Adams, N.R. (1995) Detection of the effects of phytoestrogens on sheep and cattle. *Journal of Animal Science* 73, 1509–1515.

Barnes, A.L., Croker, K.P., Allen, J.G. and Costa, N.D. (1996) Lupinosis of ewes around the time of mating reduces reproductive performance. *Australian Journal of Agricultural Research* 47, 1305–1314.

Barry, T.N., Manley, T.R. and Duncan, S.J. (1986) The role of condensed tannins in the nutritional value of *Lotus pedunculatus* for sheep. 4. Sites of carbohydrate and protein digestion as influenced by dietary reactive tannin concentration. *British Journal of Nutrition* 55, 123–137.

D'Mello, J.P.F. (1991a) Toxic amino acids. In: D'Mello, J.P.F., Duffus, C.M. and Duffus, J.H. (eds) *Toxic Substances in Crop Plants.* The Royal Society of Chemistry, Cambridge, pp. 21–48.

D'Mello, J.P.F. (1991b) Antigenic proteins. In: D'Mello, J.P.F., Duffus, C.M. and Duffus, J.H. (eds) *Toxic Substances in Crop Plants.* The Royal Society of Chemistry, Cambridge, pp. 107–125.

D'Mello, J.P.F. (1992) Chemical constraints to the use of tropical legumes in animal nutrition. *Animal Feed Science and Technology* 38, 237–261.

D'Mello, J.P.F. (1994) Amino acid imbalances, antagonisms and toxicities. In: D'Mello, J.P.F. (ed.) *Amino Acids in Farm Animal Nutrition.* CAB International, Wallingford, UK, pp. 63–97.

D'Mello, J.P.F. (1995) Anti-nutritional substances in legume seeds. In: D'Mello, J.P.F. and Devendra, C. (eds) *Tropical Legumes in Animal Nutrition.* CAB International, Wallingford, UK, pp. 135–172.

D'Mello, J.P.F., Porter, J.K. and Macdonald, A.M.C. (1997) *Fusarium* mycotoxins. In: D'Mello, J.P.F. (ed.) *Handbook of Plant and Fungal Toxicants.* CRC Press, Boca Raton, Florida, pp. 287–301.

Duncan, A.J. (1991) Condensed tannins. In: D'Mello, J.P.F., Duffus, C.M. and Duffus, J.H. (eds) *Toxic Substances in Crop Plants.* The Royal Society of Chemistry, Cambridge, pp. 126–147.

Flaoyen, A. and Froslie, A. (1997) Photosensitization disorders. In: D'Mello, J.P.F. (ed.) *Handbook of Plant and Fungal Toxicants.* CRC Press, Boca Raton, Florida, pp. 191–204.

Ford, S.P., Rosazza, J.P.N. and Short, R.E. (1997) *Pinus ponderosa* needle-induced toxicity. In: D'Mello, J.P.F. (ed.) *Handbook of Plant and Fungal Toxicants.* CRC Press, Boca Raton, Florida, pp. 219–229.

Griffiths, D.W. (1991) Condensed tannins. In: D'Mello, J.P.F., Duffus, C.M. and Duffus, J.H. (eds) *Toxic Substances in Crop Plants.* The Royal Society of Chemistry, Cambridge, pp. 180–201.

Kumar, R. and D'Mello, J.P.F. (1995) Anti-nutritional factors in forage legumes. In: D'Mello, J.P.F. and Devendra, C. (eds) *Tropical Legumes in Animal Nutrition.* CAB International, Wallingford, UK, pp. 95–133.

Marais, J.P. (1997) Nitrate and oxalates. In: D'Mello, J.P.F. (ed.) *Handbook of Plant and Fungal Toxicants.* CRC Press, Boca Raton, Florida, pp. 205–218.

Miles, C.O., Erasmuson, A.F. and Wilkins, A.L. (1996) Ovine metabolism of zearalenone to α-zearalanol (zeranol). *Journal of Agricultural and Food Chemistry* 44, 3244–3250.

Niezen, J.H., Waghorn, T.S., Charleston, W.A.G. and Waghorn, G.C. (1995) Growth and gastrointestinal nematode parasitism in lambs grazing either lucerne (*Medicago sativa*) or sulla (*Hedysarum coronarium*) which contains condensed tannins. *Journal of Agricultural Science* 125, 281–289.

Norton, G. (1991) Proteinase inhibitors. In: D'Mello, J.P.F., Duffus, C.M. and Duffus, J.H. (eds) *Toxic Substances in Crop Plants.* The Royal Society of Chemistry, Cambridge, pp. 68–106.

Pestka, J.J. and Bondy, G.S. (1994) Immunotoxic effects of mycotoxins. In: Miller, J.D. and Trenholm, H.L. (eds) *Mycotoxins in Grain. Compounds Other than Aflatoxin.* Eagan Press, St Paul, Minnesota, pp. 339–358.

Petterson, D.S., Harris, D.J. and Allen, D.G. (1991) Alkaloids. In: D'Mello, J.P.F., Duffus, C.M. and Duffus, J.H. (eds) *Toxic Substances in Crop Plants.* The Royal Society of Chemistry, Cambridge, pp. 148–179.

Pier, A.C. (1991) The influence of mycotoxins on the immune system. In: Smith, J.E. and Henderson, R.S. (eds) *Mycotoxins and Animal Foods.* CRC Press, Boca Raton, Florida, pp. 489–497.

Porter, J.K. (1997) Endophyte alkaloids. In: D'Mello, J.P.F. (ed.) *Handbook of Plant and Fungal Toxicants.* CRC Press, Boca Raton, Florida, pp. 51–62.

Smith, J.E. (1997) Aflatoxins. In: D'Mello, J.P.F. (ed.) *Handbook of Plant and Fungal Toxicants.* CRC Press, Boca Raton, Florida, pp. 269–285.

Waghorn, G.C., Shelton, I.D., McNabb, W.C. and McCutcheon, S.N. (1994) Effects of condensed tannins in *Lotus pedunculatus* on its nutritive value for sheep. 2. Nitrogenous aspects. *Journal of Agricultural Science* 123, 109–119.

Wang, Y., Waghorn, G.C., Barry, T.N. and Shelton, I.D. (1994) The effect of condensed tannins in *Lotus pedunculatus* on plasma metabolism of methionine, cystine and inorganic sulphate by sheep. *British Journal of Nutrition* 72, 923–935.

Whitten, P.L., Kudo, S. and Okubo, K.K. (1997) Isoflavonoids. In: D'Mello, J.P.F. (ed.) *Handbook of Plant and Fungal Toxicants.* CRC Press, Boca Raton, Florida, pp. 117–137.

Chapter 19

Feed Enzymes

D.I. Officer

*NSW Agriculture, Agricultural Research and Advisory Station,
Grafton, NSW, Australia*

Introduction

Early enzyme preparations included in animal diets were not formulated as animal feed additives but were produced for industrial or human food uses. Between the late 1980s and mid 1990s, enzyme products changed with the formulation of feed enzyme supplements specifically for animal diets. Over this period, feed enzyme supplementation has increased dramatically all over the world, but predominantly in pig and poultry diets. Also in recent years, renewed research interest into the potential value of feed enzymes has occurred in the fields of ruminant nutrition and aquaculture. The reliability of enzyme supplementation has improved over time, especially with respect to heat stability during pelleting and the matching of enzyme activity to anti-nutritive components in the feed.

The importance of matching enzyme activity and feed composition has become evident as our understanding of the chemistry of non-starch polysaccharides and other feed components has improved. To provide any benefit to the animal, feed enzymes must target specific feed components which are otherwise harmful or of little or no value. In doing so, a wider range of ingredients may be used in diet formulation without compromising on diet cost or animal performance. For example, feed enzymes are used to increase the amount of nutrients available from vegetable proteins so that they can be substituted for fish meal or other high-quality and expensive animal protein sources. Feed enzymes can also be used to substitute a previously unacceptable energy source for another (e.g. barley for wheat in broilers).

One of the benefits from increasing the efficiency with which nutrients are obtained from a feed ingredient is the reduction in faecal nutrient level. Reductions in nutrient excretion produced by enzyme supplementation are especially important where faeces are being applied to land with restrictions on nutrient application and for aquaculture where there is the potential to maintain or improve water quality after feeding.

Feed enzymes are also increasingly seen as 'environmentally responsible' alternatives to some hormone growth promotants and antibiotics. This is because they currently are seen as 'natural products' rather than as chemical additives. Across the world, bacteria are developing resistance to antibiotics, and in markets such as the European Community there is a ban on meat produced with hormone growth promotants. As a result, feed enzymes in specific situations have the potential to replace hormone growth promotants and antibiotics. This allows products to be marketed in a way that is more attractive to the increasing number of environmentally conscious consumers while providing growth and health benefits.

Mechanism of Feed Enzyme Action

There is evidence to support two main ways in which feed enzymes improve diet digestibility and animal performance (Pettersson and Aman, 1988, 1989; Annison, 1991). Firstly feed enzymes increase the access to nutrients previously bound in or by cell walls. For nutrients to be available at the cell level, large compounds must be broken into smaller molecules and absorbed by the intestinal wall. The role of feed enzymes is to work in combination with endogenous enzymes to degrade compounds to a size that can be utilized by the animal. Consequently, it is important to choose exogenous enzymes with complementary action to enzymes produced by the animal.

Secondly, feed enzymes must prevent increases in digesta viscosity which can impair nutrient absorption. Some compounds, once they are released from the cell walls, form gels which can increase digesta viscosity. Young animals, especially birds, are very sensitive to changes in digesta viscosity. If they eat diets containing high levels of gel-forming non-starch polysaccharides (NSPs), low digesta viscosity can be maintained with enzymes which reduce the chain length of the polysaccharides rather than remove side branches (Chesson, 1993).

If enzymes preparations are to be effective in releasing nutrients, they must have activities which degrade a range of compounds. For example, the β-glucanase-type enzymes are usually sufficient to disrupt barley endosperm walls, but both cellulase and pentosanase are required to maximize release of protein from the aleurone layer (Murison *et al.*, 1989; Mulder *et al.*, 1991). Multienzyme products, therefore, have the potential to release more nutrients than single enzyme products.

Although it may seem attractive to be able to break down all of the carbohydrate in the diet into absorbable units, not all monosaccharide sugars are well utilized by all animal species or by all parts of the gastrointestinal tract of those species. Some sugars, such as xylose, are universally well utilized by both pigs and poultry (Longstaff *et al.*, 1988; Yule and Fuller, 1992). Other sugars, such as arabinose, are poorly utilized if released prior to the terminal ileum but well utilized if broken down and absorbed in the hindgut of the pig (Yule and Fuller, 1992). Therefore feed enzymes formulations should not contain glycosidases, other than glucosidase (Chesson, 1993), if optimal utilization of energy from pentose sugars is to be achieved.

The interactions between the animal and the feed enzyme-supplemented diet are complex. For example, pentosanase supplementation of rye diets has been found to have adverse effects on digesta pH, viscosity and dry matter digestibility in piglets (Inborr *et al.*, 1991). Yet, piglets given β-glucanase-supplemented rye diets, and pentosanase- or β-glucanase-supplemented barley diets, showed no ill effects. These results show the importance of understanding how enzymes interact with different feed ingredients.

In summary:

- Feed enzymes increase nutrient availability by both releasing bound nutrients and breaking down compounds which increase digesta viscosity.
- Feed enzyme formulators need to understand how each enzyme activity interacts with the feed. Enzyme formulations must be complementary to diet composition.
- Multienzyme products have the potential to release more nutrients than single enzyme products.

Matching Enzyme Activity to Diet Composition

Role of fibre-degrading enzymes

Fibre in its various forms is a major cause of poor feed digestion especially in young animals. Even within a group of feedstuffs such as cereals, there is considerable variation in the amount and type of NSP they contain (see Tables 19.1 and 19.2).

The two main types of NSP found in cereals are the arabinoxylans (or pentosans) and the β-glucans. Arabinoxylans are made of a linear backbone of xylose substituted with arabinose (Bedford, 1995). β-Glucans are made up of a polymer of glucose which has kinks that are responsible for the anti-nutritional properties of barley and oats (Bedford, 1995).

Given the typical arabinoxylan composition of wheat (Table 19.2), the addition of a β-glucanase to a wheat-based diet will have significantly less effect than if it were added to a barley-based diet. Yet the addition of a xylanase (or pentosanase) to a wheat- or rye-based diet will have more effect than if it were added to a barley-based diet.

The amount of soluble arabinoxylan and β-glucan in a feedstuff is important because it is this fraction of the cereal which is believed to increase the viscosity of digesta (important especially in poultry). Increased digesta viscosity slows the rate of digestion and absorption, increases microbial activity, reduces feed intake and, especially in birds, increases faecal moisture content. Xylanases and β-glucanases reduce the size of the molecules of arabinoxylan and β-glucan, and in turn reduce digesta viscosity.

Two points emerge from the foregoing:

- It is important that the feed enzyme activity is matched to the ingredient composition of the diet.
- Feed enzyme supplementation is more likely to improve digestibility when β-glucanases are added to barley diets and xylanases are added to rye or wheat diets.

Role of phytase

Phosphorus is a major mineral required by animals in bone and is used in nerve and embryo development. Inorganic forms of P, although generally highly available, are

Table 19.1. Cell wall (NDF), starch, fat (acid ether extractives) and metabolizable energy (ME) for poultry content of selected feed grains (g kg^{-1} dry matter basis).

Cereal	Cell wall	Starch	Fat	ME (MJ kg^{-1})
Barley	201	562	26	14.5
Maize	117	700	42	16.1
Oats	315	469	51	14.8
Naked oats	114	590	101	16.7
Triticale	119	517	22	14.4
Wheat	124	674	21	15.5

After Chesson (1993).

Table 19.2. Arabinoxylan and β-glucan content of cereal grains (g kg^{-1}).

Cereal	Arabinoxylan			β-glucan		
	Grain total	Grain water-soluble	Endosperm (% of total)	Grain total	Grain water-soluble	Endosperm (% of total)
Barley	56.9	4.8	22	43.6	28.9	99
Oats	76.5	5.0	12	33.7	21.3	47
Rye	84.9	26.0	44	18.9	6.8	71
Wheat	66.3	11.8	35	6.5	5.2	48

After Chesson (1993).

relatively expensive. Plants store P in the form of phytic acid which cannot be broken down by monogastric animals unless there is inherent phytase activity in the feed. The enzyme phytase breaks down phytic acid releasing six phosphate molecules, and has been available commercially since the mid 1990s. Addition of phytase to the diet allows substantially less inorganic P to be included in the diet and, as a result, reduces the amount of P excreted. Lower P waste is advantageous especially in intensively farmed environments where it is viewed as a pollutant.

Phytase, according to Jongbloed (1997), is used in >80% of Dutch pig feeds and has been partly responsible for a reduction of 60% in the excretion of P by pigs in The Netherlands between 1973 and 1995. Phytase is also widely used in other parts of the world. Increasing environmental pressure for the inclusion of phytase in all animal diets is likely to continue.

Unfortunately, addition of phytase, like other enzyme products, cannot be relied upon to release a fixed amount of P from every diet. Different ingredients have varying concentrations of phytate P and an inherent level of plant phytase. This means that the availability of phytate P will be higher for ingredients with inherent phytase than would be expected from the concentration of phytate P.

As well as releasing bound P, phytase may have a role in improving the metabolizable energy content of protein meals. Rojas and Scott (1969) showed that incubation (in vitro) of both cottonseed meal and soybean meal with a phytase improved the metabolizable energy content of both meals. Rojas and Scott (1969) also demonstrated that addition of phytase decreased the amount of gossypol in cottonseed meal as well as reducing total phytate. The authors suggest part of the improvement in metabolizable energy digestibility is due to the breakdown of bonds between phytate and other compounds such as protein. Therefore, any breakdown in phytate–protein complexes is likely to increase protein digestibility.

Because enzyme products can be relatively expensive, alternative sources of phytase from plants have been sought. The intrinsic phytase activity in plant materials is higher in wheat, wheat bran, barley and triticale but lower in maize and legume seeds which have been heat treated (Eeckhout et al., 1994; Schroder et al., 1996). Of 285 samples from 51 feedstuffs tested by Eeckhout et al. (1994), only 13 were found to have >100 U kg^{-1} of intrinsic phytase activity. All other samples had zero or very small amounts of phytase (Table 19.3).

Han et al. (1998) tested the value of wheat middlings as a practical phytase source for pigs. Their experiment showed gain, feed intake, feed conversion ratio (FCR) and metatarsal bone strength were equal for a maize–soybean diet with 150 g kg^{-1} wheat middlings, maize–soybean plus 1200 U phytase or maize–soybean plus 2 g kg^{-1} inorganic P.

To reduce the diet cost, Han et al. (1998) reduced the level of phytase to 300 U kg^{-1} and added citric acid (15 g kg^{-1}) to maize–soybean diets containing either 100 or 150 g kg^{-1} wheat middlings. The addition of both phytase and citric acid improved gain and FCR compared with the diet without citric acid. The authors suggested that the additional citric acid had

Table 19.3. Feed ingredients with >100 units kg^{-1} of phytase activity.

Cereals		Wheat by-products	
Barley	582	Fine bran meal	460
Rye	5130	pellets	2573
Triticale	1688	Middlings	4381
Wheat	1193	Feed flour	3350
		Bran	2957

Source: Eeckhout et al. (1994).

reduced the gastrointestinal pH to an optimum which better suited the microbial phytase, allowing more P to be released.

In summary:

- Phytase addition allows the release of plant P that is not otherwise available to the animal. Phytase may also release other minerals and protein bound to phytate in compounds called phytate complexes. Phytase addition reduces the need for inorganic P supplementation, and in turn reduces the P content excreted by animals.
- The amount of P released by a given amount of phytase is affected by diet composition.
- Some cereals including barley, triticale, rye, wheat and wheat by-products have significant inherent phytase activity. Heat treatment of vegetable proteins deactivates inherent phytase activity. Inherent phytase activity increases the availability of P in the plant source in which it is contained but has no effect on other ingredients in the diet.
- The choice of phytase source either as a feed supplement, in feedstuffs with high intrinsic phytase or combinations of these sources with or without additional products such as organic acid will be made on the P-releasing capacity and price of each competing source.

Role of proteases

Many vegetable protein sources such as soybean contain protease inhibitors, lectins and tannins which reduce animal performance. To remove the anti-nutritive effects of these compounds, legume seed is heat treated. Unfortunately heat treatment can reduce the availability of amino acids.

As an alternative to heat treatment, enzymes have proved partially successful in deactivating anti-nutritional factors in legume seed (Bohme, 1997). For example, the addition of a protease to non-heat-treated canola meal improved broiler chick growth (Simbaya *et al.*, 1996). Yet, it is in combination with other enzyme activities where proteases have been most successful.

The inclusion of a protease in multi-enzyme supplements has proven beneficial for chicks (Ranade and Rajmane, 1992; Morgan and Bedford, 1995; Simbaya *et al.*, 1996) and layer egg yield and for piglet gain and FCR (Adams, 1989). Not all experiments have shown improved performance with proteases (Officer, 1995). In Officer (1995), two protease containing multienzyme supplements failed to improve piglet performance. It appears that both the type of protease and the complementary enzyme activities in the multienzyme supplement influence digestibility.

Antigenic effects of soybean on piglets are not always removed with heat treatment. Rooke *et al.* (1998) added an acid pH protease to soybean meal and improved piglet growth in the 7 days immediately post-weaning. No reduction in soybean-specific antibodies was observed for the acid protease-supplemented pigs. This experiment was brief in duration and there was no evidence of soybean having an antigenic effect on any of the treatments.

The fact that proteases improve performance in some circumstances is remarkable. Except for the period immediately post-weaning, ileal digestibility of protein is high as a result of endogenous protease activity.

Two points are worth noting:

- Multienzyme supplements containing protease have proven beneficial in both pigs and poultry.
- There is potential for further research into protease supplementation of non-heat-treated legume seed.

Feed enzymes are added to diets of many of the animal species we farm. The effectiveness of various types of enzymes is discussed for poultry, pigs and some aquaculture and ruminant animals.

Enzyme Supplementation of Poultry Diets

Broilers

More than any other animal industry, it has been the broiler industry which has most widely adopted feed enzyme technology. Annison (1997) suggests that feed enzymes have proved successful with broilers, for the following reasons:

1. The digestive system of the chicken is relatively simple which makes it susceptible to digestive upsets that may be overcome by specific feed enzymes.
2. Considerable research effort into the additional enzyme activities required by chickens and the composition of feed ingredients has allowed nutritionists to target dietary components which at present either impair animal performance or are of no nutritional value without enzymes.
3. Research into the effects of feed enzymes in chickens can be done inexpensively, compared with larger animals. The favourable cost of research with chickens means observations can be made based on sound scientific principals in terms of statistics, chemistry and physiology. Also, experiments with broilers produce results quickly which in turn speeds up development of new products.

Many early experiments with broilers looked at their response to enzymes from day-old chicks for just 21 days and not the whole growing period of 35–49 days. Response to enzymes is much higher over the 21-day period and does not truly reflect their response from birth to slaughter. Jeroch et al. (1995) completed a comprehensive review (1987–1995) of enzyme preparations for broilers. Over this period, there were 33 broiler experiments (from Europe and Canada) which looked at the effects of enzyme supplementation over the

whole growing period (Table 19.4). The rye and triticale diets produced the greatest weight gain and FCR response to enzymes, followed by barley diets, with the smallest improvement coming from enzyme-supplemented wheat diets. Although the magnitude of the improvement brought about by enzymes was small, the improvements are economically significant because of the large numbers of birds produced on each farm.

Broilers are particularly sensitive to the water-soluble polysaccharide content (mainly arabinoxyl) of cereals. The birds' sensitivity to water-soluble polysaccharides was detected when the apparent metabolizable energy content of approximately 25% of Australian wheat was found to be less than was predicted from proximate analysis and gross energy determinations (Rogel et al., 1987). Annison (1991) showed that there is a negative correlation between water-soluble polysaccharide content (mainly arabinoxyl) and apparent metabolizable energy content. Therefore, any genetic or growing conditions which favour water-soluble polysaccharide production will reduce broiler performance. A rapid, cheap and effective method is required to measure soluble NSP, which will allow enzyme supplementation to be based on actual NSP content not typical values.

Diets with high levels of pentosans or β-glucans can increase the digesta viscosity which in turn increases the incidence of sticky droppings. The addition of pentosanase to rye-based diets (Pettersson and Aman, 1988, 1989; Bedford et al., 1991)

Table 19.4. Effect of enzyme supplementation of barley-, rye-, triticale- and wheat-based broiler diets on final body weight and feed conversion ratio (FCR).

Cereal	No. of experiments	Inclusion (g kg^{-1})	Improvement in final weight (%)[a]	Improvement in FCR (%)
Barley	11	350–700	3.5 (0–6)	3.6 (0–6)
Rye/triticale	11	155–600	4.6–7.5 (0.5–14)	3.2–4.6 (0.5–6.5)
Wheat	11	150–660	0.6–2.3 (−3 to 7.5)	1.5–2.8 (−1 to 6.5)

[a]Mean response with a range of enzyme doses (range).
Summary of Jeroch et al. (1995) Table 3. Note: the rye experiment of Petterrson and Aman (1988) was excluded from the table as an outlier with a 34% increase in final weight and 8% improvement in FCR.

and β-glucanase to barley-based poultry diets reduces the problem of sticky droppings (Broz and Frigg, 1986; Elwinger and Sarterby, 1987; Rotter et al., 1989; Brufau et al., 1991) and can also increase the metabolizable energy content of the diet.

Apart from carbohydrases, supplementary phytase has been used to improve P digestibility in poultry diets and provide P which is similar in biological value to inorganic P (Qian et al., 1996a,b). The level of phytase required varies depending upon a number of factors, including diet composition and bird age.

The amount of total and phytate P, Ca and Zn and the concentration of inherent phytase activity all affect the amount of phytase required to release sufficient P to meet the bird's requirements. In an experiment with day-old male broilers, Kornegay et al. (1996) measured the efficiency of phytase (0–1200 U) added to maize–soybean diets with three levels of non-phytate P of 2.0, 2.7 or 3.4 g kg^{-1}. Increasing levels of phytase linearly improved body weight gain, feed intake, toe ash % and apparent retention (% of intake) of total Ca + P. Phytase linearly decreased P excretion. The size of the response to phytase was inversely related to the level of non-phytate P in the diet. In contrast to phytase, increasing supplementation of non-phytate P increased P excretion and reduced P retention. In this experiment, 939 U kg^{-1} of microbial phytase activity were required to replace 1 g of defluorinated phosphate for broilers given maize–soybean diets.

Schoner et al. (1993a) showed that the amount of phytase required increases as dietary Ca levels increase. There were three levels of Ca tested in the Schoner et al. (1993a) experiment (6, 7.5 and 9 g kg^{-1}). All diets were based on a maize–soybean combination that was P deficient (3.5 g kg^{-1} total P). In the diet with 6 g kg^{-1} Ca, 1 g of inorganic P was equivalent to 570 U phytase. Increasing Ca from 6 to 9 g kg^{-1} required more phytase to be added to meet the bird's P requirements.

Phytase supplementation not only affects/or is affected by P and Ca level, but also Zn. Thiel et al. (1993) found Zn retention in broilers increased by an amount equivalent to 15 mg kg^{-1} of supplementary Zn with the addition of 700 U kg^{-1} of phytase. This response occurred in a diet which contained 30 mg kg^{-1} Zn. As additional Zn (4, 9 and 15 mg kg^{-1}) was added, the effect of phytase on Zn retention diminished. The Zn and Ca experiments described show how important it is to know the mineral balance of a diet before recommending an optimum concentration of exogenous phytase.

Schoner et al. (1993a) also showed that the inorganic P equivalence of phytase is dependent upon broiler age (30–70 days of age). Using liveweight as the criterion, broilers at 44 days of age required 570 U of phytase to release 1 g of P. By 70 days of age, the amount of phytase required to release 1 g of P had increased to 850 U. This result suggests that phytase efficiency declines with increasing age.

Increasing the P digestibility of a diet can significantly reduce the amount of inorganic P required in the diet and reduce P pollution. In those countries where there are limits on P addition to the soil, Schoner et al. (1991) estimated that a 14% increase in P retention would allow a 50% increase in the stocking rate of broilers from 350 to 525 birds per dung unit (1 dung unit = 50 kg of P$_2$O$_5$). This means that more birds can be grown on a given area without exceeding application levels of waste P to land set by legislation.

Layers

Considerably fewer experiments have been conducted with laying hens than broilers and the measured effect of enzymes on digestibility is smaller. Enzyme supplementation of barley-rich layer diets had no significant effect on layer production or feed:egg (kg kg^{-1}) efficiency in a number of experiments (Al Bustany and Elwinger, 1988; Nasi, 1988 (experiment 1); Aimonen and Nasi, 1991; Gruzauskas et al., 1991 (two experiments); Jeroch, 1991 (experiments 1 and 2); Benabdeljelil and Arbaoui, 1994 (two experiments); Roth Maier and Kirchgessner, 1995). The lack of response to enzyme supplementation with layers may be due to the age of the bird (starting age 21–31 weeks), compared with the digestively immature broiler chick. Stevens *et al.* (1988) have also noted the effects of enzymes on production declines with age.

Although Aimonen and Nasi (1991) showed no effect of enzymes on laying performance, the multienzyme supplement used increased the apparent metabolizable energy content of oats (from 11.8 to 12.1 MJ kg^{-1}) and improved FCR by 3%. The multi-enzyme supplement only had an effect when oats provided >8% crude fibre.

Nasi (1988) showed that a β-glucanase preparation had no effect on layer perform-ance on barley-, wheat- or hulled oat-based diets. Yet when Nasi (1988) included a cel-lulase, β-glucanase and protease formula-tion, layer egg production and feed conversion were improved. Graham (1991) also measured a small improvement in egg production with the addition of another multienzyme product to a barley-based diet. Other experiments which have mea-sured improved egg production include those of Iotsius *et al.* (1986), Adams (1989), Jeroch (1991) (experiment 3) and Zang *et al.* (1995). Addition of multienzyme sup-plements has proven to be generally more effective in improving egg production than supplements which contained only one enzyme.

In addition to some experiments showing improved performance, there is a hygiene benefit from the addition of enzymes to rye, wheat and barley diets for layers. Enzyme supplementation reduces sticky droppings as a result of reduced water intake (Jeroch *et al.*, 1995) and digesta viscosity (Bedford, 1993). Less sticky droppings means fewer dirty eggs (Francesh *et al.*, 1995).

Enzyme supplementation tends to be most efficacious in layers when β-glucanase products are added to diets with significant amounts of barley. For enzyme addition to wheat-based diets to be reliably beneficial in terms of egg production, more work is required to improve our knowledge of the relationship between bird metabolism and wheat carbohydrate chemistry. A quick, cheap and reliable means of measuring the NSP in wheat is warranted to improve the reliability of adding enzymes to poultry diets containing wheat.

Even though improvements in digestibility with carbohydrase enzyme supplementation of layer diets is generally smaller than for broilers, significant improvements in P digestibility and reten-tion can be made. Schoner *et al.* (1993b) showed that P excretion in layers was reduced by 45–50% with 400–500 U kg^{-1} of phytase compared with a monocalcium phosphate-supplemented control.

Recent findings are summarized below:

- Broilers are sensitive to many anti-nutritional factors and therefore respond favourably to appropriate enzyme supplementation (i.e. β-glucanases for barley; pentosanases for rye and wheat; phytase for phytate). Multienzyme supplements tend to be more effective than single activity supplements.
- The amount of enzyme required varies with bird age and diet composition (NSP, Ca, Zn and total and phytate P).
- Layers are less responsive to enzyme supplementation than broilers. Benefits such as less sticky droppings, increased egg production and FCR have been measured, especially when the enzyme supplement has multiple activities.

Enzyme Supplementation of Pig Diets

Unlike the broiler industry, the pig indus-try has been more cautious in accepting feed enzymes because the pig's response to them is less consistent. Compared with poultry, the efficacy of feed enzymes in pig diets has been less consistent. Young pigs rely on enzymatic digestion for the release of most of their nutrients, which means that they are more susceptible to anti-nutritional factors in their diet. By the time a pig reaches 50 kg, around 30% of its energy requirements come from fermenta-tion in the hindgut (Rerat *et al.*, 1987).

Despite this two-pronged approach to digestion, some feed compounds are still not well utilized.

Poor digestion of solid feed by piglets weaned at 21–28 days of age is especially obvious in the first 2–3 weeks after weaning (Cera *et al.*, 1988). Inappropriate choice of feed ingredients at this time can produce diarrhoea, due in part to a lack of pancreatic and intestinal enzyme activity and/or by the colonization by enterotoxigenic coli bacteria (Cera *et al.*, 1988). The lack of pancreatic and intestinal enzyme activity results in more nutrients passing through the digestive system rather than being absorbed by it. These nutrients provide the substrate for pathogenic bacteria such as *Escherichia coli* which produce enterotoxins (affecting the enterocyctes in the wall of the intestine). These in turn increase intestinal secretions and further reduce digestion and absorption. Removal of dietary ingredients which may produce diarrhoea or hypersensitivity reactions often means providing diets with minimal vegetable protein meals and cereals which are low in fibre and are more expensive. Supplementation with feed enzymes has the potential to increase the use of vegetable protein meals and high-fibre cereals and reduce diet cost without compromising piglet health.

Typical endogenous protease and amylase activity levels in piglets suggest that supplementation should not be required except for a short period (1–2 weeks) immediately post-weaning (Lindemann *et al.*, 1986; Owsley *et al.*, 1986). This was confirmed by Cromwell *et al.* (1988), who showed that an amylase–protease combination was effective in improving piglet performance but not when the pigs were older or with protease alone.

The results of enzyme addition to pigs have been highly variable, with many weaner pig enzyme trials failing to demonstrate any benefit in terms of health or increased production. For example, a literature survey revealed that of 23 enzyme supplements for which growth trials were conducted between 1978 and 1993, only four improved growth rate of piglets (Officer, 1995). In growing–finishing pigs, the growth-promoting effect of NSP-degrading enzymes supplemented to cereal diets has also not been established with certainty (Chu *et al.*, 1998).

Soluble NSP does not appear to depress pig performance as it does in birds. Thacker *et al.* (1988) showed no improvement in weight gain intake or feed conversion of 20 kg pigs (given a hull-less barley high in soluble glucan). This was despite recording significant increases in dry matter and protein digestibility in pigs given the diet supplemented with β-glucanase. Unlike in birds, pentosans do not appear to be a significant cause of reduced performance in young pigs. Pentosanase supplementation of a rye-based diet given to 20–25 kg pigs (Thacker *et al.*, 1991) failed to significantly improve growth. Supplementation with β-glucanase in 80 kg pigs tended to improve dry matter and protein digestibility, but these changes were thought to be too small to improve weight gain or FCR.

In recent years, the most significant development in feed enzyme technology has been the release of phytase. Research with phytase (1000 U kg^{-1} diet) has shown that it increases P digestibility by 36–55% in maize–soybean and by 54–68% in wheat–soybean diets given to 5-week-old weaner pigs (Eeckhout *et al.*, 1992a). Jongbloed (1997) also states that no inorganic P is required in phytase-supplemented diets for grower–finisher pigs and pregnant sows. The benefits from adding phytase are significant in terms of reducing diet cost, improving mineral retention and animal performance, but unfortunately recommendations for phytase supplementation vary with class of pig and diet (Yi *et al.*, 1996). There is no standard level of phytase supplementation for all diets because the total and phytate P level of each diet varies.

These two experiments show how the P equivalence of phytase is dependent upon the diet. Yi *et al.* (1996) found that the amount of phytase required to release 1 g of phytate P varied from 785 U, for a maize–soybean diet, to 1146 U, for a semi-purified soybean diet. Piglets given a maize–oats–soybean meal diet required only 380 U of phytase to release 1 g of P (Hoppe *et al.*, 1993).

The P-releasing power of microbial phytase and wheat phytase are very different. Eeckhout *et al.* (1992b) compared the efficacy of 500 U of wheat middlings phytase and natuphos (microbial phytase) in 13 kg piglets. Although both phytase sources increased digestibility of P and Ca, the microbial phytase was 74% more efficient. The increased effectiveness of the microbial phytase was attributed to its ability to retain activity at lower pHs than wheat phytase. The additional benefit of microbial phytase was that there was 27% less P found in the faeces compared with a maize–soybean meal–heated wheat middlings diet (i.e. no phytase activity) without microbial phytase supplementation.

Eeckhout *et al.* (1992c) conducted the same experiment with 50 kg pigs. As a result, pigs given 500 U kg^{-1} of microbial phytase had 0.035% (20% of requirements) more absorbable P. There was no evidence from Eekhout *et al.* (1992c) to suggest that the efficiency of microbial phytase is affected by pig weight between 13 and 50 kg. Over a broader range in liveweight and physiological status, phytase efficacy does change (Kemme *et al.*, 1997) (Table 19.5). All pigs in this experiment were given identical diets containing Ca 6.2 g kg^{-1}, total P 4.8 g kg^{-1} and phytate P 3.7 g kg^{-1} with an intrinsic phytase activity of 120 FTU kg^{-1}. This table shows how stage of pregnancy and liveweight influence the amount of P released by phytase.

Mroz *et al.* (1994) showed the importance of feeding level and feeding frequency on the apparent digestibility of phytate P, N and Ca in grower pigs (45 kg) given supplementary phytase (800 U kg^{-1}). Phytase increased the apparent total tract digestibility of DM OM, CP, Ca, total P and all amino acids except cysteine and proline. Increasing the feeding level from 2.3 to 2.8 times maintenance improved the retention of N, Ca and P, and increasing the feeding frequency from once to seven times per day

Table 19.5. Effect of physiological status of a pig on the efficiency of P release (g) with the addition of 500 FTU kg^{-1} phytase.

Physiological status	g Extra digestible P
Lactating sows	1.03
Grower/finishing pigs	0.83
Sow (end of pregnancy)	0.74
Piglets	0.66
Sows (mid-pregnancy)	0.32

Kemme *et al.* (1997a).

increased the ileal digestibility of phytic acid and some amino acids. This experiment highlights how difficult it is to interpret and compare results between experiments as there are a large number of factors influencing the efficiency of supplementary phytase.

In summary:

- Pigs are less susceptible to dietary anti-nutritional factors than broilers and are less likely to show an economic response to enzyme supplementation. Of the classes of pig, it is the piglet that stands to benefit most from enzyme supplementation. Multienzyme supplements tend to be more effective than those with single activity.
- Microbial phytase can increase P availability, Ca + N retention and decrease P excretion in young pigs. The efficiency of phytase is affected by diet, feeding level, feeding frequency, source and amount of phytase and the physiological state of the pig.

Feed Enzymes in Aquaculture

Aquaculture has been relatively slow to adopt feed enzyme technology. This is possibly due to its reliance, until recently, on fish meal as the sole or major source of protein, especially for carnivorous species. Fish meal is highly digestible and meant there was little to be gained by adding either protease or carbohydrases.

Yet, in recent years, the world catch of wild fish has begun to decline and alternatives to fish meal protein have been sought.

Plant feed sources are cheaper than fish meal but are also higher in fibre and anti-nutritive factors such as phytin, gossypol, trypsin inhibitors, lectins, etc. Therefore, feed enzymes, now more than in the past, have a significant role to play in increasing the utilization of plant protein sources by aquaculture species.

Experience from other animal species would suggest the young animals grown under aquaculture conditions should benefit most from the inclusion of feed enzymes. However, research with small fish, as with immature land animals, has produced variable responses to enzymes. Kolkovski *et al.* (1997) found the feed intake and growth of seabass larvae (*Dicentrarchus labrax*) were unaffected by a pancreatin enzyme supplement. Yet, larvae of gilthead seabream (*Pagrus aurata*) fed a pancreatin supplemented micro-diet had 30% higher assimilation rates than larvae offered the control diet (Kolkovski *et al.*, 1993). Despite the improved assimilation rate of the enzyme-supplemented larvae, their intake was only half that of larvae given a live feed regime. This suggests that the characteristics which attract fish to feed may be as important as improvements in diet digestibility produced by enzyme supplementation.

The variable response to enzyme supplementation is also found with older fish. Neither the feed intake nor feed conversion efficiency of Atlantic salmon parr (*Salmo salar*) were affected by supplementation with an α-amylase (Carter *et al.*, 1992). Similarly, Renitz (1983) found that proteolytic enzymes did not improve weight gain or feed conversion efficiency (FCE) of rainbow trout given a standard USA Fish and Wildlife Service starter diet. Yet, carp given diets supplemented with a multienzyme pre-mix at 5 or 10 g kg^{-1} had 12.3 and 27.5% faster growth rates than control-fed fish (Ye *et al.*, 1995). Gorskova and Yu-Dvinen (1984) working with Coho salmon and Carter *et al.* (1994) working with Atlantic salmon have also measured improved animal performance with enzyme supplementation.

For fish, as for other monogastric species, phytate P is an anti-nutritive factor. The level of phytase activity required to improve P digestibility varies depending on the fish species and diet. For example, Li and Robinson (1997) showed that 250 U kg^{-1} of phytase was required to replace inorganic P in a practical channel catfish diet. Increasing the phytase level to 500 or 750 U kg^{-1} produced no improvement in intake, weight gain, FCR, bone ash or P compared with fish given the 250 U phytase kg^{-1}-supplemented treatment. Lunari *et al.* (1998) showed that 1000 U kg^{-1} of phytase increased P digestibility from 58.6 to 68.1% for rainbow trout.

Most research with feed enzymes in aquaculture species has added the enzyme supplement to the whole diet. In contrast, Cain and Garling (1995) gave rainbow trout (*Onchoryhnchus mykiss*) diets containing phytase-treated or untreated soybean meal. Phytase treatment either produced equal or better trout growth rates and FCE than those given the control diet. The efficiency of phytase action can depend on the weight of the fish. Phytase supplementation reduced effluent P by 65% with 2 g fish compared with 88% for fish weighing 17 g. These results show that inclusion of phytase can reduce the amount of inorganic P required in fish diets by increasing the availability of P in plant feed ingredients. In addition, the P concentration of fish effluent can be reduced by phytase supplementation, which may have significant implications for water quality.

Two points now emerge:

- There is an increasing trend for fish meal to be replaced in aquaculture diets by other protein sources including those from plants. This will mean that the importance of feed enzyme supplementation will continue to increase in the future.
- The response of fish to proteolytic and carbohydrase enzymes has been variable. Only phytase has proven consistently to improve digestibility in a range of situations.

Enzyme Supplementation of Ruminant Diets

Feed enzymes, although part of many bacteria-based silage starters, are not widely used as direct-fed additives in ruminant diets (Beauchemin and Rode, 1996). Research with feed enzymes in ruminant diets has found them to be unreliable (Leatherwood et al., 1960; Perry et al., 1966; Adoglabessa and Owen, 1995) and, until recently, the cost of development and production of enzymes for ruminants was prohibitive. Improvements in recombinant DNA technology (Selinger et al., 1996) and research with monogastric animals should see the development and release of direct-fed enzyme products specifically for ruminants.

Part of the slow uptake of enzyme technology by ruminant feed manufacturers is due to the fact there is no simple foolproof recipe for applying enzymes and securing a profitable response. A lack of understanding in the way enzymes act in ruminant feed and the complex digestive tract of ruminants means that there are many unidentified or misunderstood factors influencing feed enzyme efficacy in ruminant animals.

Enzyme supplementation in ruminants may be complex, but this should not deter investment in research and development. Improvements in the efficiency of feed utilization as the result of feed enzymes will increase production profitability and waste minimization in a large, and as yet relatively untapped, ruminant feed enzyme market.

Like monogastrics, ruminants can benefit from products that improve starch, protein and fibre digestibility. However, before beneficial enzymes can be included in the diet, a reliable method of applying feed enzymes to ruminant feed is required that accounts for the fermentation processes of the rumen.

Method of applying feed enzymes

Research to date has shown that the method of applying the enzymes can significantly alter their efficacy. The direct infusion of enzymes into the rumen is far less effective (Lewis, 1996) or can even reduce digestibility of forage compared with application of liquid enzyme to hay. Direct application is thought to be more effective as a result of binding of the feed enzyme to its substrate, rather than the enzyme being broken down in the rumen fluid by endogenous protease enzymes.

The effect of feed enzymes on in vivo digestibility is influenced by the moisture content of the forage prior to enzyme application. Feng et al. (1996) applied a cellulase and xylanase enzyme mixture to fresh and wilted hay with no effect. When the enzymes were added to dry forage immediately before feeding, however, they improved dry matter and neutral detergent fibre digestibility.

Given the importance of combining the enzyme with the feed prior to its entry into the rumen, it is important to know if there is an optimal enzyme treatment period. Treacher and Hunt (1996) reported on unpublished research which showed increases in gas production immediately after enzymes were added to maize silage. The maximum gas production occurred after 4 h of combining the enzymes and maize silage. The authors noted that their in vitro results do not necessarily indicate that enzyme addition was increasing volatile fatty acid (VFA) production. Yet the gas production results in combination with changes in the structure of this silage (measured by near infrared spectroscopy) suggest that as little as 2 h between enzyme application and feeding may be required to maximize the effect of the enzymes on maize silage digestibility.

Much more work is required to elucidate fully the optimum treatment period for enzyme formulations for typical dietary ingredients. This lack of knowledge is important because there are two main ways of using enzymes in ruminant feeds. In the first method, the feed is treated with an enzyme preparation well before it is offered to the animal. In the second, the feed enzyme is added to the feed within 1 h of it being offered.

The research of both Nakashima and Orskov (1989) and Beauchemin *et al.* (1995) shows the potential value of pre-processing feed with enzymes. Yet to ensile or cube feed requires capital to be invested possibly months before the feed is used. The reliability of combining ensiling or cubing with enzymes as a means of improving animal performance requires more research before the technique can be relied upon. Unlike the pre-processing approach, the addition of enzymes just prior to feeding (also known as the direct-fed approach) provides greater flexibility in the use of forages and minimizes the time and/or resources (silage bunker, etc.) required.

Pre-processing of forage with feed enzymes involves applying the enzyme supplement well before feeding. Silage, for example, is made by adding an inoculum prior to sealing up of forage in a bunker or wrapping round bales with plastic (haylage). The first silage additive based on enzymes alone appeared in the UK in 1985 (Treacher and Hunt, 1996). Improved enzyme formulations produce well-preserved silage, and around 75% of UK silage additives for grass and maize now contain enzymes. The enzyme activities found in commercial additives do not mimic the protein degradability of strained rumen fluid (Luchini *et al.*, 1996). This is probably a good feature because it means that feed enzyme activities are more likely to be complementary rather than competitive with endogenous enzyme activities.

By ensiling straw with a cellulase–xylanase mixture, Nakashima and Orskov (1989) improved the potential degradability of the straw by 10%. Beauchemin *et al.* (1995) measured improvements in the average daily gain (30%) and a 10% increase in dry matter intake of steers offered lucerne and timothy grass hay that had been treated with enzymes during the cubing process. It is encouraging to see feed pre-processed with enzymes improving ruminant growth. The economics of this technique, however, must be evaluated against application of enzymes at feeding.

The application of enzymes at or just prior to feeding is called direct-fed application. If enzymes can be added to the forage portion of the diet, at or just prior to feeding, and produce improvements in intake and digestibility, then the amount of concentrate in the diet and the diet cost can be reduced. Lewis *et al.* (1996) found that direct application of a cellulase and xylanase mix to the forage of a 70:30 grass hay:barley diet improved neutral detergent fibre digestibility. Improvements in digestibility have also resulted in increases in production.

Schingoethe *et al.* (1999) measured a 10.8% increase in milk production, a 20% increase in milk fat and a 13% increase in milk protein as a result of adding a cellulase and xylanase mixture at feeding. Enzyme supplementation increased milk production in the first 100 days of lactation but not in mid-lactation. The improved milk production was equivalent to providing the cows with a 45% forage:55% concentrate diet rather than the control diet which contained 55% forage and 45% concentrate. The simplicity of direct-fed application of enzymes should see it develop as the enzyme application technique of choice for ruminants in the future.

Other factors influencing efficacy of feed enzymes in ruminants

Apart from the method of applying feed enzymes, there are a number of factors which influence the efficacy of feed enzymes. These factors include diet composition, microbial source of enzyme activity, mixture of enzyme activities, inclusion rate, heat stability, ambient temperature at feeding and class of animal.

Obviously the ingredients in the diet influence the feed enzyme activities required to maximize improvement in digestibility. Beauchemin *et al.* (1997) measured the effect of two enzymes on the growth of feedlot cattle given either maize grain and maize silage or barley grain and barley silage diets. The enzyme with higher xylanase activity improved the FCR of cattle given the barley diets but not of those given maize. Beauchemin and Rode (1996) measured increased daily gain (6%) and feed DM:gain (11%) of cattle with an enzyme supplement containing a high xylanase:low cellulase ratio. No benefits were obtained by cattle given a low xylanase:high cellulase supplement. These results show the importance of having the correct balance of enzyme activity based on diet composition.

Not all enzyme combinations produce benefits for the enzyme-supplemented animal; some can have a negative effect on growth or feed conversion efficiency (Treacher and Hunt, 1996). Treacher and Hunt (1996) tested a range of cellulase and xylanase enzyme products and suggested that more work was required to identify useful combinations of enzymes for diets based on various crop products. Ruminants have bacteria that produce phytase activity (Yanke, 1998). Further research is required to determine if feed phytase has any potential in ruminant diets.

Not only the type of forage, but also the stage of maturity at harvest can influence the optimum enzyme concentration required to improve animal performance. Michal et al. (1996) showed that when the neutral detergent fibre content of lucerne haylage increased from 415 to 540 g kg^{-1}, the optimum enzyme (cellulase/xylanase) dose rate increased from 2.5 l t^{-1} to 5.0 l t^{-1}. Therefore, it is important to know not only the concentration of fibre in each batch of feed but also other factors such as feed pH which may influence the activity of enzymes when added to feed.

The concentration of enzymes added to the diet can be critical to maximizing improvement in animal performance. Treacher and Hunt (1996) showed that dairy cows given 5 l t^{-1} of enzyme-treated maize silage–lucerne hay (80:20) produce less milk than cows given a control diet. Yet cows given 2 l t^{-1} of enzymes produced 6.8% more milk and 7.8% more protein. Sanchez et al. (1996) also showed improvements in milk yield at 2.5 l t^{-1} of cellulose/xylanase enzyme but not at 1.25 or 5.0 l t^{-1}.

Treacher and Hunt (1996) suggested three possible explanations for reduced animal performance with excessive addition of enzymes. Firstly, it is possible that high doses of enzymes reduce the amount of neutral detergent fibre available for fermentation by rumen microorganisms which in turn reduces microbial protein and VFA production. Secondly, the presence of bound enzymes restricts the access of microorganisms to the feed. Thirdly, it is possible that enzymes release anti-nutritional by-products (e.g. phenols) which inhibit microbial growth.

Not only the rumen environment but also the external environment can influence how well feed enzymes work. It is well known in enzyme chemistry that interactions with a substrate are influenced by temperature. Treacher et al. (1996) showed there is a 1.5–2.0% increase in gas production per 10°C (from −30 to 30°C) from enzyme-treated barley silage. This result may suggest problems with the effectiveness of feed enzymes in the cooler parts of the USA, Canada and Europe, but benefits for subtropical countries.

Little is known of the differences between various classes of stock in their response to feed enzymes, but Beauchemin and Rode (1996) showed that heifers were more responsive to enzyme addition than steers. More research is required to determine if gender, age or physiological state influence the ability of feed enzymes to improve ruminant diet digestibility.

In short:

- Our understanding of the mode of action of enzymes in ruminants is poor. As a result, there is as yet no proven and reliable means of direct application of enzymes to ruminant feed. Despite this, some experiments have shown carbohydrase feed enzymes have the potential to improve ruminant production.

- Recommendations on the period between feed application and consumption and general recommendations on optimum concentrations of enzymes for different diets are also not yet available.

- Further research should prove valuable because there is considerable potential to improve digestive efficiency and/or growth rate or milk production by ruminant animals.

Effect of Feed Enzymes on Diet Formulation and Feed Preparation

Feed enzymes are known to produce variable responses even when given to the same-aged animal and in similar diets. Therefore, either variability in feed enzyme formulations between batches of the same product or variable composition of individual ingredients is altering the effectiveness of the same enzyme formulation.

Shelf life

Enzyme formulations have a shelf life that is dependent upon storage conditions. A product which has not been stored according to the manufacturer's recommendations cannot be guaranteed to maintain its enzyme activity.

Heat stability

Most feed manufactured for monogastric animals is sold in a form which has been heat processed. Therefore, any feed enzyme product must be able to withstand typical feed processing conditions. Fungal enzymes tend to be less heat stable than those derived from bacteria (Cowan, 1993). Without any form of protection, fungal enzymes rapidly lose activity above 60°C.

Fungal enzymes which have been stabilized and granulated can withstand up to 75°C and even 80°C if the granules are coated. Some bacterial enzymes are capable of tolerating between 85 and 90°C for short periods.

Loss of some enzyme activity due to heat may not always reduce animal performance. For example, the retention of β-glucanase activity was measured by Inborr and Bedford (1994) after broiler feed was conditioned at 75, 85 or 95°C for 30 s or 15 min before pelleting (Table 19.6). Enzyme activity was reduced at all temperatures and activity loss increased with the longer conditioning time. Yet, chicken performance was reduced only when pelleting temperature exceeded 85°C. This research shows it is important to know what effect feed processing conditions are having on animal performance. If processing conditions are adverse for enzyme activity and these cannot be altered, then application of liquid enzymes post-pelleting is an alternative to developing heat-stable enzymes and enzyme formulations. This technique ensures even dosing of enzymes onto the feed and near total recovery of enzyme activity (Cowan, 1993).

Once enzymes have survived feed processing they must then retain their activity inside the animal after consumption. Chesson (1993) notes that fungal polysaccharidases are not destroyed *in vitro* by porcine proteases used singly or in combination. Using solid phase markers, Chesson (1993) found that around three-quarters of ingested enzyme activity was

Table 19.6. Effect of feed processing conditions on retention of β-glucanase activity (% of non-heat-treated mash control; coefficient of variation = 13.8%, *n* = 14) and broiler gain and feed conversion ratio (FCR).

| | β-Glucanase activity | | | |
| | Conditioning period | | Broiler performance | |
Temperature °C	30 s	15 min	Gain (g)	FCR
75	66	49	547	1.54
85	56	31	556	1.53
95	16	11	517	1.64

After Inborr and Bedford (1994).

recovered from young broilers after the enzyme had passed through the crop and proventriculus. The activity recovery percentage from the terminal ileum for both broiler and 40 kg pigs was between 8 and 32% (Table 19.7). Therefore, a considerable portion of the added activity is lost in the protease-rich environment of the gut and small intestine.

Measuring feed enzyme activity

Part of the problem with the interpretation of feed enzyme experiments is that the enzyme activity level is often not expressed or, if it is noted, then the units or method of measuring activity varies from one enzyme product to the next. In addition to this, once the enzyme is added at low concentration to the feed, it is often even harder to measure the enzyme activity level. Cowan (1993) tested four methods of measuring enzyme activity in feed both before and after pelleting. The methods and results were as follows:

1. The standard assay for the enzyme in question which proved insensitive with only 400–800 fungal enzyme units added per kg.
2. The ELISA analysis was sensitive, but antisera for all the enzymes to be tested were not available.
3. Measurement of reducing sugars after enzyme action and extraction of the enzyme from the feed was inaccurate due to the high background of reducing sugars.
4. Measurement of reducing sugars after extended incubation had similar problems as 3.

Cowan (1993) found that the only accurate method of measuring enzyme activity was to extract the enzyme from the feed and measure the activity using the standard assay after an extended incubation time. Cowan's method, although it works for a number of enzymes, is much more complicated than the technique developed by Walsh *et al.* (1995) for β-glucanase.

Walsh *et al.* (1995) developed a simple radial diffusion assay for β-glucanase activity which has a precision of ±4% and is sensitive enough to measure activities as low as 0.5 kg t^{-1} supplement equivalent. The Walsh *et al.* (1995) assay requires no specialized equipment and measures diffusion of an enzyme containing feed extract through agar containing β1–4 and β1–3 linkages from the glucan lichenan. There appears to be scope for further research into the use of media suitable for other commonly used fibre-degrading feed enzymes.

Measuring anti-nutritive factors in feed

The accuracy of feed enzyme supplementation would be significantly improved if we had cheap, rapid and accurate techniques for measuring anti-nutritive factors in the feed. Book values for NSP or phytate, by their very nature, are averages, and can be significantly different from what is found in practice.

For example, both the season (winter and spring) and the year in which a crop was grown can influence the amount of β-glucan in barley (Jeroch *et al.*, 1995). Jeroch

Table 19.7. Recovery of enzyme activities (U g^{-1}) from diets and the terminal ileum of young pigs and broilers given β-glucanase- and β-xylanase-supplemented diets (values in parentheses % of total added).

Sample	β-Glucanase	β-Xylanase
Total added enzyme	104	130
Recovered from pig feed	127 (122%)	88 (68%)
Recovered from pig ileum	33 (32%)	28 (22%)
Recovered from broiler feed	83 (80%)	83 (64%)
Recovered from broiler ileum	8 (8%)	25 (19%)

After Chesson (1993).

et al. (1995) examined winter and spring β-glucan data from seven European countries in data (from nine papers) that covered a 12-year period. β-Glucan content varied from 1.0 to 5.6%, with an annual mean of 3.56%. The largest range in β-glucan percentage for Spain in 1987 and 1988 was 3%. Between countries, there were no clear seasonal trends in β-glucan content. Although seasonal differences were evident, there was no consistent pattern. This work shows the importance of being able to measure the NSP content of all feed samples in a rapid, accurate and economic way. If the NSP content of each feed sample was known, enzyme inclusion levels could be adjusted to maximize NSP degradation.

The Future of Feed Enzymes

Future feed enzyme research should continue the process of refining enzyme formulations and application techniques and the development of rapid, cheap and reliable assays for measuring enzyme activity and anti-nutritional compounds. Improvements in these four areas will see the value of feed enzymes in animal nutrition continue to rise.

Although feed enzyme research with poultry and pigs has been extensive, there is still potential to identify and refine protease activities which will break down the anti-nutritive compounds found in raw legume seeds. If compounds such as trypsin inhibitors, lectins, etc. can be broken down by enzymes and heat treatment is not required, then the availability of amino acids in these legumes will be improved.

The amount of research required to develop the feed enzyme industry for ruminants to the same degree as the pig and poultry industries is large. More work is required to develop optimum combinations of enzyme activities dependent on diet composition. Application and feeding protocols for direct-fed feed enzymes are also needed in ruminant diets.

The aquaculture industry has much to gain from research on feed enzymes conducted with pigs and poultry. Little work has been done with carbohydrases which will become increasingly important as the amount of non-fish meal protein in aquaculture diets increases. More research is required to determine the factors that influence the efficiency of phytase in aquaculture diets.

The amounts of NSP and other anti-nutritive factors change with each feedstuff and even with each consignment of the same feed. There is therefore a need to measure the concentration of these factors and know how to alter feed enzyme formulations to maximize improvement in animal production. Research to develop simple assays for anti-nutritive factors and even feed enzyme activities is required if we are to understand why some experiments produce greater improvements in animal response than others. The sustainability of feeding animals diets based on ingredients that can be used for human food will be improved if feed enzyme technology is used to maximize utilization.

References

Adams, C.A. (1989) Kemzyme and animal feed digestion. *Krmiva* 31, 139–144.

Adoglabessa, T. and Owen, E. (1995) Ensiling of whole-crop wheat with cellulase–hemicellulase based enzymes. 2. Effect of crop growth-stage and enzyme on silage intake, digestibility and live-weight gain by steers. *Animal Feed Science and Technology* 55, 349–357.

Aimonen, E.M.J. and Nasi, M. (1991) Replacement of barley by oats and enzyme supplementation in diets for laying hens. 1. Performance and balance trial results. *Acta Agriculturae Scandinavica* 41, 179–192.

Al Bustany, Z. and Elwinger, K. (1988) Whole grains, unprocessed rapeseed and beta-glucanase in diets for laying hens. *Swedish Journal of Agricultural Research* 18, 31–40.

Annison, G. (1991) Relationship between levels of soluble non starch polysaccharides and the apparent metabolizable energy of wheats assayed in broiler chickens. *Journal of Agricultural and Food Chemistry* 39, 1252–1256.

Annison, G. (1997) The use of exogenous enzymes in ruminant diets. In: Corbet, J.L., Choct, M., Nolan, J.V. and Rowe, J.B. (eds) *Recent Advances in Animal Nutrition in Australia*. University of New England, Armidale, pp. 8–16.

Beauchemin, K.A. and Rode, L.M. (1996) The potential use of feed enzymes for ruminants. *Proceedings of the Cornell Nutrition Conference for Feed Manufacturers*. Rochester, New York, pp. 131–141.

Beauchemin, K.A., Rode, L.M. and Sewalt, V.J.H. (1995) Fibrolytic enzymes increase fibre digestibility and growth rate of steers fed dry forages. *Canadian Journal of Animal Science* 75, 641–644.

Beauchemin, K.A., Jones, S.D.M., Rode, L.M. and Sewalt, V.J.H. (1997) Effects of fibrolytic enzymes in corn or barley diets on performance and carcass characteristics of feedlot cattle. *Canadian Journal of Animal Science* 77, 645–653.

Bedford, M.R. (1993) Mode of action of feed enzymes. *Journal of Applied Poultry Research* 2, 85–92.

Bedford, M.R. (1995) Mechanism of action and potential environmental benefits from the use of feed enzymes. *Animal Feed Science and Technology* 53, 145–155.

Bedford, M.R., Classen, H.L. and Campbell, G.L. (1991) The effect of pelleting, salt, and pentosanase on the viscosity of intestinal contents and performance of broilers fed rye. *Poultry Science* 70, 1571–1577.

Benabdeljelil, K. and Arbaoui, M.I. (1994) Effects of enzyme supplementation of barley-based diets on hen performance and egg quality. *Animal Feed Science and Technology* 48, 325–334.

Bohme, H. (1997) Dietary enzymes in pig feeding. *Muhle Mischfuttertechnik* 134, 295–298.

Broz, J. and Frigg, M. (1986) Effects of beta-glucanase on the feeding value of broiler diets based on barley or oats. *Archiv fur Geflugelkunde* 50, 41–47.

Brufau, J., Nogareda, C., Perez-Vendrell, A., Fransech, M. and Esteve-Garcia, E. (1991) Effect of *Trichoderma viride* enzymes in pelleted broiler diets based on barley. *Animal Feed Science and Technology* 34, 193–202.

Cain, K.D. and Garling, D.L. (1995) Pre-treatment of soybean meal with phytase for salmonoid diets to reduce phosphorus concentrations in hatchery effluent. *Progressive Fish Culturist* 57, 114–119.

Carter, C.G., Houlihan, D.F. and McArthy, I.D. (1992) Feed utilization efficiencies of altlantic salmon (*Salmo salar* L.) parr: effect of a single supplementary enzyme. *Comparative Biochemistry and Physiology* 101, 369–374.

Carter, C.G., Houlihan, D.F., Buchanan, B. and Mitchell, A.I. (1994) Growth and feed utilization efficiencies of seawater atlantic salmon, (*Salmo salar* L.) fed a diet containing supplementary enzymes. *Aquaculture and Fisheries Management* 25, 37–46.

Cera, K.R., Mahan, D.C. and Reinhart, G.A. (1988) Effects of dietary dried whey and corn oil on weanling pig performance, fat digestibility and nitrogen utilization. *Journal of Animal Science* 66, 1438–1445.

Chesson, A. (1993) Feed enzymes. *Animal Feed Science and Technology* 45, 65–79.

Chu, K.S., Kim, J.H., Chae, B.J., Chung, Y.K. and Han, I.K. (1998) Effects of processed barley on growth performance and ileal digestibility of growing pigs. *Asian Australasian Journal of Animal Sciences* 11, 249–254.

Cowan, W.D. (1993) Application systems for the application and control of enzyme products in animal feed. *Journal of the Science of Food and Agriculture* 63, 110.

Cromwell, G.L., Cantor, A.H., Stahly, T.S. and Randolph, J.H. (1988) Efficacy of beta-glucanase addition to barley-based diets on performance of weanling and growing–finishing pigs and broiler chicks. *Journal of Animal Science* 66 (Suppl. 1), 46.

Eeckhout, W., De Paepe, M. and De Paepe, M. (1992a) Effects of microbial phytase on the apparent digestibility of phosphorus in diets for piglets. *Revue de L'Agriculture* 45, 183–193.

Eeckhout, W., De Paepe, M. and De Paepe, M. (1992b) Wheat phytase, microbial phytase and apparent digestibility of phosphorus in a common diet for piglets. *Revue de L'Agriculture* 45, 195–207.

Eeckhout, W., De Paepe, M. and De Paepe, M. (1992c) Comparison of the effect of 500 units of phytase of wheat and of a microbial preparation on the apparent digestibility of phosphorus in a diet for fattening pigs. *Revue de L'Agriculture* 45, 209–216.

Eeckhout, W., De Paepe, M. and De Paepe, M. (1994) Total phosphorus, phytate-phosphorus and phytase activity in plant feedstuffs. *Animal Feed Science and Technology* 47, 19–29.

Elwinger, K. and Saterby, B. (1987) The use of β-glucanase in practical broiler diets containing barley or oats. *Swedish Journal of Agricultural Research* 17, 133–139.

Feng, P., Hunt, W.W., Pritchard, G.T. and Julien, W.E. (1996) Effect of enzyme preparations on *in situ* and *in vitro* degradation and *in vivo* digestive characteristics of mature cool-season grass forage in beef steers. *Journal of Animal Science* 74, 1349–1357.

Francesch, M., Perez Vendrell, A.M., Esteve Garcia, E. and Brufau, J. (1995) Enzyme supplementation of a barley and sunflower-based diet on laying hen performance. *Journal of Applied Poultry Research* 4, 32–40.

Gorshkova, G.L. and Dvinin Yu, F. (1984) Effect of some enzyme preparations on growth and chemical composition of tissues of two year old Coho salmon. *Rybnoe, Khozyaistvo* 8, 40–42.

Graham, H. (1991) Developments in the application of feed enzymes in layer and turkey diets. *Feed Compounder* 11, 19–21.

Gruzauskas, R., Jeroch, H., Jeroch, K., Sirvydis, V., Danius, S. and Bobina, A. (1991) Effect of different enzyme preparations on the performance of laying hens fed with a feed mixture based on barley. *Proceedings of International Conference 'Industrial Enzymes, Probiotics and Biological Additives'*. Kaunas, pp. 32–35.

Han, Y.M., Roneker, K.R., Pond, W.G. and Lei, X.G. (1988) Adding wheat middlings, microbial phytase, and citric acid to corn–soybean meal diets for growing pigs may replace inorganic phosphorus supplementation. *Journal of Animal Science* 76, 2655.

Hoppe, P.P., Schoner, F.J., Wiesche, H., Schwarz, G. and Safer, S. (1993) Phosphorus equivalency of *Aspergillus niger* phytase for piglets fed a grain soybean meal diet. *Journal of Animal Physiology and Animal Nutrition* 69, 225–234.

Inborr, J., Bedford, M.R., Patience, J.F., Classen, H.L. and Verstegen, M.W.A. (1991) The influence of supplementary feed enzymes on nutrient disappearance and digesta characteristics in the GI-tract of early weaned pigs. In: Huisman, J. and den Hartog, L.A. (eds) *Digestive Physiology in Pigs. Proceedings of the 5th International Symposium on Digestive Physiology in Pigs.* Wageningen (Doorwerth), The Netherlands, pp. 405–410.

Inborr, J. and Bedford, M.R. (1994) Stability of feed enzymes to steam pelleting during feed processing. *Animal Feed Science and Technology* 46, 179–196.

Iotsius, G.P., Vasiliauskas, I.F. and Larbier, M. (1986) The influence of enzyme preparations added to low crude protein all-mash feeds on laying hens performances. *Seventh European Poultry Conference* 1, 506–510.

Jeroch, H. (1991) Gerste als Futtermittel fur Legehennen. *Archives of Tierzucht* 34, 581–590.

Jeroch, H., Danicke, S., Ebert, K., Siebecke Strempel, H. and Keller, T. (1995) Barley in poultry nutrition especially of fowls. *Ubersichten Zur Tierernahrung* 23, 27–54.

Jongbloed, A.W. (1997) Digestibility of phosphorus in pig nutrition – experiences in The Netherlands. *Kraftfutter* 7–8, 319–324.

Kemme, P.A., Radcliffe, J.S., Jongbloed, A.W., Mroz, Z. and Beyen, A.C. (1997) The efficacy of *Aspergillus niger* phytase in rendering phytate phosphorus available for absorption in pigs is influenced by pig physiological status. *Journal of Animal Science* 75, 2129–2138.

Kolkovski, S., Tandler, A., Kissil, G.W. and Gertler, A. (1993) The effect of dietary exogenous digestive enzymes on ingestion, assimilation, growth and survival of gilthead seabream (*Sparus aurata*, Sparidae, Linnaeus) larvae. *Fish Physiology and Biochemistry* 12, 203–209.

Kolkovski, S., Tandler, A. and Izquierdo, M.S. (1997) Effects of live food and dietary digestive enzymes on the efficiency of microdiets for seabass (*Dicentrarchus labrax*) larvae. *Aquaculture* 148, 313–322.

Kornegay, E.T., Denbow, D.M., Yi, Z. and Ravindran, V. (1996) Response of broilers to graded levels of microbial phytase added to maize–soyabean meal based diets containing three levels of non-phytate phosphorus. *British Journal of Nutrition* 75, 839–852.

Leatherwood, J.M., Mochrie, R.D. and Thomas, W.E. (1960) Some effects of a supplementary cellulase preparation on feed utilization by ruminants. *Journal of Dairy Science* 43, 1460.

Lewis, G.E., Hunt, C.W., Sanchez, W.K., Treacher, R., Pritchard, G.T. and Feng, P. (1996) Effect of direct fed fibrolytic enzymes on the digestive characteristics of a forage-based diet fed to beef steers. *Journal of Animal Science* 74, 3020–3028.

Li, M.H. and Robinson, E.H. (1997) Microbial phytase can replace inorganic phosphorus supplements in channel catfish (*Ictalurus punctatus*) diets. *Journal of the World Aquaculture Society* 28, 402–406.

Lindemann, M.D., Cornelius, S.G., El Kandelgy, S.M., Moser, R.L. and Pettigrew, J.E. (1986) Effect of age, weaning and diet on digestive enzyme levels in the piglet. *Journal of Animal Science* 62, 1298–1307.

Longstaff, M.A., Knox, A. and McNab, J.M. (1988) Digestibility of pentose sugars and uronic acids and their effect on chick weight gain and caecal size. *British Poultry Science* 29, 379–393.

Luchini, N.D., Broderick, G.A. and Combs, D.K. (1996) Characterization of the proteolytic activity of commercial proteases and strained ruminal fluid. *Journal of Animal Science* 74, 685–692.

Lunari, D., D'Argaro, E., Turri, C. and Wilson, R.P. (1998) Use of nonlinear regression to evaluate the effects of phytase enzyme treatment of plant protein diets for rainbow trout (*Oncorhynchus mykiss*). *Aquaculture* 161, 345–356.

Michal, J.J., Johnson, K.A., Treacher, R.J., Gaskins, C.T. and Sears, O. (1996) The impact of direct fed fibrolytic enzymes on the growth rate and feed efficiency of growing beef steers and heifers. *Journal of Animal Science* 74 (Suppl. 1), 296.

Morgan, A.J. and Bedford, M.R. (1995) Wheat-specific feed enzymes. *Feed Compounder* 15, 25–27.

Mroz, Z., Jongbloed, A.W. and Kemme, P.A. (1994) Apparent digestibility and retention of nutrients bound to phytate complexes as influenced by microbial phytase and feeding regimen in pigs. *Journal of Animal Science* 72, 126–132.

Murison, S.D., Mulder, M.M. and Hotten, J.M. (1989) Enzymatic solubilization of aleurone cell wall and release of protein. In: Fry, S.C., Brett, C.T. and Reid, J.S.G. (eds) *Proceedings of the Fifth Cell Wall Meeting*. University of Edinburgh, Edinburgh, p. 197.

Mulder, M.M., Lomax, J.A., Hotten, P.M., Cowie, E. and Chesson, A. (1991) Digestion of wheat aleurone by commercial polysaccharidases. *Animal Feed Science and Technology* 32, 185–192.

Nakashima, Y. and Orskov, E.R. (1989) Rumen degradation of straw – 7. Effects of chemical pre-treatment and addition of propionic acid on degradation characteristics of botanical fractions of barley straw treated with cellulase preparation. *Animal Production* 48, 543–551.

Nasi, M. (1988) Enzyme supplementation of laying hen diets based on barley and oats. In: Lyons, T.P. (ed.) *Biotechnology in the Feed Industry, Proceedings of Alltech's 7th Annual Symposium*. Alltech Technical Publications, Kentucky, pp. 169–177.

Nasi, M. and Lyons, T.P. (1988) Enzyme supplementation of laying hen diets based on barley and oats. In: Lyons, T.P. (ed.) *Biotechnology in the Feed Industry. Proceedings of Alltech's Fourth Annual Symposium*. Alltech Technical Publications, Kentucky, pp. 199–204.

Officer, D.I. (1995) Effect of multi-enzyme supplements on the growth performance of piglets during the pre- and post-weaning periods. *Animal Feed Science and Technology* 56, 55–65.

Owsley, W.F., Orr, D.E. and Tribble, L.F. (1986) Effect of age and diet on the development of the pancreas and the synthesis and secretion of pancreatic enzymes in the young pig. *Journal of Animal Science* 63, 497–504.

Perry, T.W., Purkhiser, E.D. and Beeson, W.M. (1966) Effects of supplemental enzymes on nitrogen balance digestibility of energy and nutrients on growth and feed efficiency of cattle. *Journal of Animal Science* 25, 760–764.

Pettersson, D. and Aman, P. (1988) Effects of enzyme supplementation of diets based on wheat, rye, or triticale on their productive value for broiler chickens. *Animal Feed Science and Technology* 20, 313–324.

Pettersson, D. and Aman, P. (1989) Enzyme supplementation of a poultry diet containing rye and wheat. *British Journal of Nutrition* 62, 139–149.

Qian, H., Kornegay, E.T. and Veit, H.P. (1996a) Effects of supplemental phytase and phosphorus on histological, mechanical and chemical traits of tibia and performance of turkeys fed on soyabean-meal-based semi-purified diets high in phytate phosphorus. *British Journal of Nutrition* 76, 263–272.

Qian, H., Veit, H.P., Kornegay, E.T., Ravindran, V. and Denbow, D.M. (1996b) Effects of supplemental phytase and phosphorous on histological and the tibial bone characteristics and performances of broilers fed semi-purified diets. *Poultry Science* 75, 618–626.

Ranade, A.S. and Rajmane, B.V. (1992) Effect of enzyme feed supplement on commercial broilers. *Proceedings of the 19th World's Poultry Congress*. Amsterdam, The Netherlands, Vol. 2, World's Poultry Science Association, Beekbergen, The Netherlands, pp. 485–487.

Reinitz, G. (1983) Supplementation of rainbow trout starter diets with proteolytic enzyme formulas. *Feedstuffs* 55, 18.

Rerat, A., Fiszlewicz, M., Giusi, A. and Vaugelade, P. (1987) Influence of meal frequency on post-prandial variations in the production and absorption of volatile fatty acids in the digestive tract of conscious pigs. *Journal of Animal Science* 64, 448–456.

Rogel, A.M., Annison, E.F., Bryden, W.L. and Balnave, D. (1987) The digestion of wheat starch in broiler chickens. *Australian Journal of Agricultural Research* 38, 639–649.

Rojas, S.W. and Scott, M.L. (1968) Factors affecting the nutritive value of cottonseed meal as a protein source in chick diets. *Poultry Science* 47, 819–835.

Rooke, J.A., Slessor, M., Fraser, H. and Thomson, J.R. (1998) Growth performance and gut function of piglets weaned at four weeks of age and fed protease-treated soya-bean meal. *Animal Feed Science and Technology* 70, 175–190.

Roth Maier, D.A. and Kirchgessner, M. (1995) White lupins (*Lupinus albus* L.) and enzyme supplements for layers. *Archiv für Geflugelkunde* 59, 186–189.

Rotter, B.A., Nesker, M., Marquardt, R.R. and Guenter, W. (1989) Effects of different enzyme preparations on the nutritional value of barley in chicken diets. *Nutrition Reports International* 39, 107–120.

Sanchez, W.K., Hunt, C.W., Guy, M.A., Pritchard, G.T., Swanson, B., Warner, T. and Treacher, R.J. (1996) Effect of fibrolytic enzymes on lactational performance of dairy cows. *Proceedings of American Dairy Science Association*. Corvallis, Oregon.

Schingoethe, D.J., Stegeman, G.A. and Treacher, R.J. (1999) Response of lactating dairy cows to a cellulase and xylanase enzyme mixture applied to forages at the time of feeding. *Journal of Dairy Science* 82, 996–1003.

Schoner, F.J., Hoppe, P.P. and Schwarz, G. (1991) Reduction of phosphorus excretion in broiler production by supplementing microbial phytase. *Journal of Animal Physiology and Animal Nutrition* 33, 481–486.

Schoner, F.J., Hoppe, P.P., Schwarz, G. and Wiesche, H. (1993a) Comparison of microbial phytase and inorganic phosphate in male chickens: the influence on performance data, mineral retention and dietary calcium. *Journal of Animal Physiology and Animal Nutrition* 69, 235–244.

Schoner, F.J., Hoppe, P.P., Schwarz, G. and Wiesche, H. (1993b) Phosphorus balance of layers supplied with phytase from *Aspergillus niger*. In: Flachowsky, G. and Schubert, R. (eds) *Vitamine und weitere Zusatzstoffe bei Mensch und Tier: 4th Symposium*. Jena, Germany, pp. 371–376.

Schroder, B., Breves, G. and Rodehutscord, M. (1996) Mechanisms of intestinal phosphorus absorption and availability of dietary phosphorus in pigs. *Deutsche Tierarztliche Wochenschrift* 103, 209–214.

Selinger, L.B., Forsberg, C.W. and Cheng, K.J. (1996) The rumen: a unique source of enzymes for enhancing livestock production. *Anaerobe* 2, 263–284.

Simbaya, J., Slominski, B.A., Guenter, W., Morgan, A. and Campbell, L.D. (1996) The effects of protease and carbohydrase supplementation on the nutritive value of canola meal for poultry: *in vitro* and *in vivo* studies. *Animal Feed Science and Technology* 61, 219–234.

Stevens, V.I., Salmon, R.E., Classen, H.L. and Campbell, G.L. (1988) Effects of dietary beta-glucanase, vitamin D3 and available phosphorus on the utilization of hulless barley by broiler turkeys. *Nutrition Reports International* 38, 283–290.

Thacker, P.A., Campbell, G.L. and Groot-Wassink, J.W.D. (1988) The effect of beta-glucanase supplementation on the performance of pre-fed hulless barley. *Nutrition Reports International* 38, 91–99.

Thacker, P.A., Campbell, G.L. and Groot-Wassink, J.W.D. (1991) The effect of enzyme supplementation on the nutritive value of rye-based diets for swine. *Canadian Journal of Animal Science* 71, 489–496.

Thiel U., Weigand, E., Hoppe, P.P., Schoner, F.J. and Anke, M. (1993) Zinc retention of broiler chickens as affected by dietary supplementation of zinc and microbial phytase. In: Meissner, D. and Mills, C.F. (eds) *Proceedings of the Eighth International Symposium on Trace Elements in Man and Animals*, Verlag Media Touristik, Gersdorf, Germany, pp. 658–659.

Treacher, R.J. and Hunt, C.W. (1996) Recent developments in feed enzymes for ruminant rations with special reference to direct fed applications. *Northwest Animal Nutrition Conference*. Seattle, Washington, Vol. 31, pp. 37–54.

Treacher, R.J., McAllister, T.A., Popp, J.D., Mir, Z., Mir, P. and Cheng, K.J. (1996) Effect of exogenous cellulases and xylanases on feed utilization and growth performance of ruminants. *Proceedings of the Canadian Society of Animal Science Annual Meeting*. Lethbridge, Alberta.

Walsh, G.A., Murphy, R.A., Killeen, G.F., Headon, D.R. and Power, R.F. (1995) Technical note: detection and quantification of supplemental fungal beta-glucanase activity in animal feed. *Journal of Animal Science* 73, 1074–1076.

Yanke, L.J., Bae, H.D., Selinger, L.B. and Cheng, K.J. (1998) Phytase activity of anaerobic ruminal bacteria. *Microbiology Reading* 144, 1565–1573.

Ye, Y.T., Chen, C.Q., Li, X.P., Xiao, L.R. and Zheng, Y.H. (1995) The effect of multi-enzyme premix EA-2 on the growth of carp (*Cyprinus carpio*). *Acta Hydrobiologica Sinica* 19, 299–303.

Yi, Z., Kornegay, E.T., Ravindran, V., Lindemann, M.D. and Wilson, J.H. (1996) Effectiveness of Natuphos R phytase in improving the bioavailabilities of phosphorus and other nutrients in soybean meal-based semipurified diets for young pigs. *Journal of Animal Science* 74, 1601–1611.

Yule, M.A. and Fuller, M.F. (1992) The utilisation of orally administered D-xylose, L-arabinose and D-galacturonic acid in the pig. *International Journal of Food Science and Nutrition* 43, 31–40.

Zang, S.M., Zhao, G.X., Zhang, B.Q. and Li, T.Z. (1995) Study on the influence of compound enzyme preparation on laying performance of layers. *Journal of Hebei Agricultural University* 18, 62–65.

Index

___